disha
Nurturing Ambitions

43 JEE MAIN PHYSICS

ONLINE & OFFLINE

2019-2012 2018-2002

CHAPTER-WISE + TOPIC-WISE SOLVED PAPERS

AF519265

• **Corporate Office :** 45, 2nd Floor, Maharishi Dayanand Marg, Corner Market,
Malviya Nagar, New Delhi-110017
Tel. : 011-49842349 / 49842350

By
Sanjeev Kumar Jha

Typeset by Disha DTP Team

DISHA PUBLICATION

For further information about the books from DISHA,
Log on to www.dishapublication.com or email to info@dishapublication.com

Contents

JEE Main Solved Paper 2019

CHAPTER-1 : Physical World, Units and Measurements

TOPIC-1 : Unit of Physical Quantities

1. The density of a material in SI unit of is 128 kg m^{-3} In certain units in which the unit of length is 25 cm and the unit of mass is 50 g, the numerical value of density of the material is: **[Set-II, Jan. 2019]**

(a) 40 (b) 16 (c) 640 (d) 410

TOPIC-2 : Dimensions of Physical Quantities

2. In SI units, the dimensions of $\sqrt{\frac{\epsilon_0}{\mu_0}}$ is : **[Set I, April 2019]**

(a) $A^{-1}TML^3$ (b) $AT^2 M^{-1}L^{-1}$

(c) $AT^{-3}ML^{3/2}$ (d) $A^2T^3 M^{-1}L^{-2}$

TOPIC-3 : Errors in Measurements

3. In the density measurement of a cube, the mass and edge length are measured as (10.00 ± 0.10) kg and (0.10 ± 0.01) m, respectively. The error in the measurement of density is: **[Set II, April 2019]**

(a) 0.01 kg/m^3 (b) 0.10 kg/m^3

(c) 0.31 kg/m^3 (d) 0.07 kg/m^3

CHAPTER-3 : Motion in a Plane

Topic-1 : Vectors

4. In the cube of side 'a' shown in the figure, the vector from the central point of the face ABOD to the central point of the face BEFO will be: **[Set-II, Jan. 2019]**

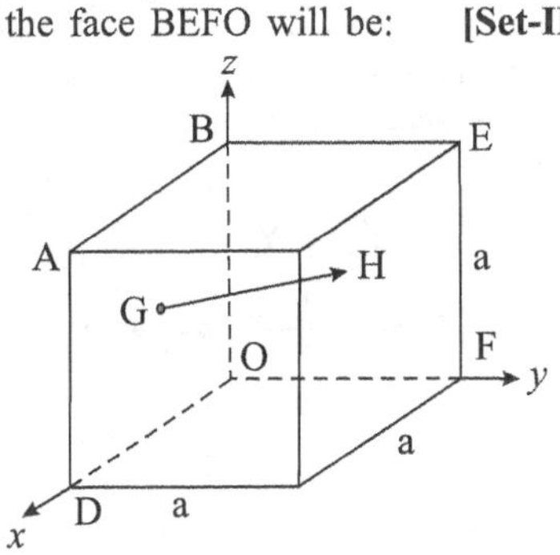

(a) $\frac{1}{2}a\left(\hat{k}-\hat{i}\right)$ (b) $\frac{1}{2}a\left(\hat{i}-\hat{k}\right)$

(c) $\frac{1}{2}a\left(\hat{j}-\hat{i}\right)$ (d) $-\left(\hat{j}\ \hat{k}\right)$

TOPIC-2 : Motion in a Plane with Constant Acceleration

5. A particle is moving with a velocity $\vec{v} = K(y\hat{i} + x\hat{j})$, where K is a constant. The general equation for its path is: **[Set I, Jan. 2019]**

(a) $y = x^2$ + constant (b) $y^2 = x$ + constant

(c) $y^2 = x^2$ + constant (d) xy = constant

TOPIC-3 : Projectile Motion

6. Two guns A and B can fire bullets at speeds 1 km/s and 2 km/s respectively. From a point on a horizontal ground, they are fired in all possible directions. The ratio of maximum areas covered by the bullets fired by the two guns, on the ground is: **[Set-II, Jan. 2019]**

(a) 1 : 16 (b) 1 : 2 (c) 1 : 4 (d) 1 : 8

TOPIC-4 : Relative Velocity in Two Dimensions & Uniform Circular Motion

7. Ship A is sailing towards north-east with velocity $\vec{v} = 30\hat{i} + 50\hat{j}$ km/hr where $\hat{i}$ points east and $\hat{j}$, north. Ship B is at a distance of 80 km east and 150 km north of Ship A and is sailing towards west at 10 km/hr. A will be at minimum distance from B in: **[Set I, April 2019]**

(a) 4.2 hrs. (b) 2.6 hrs. (c) 3.2 hrs. (d) 2.2 hrs.

8. The stream of a river is flowing with a speed of 2 km/h. A swimmer can swim at a speed of 4 km/h. What should be the direction of the swimmer with respect to the flow of the river to cross the river straight? **[Set II, April 2019]**

(a) 90° (b) 150° (c) 120° (d) 60°

CHAPTER-4 : Laws of Motion

TOPIC-1 : Ist, IInd & IIIrd Laws of Motion

9. A ball is thrown vertically up (taken as + z-axis) from the ground. The correct momentum-height (p-h) diagram is: **[Set II, April 2019]**

(a) 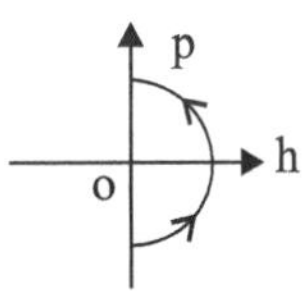

(b) 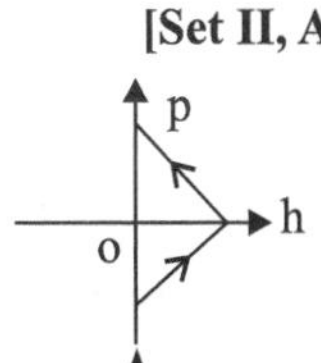

(c) 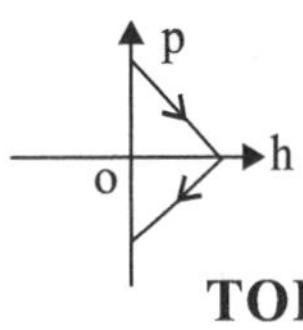

(d) 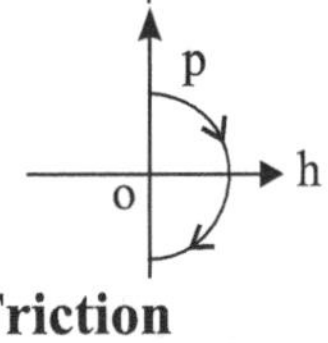

TOPIC-3 : Friction

10. A block of mass 10 kg is kept on a rough inclined plane as shown in the figure. A force of 3 N is applied on the block. The coefficient of static friction between the plane and the block is 0.6. What should be the minimum value of force P, such that the block doesnot move downward? (take g = 10 ms^{-2}) **[Set I, Jan. 2019]**

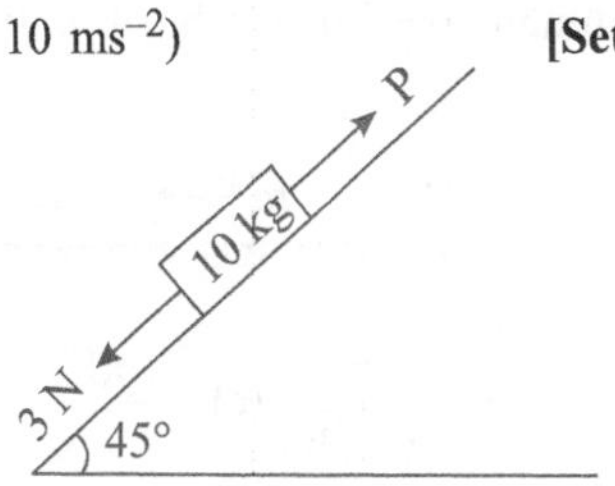

(a) 32 N (b) 18 N (c) 23 N (d) 25 N

CHAPTER-5 : Work, Energy and Power

TOPIC-1 : Work

11. A uniform cable of mass 'M' and length 'L' is placed on a horizontal surface such that its $\left(\frac{1}{n}\right)^{th}$ part is hanging below the edge of the surface. To lift the hanging part of the cable upto the surface, the work done should be: **[Set II, April 2019]**

(a) $\frac{MgL}{2n^2}$ (b) $\frac{MgL}{n^2}$

(c) $\frac{2MgL}{n^2}$ (d) nMgL

12. A block of mass m is kept on a platform which starts from rest with constant acceleration g/2 upward, as shown in fig. work done by normal reaction on block in time t is: **[Set-II, Jan. 2019]**

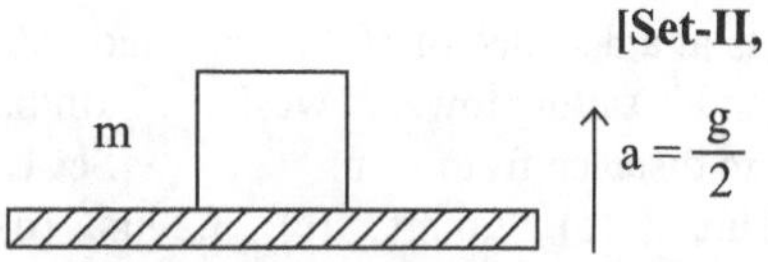

(a) $-\frac{m g^2 t^2}{8}$ (b) $\frac{m g^2 t^2}{8}$

(c) 0 (d) $\frac{3m g^2 t^2}{8}$

TOPIC-2 : Energy

13. A particle moves in one dimension from rest under the influence of a force that varies with the distance travelled by the particle as shown in the figure. The kinetic energy of the particle after it has travelled 3 m is : **[Set I, April 2019]**

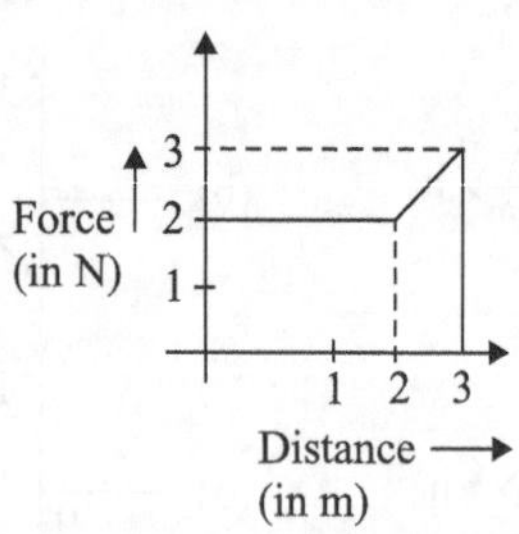

(a) 4 J (b) 2.5 J (c) 6.5 J (d) 5 J

14. A block of mass m, lying on a smooth horizontal surface, is attached to a spring (of negligible mass) of spring constant k. The other end of the spring is fixed, as shown in the figure. The block is initally at rest in its equilibrium position. If now the block is pulled with a constant force F, the maximum speed of the block is: **[Set I, Jan. 2019]**

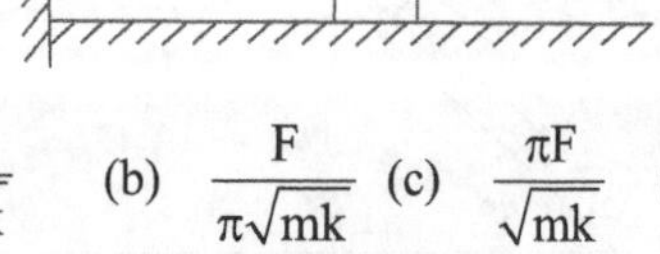

(a) $\frac{2F}{\sqrt{mk}}$ (b) $\frac{F}{\pi\sqrt{mk}}$ (c) $\frac{\pi F}{\sqrt{mk}}$ (d) $\frac{F}{\sqrt{mk}}$

TOPIC-4 : Collisions

15. A body of mass 2 kg makes an elastic collision with a second body at rest and continues to move in the original direction but with one fourth of its original speed. What is the mass of the second body? **[Set II, April 2019]**

(a) 1.0 kg (b) 1.5 kg (c) 1.8 kg (d) 1.2 kg

16. There block A, B and C are lying on a smooth horizontal surface, as shown in the figure. A and B have equal masses, m while C has mass M. Block A is given an inital speed v towards B due to which it collides with B perfectly inelastically. The combined mass collides with C, also perfectly inelastically $\frac{5}{6}$ th of the initial kinetic energy is lost in whole process. What is value of M/m? **[Set I, Jan. 2019]**

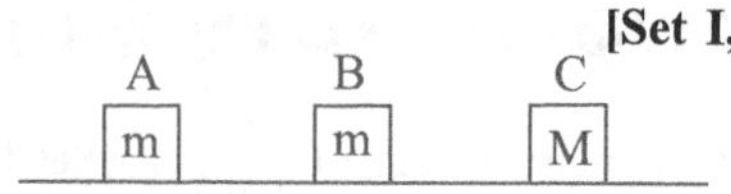

(a) 5 (b) 2 (c) 4 (d) 3

17. A piece of wood of mass 0.03 kg is dropped from the top of a 100 m height building. At the same time, a bullet of mass 0.02 kg is fired vertically upward, with a velocity 100 ms^{-1}, from the ground. The bullet gets embedded in the wood. Then the maximum height to which the combined system reaches above the top of the building before falling below is: (g = 10 ms^{-2}) **[Set-II, Jan. 2019]**

(a) 20 m (b) 30 m (c) 40 m (d) 10 m

CHAPTER-6 : System of Particles and Rotational Motion

TOPIC-1 : Centre of Mass, Centre of Gravity and Principle of moments

18. Four particles A, B, C and D with masses $m_A = m$, $m_B = 2m$, $m_C = 3m$ and $m_D = 4m$ are at the corners of a square. They have accelerations of equal magnitude with directions as shown. The acceleration of the centre of mass of the particles is : **[Set I, April 2019]**

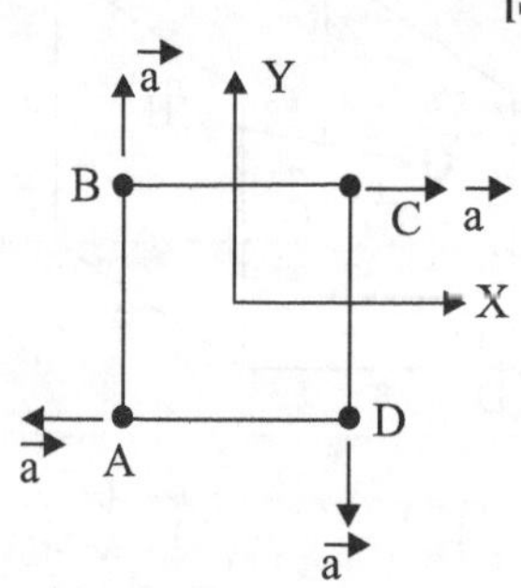

(a) $\frac{a}{5}(\hat{i}-\hat{j})$ (b) $a(\hat{i}+\hat{j})$ (c) Zero (d) $\frac{a}{5}(\hat{i}+\hat{j})$

TOPIC-3 : Torque, Couple and Angular Momentum

19. An L-shaped object, made of thin rods of uniform mass density, is suspended with a string as shown in figure. If AB = BC, and the angle made by AB with downward vertical is θ, then: **[Set I, Jan. 2019]**

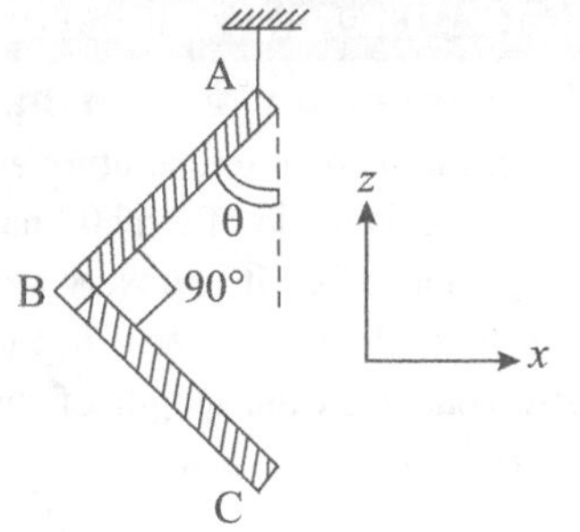

(a) $\tan\theta = \frac{1}{2\sqrt{3}}$ (b) $\tan\theta = \frac{1}{2}$

(c) $\tan\theta = \frac{2}{\sqrt{3}}$ (d) $\tan\theta = \frac{1}{3}$

20. To mop-clean a floor, a cleaning machine presses a circular mop of radius R vertically down with a total force F and rotates it with a constant angular speed about its axis. If the force F is distributed uniformly over the mop and if coefficient of friction between the mop and the floor is μ, the torque, applied by the machine on the mop is: **[Set-II, Jan. 2019]**

(a) μ FR/3 (b) μ FR/6

(c) μ FR/2 (d) $\frac{2}{3}$ μFR

TOPIC-4 : Moment of Inertia and Rotational K.E.

21. A thin circular plate of mass M and radius R has its density varying as $\rho(r) = \rho_0 r$ with ρ_0 as constant and r is the distance from its center. The moment of Inertia of the circular plate about an axis perpendicular to the plate and passing through its edge is $I = a\,MR^2$. The value of the coefficient a is: **[Set I, April 2019]**

(a) $1/2$ (b) $3/5$ (c) $8/5$ (d) $3/2$

22. A stationary horizontal disc is free to rotate about its axis. When a torque is applied on it, its kinetic energy as a function of θ, where θ is the angle by which it has rotated, is given as $k\theta^2$. If its moment of inertia is I then the angular acceleration of the disc is: **[Set II, April 2019]**

(a) $\frac{k}{4I}\theta$ (b) $\frac{k}{I}\theta$ (c) $\frac{k}{2I}\theta$ (d) $\frac{2k}{I}\theta$

23. Two masses m and $\frac{m}{2}$ are connected at the two ends of a massless rigid rod of length l. The rod is suspended by a thin wire of torsional constant k at the centre of mass of the rod-mass system (see figure). Because of torsional constant k, the restoring toruque is $\tau = k\theta$ for angular displacement θ. If the rod is rotated by θ_0 and released, the tension in it when it passes through its mean position will be: **[Set I, Jan. 2019]**

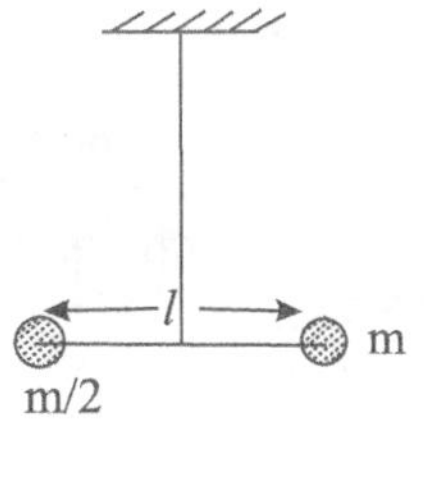

(a) $\frac{3k\theta_0^2}{l}$ (b) $\frac{2k\theta_0^2}{l}$ (c) $\frac{k\theta_0^2}{l}$ (d) $\frac{k\theta_0^2}{2l}$

TOPIC-5 : Rolling Motion

24. The following bodies are made to roll up (without slipping) the same inclined plane from a horizontal plane : (i) a ring of radius R, (ii) a solid cylinder of radius $\frac{R}{2}$ and (iii) a solid sphere of radius $\frac{R}{4}$. If, in each case, the speed of the center of mass at the bottom of the incline is same, the ratio of the maximum heights they climb is : **[Set II, April 2019]**

(a) 4 : 3 : 2 (b) 10 : 15 : 7

(c) 14 : 15 : 20 (d) 2 : 3 : 4

25. A homogeneous solid cylindrical roller of radius R and mass M is pulled on a cricket pitch by a horizontal force. Assuming rolling without slipping, angular acceleration of the cylinder is: **[Set-II, Jan. 2019]**

(a) $\frac{3F}{2mR}$ (b) $\frac{F}{3mR}$ (c) $\frac{F}{2mR}$ (d) $\frac{2F}{3mR}$

CHAPTER-7 : Gravitation

TOPIC-1 : Kepler's Laws of Planetary Motion

26. If the angular momentum of a planet of mass m, moving around the Sun in a circular orbit is L, about the center of the Sun, its areal velocity is: **[Set I, Jan. 2019]**

(a) $\frac{L}{m}$ (b) $\frac{4L}{m}$ (c) $\frac{L}{2m}$ (d) $\frac{2L}{m}$

TOPIC-4 : Gravitational Field and Potential Energy

27. Four identical particles of mass M are located at the corners of a square of side 'a'. What should be their speed if each of them revolves under the influence of others' gravitational field in a circular orbit circumscribing the square ? **[Set I, April 2019]**

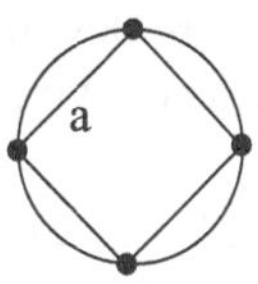

(a) $1.35\sqrt{\frac{GM}{a}}$ (b) $1.16\sqrt{\frac{GM}{a}}$

(c) $1.21\sqrt{\frac{GM}{a}}$ (d) $1.41\sqrt{\frac{GM}{a}}$

28. A solid sphere of mass 'M' and radius 'a' is surrounded by a uniform concentric spherical shell of thickness 2a and mass 2M. The gravitational field at distance '3a' from the centre will be: **[Set II, April 2019]**

(a) $\frac{2GM}{9a^2}$ (b) $\frac{GM}{9a^2}$ (c) $\frac{GM}{3a^2}$ (d) $\frac{2GM}{3a^2}$

TOPIC-5 : Motion of Satellites, Escape speed and Orbital Velocities

29. A satellite is moving with a constant speed v in circular orbit around the earth. An object of mass 'm' is ejected from the satellite such that it just escapes from the gravitational pull of the earth. At the time of ejection, the kinetic energy of the object is: **[Set-II, Jan. 2019]**

(a) $2\ m\ v^2$ (b) $m\ v^2$ (c) $\frac{1}{2}\ m\ v^2$ (d) $\frac{3}{2}\ m\ v^2$

CHAPTER-8 : Mechanical Properties of Solids

TOPIC-1 : Hooke's and Young's Modulus

30. A steel wire having a radius of 2.0 mm, carrying a load of 4kg, is hanging from a ceiling. Given that $g = 3.1\ \pi\ ms^{-2}$, what will be the tensile stress that would be developed in the wire? **[Set I, April 2019]**

(a) $6.2 \times 10^6\ Nm^{-2}$ (b) $5.2 \times 10^6\ Nm^{-2}$
(c) $3.1 \times 10^6\ Nm^{-2}$ (d) $4.8 \times 10^6\ Nm^{-2}$

TOPIC-2 : Bulk and Rigidity Modulus and Work done in stretching a wire

31. A boy's catapult is made of rubber cord which is 42 cm long, with 6 mm diameter of cross-section and of negligible mass. The boy keeps a stone weighing 0.02 kg on it and stretches the cord by 20 cm by applying a constant force. When released, the stone flies off with a velocity of 20 ms^{-1}. Neglect the change in the area of cross-section of the cord while stretched. The Young's modulus of rubber is closest to : **[Set I, April 2019]**

(a) $10^6\ N/m^{-2}$ (b) $10^4\ N/m^{-2}$
(c) $10^8\ N/m^{-2}$ (d) $10^3\ N/m^{-2}$

CHAPTER-9 : Mechanical Properties of Fluids

TOPIC-2 : Fluid Flow, Reynold's Number and Bernoulli's Principle

32. Water from a pipe is coming at a rate of 100 liters per minute. If the radius of the pipe is 5 cm, the Reynolds number for the flow is of the order of : (density of water = 1000 kg/m^3, coefficient of viscosity of water = 1 mPa *s*) **[Set I, April 2019]**

(a) 10^3 (b) 10^4 (c) 10^2 (d) 10^6

33. Water flows into a large tank with flat bottom at the rate of $10^{-4}\ m^3\ s^{-(1)}$ Water is also leaking out of a hole of area 1 cm^2 at its bottom. If the height of the water in the tank remains steady, then this height is: **[Set-II, Jan. 2019]**

(a) 5.1 cm (b) 7 cm (c) 4 cm (d) 9 cm

TOPIC-4 : Surface Tension, Surface Energy and Capillarity

34. If 'M' is the mass of water that rises in a capillary tube of radius 'r', then mass of water which will rise in a capillary tube of radius '2r' is : **[Set II, April 2019]**

(a) M (b) $\frac{M}{2}$ (c) 4 M (d) 2 M

CHAPTER-10 : Thermal Properties of Matter

TOPIC-1 : Thermometer & Thermal Expansion

35. A rod, of length L at room temperature and uniform area of cross section A, is made of a metal having coefficient of linear expansion α/°C. It is observed that an external compressive force F, is applied on each of its ends, prevents any change in the length of the rod, when its temperature rises by ΔT K. Young's modulus, Y, for this metal is: **[Set I, Jan. 2019]**

(a) $\frac{F}{A\alpha\Delta T}$ (b) $\frac{F}{A\alpha(\Delta T - 273)}$
(c) $\frac{F}{2A\alpha\Delta T}$ (d) $\frac{2F}{A\alpha\Delta T}$

TOPIC-2 : Calorimetry and Heat Transfer

36. Temperature difference of 120°C is maintained between two ends of a uniform rod AB of length 2L. Another bent rod PQ, of same cross-section as AB and length $\frac{3L}{2}$, is connected across AB (See figure). In steady state, temperature difference between P and Q will be close to: **[Set I, Jan. 2019]**

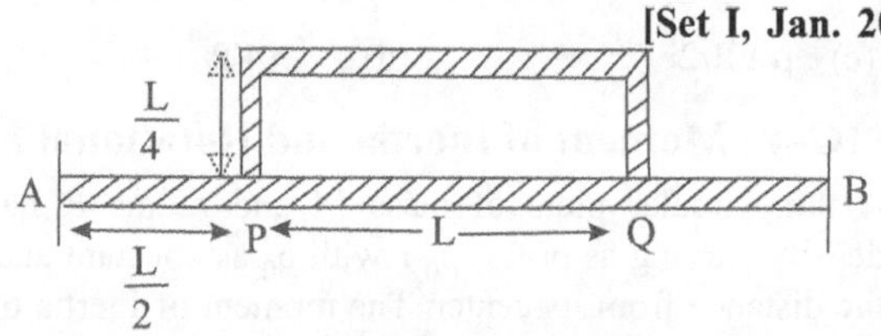

(a) 45°C (b) 75°C (c) 60°C (d) 35°C

37. A heat source at T = 10^3 K is connected to another heat reservoir at T = 10^2 K by a copper slab which is 1 m thick. Given that the thermal conductivity of copper is 0.1 $WK^{-1}\ m^{-1}$, the energy flux through it in the steady state is: **[Set-II, Jan. 2019]**

(a) 90 Wm^{-2} (b) 120 Wm^{-2}
(c) 65 Wm^{-2} (d) 200 Wm^{-2}

TOPIC-3 : Newton's Law of Cooling

38. Two identical beakers A and B contain equal volumes of two different liquids at 60°C each and left to cool down. Liquid in A has density of $8 \times 10^2\ kg/m^3$ and specific heat of 2000 J $kg^{-1}\ K^{-1}$ while liquid in B has density of $10^3\ kg\ m^{-3}$ and specific heat of 4000 J $kg^{-1}\ K^{-1}$. Which of the following best describes their temperature versus time graph schematically ? (assume the emissivity of both the beakers to be the same) **[Set I, April 2019]**

(a)
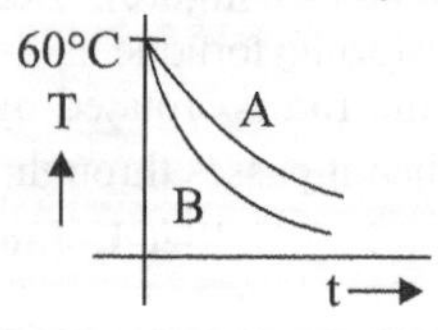

(b)
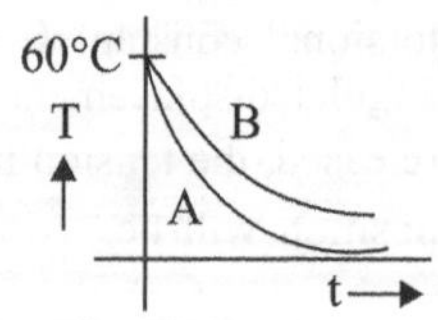

(c)
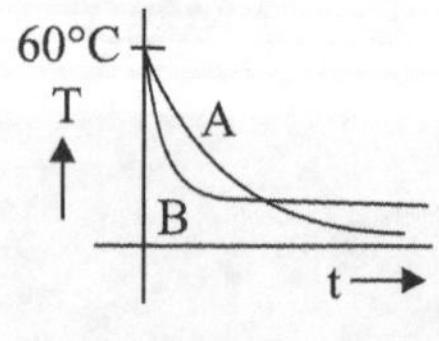

(d)
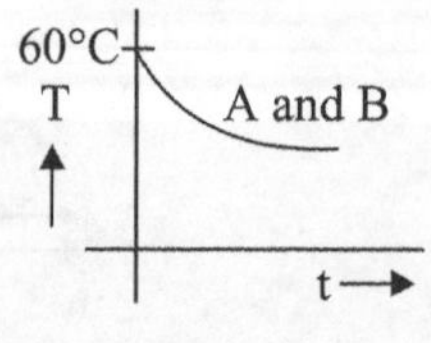

CHAPTER-11 : Thermodynamics

TOPIC-1 : First Law of Thermodynamics

39. A gas can be taken from A to B via two different processes ACB and ADB.

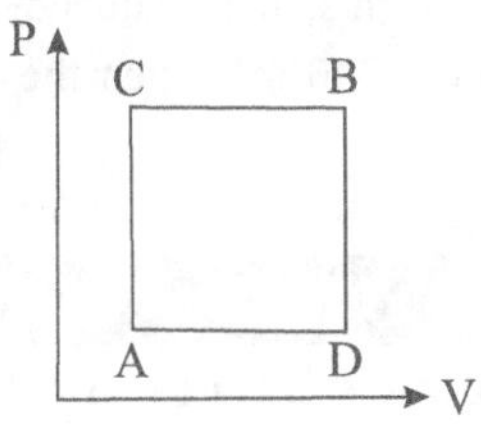

When path ACB is used 60 J of heat flows into the system and 30J of work is done by the system. If path ADB is used work done by the system is 10 J. The heat Flow into the system in path ADB is : **[Set I, Jan. 2019]**

(a) 40 J (b) 80 J (c) 100 J (d) 20 J

TOPIC-2 : Specific Heat Capacity and Thermodynamical Processes

40. A thermally insulted vessel contains 150 g of water at 0°C. Then the air from the vessel is pumped out adiabatically. A fraction of water turns into ice and the rest evaporates at 0°C itself. The mass of evaporated water will be closed to : (Latent heat of vaporization of water = 2.10×10^6 J kg^{-1} and Latent heat of Fusion of water = 3.36×10^5 J kg^{-1}) **[Set I, April 2019]**

(a) 150 g (b) 20 g (c) 130 g (d) 35 g

41. Following figure shows two processes A and B for a gas. If ΔQ_A and ΔQ_B are the amount of heat absorbed by the system in two cases, and ΔU_A and ΔU_B are changes in internal energies, respectively, then: **[Set II, April 2019]**

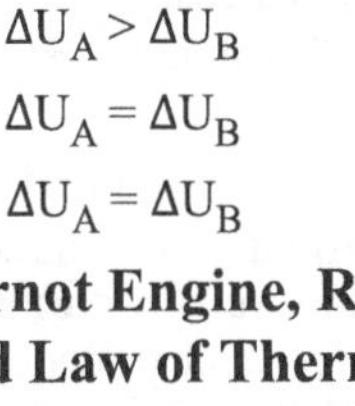

(a) $\Delta Q_A < \Delta Q_B, \Delta U_A < \Delta U_B$

(b) $\Delta Q_A > \Delta Q_B, \Delta U_A > \Delta U_B$

(c) $\Delta Q_A > \Delta Q_B, \Delta U_A = \Delta U_B$

(d) $\Delta Q_A = \Delta Q_B; \Delta U_A = \Delta U_B$

TOPIC-3 : Carnot Engine, Refrigerators and Second Law of Thermodynamics

42. Three Carnot engines operate in series between a heat source at a temperature T_1 and a heat sink at temperature T_4 (see figure). There are two other reservoirs at temperature T_2 and T_3, as shown, with $T_1 > T_2 > T_3 > T(4)$ The three engines are equally efficient if: **[Set-II, Jan. 2019]**

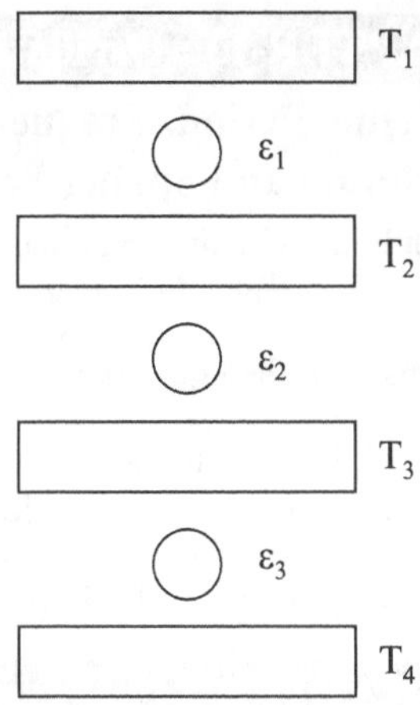

(a) $T_2 = (T_1 T_4)^{1/2}; T_3 = \left(T_1^2 T_4\right)^{1/3}$

(b) $T_2 = \left(T_1^2 T_4\right)^{1/3}; T_3 = \left(T_1 T_4^2\right)^{1/3}$

(c) $T_2 = \left(T_1 T_4^2\right)^{1/3}; T_3 = \left(T_1^2 T_4\right)^{1/3}$

(d) $T_2 = \left(T_1^3 T_4\right)^{1/4}; T_3 = \left(T_1 T_4^3\right)^{1/4}$

CHAPTER-12 : Kinetic Theory

TOPIC-2 : Speed of Gas, Pressure and Kinetic Energy

43. If 10^{22} gas molecules each of mass 10^{-26} kg collide with a surface (perpendicular to it) elastically per second over an area 1 m^2 with a speed 10^4 m/s, the pressure exerted by the gas molecules will be of the order of : **[Set I, April 2019]**

(a) 10^4 N/m^2 (b) 10^8 N/m^2
(c) 10^3 N/m^2 (d) 10^{16} N/m^2

44. For a given gas at 1 atm pressure, rms speed of the molecules is 200 m/s at 127°C. At 2 atm pressure and at 227°C, the rms speed of the molecules will be: **[Set II, April 2019]**

(a) 100 m/s (b) $80\sqrt{5}$ m/s
(c) $100\sqrt{5}$ m/s (d) 80 m/s

45. A mixture of 2 moles of helium gas (atomic mass = 4u), and 1 mole of argon gas (atomic mass = 40u) is kept at 300 K in a container. The ratio of their rms speeds $\left[\dfrac{V_{rms}(\text{helium})}{V_{rms}(\text{argon})}\right]$ is close to : **[Set I, Jan. 2019]**

(a) 3.16 (b) 0.32 (c) 0.45 (d) 2.24

TOPIC-3 : Degree of Freedom, Specific Heat Capacity and Mean free path

46. An HCl molecule has rotational, translational and vibrational motions. If the rms velocity of HCl molecules in its gaseous phase is $\bar{v}$, m is its mass and k_B is Boltzmann constant, then its temperature will be: **[Set II, April 2019]**

(a) $\dfrac{m\bar{v}^2}{6k_B}$ (b) $\dfrac{m\bar{v}^2}{3k_B}$ (c) $\dfrac{m\bar{v}^2}{7k_B}$ (d) $\dfrac{m\bar{v}^2}{5k_B}$

CHAPTER-13 : Oscillations

TOPIC-3 : Time Period, Frequency, Simple Pendulum and Spring Pendulum

47. A simple pendulum oscillating in air has period T. The bob of the pendulum is completely immersed in a non-viscous liquid. The density of the liquid is $\frac{1}{16}$th of the material of the bob. If the bob is inside liquid all the time, its period of oscillation in this liquid is : **[Set II, April 2019]**

(a) $2T\sqrt{\frac{1}{10}}$ (b) $2T\sqrt{\frac{1}{14}}$ (c) $4T\sqrt{\frac{1}{15}}$ (d) $4T\sqrt{\frac{1}{14}}$

CHAPTER-14 : Waves

TOPIC-1 : Basic of Mechanical Waves, Progressive and Stationary Waves

48. The pressure wave,
$P = 0.01 \sin[1000t - 3x]$ Nm^{-2}, corresponds to the sound produced by a vibrating blade on a day when atmospheric temperature is 0°C. On some other day when temperature is T, the speed of sound produced by the same blade and at the same frequency is found to be 336 ms^{-1}. Approximate value of T is : **[Set II, April 2019]**

(a) 4°C (b) 11°C (c) 12°C (d) 15°C

49. A heavy ball of mass M is suspended from the ceiling of a car by a light string of mass m (m<<M). When the car is at rest, the speeed of transverse waves in the string is 60 ms^{-1}. when the car has acceleration a, the wave-speed increases to 60.5 ms^{-1}. The value of a, in terms of gravitational acceleration g, is closest to: **[Set I, Jan. 2019]**

(a) $\frac{g}{30}$ (b) $\frac{g}{5}$ (c) $\frac{g}{10}$ (d) $\frac{g}{20}$

TOPIC-2 : Vibration of String and Organ pipe

50. A wire of length 2L, is made by joining two wires A and B of same length but different radii r and $2r$ and made of the same material. It is vibrating at a frequency such that the joint of the two wires forms a node. If the number of antinodes in wire A is p and that in B is q then the ratio $p : q$ is : **[Set I, April 2019]**

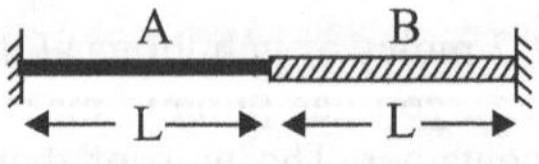

(a) 3 : 5 (b) 4 : 9 (c) 1 : 2 (d) 1 : 4

51. A string is clamped at both the ends and it is vibrating in its 4th harmonic. The equation of the stationary wave is $Y = 0.3 \sin(0.157x) \cos(200\pi t)$. The length of the string is: (All quantities are in SI units.) **[Set II, April 2019]**

(a) 20 m (b) 80 m (c) 40 m (d) 60 m

52. A string of length 1 m and mass 5 g is fixed at both ends. The tension in the string is 8.0 N. The string is set into vibration using an external vibrator of frequency 100 Hz. The separation between successive nodes on the string is close to: **[Set-II, Jan. 2019]**

(a) 10.0 cm (b) 33.3 cm (c) 16.6 cm (d) 20.0 cm

TOPIC-3 : Beats, Interference and Superposition of Waves

53. A train moves towards a stationary observer with speed 34 m/s. The train sounds a whistle and its frequency registered by the observer is f_1 If the speed of the train is reduced to 17 m/s, the frequency registered is f_2 If speed of sound is 340 m/s, then the ratio f_1/f_2 is: **[Set-II, Jan. 2019]**

(a) 18/17 (b) 19/18 (c) 20/19 (d) 21/20

CHAPTER-15 : Electric Charges and Fields

TOPIC - 1: Electric Charges and Coulomb's Law

54. Three charges + Q, q, + Q are placed respectively, at distance, d/2 and d from the origin, on the x-axis. If the net force experienced by + Q, placed at $x = 0$, is zero, then value of q is: **[Set I, Jan. 2019]**

(a) – Q/4 (b) + Q/2 (c) + Q/4 (d) – Q/2

TOPIC-2: Electric Field and Electric Field Lines

55. The bob of a simple pendulum has mass 2 g and a charge of 5.0 μC. It is at rest in a uniform horizontal electric field of intensity 2000 V/m. At equilibrium, the angle that the pendulum makes with the vertical is : **[Set I, April 2019]** (take $g = 10$ m/s^2)

(a) $\tan^{-1}(2.0)$ (b) $\tan^{-1}(0.2)$
(c) $\tan^{-1}(5.0)$ (d) $\tan^{-1}(0.5)$

56. For a uniformly charged ring of radius R, the electric field on its axis has the largest magnitude at a distance h from its centre. Then value of h is: **[Set I, Jan. 2019]**

(a) $\frac{R}{\sqrt{5}}$ (b) $\frac{R}{\sqrt{2}}$ (c) R (d) $R\sqrt{2}$

CHAPTER-16 : Electrostatic Potential and Capacitance

TOPIC - 1: Electrostatic Potential and Equipotential Surfaces

57. A solid conducting sphere, having a charge Q, is surrounded by an uncharged conducting hollow spherical shell. Let the potential difference between the surface of the solid sphere and that of the outer surface of the hollow shell be V. If the shell is now given a charge of – 4 Q, the new potential difference between the same two surfaces is : **[Set I, April 2019]**

(a) – 2V (b) 2 V (c) 4 V (d) V

58. A charge Q is distributed over three concentric spherical shells of radii a, b, c (a < b < c) such that their surface charge densities are equal to one another.
The total potential at a point at distance r from their common centre, where r < a, would be: **[Set-II, Jan. 2019]**

(a) $\frac{Q}{12\pi\epsilon_0}\frac{ab+bc+ca}{abc}$ (b) $\frac{Q(a^2+b^2+c^2)}{4\pi\epsilon_0(a^3+b^3+c^3)}$

(c) $\frac{Q}{4\pi\epsilon_0(a+b+c)}$ (d) $\frac{Q(a+b+c)}{4\pi\epsilon_0(a^2+b^2+c^2)}$

59. Two electric dipoles, A, B with respective dipole moments $\vec{d}_A = -4\,qa\,\hat{i}$ and $\vec{d}_B = -2\,qa\,\hat{i}$ are placed on the x-axis with a separation R, as shown in the figure

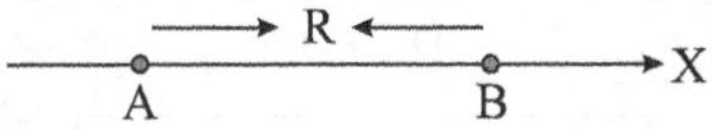

The distance from A at which both of them produce the same potential is: **[Set-II, Jan. 2019]**

(a) $\frac{R}{\sqrt{2}+1}$ (b) $\frac{\sqrt{2}R}{\sqrt{2}+1}$ (c) $\frac{R}{\sqrt{2}-1}$ (d) $\frac{\sqrt{2}R}{\sqrt{2}-1}$

TOPIC - 2 : Electric Potential Energy and Work done in Carrying a charge

60. A system of three charges are placed as shown in the figure:

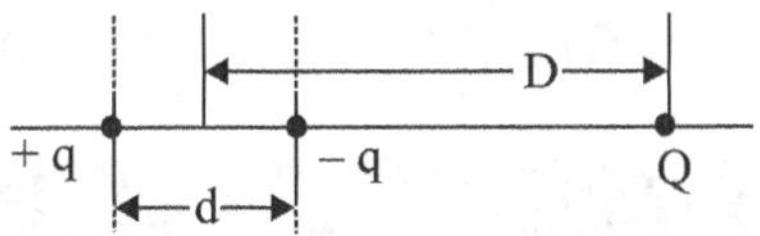

If D >> d, the potential energy of the system is best given by **[Set II, April 2019]**

(a) $\frac{1}{4\pi\epsilon_0}\left[\frac{-q^2}{d}-\frac{qQd}{2D^2}\right]$ (b) $\frac{1}{4\pi\epsilon_0}\left[\frac{-q^2}{d}+\frac{2qQd}{D^2}\right]$

(c) $\frac{1}{4\pi\epsilon_0}\left[+\frac{q^2}{d}+\frac{qQd}{D^2}\right]$ (d) $\frac{1}{4\pi\epsilon_0}\left[-\frac{q^2}{d}-\frac{qQd}{D^2}\right]$

TOPIC - 3: Capacitors, Grouping of Capacitor and Energy Stored in a Capacitor

61. Voltage rating of a parallel plate capacitor is 500 V. Its dielectric can withstand a maximum electric field of 10^6 V/m. The plate area is 10^{-4} m^2. What is the dielectric constant if the capacitance is 15 pF ? **[Set I, April 2019]** (given $\epsilon_0 = 8.86 \times 10^{-12}$ C^2/Nm^2)

(a) 3.8 (b) 8.5 (c) 4.5 (d) 6.2

62. Determine the charge on the capacitor in the following circuit: **[Set II, April 2019]**

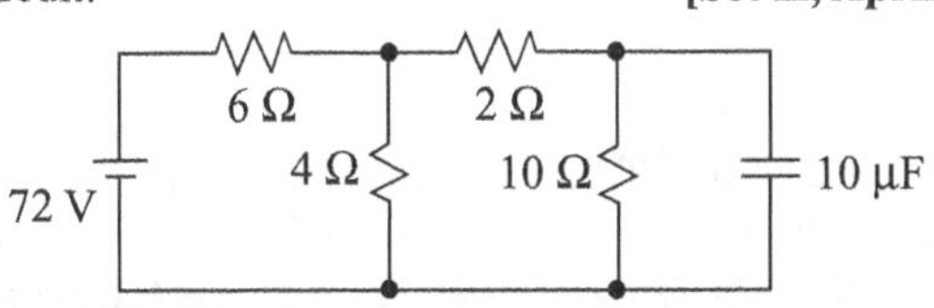

(a) 60 μC (b) 2 μC (c) 10 μC (d) 200 μC

63. A capacitor with capacitance 5 μF is charged to 5 μC. If the plates are pulled apart to reduce the capacitance to 2 μF, how much work is done? **[Set II, April 2019]**

(a) 6.25×10^{-6} J (b) 3.75×10^{-6} J
(c) 2.16×10^{-6} J (d) 2.55×10^{-6} J

64. A parallel plate capacitor is made of two square plates of side 'a', separated by a distance d (d<<a). The lower triangular portion is filled with a dielectric of dielectric constant K, as shown in the figure. Capacitance of this capacitor is: **[Set I, Jan. 2019]**

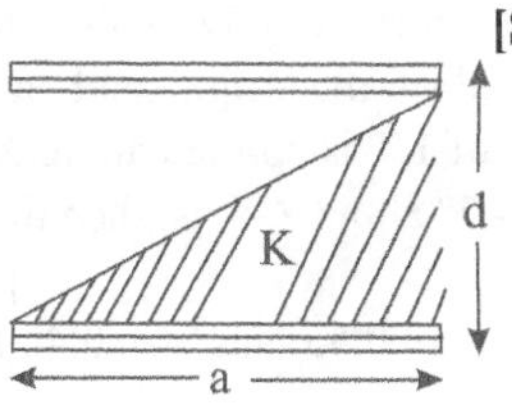

(a) $\frac{K\epsilon_0 a^2}{2d(K+1)}$ (b) $\frac{K\epsilon_0 a^2}{d(K-1)}\ln K$

(c) $\frac{K\epsilon_0 a^2}{d}\ln K$ (d) $\frac{1}{2}\frac{K\epsilon_0 a^2}{d}$

65. A parallel plate capacitor is of area 6 cm^2 and a separation 3 mm. The gap is filled with three dielectric materials of equal thickness (see figure) with dielectric constants $K_1 = 10$, $K_2 = 12$ and $K_3 = 1(4)$ The dielectric constant of a material which when fully inserted in above capacitor, gives same capacitance would be: **[Set-II, Jan. 2019]**

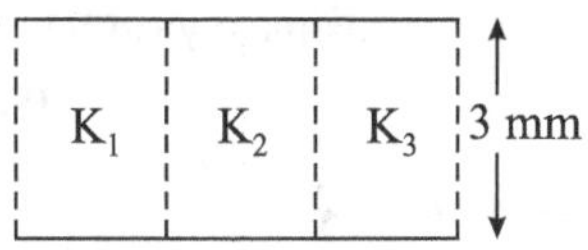

(a) 4 (b) 14 (c) 12 d) 36

CHAPTER-17 : Current Electricity

TOPIC - 1: Electric Current, Drift of Electrons, Ohm's Law, Resistance and Resistivity

66. A 200 Ω resistor has a certain color code. If one replaces the red color by green in the code, the new resistance will be : **[Set I, April 2019]**

(a) 100 Ω (b) 400 Ω (c) 300 Ω (d) 500 Ω

67. A resistance is shown in the figure. Its value and tolerance are given respectively by: **[Set I, Jan. 2019]**

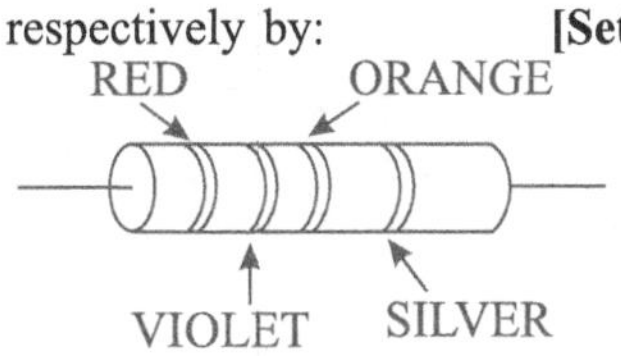

(a) 270 Ω, 10% (b) 27 kΩ, 10%
(c) 27 kΩ, 20% (d) 270 Ω, 5%

68. Drift speed of electrons, when 1.5 A of current flows in a copper wire of cross section 5 mm^2, is v. If the electron density in copper is 9×10^{28}/m^3 the value of v in mm/s close to (Take charge of electron to be = 1.6×10^{-19}C) **[Set I, Jan. 2019]**

(a) 0.02 (b) 3 (c) 2 (d) 0.2

69. A copper wire is stretched to make it 0.5% longer. The percentage change in its electrical resistance if its volume remains unchanged is: **[Set I, Jan. 2019]**

(a) 2.0% (b) 2.5% (c) 1.0% (d) 0.5%

TOPIC - 2: Combination of Resistances

70. A wire of resistance R is bent to form a square ABCD as shown in the figure. The effective resistance between E and C is: (E is mid-point of arm CD) **[Set II, April 2019]**

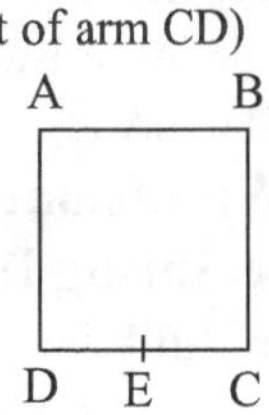

(a) R (b) $\frac{7}{64}R$ (c) $\frac{3}{4}R$ (d) $\frac{1}{16}R$

71. A uniform metallic wire has a resistance of 18 Ω and is bent into an equilateral triangle. Then, the resistance between any two vertices of the triangle is: **[Set-II, Jan. 2019]**

(a) 4 Ω (b) 8 Ω (c) 12 W (d) 2 W

TOPIC - 3: Kirchoff 's Laws, Cells, Thermo e.m.f. Electrolysis

72. For the circuit shown, with $R_1 = 1.0\ \Omega$, $R_2 = 2.0\ \Omega$, $E_1 = 2$ V and $E_2 = E_3 = 4$ V, the potential difference between the points '*a*' and '*b*' is approximately (in V) : **[Set I, April 2019]**

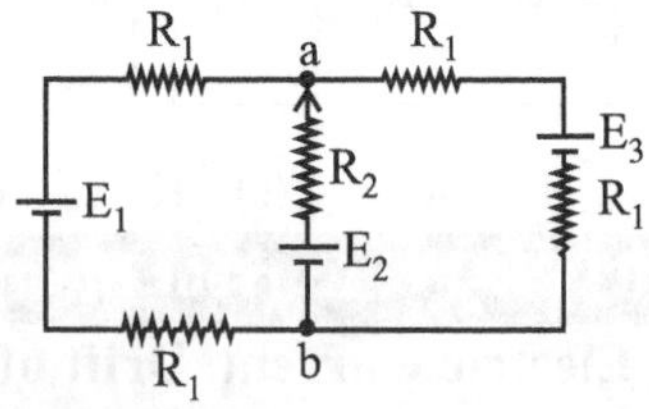

(a) 2.7 (b) 2.3 (c) 3.7 (d) 3.3

73. When the switch S, in the circuit shown, is closed then the valued of current *i* will be: **[Set I, Jan. 2019]**

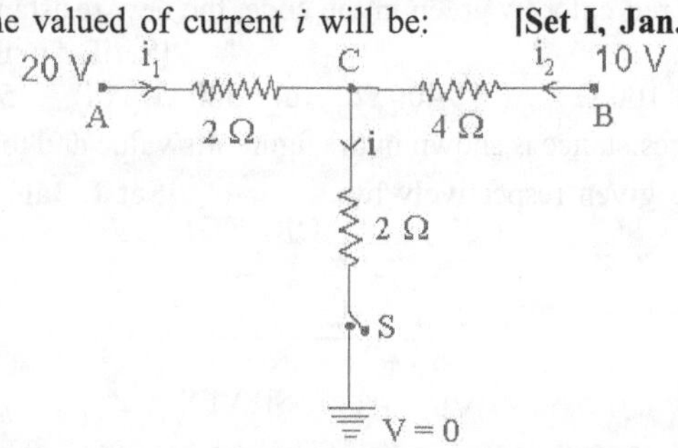

(a) 3A (b) 5A (c) 4A (d) 2A

74. In the given circuit the cells have zero internal resistance. The currents (in Amperes) passing through resistance R_1 and R_2 respectively, are: **[Set-II, Jan. 2019]**

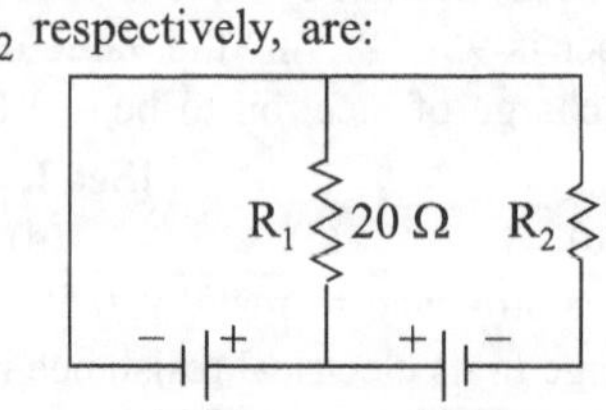

(a) 1, 2 (b) 2, 2 (c) 0.5, 0 (d) 0, 1

TOPIC - 4: Heating Effects of Current

75. A 2 W carbon resistor is color coded with green, black, red and brown respectively. The maximum current which can be passed through this resistor is: **[Set-II, Jan. 2019]**

(a) 20 mA (b) 100 mA (c) 0.4 mA (d) 63 mA

TOPIC - 5: Wheatstone Bridge and Different Measuring Instruments

76. A potentiometer wire AB having length L and resistance 12 r is joined to a cell D of emf ε and internal resistance r. A cell C having emf ε/2 and internal resistance 3r is connected. The length AJ at which the galvanometer as shown in fig. shows no deflection is: **[Set-II, Jan. 2019]**

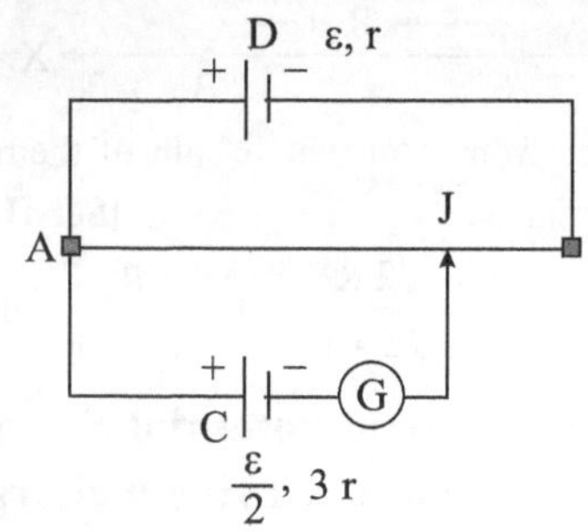

(a) $\frac{11}{12}L$ (b) $\frac{11}{24}L$ (c) $\frac{13}{24}L$ (d) $\frac{5}{12}L$

CHAPTER-18 : Moving Charges and Magnetism

TOPIC - 2: Magnetic Field Lines, Biot-Savart's Law and Ampere's Circuital Law

77. A current loop, having two circular arcs joined by two radial lines is shown in the figure. It carries a current of 10 A. The magnetic field at point O will be close to: **[Set I, Jan. 2019]**

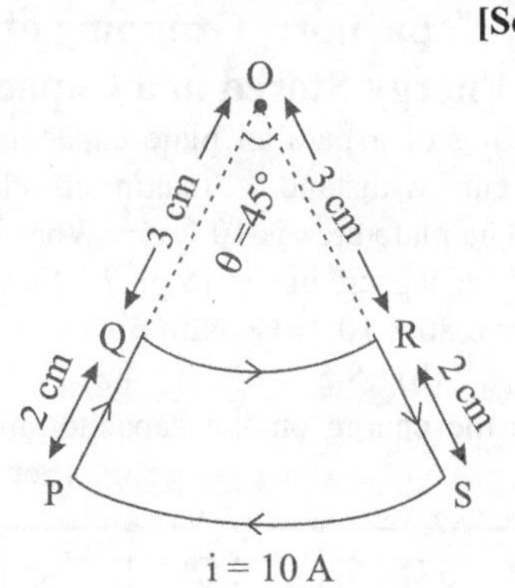

(a) 1.0×10^{-7} T (b) 1.5×10^{-7} T
(c) 1.5×10^{-5} T (d) 1.0×10^{-5} T

TOPIC - 3: Force and Torque on Current Carrying Conductor

78. A circular coil having N turns and radius *r* carries a current *I*. It is held in the XZ plane in a magnetic field $B\hat{i}$. The torque on the coil due to the magnetic field is : **[Set I, April 2019]**

(a) $\frac{Br^2 I}{\pi N}$ (b) $B\pi r^2 I N$ (c) $\frac{B\pi r^2 I}{N}$ (d) Zero

79. A rectangular coil (Dimension 5 cm × 2.5 cm) with 100 turns, carrying a current of 3 A in the clock-wise direction, is kept centered at the origin and in the X-Z plane. A magnetic field of 1 T is applied along X-axis. If the coil is tilted through 45° about Z-axis, then the torque on the coil is: **[Set II, April 2019]**

(a) 0.38 Nm (b) 0.55 Nm (c) 0.42 Nm (d) 0.27 Nm

80. A rigid square of loop of side 'a' and carrying current I_2 is lying on a horizontal surface near a long current I_1 carrying wire in the same plane as shown in figure. The net force on the loop due to the wire will be: **[Set II, April 2019]**

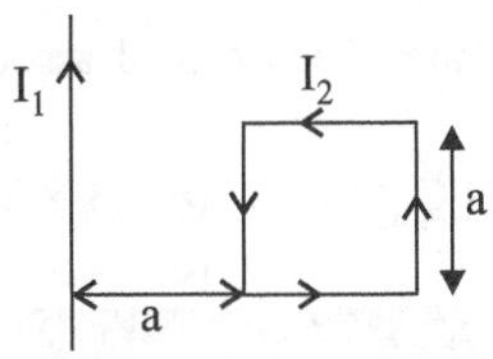

(a) Repulsive and equal to $\frac{\mu_0 I_1 I_2}{2\pi}$
(b) Attractive and equal to $\frac{\mu_0 I_1 I_2}{3\pi}$
(c) Repulsive and equal to $\frac{\mu_0 I_1 I_2}{4\pi}$
(d) Zero

81. An infinitely long current carrying wire and a small current carrying loop are in the plane of the paper as shown. The redius of the loop is a and distance of its centre from the wire is d (d>>a). If the loop applies a force F on the wire then: **[Set I, Jan. 2019]**

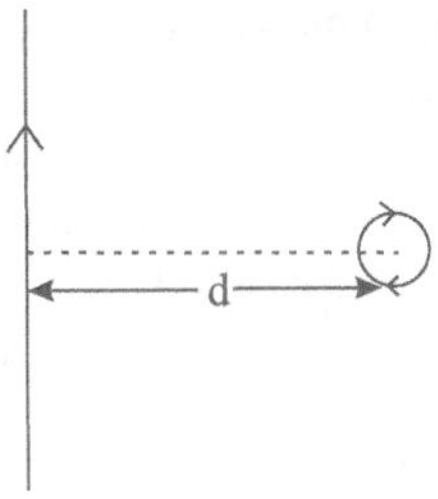

(a) F = 0 (b) $F \propto \left(\frac{a}{d}\right)$
(c) $F \propto \left(\frac{a^2}{d^3}\right)$ (d) $\propto \left(-\right)$

TOPIC - 4: Galvanometer and its Conversion into Ammeter and Voltmeter

82. A moving coil galvanometer has resistance 50 Ω and it indicates full deflection at 4 mA current. A voltmeter is made using this galvanometer and a 5 k Ω resistance. The maximum voltage, that can be measured using this voltmeter, will be close to: **[Set II, April 2019]**
(a) 40 V (b) 15 V (c) 20 V (d) 10 V

CHAPTER-19 : Magnetism and Matter

TOPIC - 1: Magnetism, Gauss's Law, Magnetic Moment, Properties of Magnet

83. A magnet of total magnetic moment $10^{-2}\hat{i}$ A-m^2 is placed in a time varying magnetic field, $B\hat{i}$ (cosωt)where B = 1 Tesla and ω = 0.125 rad/s. The work done for reversing the direction of the magnetic moment at t = 1 second, is: **[Set-II, Jan. 2019]**
(a) 0.01 J (b) 0.007 J (c) 0.028 J (d) 0.014 J

TOPIC - 2: The Earth Magnetism, Magnetic Materials and their properties

84. A bar magnet is demagnetized by inserthing it inside a solenoid of length 0.2 m, 100 turns, and carrying a current of 5.2 A. The coercivity of the bar magnet is: **[Set I, Jan. 2019]**
(a) 285 A/m (b) 2600 A/m
(c) 520 A/m (d) 1200 A/m

CHAPTER-20 : Electromagnetic Induction

TOPIC - 1: Magnetic Flux, Faraday's and Lenz's Law

85. A conducting circular loop made of a thin wire, has area 3.5×10^{-3}m^2 and resistance 10Ω. It is placed perpendicular to a time dependent magnetic field B (t) = (0.4T) sin (50πt). The the net charge flowing through the loop during t = 0 s and t = 10 ms is close to: **[Set I, Jan. 2019]**
(a) 14 mC (b) 7 mC (c) 21 mC (d) 6 mC

TOPIC - 2: Motional and Static EMI and Application of EMI

86. A thin strip 10 cm long is on a U shaped wire of negligible resistance and it is connected to a spring of spring constant 0.5 Nm^{-1} (see figure). The assembly is kept in a uniform magnetic field of 0.1 T. If the strip is pulled from its equilibrium position and released, the number of oscillations it performs before its amplitude decreases by a factor of e is N. If the mass of strip is 50 grams, its resistance 10Ω and air drag negligible, N will be close to :

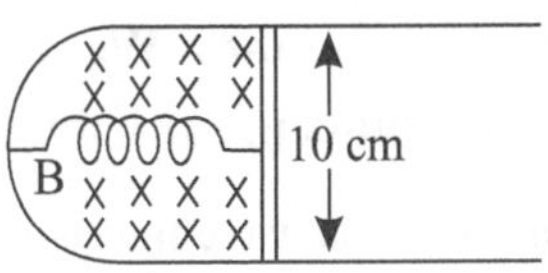

[Set I, April 2019]
(a) 1000 (b) 50000 (c) 5000 (d) 10000

87. The total number of turns and cross-section area in a solenoid is fixed. However, its length L is varied by adjusting the separation between windings. The inductance of solenoid will be proportional to: **[Set II, April 2019]**
(a) L (b) L^2 (c) $1/L^2$ (d) 1/L

88. A solid metal cube of edge length 2 cm is moving in a positive y-direction at a constant speed of 6 m/s. There is a uniform magnetic field of 0.1 T in the positive z-direction. The potential difference between the two faces of the cube perpendicular to the x-axis, is: **[Set-II, Jan. 2019]**
(a) 12 mV (b) 6 mV (c) 1 mV (d) 2 mV

89. An insulating thin rod of length l has a linear charge density $\rho(x) = \rho_0 \frac{x}{l}$ on it. The rod is rotated about an axis passing through the origin (x = 0) and perpendicular to the rod. If the rod makes n rotations per second, then the time averaged magnetic moment of the rod is: **[Set-II, Jan. 2019]**
(a) $\pi n \rho l^3$ (b) $\frac{\pi}{3} n \rho l^3$ (c) $\frac{\pi}{4} n \rho l^3$ (d) $n \rho l^3$

CHAPTER-21 : Alternating Current

TOPIC - 1: Alternating Current, Voltage and Power

90. An alternating voltage $v(t) = 220 \sin 100\pi t$ volt is applied to a purely resistive load of 50Ω. The time taken for the current to rise from half of the peak value to the peak value is : **[Set I, April 2019]**

(a) 5 ms (b) 2.2 ms
(c) 7.2 ms (d) 3.3 ms

TOPIC - 2: AC Circuit, LCR Circuit, Quality and Power Factor

91. A 20 Henry inductor coil is connected to a 10 ohm resistance in series as shown in figure. The time at which rate of dissipation of energy (Joule's heat) across resistance is equal to the rate at which magnetic energy is stored in the inductor, is : **[Set I, April 2019]**

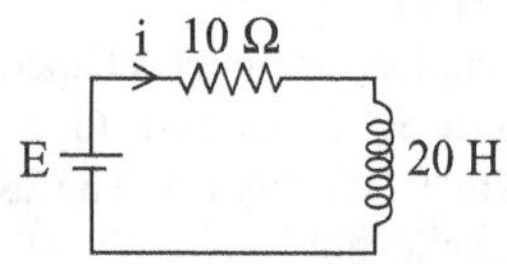

(a) $\frac{2}{ln\,2}$ (b) $\frac{1}{2} ln\,2$ (c) $2\,ln\,2$ (d) $ln\,2$

CHAPTER-22 : Electromagnetic Waves

TOPIC-1 : Electromagnetic Waves, Conduction and Displacement Current

92. A plane electromagnetic wave travels in free space along the x-direction. The electric field component of the wave at a particular point of space and time is $E = 6\ Vm^{-1}$ along y-direction. Its corresponding magnetic field component, B would be: **[Set I, April 2019]**

(a) 2×10^{-8} T along z-direction
(b) 6×10^{-8} T along x-direction
(c) 6×10^{-8} T along z-direction
(d) 2×10^{-8} T along y-direction

93. The magnetic field of a plane electromagnetic wave is given by:

$$\vec{B} = B_0\hat{i}[\cos(kz - \omega t)] + B_1\hat{j}\cos(kz + \omega t)$$

Where $B_0 = 3 \times 10^{-5}$ T and $B_1 = 2 \times 10^{-6}$ T.

The rms value of the force experienced by a stationary charge $Q = 10^{-4}$ C at $z = 0$ is closest to: **[Set II, April 2019]**

(a) 0.6 N (b) 0.1 N
(c) 0.9 N (d) 3×10^{-2} N

94. A plane electromagnetic wave of frequency 50 MHz travels in free space along the positive x-direction. At a particular point in space and time, $\vec{E} = 6.3\,\hat{j}\ V/m$. The corresponding magnetic field $\vec{B}$, at that point will be: **[Set II, April 2019]**

(a) $18.9 \times 10^{-8}\ \hat{k}T$ (b) $2.1 \times 10^{-8}\ \hat{k}T$
(c) $6.3 \times 10^{-8}\ \hat{k}T$ (d) $18.9 \times 10^{8}\ \hat{k}T$

95. If the magnetic field of a plane electromagnetic wave is given by (The speed of light = 3×10^8 m/s)

$$B = 100 \times 10^{-6} \sin\left[2\pi \times 2 \times 10^{15}\left(t - \frac{x}{c}\right)\right]$$

then the maximum electric field associated with it is: **[Set-II, Jan. 2019]**

(a) 6×10^4 N/C (b) 3×10^4 N/C
(c) 4×10^4 N/C (d) $4.5\ 10^4$ N/C

CHAPTER-23 : Ray Optics and Optical Instruments

TOPIC - 1: Plane Mirror, Spherical Mirror and Reflection of Light

96. A concave mirror for face viewing has focal length of 0.4 m. The distance at which you hold the mirror from your face in order to see your image upright with a magnification of 5 is: **[Set II, April 2019]**

(a) 0.24 m (b) 1.60 m (c) 0.32 m (d) 0.16 m

TOPIC - 2: Refraction of Light at Plane Surface and Total Internal Reflection

97. In figure, the optical fiber is $l = 2$ m long and has a diameter of $d = 20$ μm. If a ray of light is incident on one end of the fiber at angle $\theta_1 = 40°$, the number of reflections it makes before emerging from the other end is close to : (refractive index of fiber is 1.31 and sin 40° = 0.64) **[Set I, April 2019]**

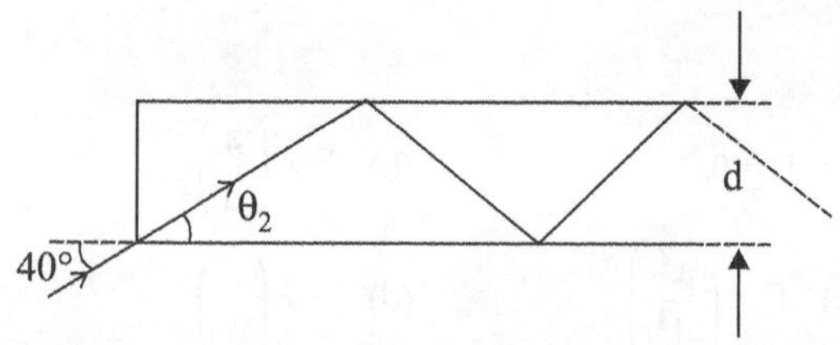

(a) 55000 (b) 66000 (c) 45000 (d) 57000

TOPIC - 3: Refraction at Curved Surface Lenses and Power of Lens

98. An upright object is placed at a distance of 40 cm in front of a convergent lens of focal length 20 cm. A convergent mirror of focal length 10 cm is placed at a distance of 60 cm on the other side of the lens. The position and size of the final image will be : **[Set I, April 2019]**

(a) 20 cm from the convergent mirror, same size as the object
(b) 40 cm from the convergent mirror, same size as the object
(c) 40 cm from the convergent lens, twice the size of the object
(d) 20 cm from the convergent mirror, twice the size of the object

99. A convex lens is put 10 cm from a light source and it makes a sharp image on a screen, kept 10 cm from the lens. Now a glass block (refractive index 1.5) of 1.5 cm thickness is placed in contact with the light source. To get the sharp image again, the screem is shifted by a distance d. Then d is: **[Set I, Jan. 2019]**

(a) 1.1 cm away from the lens
(b) 0
(c) 0.55 cm towards the lens
(d) 0.55 cm away from the lens

100. A plano convex lens of refractive index μ_1 and focal length f_1 is kept in contact with another plano concave lens of refractive index μ_2 and focal length f_2 If the radius of curvature of their spherical faces is R each and $f_1 = 2f_2$, then μ_1 and μ_2 are related as: **[Set-II, Jan. 2019]**

(a) $\mu_1 + \mu_2 = 3$ (b) $2\mu_1 - \mu_2 = 1$
(c) $3\mu_2 - 2\mu_1 = 1$ (d) $2\mu_2 - \mu_1 = 1$

CHAPTER-24 : Wave Optics

TOPIC - 1: Wavefront, Interference of Light, Coherent and Incoherent Sources

101. In an interference experiment the ratio of amplitudes of coherent waves is $\frac{a_1}{a_2} = \frac{1}{3}$. The ratio of maximum and minimum intensities of fringes will be :**[Set I, April 2019]**

(a) 2 (b) 18
(c) 4 (d) 9

102. Two coherent sources produce waves of different intensities which interfere. After interference, the ratio of the maximum intensity to the minimum intensity is 16. The intensity of the waves are in the ratio: **[Set I, Jan. 2019]**

(a) 16 : 9 (b) 25 : 9 (c) 4 : 1 (d) 5 : 3

TOPIC - 2: Young's Double Slit Experiment

103. The figure shows a Young's double slit experimental setup. It is observed that when a thin transparent sheet of thickness t and refractive index μ is put in front of one of the slits, the central maximum gets shifted by a distance equal to n fringe widths. If the wavelength of light used is λ, t will be: **[Set II, April 2019]**

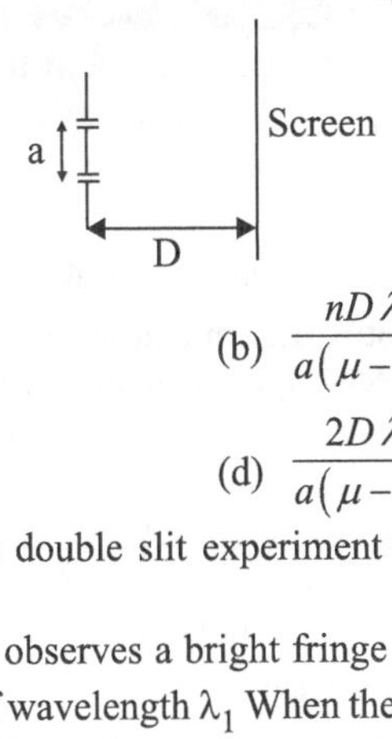

(a) $\frac{2nD\lambda}{a(\mu-1)}$ (b) $\frac{nD\lambda}{a(\mu-1)}$
(c) $\frac{D\lambda}{a(\mu-1)}$ (d) $\frac{2D\lambda}{a(\mu-1)}$

104. In a Young's double slit experiment with slit separation 0.1 mm, one observes a bright fringe at angle $\frac{1}{40}$ rad by using light of wavelength λ_1 When the light of wavelength λ_2 is used a bright fringe is seen at the same angle in the same set up. Given that λ_1 and λ_2 are in visible range (380 nm to 740 nm), their values are: **[Set-II, Jan. 2019]**

(a) 625 nm, 500 nm (b) 380 nm, 525 nm
(c) 380 nm, 500 nm (d) 400 nm, 500 nm

TOPIC - 3: Diffraction, Polarisation of Light and Resolving Power

105. Consider a tank made of glass (refractive index 1.5) with a thick bottom. It is filled with a liquid of refractive index μ. A student finds that, irrespective of what the incident angle i (see figure) is for a beam of light entering the liquid, the light reflected from the liquid glass interface is never completely polarized. For this to happen, the minimum value of μ is: **[Set I, Jan. 2019]**

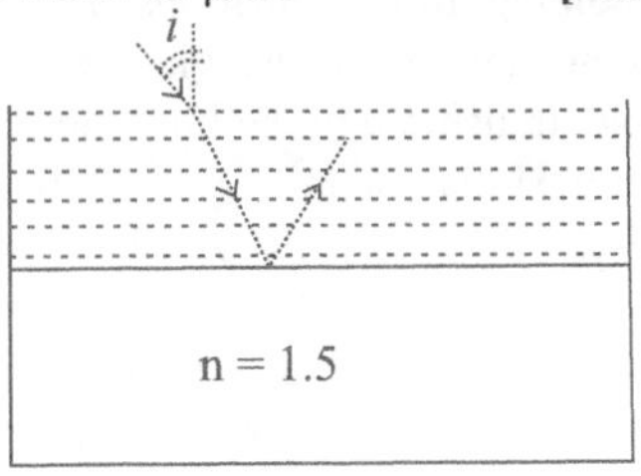

(a) $\sqrt{\frac{5}{3}}$ (b) $\frac{3}{\sqrt{5}}$ (c) $\frac{5}{\sqrt{3}}$ (d) $\frac{4}{3}$

CHAPTER-25 : Dual Nature of Radiation and Matter

TOPIC - 1: Matter Waves, Cathode and Positive Rays

106. Two particles move at right angle to each other. Their de Broglie wavelengths are λ_1 and λ_2 respectively. The particles suffer perfectly inelastic collision. The de Broglie wavelength λ, of the final particle, is given by : **[Set I, April 2019]**

(a) $\frac{1}{\lambda^2} = \frac{1}{\lambda_1^2} + \frac{1}{\lambda_2^2}$ (b) $\lambda = \sqrt{\lambda_1\lambda_2}$

(c) $\lambda = \frac{\lambda_2 + \lambda_2}{2}$ (d) $\frac{2}{\lambda} = \frac{1}{\lambda_1} + \frac{1}{\lambda_2}$

107. In an electron microscope, the resolution that can be achieved is of the order of the wavelength of electrons used. To resolve a width of 7.5×10^{-12} m, the minimum electron energy required is close to: **[Set-II, Jan. 2019]**

(a) 500 keV (b) 100 keV (c) 1 keV (d) 25 keV

TOPIC - 2: Photon, Photoelectric Effect X-rays and Davisson-Germer Experiment

108. The electric field of light wave is given as

$$\vec{E} = 10^3 \cos\left(\frac{2\pi x}{5\times10^{-7}} - 2\pi\times6\times10^{14}t\right)\hat{x}\,\frac{N}{C}$$

This light falls on a metal plate of work function 2eV. The stopping potential of the photo-electrons is:

Given, E (in eV) = $\frac{12375}{\lambda(\text{in A})}$ **[Set II, April 2019]**

(a) 2.0 V (b) 0.72 V (c) 0.48 V (d) 2.48 V

109. Surface of certain metal is first illuminated with light of wavelength λ_1 = 350 nm and then, by light of wavelength λ_2 = 540 nm. It is found that the maximum speed of the photo electrons in the two cases differ by a factor of (2) The work function of the metal (in eV) is close to: **[Set I, Jan. 2019]**

(Energy of photon = $\frac{1240}{\lambda\,(\text{in nm})}$ eV)

(a) 1.8 (b) 2.5 (c) 5.6 (d) 1.4

CHAPTER-26 : Atoms

TOPIC - 2 : Bohr's Model and the Spectra of the Hydrogen atom

110. Radiation coming from transitions $n = 2$ to $n = 1$ of hydrogen atoms fall on He^+ ions in $n = 1$ and $n = 2$ states. The possible transition of helium ions as they absorb energy from the radiation is : **[Set I, April 2019]**

(a) $n = 2 \rightarrow n = 3$ (b) $n = 1 \rightarrow n = 4$
(c) $n = 2 \rightarrow n = 5$ (d) $n = 2 \rightarrow n = 4$

111. Taking the wavelength of first Balmer line in hydrogen spectrum (n = 3 to n = 2) as 660 nm, the wavelength of the 2nd Balmer line (n = 4 to n = 2) will be; **[Set II, April 2019]**

(a) 889.2 nm (b) 488.9 nm (c) 642.7 nm (d) 388.9 nm

CHAPTER-27 : Nuclei

TOPIC - 3: Radioactivity

112. A sample of radioactive material A, that has an activity of 10 mCi (1 Ci = 3.7×10^{10} decays/s), has twice the number of nuclei as another sample of a different radioactive material B which has an acitvity of 20 mCi. The correct choices for half-lives of A and B would then be respectively: **[Set I, Jan. 2019]**

(a) 5 days and 10 days (b) 10 days and 40 days
(c) 20 days and 5 days (d) 20 days and 10 days

113. Using a nuclear counter the count rate of emitted particles from a radioactive source is measured. At t = 0 it was 1600 counts per second and t = 8 seconds it was 100 counts per second. The count rate observed, as counts per second, at t = 6 seconds is close to: **[Set-II, Jan. 2019]**

(a) 200 (b) 150 (c) 400 (d) 360

CHAPTER-28 : Semiconductor Electronics : Materials, Devices and Simple Circuits

TOPIC - 1: Solids, Semiconductors and P-N Junction Diode

114. The reverse breakdown voltage of a Zener diode is 5.6 V in the given circuit.

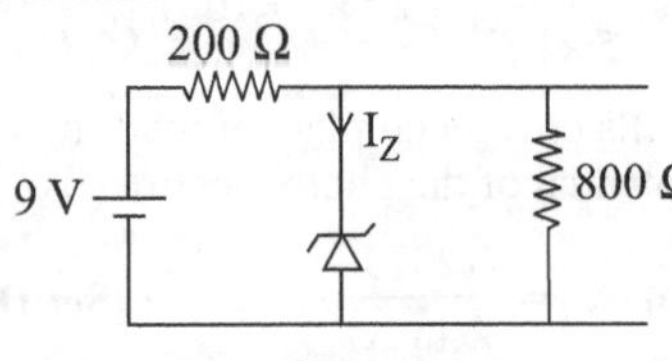

The current I_z through the Zener is : **[Set I, April 2019]**

(a) 10 mA (b) 17 mA (c) 15 mA (d) 7 mA

115. Mobility of electrons in a semiconductor is defined as the ratio of their drift velocity to the applied electric field. If, for an n-type semiconductor, the density of electrons is 10^{19} m^{-3} and their mobility is 1.6m^2/(V.s) then the resistivity of the semiconductor (since it is an n-type semiconductor contribution of holes is ignored) is close to: **[Set I, Jan. 2019]**

(a) 2 Ωm (b) 4 Ωm (c) 0.4 Ωm (d) 0.2 Ωm

TOPIC - 2: Junction Transistor

116. An NPN transistor is used in common emitter configuration as an amplifier with 1 k Ω load resistance. Signal voltage of 10 mV is applied across the base-emitter. This produces a 3 mA change in the collector current and 15 μA change in the base current of the amplifier. The input resistance and voltage gain are: **[Set II, April 2019]**

(a) 0.33 kΩ, 1.5 (b) 0.67 kΩ, 300
(c) 0.67 kΩ, 200 (d) 0.33 kΩ, 300

TOPIC - 3: Digital Electronics and Logic Gates

117. To get output '1' at R, for the given logic gate circuit the input values must be: **[Set-II, Jan. 2019]**

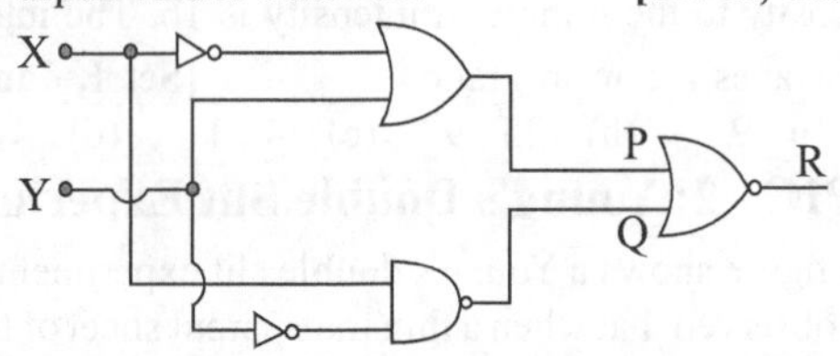

(a) X = 0, Y = 1 (b) X = 1, Y = 1
(c) X = 1, Y = 0 (d) X = 0, Y = 0

CHAPTER-29 : Communication Systems

TOPIC-1 : Communication Systems

118. The wavelength of the carrier waves in a modern optical fiber communication network is close to : **[Set I, April 2019]**

(a) 2400 nm (b) 1500 nm (c) 600 nm (d) 900 nm

119. A signal Acosωt is transmitted using $v_0 \sin \omega_0 t$ as carrier wave. The correct amplitude modulated (AM) signal is: **[Set II, April 2019]**

(a) $v_0 \sin\omega_0 t + \frac{A}{2}\sin(\omega_0 - \omega)t + \frac{A}{2}\sin(\omega_0 + \omega)t$

(b) $v_0 \sin[\omega_0(1 + 0.01 A\sin\omega t)t]$

(c) $v_0 \sin\omega_0 t + A\cos\omega t$

(d) $(v_0 + A)\cos\omega t \sin\omega_0 t$

120. A TV transmission tower has a height of 140 m and the height of the receiving antenna is 40 m. What is the maximum distance upto which signals can be broadcasted from this tower in LOS (Line of Sight) mode? (Given : radius of earth = 6.4×10^6 m). **[Set-II, Jan. 2019]**

(a) 65 km (b) 48 km (c) 80 km (d) 40 km

Hints and Solutions

CHAPTER-1 : Physical World, Units and Measurements

TOPIC-1 : Unit of Physical Quantities

1. **(a)** Density of material in SI unit,

$$= \frac{128\text{kg}}{\text{m}^3}$$

Density of material in new system

$$= \frac{128(50\,\text{g})(20)}{(25\,\text{cm})^3(4)^3}$$

$$= \frac{128}{64} \times (20) = 40\,\text{units}$$

TOPIC-2 : Dimensions of Physical Quantities

2. **(d)** $$\left[\sqrt{\frac{\varepsilon_0}{\mu_0}}\right] = \sqrt{\frac{\varepsilon_0^2}{\mu_0\varepsilon_0}} = \left[\frac{\varepsilon_0}{\sqrt{\mu_0\varepsilon_0}}\right] = \varepsilon_0 C[LT^{-1}] \times [\varepsilon_0]$$

$$\left[\because \frac{1}{\sqrt{\mu_0\varepsilon_0}} = C\right]$$

$$\because F = \frac{q^2}{4\pi\varepsilon_0 r^2}$$

$$\Rightarrow [\varepsilon_0] = \frac{[AT]^2}{[MLT^{-2}] \times [L^2]} = [A^2M^{-1}L^{-3}T^4]$$

$$\therefore \left[\sqrt{\frac{\varepsilon_0}{\mu_0}}\right] = [LT^{-1}] \times [A^2M^{-1}L^{-3}T^4]$$

$$= [M^{-1}L^{-2}T^3A^2]$$

TOPIC-3 : Errors in Measurements

3. **(Bonus)** $\delta = \frac{M}{V} = \frac{M}{2^3} = Ml^{-3}$

$$\frac{\Delta\delta}{3} = \frac{\Delta M}{M} + 3\frac{\Delta l}{2}$$

$$= \frac{0.10}{10.00} + 3\left(\frac{0.01}{0.10}\right)$$

$= 0.013\ \text{kg/m}^3$

CHAPTER-3 : Motion in a Plane

TOPIC-1 : Vectors

4. **(c)** From figure,

$$\vec{r}_G = \frac{a}{2}\hat{i} + \frac{a}{2}\hat{k}$$

$$\vec{r}_H = \frac{a}{2}\hat{j} + \frac{a}{2}\hat{k}$$

$$\therefore \vec{r}_H - \vec{r}_G = \left(\frac{a}{2}\hat{j} + \frac{a}{2}\hat{k}\right) - \left(\frac{a}{2}\hat{i} + \frac{a}{2}\hat{k}\right) = \frac{a}{2}\left(\hat{j} - \hat{i}\right)$$

TOPIC-2 : Motion in a Plane with Constant Acceleration

5. **(c)** From given equation,

$$\vec{V} = K\left(y\hat{i} + x\hat{j}\right)$$

$$\frac{dx}{dt} = ky \text{ and } \frac{dy}{dt} = kx$$

$$\text{Now, } \frac{\frac{dy}{dt}}{\frac{dx}{dt}} = \frac{x}{y} = \frac{dy}{dx} \Rightarrow ydy = xdx$$

Integrating both side

$y^2 = x^2 + c$

TOPIC-3 : Projectile Motion

6. **(a)** As we know, range $R = \frac{u^2 \sin 2\theta}{g}$

and, area $A = \pi R^2$

$\therefore\ A \propto R^2$ or, $A \propto u^4$

$$\therefore \frac{A_1}{A_2} = \frac{u_1^4}{u_2^4} = \left[\frac{1}{2}\right]^4 = \frac{1}{16}$$

TOPIC-4 : Relative Velocity in Two Dimensions & Uniform Circular Motion

7. **(b)**

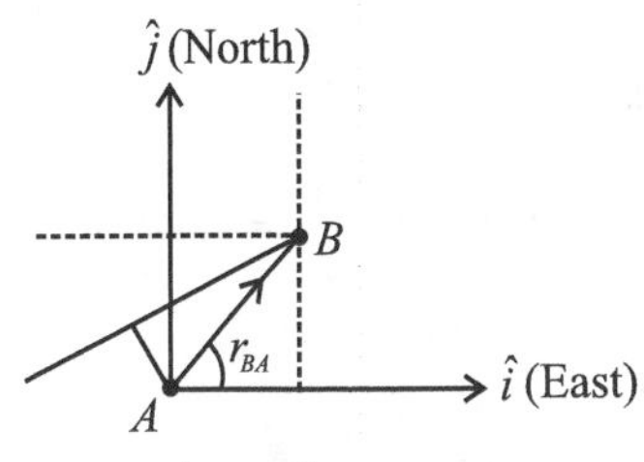

$$\vec{v}_A = 30\hat{i} + 50\hat{j}\ \text{km/hr}$$

$$\vec{v}_B = (-10\hat{i})\ \text{km/hr}$$

$$r_{BA} = (80\hat{i} + 150\hat{j})\ \text{km}$$

$$\vec{v}_{BA} = \vec{v}_B - \vec{v}_A = -10\hat{i} - 30\hat{i} - 50\hat{i} = 40\hat{i} - 50\hat{j}$$

$$t_{\text{minimum}} = \frac{\left|(\vec{r}_{BA}) \cdot (\vec{v}_{BA})\right|}{\left|(\vec{v}_{BA})\right|^2}$$

$$= \frac{|(80\hat{i} + 150\hat{j})(-40\hat{i} - 50\hat{j})|}{(10\sqrt{41})^2}$$

$$\therefore\ t = \frac{10700}{10\sqrt{41} \times 10\sqrt{41}} = \frac{107}{41} = 2.6 \text{ Hrs.}$$

8. (c) $\sin\theta = \frac{u}{v} = \frac{2}{4} = \frac{1}{2}$

or $\theta = 30°$

with respect to flow,

$= 90° + 30° = 120°$

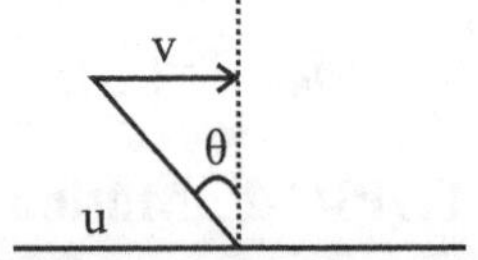

CHAPTER-4 : Laws of Motion

TOPIC-1 : Ist, IInd & IIIrd Laws of Motion

9. (d) $v^2 = u^2 - 2gh$

or $v = \sqrt{u^2 - 2gh}$

Momentum, $P = mv$

$= m\sqrt{u^2 - 2gh}$

At h = 0, P = mu and at $h = \frac{u^2}{f}, P = 0$

upward direction is positive and downward direction is negative.

TOPIC-3 : Friction

10. (a)

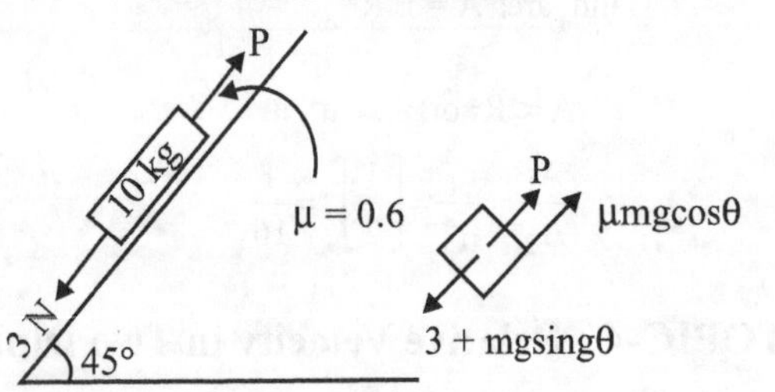

$\text{mg sin } 45° = \frac{100}{\sqrt{2}} = 50\sqrt{2}$

$[\because m = 10\text{kg}, g = 9.8\text{ms}^{-2}]$

$\mu\text{mg cos}\theta = 0.6 \times \text{mg} \times \frac{1}{\sqrt{2}} = 0.6 \times 50\sqrt{2}$

$3 + \text{mg sin}\theta = P + \mu\text{mg cos}\theta$

$3 + 50\sqrt{2} = P + 30\sqrt{2}$

$\therefore P = 31.28 = 32$ N

CHAPTER-5 : Work, Energy and Power

TOPIC-1 : Work

11. (a) $W = u_f - u_i$

$= 0 - \left(-\frac{mg}{n} \times \frac{L}{2n}\right)$

$= \frac{MgL}{2n^2}.$

12. (d) Here, $N - mg = ma = \frac{mg}{2} \Rightarrow N = \frac{3mg}{2}$

N = normal reaction

Now, work done by normal reaction 'N' on block in time t, $W = \vec{N}\vec{S} = \left(\frac{3mg}{2}\right)\left(\frac{1}{2}g/_2 t^2\right)$

or, $W = \frac{3mg^2t^2}{8}$

TOPIC-2 : Energy

13. (c) We know area under F-x graph gives the work done by the body

$\therefore\ W = \frac{1}{2} \times (3+2) \times (3-2) + 2 \times 2$

$= 2.5 + 4$

$= 6.5$ J

Using work energy theorem,

Δ K.E = work done

$\therefore\ \Delta$ K.E = 6.5 J

14. (d) Maximum speed is at mean position or equilibrium

At equilibrium Position

$F = kx \Rightarrow x = \frac{F}{k}$

From work-energy theorem,

$W_F + W_{sp} = \Delta KE$

$F(x) - \frac{1}{2}kx^2 = \frac{1}{2}mv^2 - 0$

$F\left(\frac{F}{k}\right) - \frac{1}{2}k\left(\frac{F}{k}\right)^2 = \frac{1}{2}mv^2$

$\Rightarrow \frac{1}{2}\frac{F^2}{K} = \frac{1}{2}mv^2$

or, $v_{max} = \frac{F}{\sqrt{mk}}$

TOPIC-4 : Collisions

15. (b) $2u + 0 = 2\left(\frac{u}{4}\right) + mv_2$

and $\frac{1}{2} \times 2 \times u^2 + 0 = \frac{1}{2} \times 2 \times \left(\frac{u}{4}\right)^2 + \frac{1}{2}mv_2^2$

On solving, we get

m = 1.5 kg

16. (c) Kinetic energy of block A

$k_1 = \frac{1}{2}mv_0^2$

$\therefore$ From principle of linear momentum conservation

$mv_0 = (2m + M)v_f \Rightarrow v_f = \frac{mv_0}{2m + M}$

According to question, of $\frac{5}{6}$ th the initial kinetic energy is lost in whole process.

$$\therefore \frac{k_i}{k_f} = 6 \Rightarrow \frac{\frac{1}{2}mv_0^2}{\frac{1}{2}(2m+M)\left(\frac{mv_0}{2m+M}\right)^2} = 6$$

$$\Rightarrow \frac{2m+M}{m} = 6 \therefore \frac{M}{m} = 4$$

17. **(c)**

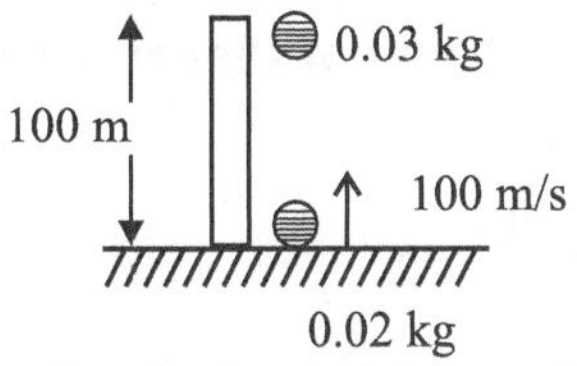

Time taken for the particles to collide,

$$t = \frac{d}{V_{rel}} = \frac{100}{100} = 1\,\text{sec}$$

Speed of wood just before collision = gt = 10 m/s and speed of bullet just before collision = v – gt

= 100 – 10 = 90 m/s

$$S = 100 \times 1 - \frac{1}{2} \times 10 \times 1 = 95 \text{ m}$$

Now, using conservation of linear momentum just before and after the collision

$-(0.03)(10) + (0.02)(90) = (0.05)v$

$\Rightarrow 150 = 5v$ $\therefore v = 30$ m/s

Max. height reached by body

$$h = \frac{v^2}{2g} = \frac{30\times 30}{2\times 10} = 45\,\text{m}$$

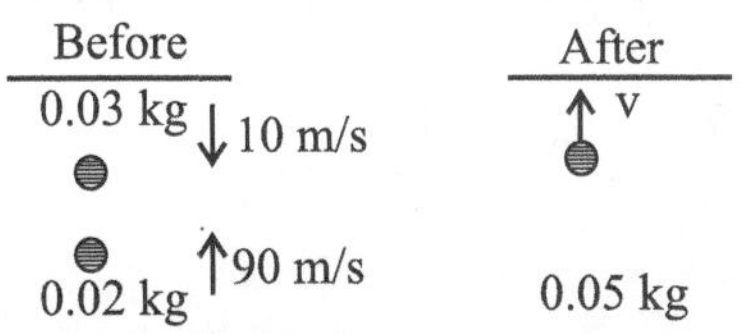

$\therefore$ Height above tower = 40 m

CHAPTER-6 : System of Particles and Rotational Motion

TOPIC-1 : Centre of Mass, Centre of Gravity & Principle of Moments

18. **(a)** Acceleration of centre of mass (a_{cm}) is given by

$$\therefore \vec{a}_{cm} = \frac{m_1\vec{a}_1 + m_2\vec{a}_2 + \ldots\ldots}{m_1 + m_2 + \ldots\ldots}$$

$$= \frac{(2m)a\hat{j} + 3m\times a\hat{i} + ma(-\hat{i}) + 4m\times a(-\hat{j})}{2m+3m+4m+m}$$

$$= \frac{2a\hat{i} - 2a\hat{j}}{10} = \frac{a}{5}(\hat{i} - \hat{j})$$

TOPIC-3 : Torque, Couple and Angular Momentum

19. **(d)** Given that, the rod is of uniform mass density and AB = BC

Let mass of one rod is m.

Balancing torque about hinge point.

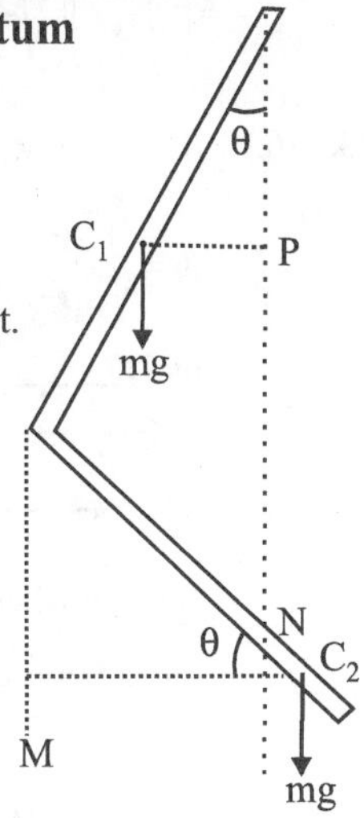

$$mg(C_1P) = mg(C_2N)$$

$$mg\left(\frac{L}{2}\sin\theta\right) = mg\left(\frac{L}{2}\cos\theta - L\sin\theta\right)$$

$$\Rightarrow \frac{3}{2}mgL\sin\theta = \frac{mgL}{2}\cos\theta \Rightarrow \frac{\sin\theta}{\cos\theta} = \frac{1}{3} \text{ or, } \tan\theta = \frac{1}{3}$$

20. **(d)** Consider a strip of radius x and thickness dx,

Torque due to friction on this strip

Net torque = Σ Torque on ring

$$\int d\tau = \int_0^R \frac{\mu F.2\pi x dx}{\pi R^2}$$

$$\Rightarrow \tau = \frac{2\mu F}{R^2}\cdot\frac{R^3}{3}$$

$$\tau = \frac{2\mu FR}{3}$$

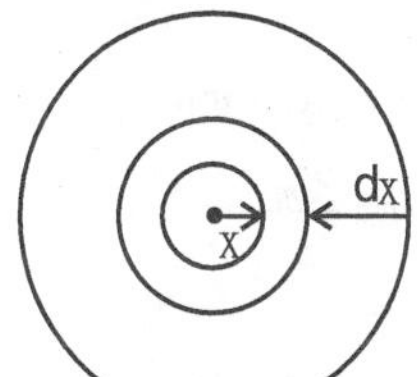

TOPIC-4 : Moment of Inertia and Rotational K.E.

21. **(c)** Taking a circular ring of radius *r* and thickness *dr* as a mass element, so total mass,

$$M = \int_0^R \rho_0 r \times 2\pi r dr = \frac{2\pi\rho_0 R^3}{3}$$

$$_C = \int_0^R \rho_0 r \times 2\pi r dr \times r^2 = \frac{2\pi\rho_0 R^5}{5}$$

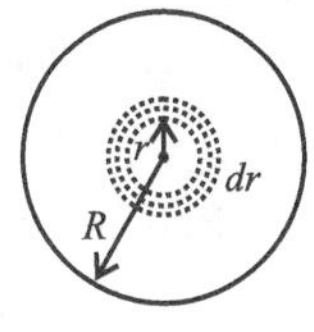

Using parallel axis theorem

$$\therefore I = I_C + MR^2 = 2\pi\rho_0 R^5\left(\frac{1}{3} + \frac{1}{5}\right) = \frac{16\pi\rho_0 R^5}{15}$$

$$= \frac{8}{5}\left[\frac{2}{3}\pi\rho_0 R^3\right]R^2 = \frac{8}{5}MR^2$$

22. **(d)** $\frac{1}{2}I\omega^2 = kQ^2$

$$\text{or } \omega = \left(\sqrt{\frac{2k}{I}}\right)Q$$

$$\text{or } \alpha = \frac{d\omega}{\pi} = \sqrt{\frac{2K}{I}}\left(\frac{dQ}{dt}\right) = \left(\sqrt{\frac{2k}{I}}\right)\omega$$

$$=\left(\sqrt{\frac{2k}{I}}\right)\left(\sqrt{\frac{2k}{I}}\right)\theta \;=\frac{2k\theta}{I}$$

23. (c) As we know, $\omega=\sqrt{\frac{k}{I}}$

$$\omega=\sqrt{\frac{3k}{m\ell^2}} \quad \left[\because\ I_{rod}=\frac{1}{3}m\ell^2\right]$$

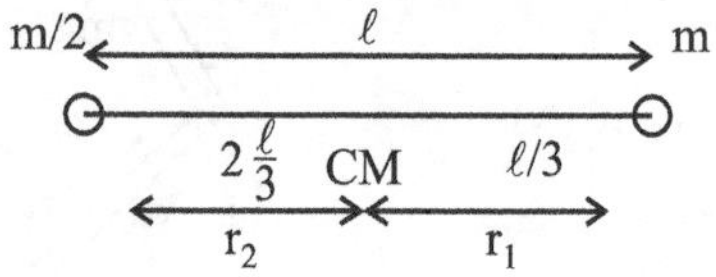

Tension when it passes through the mean position,

$$=m\omega^2\theta_0^2\frac{\ell}{3}=m\frac{3k}{m\ell^2}\theta_0^2\frac{\ell}{3}=\frac{k\theta_0^2}{\ell}$$

TOPIC-5 : Rolling Motion

24. (Bonus) $mgh=\frac{1}{2}mv_{cm}^2+\frac{1}{2}I_{cm}\omega^2$

$$=\frac{1}{2}mv_{cm}^2+\frac{1}{2}I_{cm}\left(\frac{v_{cm}}{R}\right)^2$$

$$=\frac{1}{2}\left(m+\frac{I_{cm}}{R^2}\right)v_{cm}^2$$

For ring : mgh $=\frac{1}{2}\left(m+\frac{mR^2}{R^2}\right)v_{cm}^2$

$\therefore h=\frac{v_{cm}^2}{g}$.

For solid cylinder, $mgh=\frac{1}{2}\left(m+\frac{mR^2}{2R^2}\right)v_{cm}^2$

$\therefore h=\frac{3v_{cm}^2}{4g}$

For sphere, $mgh=\frac{1}{2}\left(m+\frac{2}{5}\frac{mR^2}{R^2}\right)v_{cm}^2$

$\therefore h=\frac{7v_{cm}^2}{10g}$

Ratio of heights $1:\frac{3}{4}:\frac{7}{10}\Rightarrow 20:15:14$

25. (d)

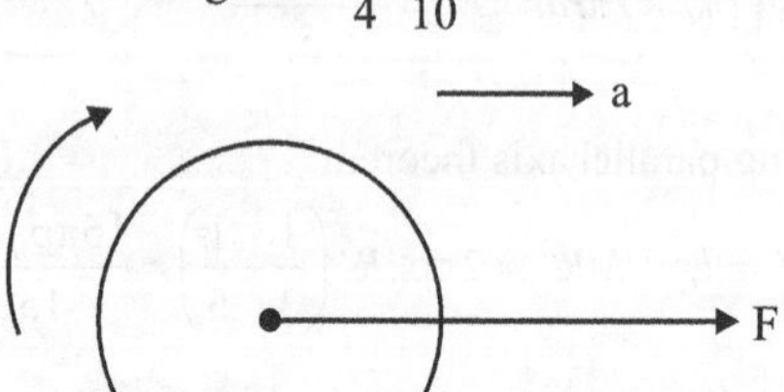

$F-fr=ma$ ...(i)

$f_rR=I\alpha=\frac{mR^2}{2}\alpha$ ...(ii)

for pure rolling

$a=\alpha R$ ...(iii)

from (1) (2) and (3)

$$F-\frac{mR\alpha}{2}=m\alpha R$$

$$F=\frac{3}{2}mR\alpha$$

$$\alpha=\frac{2F}{3mR}$$

CHAPTER-7 : Gravitation

TOPIC-1 : Kepler's Laws of Planetary Motion

26. (c) Areal velocity $\frac{dA}{dt}$;

$$dA=\frac{1}{2}r^2d\theta$$

$$\Rightarrow\frac{dA}{dt}=\frac{1}{2}r^2\frac{d\theta}{dt}$$

$$\frac{1}{2}r^2\omega$$

Also, $L=mvr$
$=mr^2\omega$

$$\Rightarrow\frac{dA}{dt}=\frac{1}{2}\frac{L}{m}$$

TOPIC-4 : Gravitational Field and Potential Energy

27. (b) $AC=a\sqrt{2}\quad\because\ r=\frac{AC}{2}=\frac{a\sqrt{2}}{2}=\frac{a}{\sqrt{2}}$

Resultant force on the body

$$B=\frac{GM^2}{a^2}\hat{i}+\frac{GM^2}{a^2}\hat{j}+\frac{GM^2}{(a\sqrt{2})^2}(\cos 45°\hat{i}+\sin 45°\hat{j})$$

$$\Rightarrow |F|=\frac{GM^2}{a^2}(\sqrt{2})+\frac{GM^2}{2a^2}$$

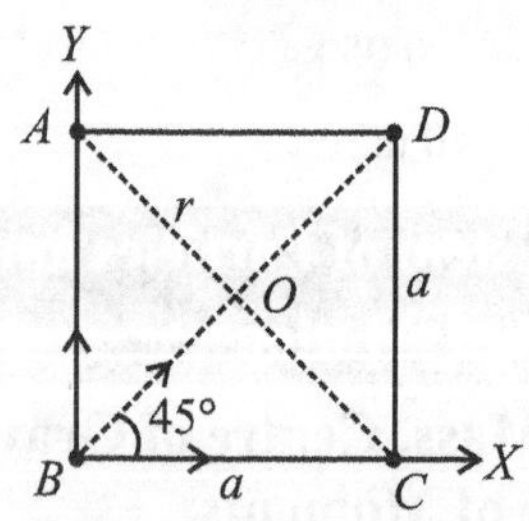

$\frac{Mv^2}{r}$ = Resultant force towards centre

$$\therefore\ \frac{Mv^2}{\left(\frac{a}{\sqrt{2}}\right)}=\frac{GM^2}{a^2}\left(\sqrt{2}+\frac{1}{2}\right)$$

$$\Rightarrow v^2=\frac{GM}{a}\left(1+\frac{1}{2\sqrt{2}}\right)$$

$$\Rightarrow v=\sqrt{\frac{GM}{a}\left(1+\frac{1}{2\sqrt{2}}\right)}=1.16\sqrt{\frac{GM}{a}}$$

28. (c) $E_g = \frac{GM}{(3a)^2} + \frac{G(2M)}{(3a)^2} = \frac{GM}{3a^2}$

TOPIC-5 : Motion of Satellites, Escape Speed and Orbital Velocity

29. (b) At height r from center of earth, orbital velocity

$v = \sqrt{\frac{GM}{r}}$

By principle of energy conservation

KE of 'm' + $\left(-\frac{GMm}{r}\right) = 0 + 0$

($\because$ At infinity, PE = KE = 0)

or KE of 'm' = $\frac{GMm}{r} = \left(\sqrt{\frac{GM}{r}}\right)$ m = mv

CHAPTER-8 : Mechanical Properties of Solids

TOPIC-1 : Hooke's Law & Young's Modulus

30. (c) Given,

Radius of wire, $r = 2$ mm

Mass of the load m = 4 kg

Stress $= \frac{F}{A} = \frac{mg}{\pi(r)^2} = \frac{4 \times 3.1\pi}{\pi \times (2 \times 10^{-3})^2} = 3.1 \times 10^6 \text{ N/m}^2$

TOPIC-2 : Bulk and Rigidity Modulus and Work Done in Stretching a Wire

31. (a) When a catapult is stretched up to length ℓ, then the stored energy in it = Δk. E $\Rightarrow$

$\frac{1}{2} \cdot \left(\frac{YA}{L}\right)(\Delta l)^2 = \frac{1}{2} mv^2$

$\Rightarrow y = \frac{mv^2 L}{A(\Delta l)^2}$

m = 0.02 kg

v = 20 ms^{-1}

L = 0.42 m

A = (π d^2)/(4)

d = 6 × 10^{-3} m

$\Delta \ell$ = 0.2 m

$= \frac{0.02 \times 400 \times 0.42 \times 4}{\pi \times 36 \times 10^{-6} \times 0.04}$

= 2.3 × 10^6 N/m^2

So, order is 10^6.

CHAPTER-9 : Mechanical Properties of Fluids

TOPIC-2 : Fluid Flow, Reynold's Number and Bernoulli's Principle

32. (b) Rate of flow of water (V) = 100 lit/min

$= \frac{100 \times 10^{-3}}{60} \times \frac{5}{3} \times 10^{-3} \text{m}^3$

$\therefore$ Velocity of flow of water (v) $= \frac{V}{A} = \frac{5 \times 10^{-3}}{3 \times \times (5 \times 10^{-2})^2}$

$= \frac{10}{15\pi} = \frac{2}{3\pi}$ m/s

= 0.2 m/s

$\therefore$ Reynold number (N_R) $= \frac{Dv\rho}{\eta}$

$= \frac{(10 \times 10^{-2}) \times \frac{2}{3\pi} \times 1000}{1} = 2 \times 10^4$

Order of $N_R = 10^4$

33. (a)

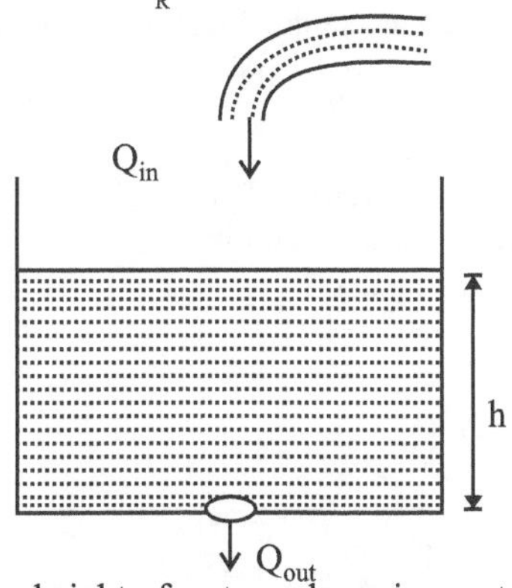

Since height of water column is constant therefore, water inflow rate (Q_{in})

= water outflow rate

$Q_{in} = 10^{-4} \text{ m}^3\text{s}^{-1}$

$Q_{out} = Au = 10^{-4} \times \sqrt{2gh}$

$\therefore 10^{-4} = 10^{-4} \times \sqrt{20 \times h}$

$\therefore h = \frac{1}{20}$ m = 5 cm

TOPIC-4 : Surface Tension, Surface Energy and Capillarity

34. (d) We have, $h = \frac{2T\cos\theta}{r\rho g}$

Mass of the water in the capillary

$m = \rho V = \rho \times \pi r^2 h = \rho \times \pi r^2 \times \frac{2T\cos\theta}{r\rho g}$

$\Rightarrow m \alpha r$

$\therefore \frac{m_1}{m_2} = \frac{r}{2r}$

or $m_2 = 2m_1 = 2m$.

CHAPTER-10 : Thermal Properties of Matter

TOPIC-1 : Thermometer & Thermal Expansion

35. (a) Young's modulus $Y = \frac{\text{stress}}{\text{strain}} = \frac{F/A}{A(\Delta\ell/\ell)}$

Using, coefficient of linear expansion,

$\alpha = \frac{\Delta\ell}{\ell\Delta T} \Rightarrow \frac{\Delta\ell}{\ell} = \alpha\Delta T$

$\therefore Y = \frac{F}{A(\alpha\Delta T)}$

TOPIC-2 : Calorimetry and Heat Transfer

36. (a) $\frac{\Delta T_{AB}}{R_{AB}} = \frac{120}{\frac{8}{5}R} = \frac{120 \times 5}{8R}$

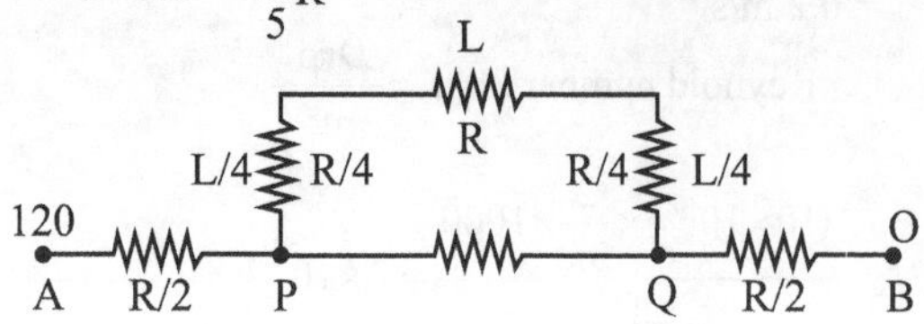

In steady state temperature difference between P and Q,

$\Delta T_{PQ} = \frac{120 \times 5}{8R} \times \frac{3}{5}R = \frac{360}{8} = 45^\circ C$

37. (a)

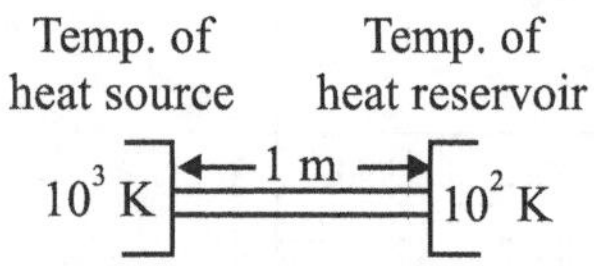

$\left(\frac{dQ}{dt}\right) = \frac{kA\Delta T}{\ell}$

Energy flux, $\frac{1}{A}\left(\frac{dQ}{dt}\right) = \frac{k\Delta T}{\ell}$

$= \frac{(0.1)(900)}{1} = 90\ W/m^2$

TOPIC-3 : Newton's Law of Cooling

38. (b) Rate of Heat loss = $mS\left(\frac{dT}{dt}\right) = e\sigma AT^4$

$-\frac{dT}{dt} = \frac{e\sigma \times A \times T^4}{\rho \times Vol. \times S} \Rightarrow -\frac{dT}{dt} \propto \frac{1}{\rho S}$

$\frac{\left(-\frac{dT}{dt}\right)_A}{\left(-\frac{dT}{dt}\right)_B} = \frac{\rho_B}{\rho_A} \times \frac{S_B}{S_A} = \frac{10^3}{8 \times 10^2} \times \frac{4000}{2000} = 2.5 > 1$

$\Rightarrow \left(-\frac{dT}{dt}\right)_A > \left(-\frac{dT}{dt}\right)_B$

So, A cools down at faster rate.

CHAPTER-11 : Thermodynamics

TOPIC-1 : First Law of Thermodynamics

39. (a)

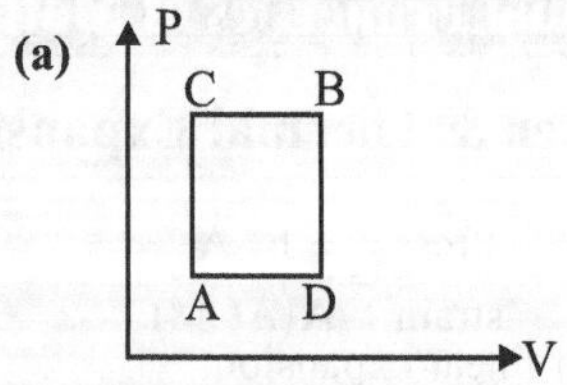

ΔU remains same for both paths ACB and ADB

$\Delta Q_{ACB} = \Delta W_{ACB} + \Delta U_{ACB}$

$\Rightarrow 60\ J = 30\ J + \Delta U_{ACB}$

$\Rightarrow U_{ACB} = 30\ J$

$\therefore \Delta U_{ADB} = \Delta U_{ACB} = 30\ J$

$\Delta Q_{ADB} = \Delta U_{ADB} + \Delta W_{ADB}$

$= 10\ J + 30\ J = 40\ J$

TOPIC-2 : Specific Heat Capacity and Thermodynamical Processes

40. (b) Suppose amount of water evaporated be M gram.
Then (150 – M) gram water converted into ice.
so, heat consumed in evoporation = Heat released in fusion

$M \times L_v = (150 - M) \times L_s$

$M \times 2.1 \times 10^6 = (150 - M) \times 3.36 \times 10^5$

$\Rightarrow M \simeq 20\ g$

41. (c) Internal energy depends only on initial and final state
So, $\Delta U_A = \Delta U_B$
Also $\Delta Q = \Delta U + W$
As $W_A > W_B \Rightarrow \Delta Q_A > \Delta Q_B$

TOPIC-3 : Carnot Engine, Refrigerators and Second Law of Thermodynamics

42. (b) According to question, $\eta_1 = \eta_2 = \eta_3$

$\therefore 1 - \frac{T_2}{T_1} = 1 - \frac{T_3}{T_2} = 1 - \frac{T_4}{T_3}$

[∵ Three engines are equally efficient]

$\Rightarrow \frac{T_2}{T_1} = \frac{T_3}{T_2} = \frac{T_4}{T_3}$

$\Rightarrow T_2 = \sqrt{T_1 T_3}$ ...(i)

$T_3 = \sqrt{T_2 T_4}$ ...(ii)

From (i) and (ii)

$T_2 = (T_1^2 T_4)^{1/3}$

$T_3 = (T_1 T_4^2)^{1/3}$

CHAPTER-12 : Kinetic Theory

TOPIC-2 : Speed of Gas, Pressure and Kinetic Energy

43. (Bouns)

Rate of change of momentum during collision

$= \frac{mv - (-mv)}{\Delta t}$

$= \frac{2mv}{\Delta t} N$

so pressure

$P = \frac{N \times (2mv)}{\Delta t \times A}$

$= \frac{10^{22} \times 2 \times 10^{-26} \times 10^4}{1 \times 1} = 2\ N/m^2$

44. (c) $V_{rms} = \sqrt{\frac{3RT}{M}}$

$$\frac{v_1}{v_2} = \sqrt{\frac{T_1}{T_2}} = \frac{(273+127)}{(273+237)} = \sqrt{\frac{400}{500}} = \sqrt{\frac{4}{5}} = \frac{2}{\sqrt{5}}$$

$$\therefore v_2 = \frac{\sqrt{5}}{2} v_1 = \frac{\sqrt{5}}{2} \times 200 = 100\sqrt{5} \text{ m/s.}$$

45. (a) Using $\frac{V_{1rms}}{V_{2rms}} = \sqrt{}$

$$\frac{V_{rms}(He)}{V_{rms}(Ar)} = \sqrt{\frac{M_{Ar}}{M_{He}}} = \sqrt{\frac{40}{4}} = 3.16$$

TOPIC-3 : Degree of Freedom, Specific Heat Capacity, and Mean Free Path

46. (a) $\frac{1}{2} m\bar{v}^2 = 3k_B T$

or $T = \frac{m\bar{v}^2}{6k_B}$

CHAPTER-13 : Oscillations

TOPIC-3 : Time Period, Frequency, Simple Pendulum and Spring Pendulum

47. (c) $T = 2\pi\sqrt{\frac{l}{g}}$

When immersed non viscous liquid

$$a_{mt} = \left(g - \frac{g}{16}\right) = \frac{15g}{16}$$

Now $T' = 2\pi\sqrt{\frac{l}{0_{net}}} = 2\pi\sqrt{\frac{l}{\sqrt{\frac{15g}{16}}}} = \frac{4}{\sqrt{15}}T$

CHAPTER-14 : Waves

TOPIC-1 : Basic of Mechanical Waves, Progressive and Stationary Waves

48. (a) On comparing with $P = P_0 \sin(wt - kx)$, we have $w = 1000$ rad/s, $K = 3\ m^{-1}$

$$\therefore v_0 = \frac{w}{k} = \frac{1000}{3} = 333.3 \text{m/s}$$

$$\frac{v_1}{v_2} = \sqrt{\frac{T_1}{T_2}}$$

or $\frac{333.3}{336} = \sqrt{\frac{273+0}{273+t}}$

$\therefore t = 4°C$

49. (b) Wave speed $V = \sqrt{\frac{T}{\mu}}$

when car is at rest a = 0

$$\therefore 60 = \sqrt{\frac{Mg}{\mu}}$$

Similarly when the car is moving with acceleration a,

$$60.5 = \sqrt{\frac{M\left(g^2+a^2\right)^{1/2}}{\mu}}$$

$$\frac{60.5}{60} = \sqrt{\sqrt{\frac{g^2+a^2}{g^2}}}$$

$$\left(1+\frac{0.5}{60}\right)^4 = \frac{g^2+a^2}{g^2} = 1+\frac{2}{60}$$

$$\Rightarrow g^2+a^2 = g^2+g^2\times\frac{2}{60}$$

$a = g\sqrt{\frac{2}{60}} = \frac{g}{\sqrt{30}}$ [which is closest to g/5]

TOPIC-2 : Vibration of String and Organ pipe

50. (c) As there must be node at both ends and at the joint of the wire *A* and *B* so

$$\frac{V_A}{V_B} = \sqrt{\frac{u_B}{u_A}} = \frac{r_B}{r_A} = 2 = \frac{\lambda_A}{\lambda_B}$$

$$\Rightarrow \lambda_A = 2\lambda_B$$

$$\Rightarrow \frac{P}{q} = \frac{1}{2}$$

51. (b) Given, $y = 0.3 \sin(0.157x)\cos(200\pi t)$
So $k = 0.157$ and $w = 200\pi$

or f = 100 Hz, $v = \frac{w}{k} = \frac{200\pi}{0.157} = 4000$m/s

Now, using $f = \frac{nv}{2l} = \frac{4v}{2l} = \frac{2v}{l}$

$$\therefore l = \frac{2v}{f} = \frac{2\times4000}{100} = 80m$$

52. (d) Velocity of wave on string

$$V = \sqrt{\frac{T}{\mu}} = \sqrt{\frac{8}{5}\times1000} = 40\text{m/s}$$

Here, T = tension and μ = mass/length

Wavelength of wave $\lambda = \frac{v}{n} = \frac{40}{100}$m

Separation b/w successive nodes,

$$\frac{\lambda}{2} = \frac{40}{2\times100} = \frac{20}{100}\text{m} = 20 \text{ cm}$$

TOPIC-3 : Beats, Interference and Superposition of Waves

53. (b) According to Doppler's effect, when source is moving but observer at rest

$$f_{app} = f_0\left[\frac{V}{V-V_s}\right] \Rightarrow f_1 = f_0\left[\frac{340}{340-34}\right]$$

and, $f_2 = f_0\left[\frac{340}{340-17}\right]$

$$\therefore \frac{f_1}{f_2} = \frac{340-17}{340-34} = \frac{323}{306} \text{ or, } \frac{f_1}{f_2} = \frac{19}{18}$$

CHAPTER-15 : Electric Charges and Fields

TOPIC - 1: Electric Charges and Coulomb's Law

54. (a)

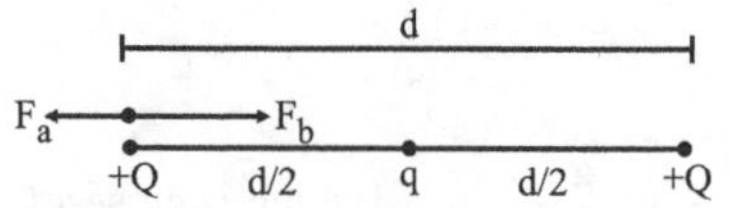

Force due to charge + Q,

$$F_a = \frac{KQQ}{d^2}$$

Force due to charge q,

$$F_b = \frac{KQq}{\left(\frac{d}{2}\right)^2}$$

For equilibrium,

$$\vec{F}_a + \vec{F}_b = 0$$

$$\Rightarrow \frac{kQQ}{d^2} + \frac{kQq}{(d/2)^2} = 0 \quad \therefore q = -\frac{Q}{4}$$

TOPIC - 2: Electric Field and Electric Field Lines

55. (d) At equilibrium resultant force on bob must be zero, so

$T\cos\theta = mg$ ..... (i)

$T\sin\theta = qE$ ..... (ii)

Solving (i) and (ii) we get

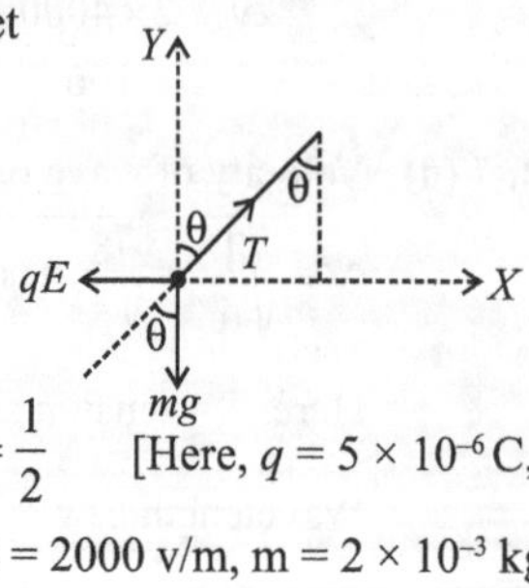

$$\tan\theta = \frac{qE}{mg}$$

$$\tan\theta = \frac{5\times10^{-6}\times2000}{2\times10^{-3}\times10} = \frac{1}{2}$$

[Here, $q = 5 \times 10^{-6}$ C, E = 2000 v/m, $m = 2 \times 10^{-3}$ kg]

$$\Rightarrow \tan^{-1}\left(\frac{1}{2}\right)$$

56. (b) Electric field on the axis of a ring of radius R at a distance h from the centre,

$$E = \frac{kQh}{\left(h^2+R^2\right)^{3/2}}$$

Condition: for maximum electric field $\frac{dE}{dh} = 0$

$$\Rightarrow \frac{d}{dh}\left[\frac{kQh}{\left(R^2+h^2\right)^{3/2}}\right] = 0$$

By using the concept of maxima and minima we get,

$$h = \frac{R}{\sqrt{2}}$$

CHAPTER-16 : Electrostatic Potential and Capacitance

TOPIC - 1: Electrostatic Potential and Equipotential Surfaces

57. (d) When charge Q is on inner solid conducting sphere

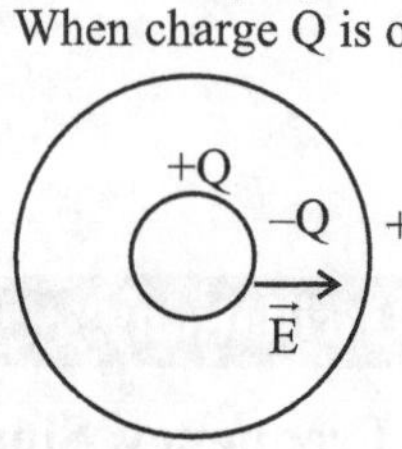

Electric field between spherical surface

$\vec{E} = \frac{KQ}{r^2}$ So $\int \vec{E}.d\vec{r} = V$ given

Now when a charge – 4Q is given to hollow shell

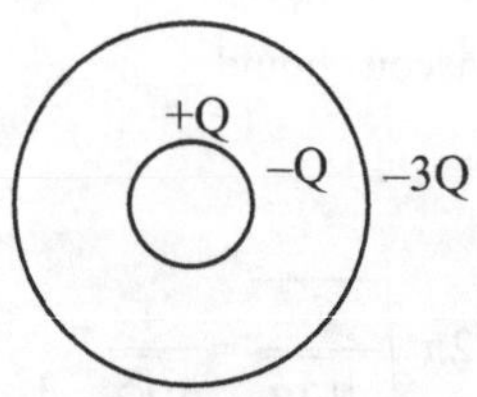

Electric field between surface remain unchanged.

$$\vec{E} = \frac{KQ}{r^2}$$

as, field inside the hollow spherical shell = 0

∴ Potential difference between them remain unchanged

i.e. $\int \vec{E}.d\vec{r} = V$

58. (d)

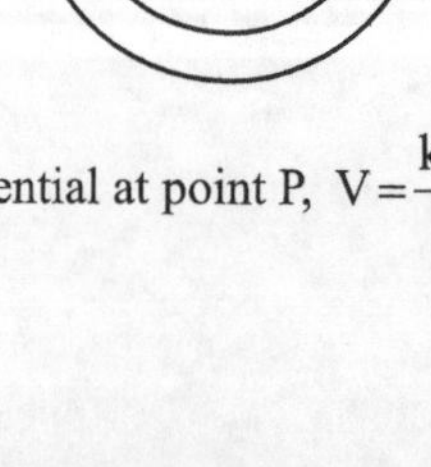

Potential at point P, $V = \frac{kQ_a}{a} + \frac{kQ_b}{b} + \frac{kQ_c}{c}$

Since surface charge densities are equal to one another i.e.,

$\sigma_a = \sigma_b = \sigma_c$

$\therefore Q_a : Q_b : Q_c :: a^2 : b^2 : c^2$

$$\therefore Q_a = \left[\frac{a^2}{a^2 + b^2 + c^2}\right]Q$$

$$Q_b = \left[\frac{b^2}{a^2 + b^2 + c^2}\right]Q$$

$$Q_c = \left[\frac{c^2}{a^2 + b^2 + c^2}\right]Q$$

$$\therefore V = \frac{Q}{4\pi\epsilon_0}\left[\frac{(a+b+c)}{a^2 + b^2 + c^2}\right]$$

59. (d) Let at a distance 'x' from point B, both the dipoles produce same potential

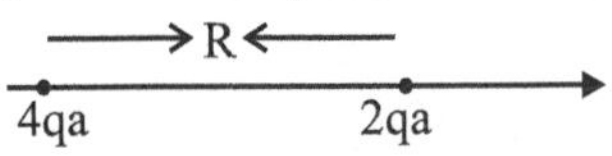

$$\therefore \frac{4qa}{(R+x)} = \frac{2qa}{(x^2)}$$

$$\Rightarrow \sqrt{2x} = R + x \Rightarrow x = \frac{R}{\sqrt{2}-1}$$

Therefore distance from A at which both of them produce the same potential

$$= \frac{R}{\sqrt{2}-1} + R = \frac{\sqrt{2}R}{\sqrt{2}-1}$$

TOPIC - 2 : Electric Potential Energy and Work done in Carrying a charge

60. (d) $$U = \frac{1}{4\pi\epsilon_0}\left[\frac{q(-q)}{d} + \frac{qQ}{\left(D + \frac{d}{2}\right)} + \frac{(-q)Q}{\left(D - \frac{d}{2}\right)}\right]$$

$$= \frac{1}{4\pi\epsilon_0}\left[-\frac{q^2}{d} - \frac{qQd}{D^2}\right], \text{ Ignoring } \frac{d^2}{4}$$

TOPIC - 3: Capacitors, Grouping of Capacitor and Energy Stored in a Capacitor

61. (b) Capacitance of a capacitor with a dielectric of dielectric constant k is given by

$$C = \frac{k\epsilon_0 A}{d}$$

$$\because E = \frac{V}{d} \qquad \therefore C = \frac{k\epsilon_0 AE}{V}$$

$$15 \times 10^{-12} = \frac{k \times 8.86 \times 10^{-12} \times 10^{-4} \times 10^6}{500}$$

$k = 8.5$

62. (d) At steady state, there is no current in capacitor. Current down from battery

$$i = \frac{V}{R} = \left(\frac{72}{6 + \frac{12 \times 4}{12 + 4}}\right) = 8A$$

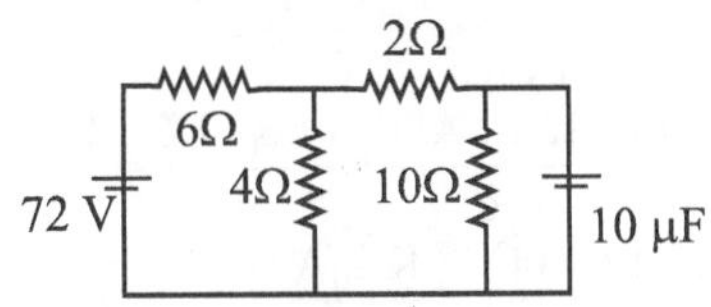

Current in 10Ω senstor,

$$i' = \frac{8 \times 4}{4 + 12} = 2A$$

Pd across capacitor, $V = iR = 2 \times 10 = 20V$

Charge on the capacitor, $q = CV$

$= 10 \times 20 = 200\ \mu C$.

63. (b) $$\omega = \omega_f - v_i = \frac{q}{2}\left(\frac{1}{C_f} - \frac{1}{C_i}\right)$$

$$= \frac{(5 \times 10)^2}{2}\left(\frac{1}{2} - \frac{1}{5}\right) \times 10^6$$

$= 3.75 \times 10^{-6} J$

64. (b)

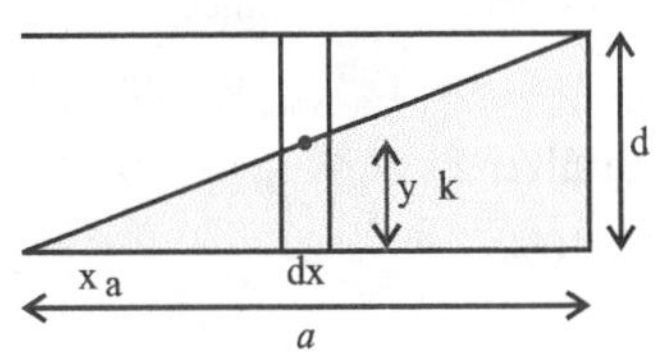

From figure, $\frac{y}{x} = \frac{d}{a} \Rightarrow y = \frac{d}{a}x$

$$dy = \frac{d}{a}(dx) \Rightarrow \frac{1}{dc} = \frac{y}{K\varepsilon_0 adx} + \frac{(d-y)}{\varepsilon_0 adx}$$

$$\frac{1}{dc} = \frac{y}{\varepsilon_0 abx}\left(\frac{y}{k} + d - y\right)$$

$$\int dc = \int \frac{\varepsilon_0 adx}{\frac{y}{k} + d - y}$$

$$\text{or, } c = \varepsilon_0 a.\frac{a}{d}\int_0^d \frac{dy}{d + y\left(\frac{1}{k} - 1\right)}$$

$$= \frac{\varepsilon_0 a^2}{\left(\frac{1}{k} - 1\right)d}\left[\ell n\left(d + y\left(\frac{1}{k} - 1\right)\right)\right]_0^d$$

$$= \frac{k \in_0 a^2}{(1-k)d} \ell n\left(\frac{d+d\left(\frac{1}{k}-1\right)}{d}\right)$$

$$= \frac{k \in_0 a^2}{(1-k)d} \ell n\left(\frac{1}{k}\right) = \frac{k \in_0 a^2 \ell nk}{(k-1)d}$$

65. (c) Let dielectric constant of material used be K.

$$\frac{k_1 \in_0 A_1}{d} + \frac{k_2 \in_0 A_2}{d} + \frac{k_3 \in_0 A_3}{d} = \frac{k \in_0 A}{d}$$

or $\frac{10 \in_0 A/3}{d} + \frac{12 \in_0 A/3}{d} + \frac{14 \in_0 A/3}{d} = \frac{K \in_0 A}{d}$

$$\frac{\in_0 A}{d}\left(\frac{10}{3} + \frac{12}{3} + \frac{14}{3}\right) = \frac{K \in_0 A}{d}$$

$\therefore K = 12$

CHAPTER-17 : Current Electricity

TOPIC - 1: Electric Current, Drift of Electrons, Ohm's Law, Resistance and Resistivity

66. (d) Number 2 is associated with the red colour. This colour is replaced by green.

$\because$ Colour code figure for green is 5

$\therefore$ New resistance = 500 Ω

67. (b) Color code : Bl, Br, R, O, Y, G, B, V, Gr, W

0, 1, 2, 3, 4, 5, 6, 7, 8 9

R = AB × C ± D% where D = tolerance

$D_{gold} = \pm 5\%$, $D_{silver} = \pm 10\%$; $D_{no\ colour} = \pm 20\%$

Red voilet orange silver

$R = 27 \times 10^3\ \Omega \pm 10\%$

$i = 27\ k\Omega \pm 10\%$

68. (a) Using, $I = neAv_d$

? ? $\therefore$ Drift speed $v_d = \frac{1}{neA}$

$$\frac{1.5}{9 \times 10^{28} \times 1.6 \times 10^{-19} \times 5 \times 10^{-6}} = 0.02\ mms^{-1}$$

69. (c) Resistance, $R = \frac{\rho \ell}{A}$

$R = \rho \frac{\ell}{A} \times - = \frac{\ell}{V}$ [$\because$ Volume (V) = A ℓ.]

Since resistivity and volume remains constant therefore % change in resistance

$$\frac{\Delta R}{R} = \frac{2\Delta \ell}{\ell} = 2 \times (0.5) = 1\%$$

TOPIC - 2: Combination of Resistances

70. (b) $R_{eq} = \frac{\left(\frac{7R}{8}\right)\left(\frac{R}{8}\right)}{R} = \frac{7R}{64}$

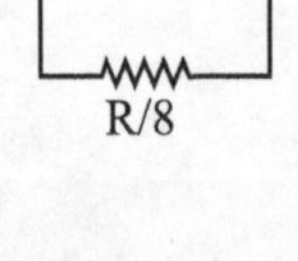

71. (a)

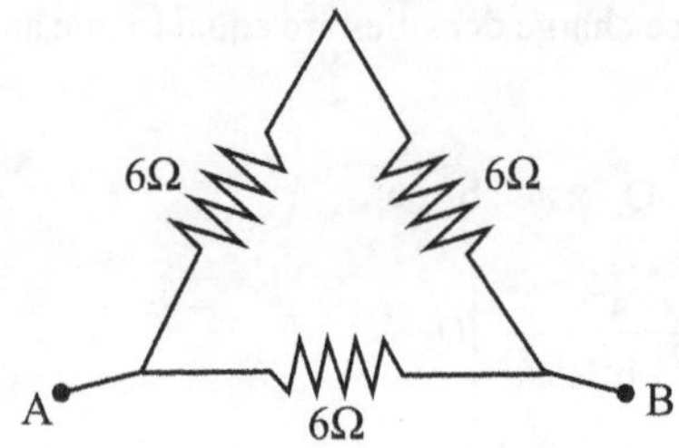

Resistance, R ∝ l so resistance of each side of the equilateral triangle = 6 Ω

Resistance R_{eq} between any two vertices

$$\frac{1}{R_{eq}} = \frac{1}{12} + \frac{1}{6} \Rightarrow R_{eq.} = 4\Omega$$

TOPIC - 3: Kirchoff's Laws, Cells, Thermo e.m.f. Electrolysis

72. (d) Applying parallel combination of batteries

$$\frac{\frac{E_1}{1+1} + \frac{E_2}{2} + \frac{E_3}{1+1}}{\frac{1}{1+1} + \frac{1}{2} + \frac{1}{1+1}}$$

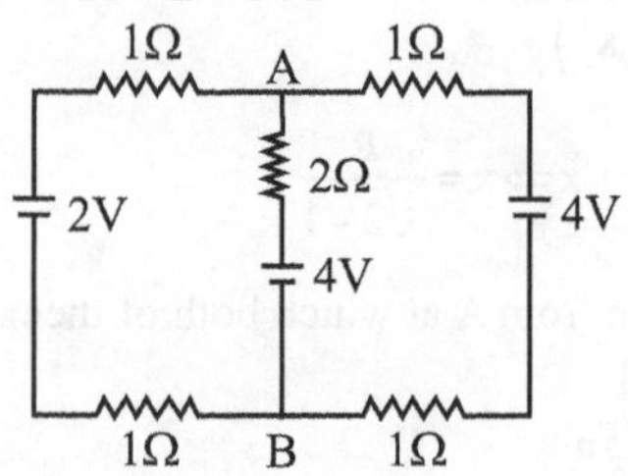

$$\frac{\frac{2}{2} + \frac{4}{2} + \frac{4}{2}}{\frac{1}{2} + \frac{1}{2} + \frac{1}{2}} = \frac{5 \times 2}{3}$$

$= \frac{10}{3} = 3.3$ Volt

73. (b)

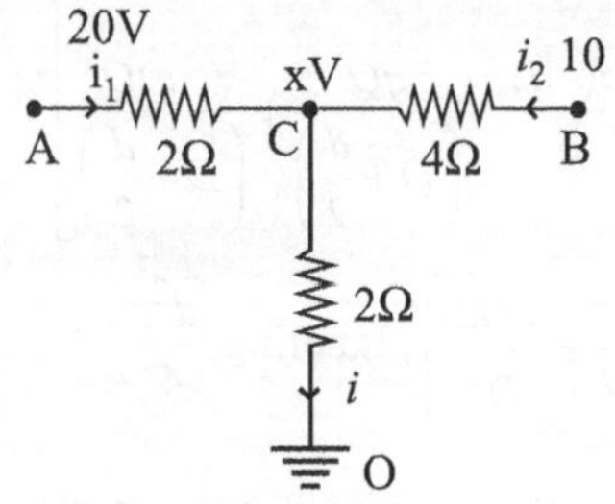

Let voltage at C = xV

From kirchhoff's current law,

KCL : $i_1 + i_2 = i$

$$\frac{20-x}{2} + \frac{10-x}{4} = \frac{x-0}{2} \Rightarrow x = 10$$

$$\therefore i = \frac{V}{R} = \frac{X}{R} = \frac{10}{2} = 5A$$

74. **(c)** Current passing through resistance R_1,

$$i_1 = \frac{v}{R_1} = \frac{10}{20} = 0.5A$$

and, $i_2 = 0$

TOPIC - 4: Heating Effects of Current

75. **(a)** Colour code for carbon resistor

Bl,	Br,	R,	O,	Y,	G,	Blue,	V,	Gr,	W
0	1	2	3	4	5	6	7	8	9

Resistance, R = AB × C ± D

∴ Resistance, $R = 50 \times 10^2 \Omega$

Now using formula, Power, $P = i^2R$

$$\therefore i = \sqrt{\frac{P}{R}} = \sqrt{\frac{2}{50 \times 10^2}} = 20mA$$

TOPIC - 5: Wheatstone Bridge and Different Measuring Instruments

76. **(c)** Let x be the length AJ at which galvanometer shows null deflection current,

$$i = \frac{\varepsilon}{12r + r} = \frac{3}{13r}$$

$$\text{or, } i\left(\frac{x}{L}12r\right) = \frac{\varepsilon}{2}$$

$$\Rightarrow \frac{\varepsilon}{13r}\left[\frac{x}{L} \cdot 12r\right] = \frac{\varepsilon}{2}$$

$$\text{or, } x = \frac{13L}{24}$$

CHAPTER-18 : Moving Charges and Magnetism

TOPIC - 2: Magnetic Field Lines, Biot-Savart's Law and Ampere's Circuital Law

77. **(d)**

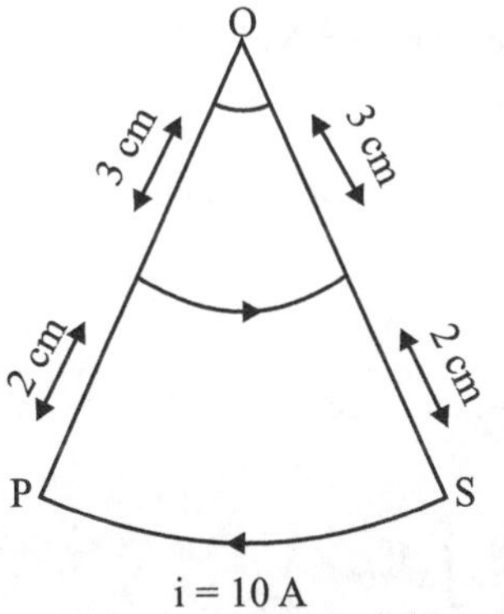

There will be no magnetic field at O due to wire PQ and RS

Magnetic field at 'O' due to arc QR

$$= \frac{\mu_0}{4\pi} \frac{\left(\frac{\pi}{4}\right).I}{r_1}$$

Magnetic field at 'O' due to are PS

$$= \frac{\mu_0}{4\pi} \frac{\left(\frac{\pi}{4}\right).I}{r_2}$$

∴ Net magnetic field at 'O'

$$B = \frac{\mu_0}{4\pi}(\pi/4) \times 10\left[\frac{1}{\left(3\times10^{-2}\right)} - \frac{1}{\left(5\times10^{-2}\right)}\right]$$

$$\Rightarrow |\vec{B}| = \frac{\pi}{3} \times 10^{-5}T \approx 1 \times 10^{-5}T$$

TOPIC - 3: Force and Torque on Current Carrying Conductor

78. **(b)** $|\vec{\tau}| = |\vec{\mu} \times \vec{B}|$ $[\mu = NIA]$

$= NIA \times B \sin 90°$ $[A = \pi r^2]$

$\Rightarrow \tau = NI\pi r^2 B$

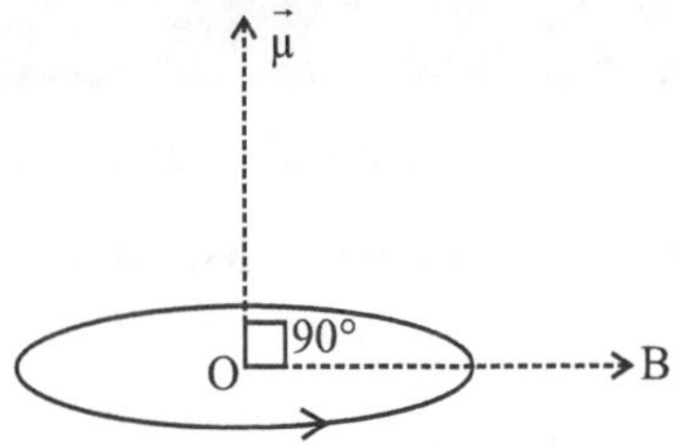

79. **(d)** $\tau = MB \sin 45° = N\,(iA)\,B \sin 45°$

$$= 100 \times 3(5 \times 2.5) \times 10^{-4} \times 1 \times \frac{1}{\sqrt{2}}$$

= 0.27 N–M

80. **(c)** $F = \frac{\mu_0}{2\pi}\left(\frac{i_1 i_2}{a} - \frac{i_1 i_2}{2a}\right) \times a = \frac{\mu_0 i_1 i_2}{4\pi}$

81. **(d)**

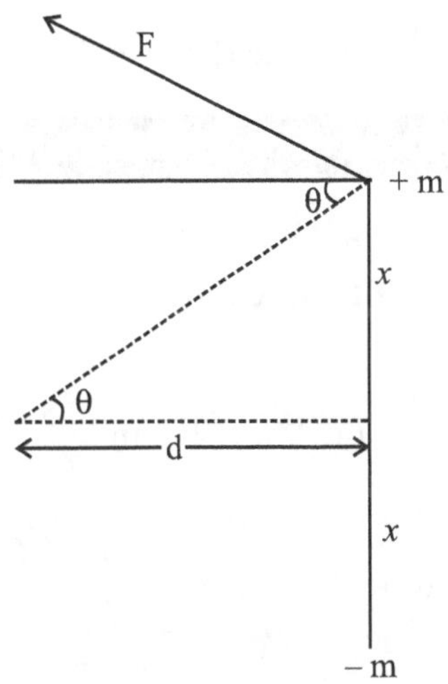

Force on one pole,

$$F = m \times \frac{\mu_0 I}{2\pi\sqrt{d^2 + x^2}}$$

Total force, $F_{total} = 2F \sin\theta$

$$= 2 \times \frac{\mu_0 Im}{2\pi\sqrt{d^2 + a^2}} \times \frac{x}{\sqrt{d^2 + a^2}}$$

$$= \frac{\mu_0 Im x}{\pi(d^2 + a^2)}$$

Magnetic moment, $M = I\pi a^2 = m \times 2$

or, Total force, $F_{total} = \frac{\mu_0 Ia^2}{2(d^2 + a^2)}$

$$= \frac{\mu_0 Ia^2}{2d^2} \quad [\because d >> a]$$

Clearly $F_{total} \propto \frac{a^2}{d^2}$

Topic - 4: Galvanometer and its Conversion into Ammeter and Voltmeter

82. (c) $V = i_g(G + R) = 4 \times 10^{-3}(50 + 5000) = 20V$

CHAPTER-19 : Magnetism and Matter

TOPIC - 1: Magnetism, Gauss's Law, Magnetic Moment, Properties of Magnet

83. (Bonus)

Work done, $W = 2\, m B$

$= 2 \times 10^{-2} \times 1 \cos(0.125)$

$= 0.02$ J

TOPIC - 2: The Earth Magnetism, Magnetic Materials and their properties

84. (b) Corecivity, $H = \frac{B}{\mu_0}$ and $B = \mu_0 ni \left(n = \frac{N}{\ell}\right)$

or, $H = \frac{N}{\ell} i = \frac{100}{0.2} \times 5.2 = 2600$ A/m

CHAPTER-20 : Electromagnetic Induction

TOPIC - 1: Magnetic Flux, Faraday's and Lenz's Law

85. [Bonus]

Net charge $Q = \frac{\Delta\phi}{R} = \frac{1}{10} A(B_f - B_i) = \frac{1}{10} \times 3.5 \times 10^{-3} \left(0.4 \sin\frac{\pi}{2} - 0\right)$

$$= \frac{1}{10}(3.5 \times 10^{-3})(0.4 - 0)$$

$= 1.4 \times 10^{-4}$

No option matches, So it should be a bonus.

TOPIC - 2: Motional and Static EMI and Application of EMI

86. (c) Force on the strip when it is at stretched position x from mean position is

$$F = -kx - iIB = -kx - \frac{BIv}{R} \times IB$$

$$F = -kx - \frac{B^2 I^2}{R} \times v$$

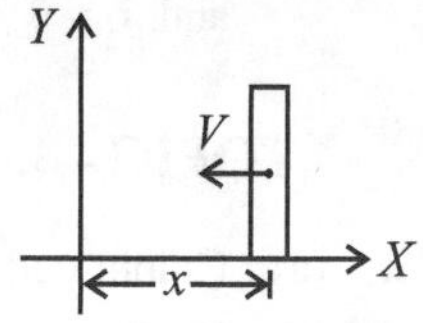

Above expression shows that it is case of damped oscillation, so its amplitude can be given by

$$\Rightarrow A = A_0 e^{-\frac{bt}{2m}}$$

$$\Rightarrow \frac{A_0}{e} = A_0 e^{-\frac{bt}{2m}} \quad \left[\text{as per question } A = \frac{A_0}{e}\right]$$

$$\Rightarrow t = \frac{2m}{\left(\frac{B^2 I^2}{R}\right)} = \frac{2 \times 50 \times 10^{-3} \times 10}{0.01 \times 0.01} = 10000 \text{ s}$$

Given, $m = 50 \times 10^{-3}$ kg

$B = 0.1$ T

$l = 0.1$ m

$R = 10\ \Omega$

$k = 0.5$ N

Time period, $T = 2\pi\sqrt{\frac{m}{k}} \simeq 2$ s

so, required number of oscillations,

$$N = \frac{10000}{2} = 5000$$

87. (d) Inductance $= \frac{\mu_0 N^2 A}{L}$

88. (a) Potential difference between two faces perpendicular to x-axis

$= \lambda\, V.B = 2 \times 10^{-2}(6 \times 0.1) = 12$mV

89. (c)

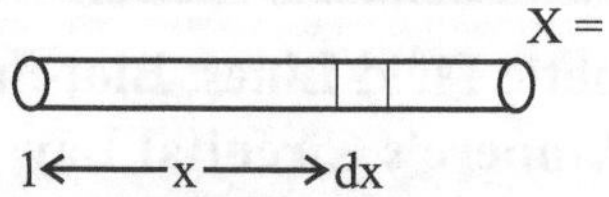

Magnetic moment, $M = NIA$

$dQ = \rho\, dx$

$$dI = \frac{dQ}{2\pi}.\omega$$

$dM = dI \times A$

$$= \frac{\omega}{2\pi}.\frac{\rho_0}{\ell}.x\pi x^2\, dx$$

$$\Rightarrow M = \frac{\rho_0}{\ell} n\pi \int_0^{\ell} x^3\, dx$$

$$= \frac{\pi}{4}.n\rho\ell^3$$

CHAPTER-21 : Alternating Current

TOPIC - 1: Alternating Current, Voltage and Power

90. (d) As $V(t) = 220 \sin 100 \pi t$

so, $I(t) = \frac{220}{50} \sin 100 \pi t$

i.e., $I = I_m = \sin(100 \pi t)$

For $I = I_m$

$t_1 = \frac{\pi}{2} \times \frac{1}{100\pi} = \frac{1}{200}$ sec.

and for $I = \frac{I_m}{2}$

$\Rightarrow \frac{I_m}{2} = I_m \sin(100 \pi t_2)$

$\Rightarrow \frac{\pi}{6} = 100 \pi t_2$

$\Rightarrow t_2 = \frac{1}{600} s$

$\therefore t_{req} = \frac{1}{200} - \frac{1}{600} = \frac{2}{600} = \frac{1}{300} s = 3.3$ ms

TOPIC - 2: AC Circuit, LCR Circuit, Quality and Power Factor

91. (c) $i^2 R = \left(\tau \frac{di}{dt}\right) i$

$\Rightarrow \frac{di}{dt} = \frac{i}{\tau}$

$\Rightarrow t = \tau \ln 2 = 2 \ln 2 \left[\text{as } \tau = \frac{L}{R} = \frac{20}{10} = 2\right]$

CHAPTER-22 : Electromagnetic Waves

TOPIC-1 : Electromagnetic Waves, Conduction and Displacement Current

92. (a) The relation between amplitudes of electric and magnetic field in free space is given by

$B_0 = \frac{E_0}{c} = \frac{6}{3 \times 10^8} = 2 \times 10^{-8} T$

Propagation direction $= \hat{E} \times \hat{B}$

$\hat{i} = \hat{j} \times \hat{B}$

$\Rightarrow \hat{B} = \hat{k}$

$\therefore$ The magnetic field component will be along z direction.

93. (a) $B_0 = \sqrt{B_0^2 + B_1^2} = \sqrt{30^2 + 2^2} \times 10^{-6}$

$= 30 \times 10^{-6}$T

$\therefore E_0 = CB = 3 \times 10^8 \times 30 \times 10^{-6}$

$= 9 \times 10^3$ V/m

$\frac{E_0}{V_2} = \frac{9}{\sqrt{2}} \times 10^3 V/m$

Force on the charge,

$F = EQ = \frac{9}{\sqrt{2}} \times 10^3 \times 10^{-4} \simeq 0.64 N.$

94. (b) As we know,

$|\vec{B}| = \frac{|\vec{E}|}{C} = \frac{6.3}{3 \times 10^8} = 2.1 \times 10^{-8}$T

and $\hat{E} \times \hat{B} = \hat{C}$

$\hat{j} \times \hat{B} = \hat{i}$ [$\because$ EM wave travels along +(ve) x-direction.]

$\therefore \hat{B} = \hat{k}$ or $\vec{B} = 2.1 \times 10^{-8} \hat{k}$T

95. (b) Using, formula $E_0 = B_0 \times C$

$= 100 \times 10^{-6} \times 3 \times 10^8$

$= 3 \times 10^4$ N/C

Here we assumed that

$B_0 = 100 \times 10^{-6}$ is in tesla (T) units

CHAPTER-23 : Ray Optics and Optical Instruments

TOPIC - 1: Plane Mirror, Spherical Mirror and Reflection of Light

96. (c) $+5 = -\frac{v}{u} \Rightarrow v = -5u$

Using $\frac{1}{v} + \frac{1}{u} = \frac{1}{f}$

or $\frac{1}{-5u} + \frac{1}{u} = \frac{1}{0.4}$

$\therefore$ u = 0.32 m.

TOPIC - 2: Refraction of Light at Plane Surface and Total Internal Reflection

97. (d) Using Snell's law of refraction,

$1 \times \sin 40° = 1.31 \sin \theta$

$\Rightarrow \sin \theta = \frac{0.64}{1.31} = 0.49 \approx 0.5$

$\Rightarrow \theta = 30°$

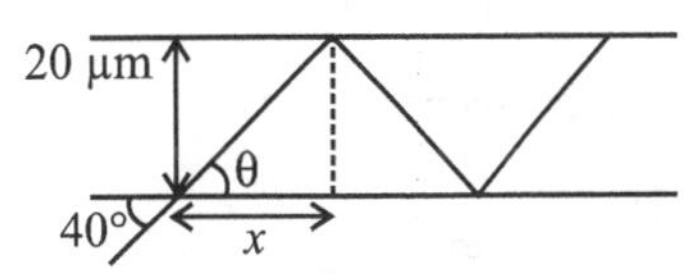

$x = 20\ \mu m \times \cot \theta$

$\therefore$ Number of reflections $= \frac{2}{20 \times 10^{-6} \times \cot\theta}$

$= \frac{2 \times 10^6}{20 \times \sqrt{3}} = 57735 \approx 57000$

TOPIC - 3: Refraction at Curved Surface Lenses and Power of Lens

98. (Bouns) $v_1 = \dfrac{40\times 20}{(40-20)} = 40\,cm$

$u_2 = 60 - 40 = 20$ cm

$\therefore v_2 = \dfrac{20\times 10}{(20-10)} = 20\,cm$

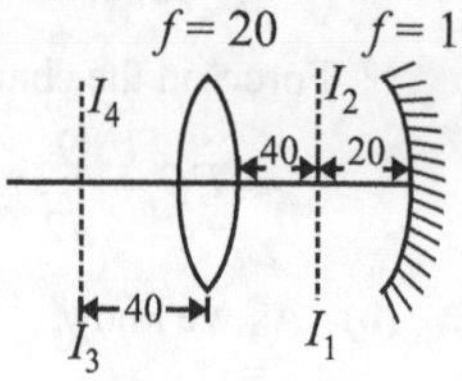

$\therefore$ Image traces back to object itself as image formed by lens is a centre of curvature of mirror.

99. (d)

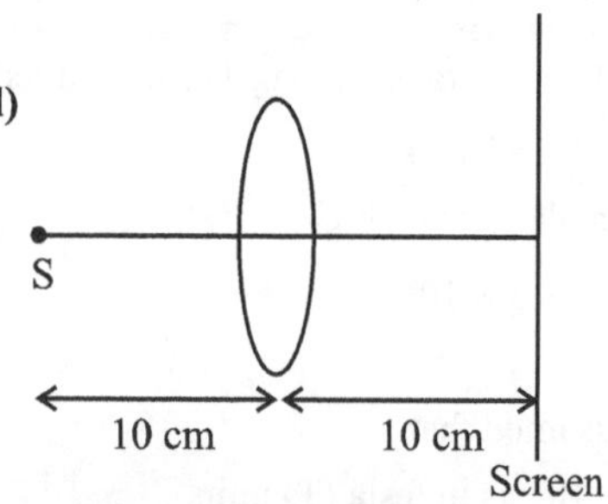

Using lens formula

$\dfrac{1}{v} - \dfrac{1}{u} = \dfrac{1}{f} \Rightarrow \dfrac{1}{10} - \dfrac{1}{-10} = \dfrac{1}{f} \Rightarrow f = 5\text{cm}$

Shift due to slab, $= t\left(1 - \dfrac{1}{\mu}\right)$ in the direction of incident ray

or, $d = 1.5\left(1 - \dfrac{2}{3}\right) = 0.5$

Now, $u = -9.5$

Again using lens formulas $\dfrac{1}{v} - \dfrac{1}{-9.5} = \dfrac{1}{5}$

$\Rightarrow \dfrac{1}{v} = \dfrac{1}{5} - \dfrac{2}{19} = \dfrac{9}{95}$

or, $v = \dfrac{95}{9} = 10.55\,\text{cm}$

Thus, screen is shifted by a distance $d = 10.55 - 10 = 0.55$ cm away from the lens.

100. (b) From lens maker's formula,

$$\frac{1}{f} = (\mu - 1)\left(\frac{1}{R_1} - \frac{1}{R_2}\right)$$

$$\frac{1}{f_1} = (\mu_1 - 1)\left(\frac{1}{\infty} - \frac{1}{-R}\right) = \frac{1}{2f_2}$$

Similarly, for plano-concave lens

$$\frac{1}{f_2} = (\mu_2 - 1)\left(\frac{1}{-R} - \frac{1}{\infty}\right)$$

Dividing $\dfrac{1}{f_1}$ by $\dfrac{1}{f_2}$ we get,

$$\frac{(\mu_1 - 1)}{R} = \frac{(\mu_2 - 1)}{2R}$$

or, $2\mu_1 - \mu_2 = 1$

CHAPTER-24 : Wave Optics

TOPIC - 1: Wavefront, Interference of Light, Coherent and Incoherent Sources

101. (c) Given amplitude ratio of waves is $\dfrac{a_1}{a_2} = \dfrac{3}{1}$

so, $\dfrac{I_{max}}{I_{min}} - \left(\dfrac{a_2 + a_1}{a_2 - a_1}\right)^2 = \left(\dfrac{3+1}{3-1}\right)^2 = \left(\dfrac{4}{2}\right)^2 = \dfrac{4}{1} = 4$

102. (b) As we know, $\dfrac{I_{max}}{I_{min}} = \left(\dfrac{A_1 + A_2}{A_1 - A_2}\right)^2$

and $\sqrt{\dfrac{I_1}{I_2}} = \dfrac{A_1}{A_2}$

$\dfrac{I_{max}}{I_{min}} = 16 \Rightarrow \dfrac{A_{max}}{A_{min}} = 4 \Rightarrow \dfrac{A_1 + A_2}{A_1 - A_2} = \dfrac{4}{1}$

Using componendo and dividendo.

$\dfrac{A_1}{A_2} = \dfrac{5}{3} \Rightarrow \dfrac{I_1}{I_2} = \left(\dfrac{5}{3}\right)^2 = \dfrac{25}{9}$

TOPIC - 2: Young's Double Slit Experiment

103. (Bonus) $n\beta = \Delta$

or $n\dfrac{D\lambda}{a} = D\dfrac{(\mu - 1)t}{a}$

or $t = \dfrac{n\lambda}{(\mu - 1)}$

104. (a) Path difference = $d \sin\theta \approx d\theta$

$= 0.1 \times \dfrac{1}{40}\text{mm} = 2500\text{nm}$

For bright fringe, path difference must be integral multiple of λ.

$\therefore 2500 = n\lambda_1 = m\lambda_2$

$\therefore \lambda_1 = 625$ (for n = 4), $\lambda_2 = 500$ (for m = 5)

TOPIC - 3: Diffraction, Polarisation of Light and Resolving Power

105. (b) According to Brewster's law, refractive index of material (μ) is equal to tangent of polarising angle

$\because \tan i_b = \mu = \dfrac{1.5}{\mu}$

$\dfrac{1}{\mu} < \dfrac{1.5}{\sqrt{\mu^2 + (1.5)^2}}$ $(\because \sin i_c < \sin i_b)$

$\therefore \sin i_b = \dfrac{1.5}{\sqrt{\mu^2 + (1.5)^2}}$

or, $\sqrt{\mu + (1.5)} < 1.5 \times \mu$

$\Rightarrow \mu^2 + (1.5)^2 < (\mu \times 1.5)^2$

$\Rightarrow \mu < \dfrac{3}{\sqrt{5}}$ i.e. minimum value of μ should be $\dfrac{3}{\sqrt{5}}$

PTER-25 : Dual Nature of Radiation and Matter

TOPIC - 1: Matter Waves, Cathode and Positive Rays

106. (a) From the de-Broglie relation,

$$p_1 = \frac{h}{\lambda_1}$$

$$p_2 = \frac{h}{\lambda_2}$$

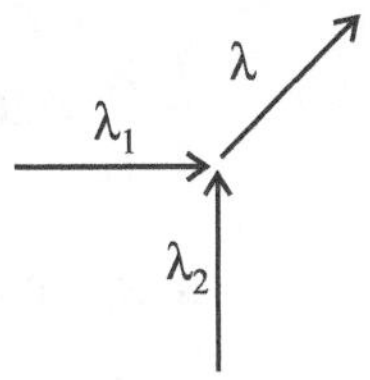

Momentum of the final particle (p_f) is given by

$$\therefore\ p_f = \sqrt{p_1^2 + p_2^2}$$

$$\Rightarrow \frac{h}{\lambda} = \sqrt{\frac{h^2}{\lambda_1^2} + \frac{h^2}{\lambda_2^2}}$$

$$\Rightarrow \frac{1}{\lambda^2} = \frac{1}{\lambda_1^2} + \frac{1}{\lambda_2^2}$$

107. (d) Using, $\lambda = \frac{h}{p}$ {given: $\lambda = 7.5 \times 10^{-12}$}

$$\Rightarrow P = \frac{h}{\lambda}$$

Minimum energy required,

$$KE = \frac{P^2}{2m} = \frac{(h/\lambda)^2}{2m} = \frac{\left\{\frac{6.6\times10^{-34}}{7.5\times10^{-12}}\right\}^2}{2\times9.1\times10^{-31}} J = 25 keV$$

TOPIC - 2: Photon, Photoelectric Effect X-rays and Davisson-Germer Experiment

108. (c) Here $w = 2\pi \times 6 \times 10^{14}$ or $f = 6 \times 10^{14}$ Hz

Wavelength $\lambda = \frac{C}{f} = \frac{3\times10^8}{6\times10^{14}} = 0.5\times10^{-6} m = 5000A^o$

Now $E = \frac{12374}{5000} = 2.48 eV$

Using $E = w + eV_s$

$2.48 = 2 + eV_s$

or $V_s = 0.48$ V

109. (a) From Einstein's photoelectric equation,

$$\frac{hc}{\lambda_1} = \phi + \frac{1}{2}m(2v)^2 \quad ....(i)$$

and $$\frac{hc}{\lambda_2} = \phi + \frac{1}{2}mv^2 \quad ....(ii)$$

As per question, maximum speed of photoelectrons in two cases differ by a factor 2

From eqn. (i) & (ii)

$$\Rightarrow \frac{\frac{hc}{\lambda_1} - \phi}{\frac{hc}{\lambda_2} - \phi} = 4 \Rightarrow \frac{hc}{\lambda_1} - \phi = \frac{4hc}{\lambda_2} - 4\phi$$

$$\Rightarrow \frac{4hc}{\lambda_2} - \frac{hc}{\lambda_1} = 3\phi \Rightarrow \phi = \frac{1}{3}hc\left(\frac{4}{\lambda_2} - \frac{1}{\lambda_1}\right)$$

$$= \frac{1}{3}\times1240\left(\frac{4\times350-540}{350\times540}\right) = 1.8 \text{ eV}$$

CHAPTER-26 : Atoms

TOPIC - 2 : Bohr's Model and the Spectra of the Hydrogen atom

110. (d) Energy released by hydrogen atom for transition $n = 2$ to $n = 1$

$$\therefore\ \Delta E_1 = 13.6\times\left(\frac{1}{1^2} - \frac{1}{2^2}\right) = \frac{3}{4}\times13.6 \text{ eV}$$

$= 10.2$ eV

This energy is absorbed by He^+ ion in transition from $n = 2$ to $n = n_1$ (say)

$$\therefore\ \Delta E_2 = 13.6\times4\times\left(\frac{1}{4} - \frac{1}{n_1^2}\right) = 10.2 \text{ eV}$$

$\Rightarrow\ n_1 = 4$

So, possible transition is $n = 2 \rightarrow n = 4$

111. (b) $$\frac{1}{\lambda_1} = -R\left(\frac{1}{2^2} - \frac{1}{3^2}\right) = \frac{5R}{36}$$

$$\frac{1}{\lambda_2} = R\left(\frac{1}{2^2} - \frac{1}{4^2}\right) = \frac{3R}{16}$$

$$\therefore \frac{\lambda_2}{\lambda_1} = \frac{80}{108}$$

$$\lambda_2 = \frac{80}{108}\lambda_1 = \frac{80}{108}\times660$$

$= 488.9$ nm.

CHAPTER-27 : Nuclei

TOPIC - 3: Radioactivity

112. (c) Activity $A = \lambda N$

For material, A $\quad 10 = (2 N_0)\lambda_A$

For material, B $\quad 20 = N_0\lambda_B$

$$\Rightarrow \lambda_B = 4\lambda_A\ \therefore T_{½A} = 4T_{½B}\left[\because T_{½} = \frac{0.693}{\lambda}\right]$$

i.e. 20 days half-lives for A and 5 days $(T_{½})_B$ For material B.

113. (a) According to question, at t = 0, $A_0 = \frac{dN}{dt} = 1600$ C/s and at t = 8s, A = 100 C/s

$\therefore \frac{A}{A_0} = \frac{1}{16}$ in 8s

Therefore half life period, $t_{1/2} = 2s$

$\therefore$ Activity at t = 6s = $1600\left(\frac{1}{2}\right)^3 = 200C/s$

CHAPTER-28 : Semiconductor Electronics : Materials, Devices and Simple Circuits

TOPIC - 1: Solids, Semiconductors and P-N Junction Diode

114. (a)

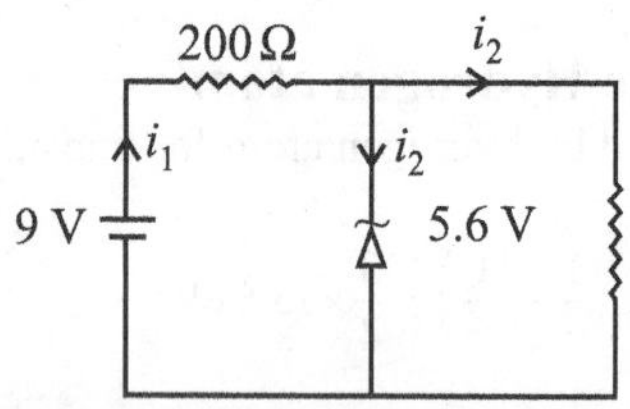

P.D. across 800Ω resistors = 5.6 V

so, $I_{800\Omega} = \frac{5.6}{800}A = 7$ mA

Now, P.D. across 200Ω resistors = 9 – 5.6 V = 3.4 V

so, $I_{200\Omega} = \frac{9-5.6}{200} = 17$ mA

so, current through zener diode = I_z = 17 – 7 = 10 mA

115. (c) As we know, current density,

$j = \sigma E = nev_d$

$\sigma = ne\frac{v_d}{E} = ne\mu$

$\frac{1}{\sigma} = \rho = \frac{1}{n_e e\mu_e}$ =Resistivity

$= \frac{1}{10^{19} \times 1.6 \times 10^{19} - 19 \times 1.6}$

or $P = 0.4\ \Omega m$

TOPIC - 2: Junction Transistor

116. (b) $\beta = \frac{\Delta Ic}{\Delta Ib} = \frac{3\times10^{-3}}{15\times10^{-6}} = 200$

We have $\frac{V_0}{V_i} = \beta\frac{R^2}{R_1}$

or $\frac{V_0}{V_i} = 200\left(\frac{1000}{R_1}\right)$

If $R_1 = 0.67k\Omega, \frac{V_0}{V_i} = 300$

TOPIC - 3: Digital Electronics and Logic Gates

117. (c) From the given logic circuit,

$p = \overline{x} + y$

$Q = \overline{\overline{y}.x} = y + \overline{x}$

Output, R = $\overline{P+Q}$

To make output 1

P + Q must be '0'

So, x = 1, y = 0

CHAPTER-29 : Communication Systems

TOPIC-1 : Communication Systems

118. (b) Carrier waves of wavelength 1500 nm is used in modern optical fiber communication.

119. (a)

120. (a) Maximum distance upto which signal can be broadcasted

$d_{max} = \sqrt{2Rh_T} + \sqrt{2Rh_R}$

where h_T and h_R are heights of transmission tower and receiving antenna respectively.

Putting values R, h_T and h_R

$d_{max} = \sqrt{2\times6.4\times106}\left[\sqrt{140}+\sqrt{40}\right]$

or, $d_{max} \simeq 65$ km

JEE Main Solved Paper 2018
Offline + Online

CHAPTER-1 : Physical World, Units and Measurements

TOPIC-2 : Dimensions of Physical Quantities

1. The characteristic distance at which quantum gravitational effects are significant, the Planck length, can be determined from a suitable combination of the fundamental physical constants G, h and c . Which of the following correctly gives the Planck length? **[Online April 15, 2018]**

(a) G^2hc (b) $\left(\frac{Gh}{c^3}\right)^{\frac{1}{2}}$ (c) $G^{\frac{1}{2}}h^2c$ (d) Gh^2c^3

TOPIC-3 : Errors in Measurements

2. The density of a material in the shape of a cube is determined by measuring three sides of the cube and its mass. If the relative errors in measuring the mass and length are respectively 1.5% and 1%, the maximum error in determining the density is: **[2018]**

(a) 2.5% (b) 3.5% (c) 4.5% (d) 6%

3. The percentage errors in quantities P, Q, R and S are 0.5%, 1%, 3% and 1.5% respectively in the measurement of a physical quantity $A = \frac{P^3Q^2}{\sqrt{RS}}$.

The maximum percentage error in the value of A will be **[Online April 16, 2018]**

(a) 8.5% (b) 6.0% (c) 7.5% (d) 6.5%

4. The relative uncertainty in the period of a satellite orbiting around the earth is 10^{-2}. If the relative uncertainty in the radius of the orbit is negligible, the relative uncertainty in the mass of the earth is **[Online April 16, 2018]**

(a) 3×10^{-2} (b) 10^{-2} (c) 2×10^{-2} (d) 6×10^{-2}

5. The relative error in the determination of the surface area of a sphere is α. Then the relative error in the determination of its volume is **[Online April 15, 2018]**

(a) $\frac{2}{3}\alpha$ (b) $\frac{2}{3}\alpha$ (c) $\frac{3}{2}\alpha$ (d) α

6. In a screw gauge, 5 complete rotations of the screw cause it to move a linear distance of 0.25 cm. There are 100 circular scale divisions. The thickness of a wire measured by this screw gauge gives a reading of 4 main scale divisions and 30 circular scale divisions. Assuming negligible zero error, the thickness of the wire is: **[Online April 15, 2018]**

(a) 0.0430 cm (b) 0.3150 cm
(c) 0.4300 cm (d) 0.2150 cm

CHAPTER-2 : Motion in a Straight Line

TOPIC-1 : Distance, Displacement & Uniform Motion

7. All the graphs below are intended to represent the same motion. One of them does it incorrectly. Pick it up. **[2018]**

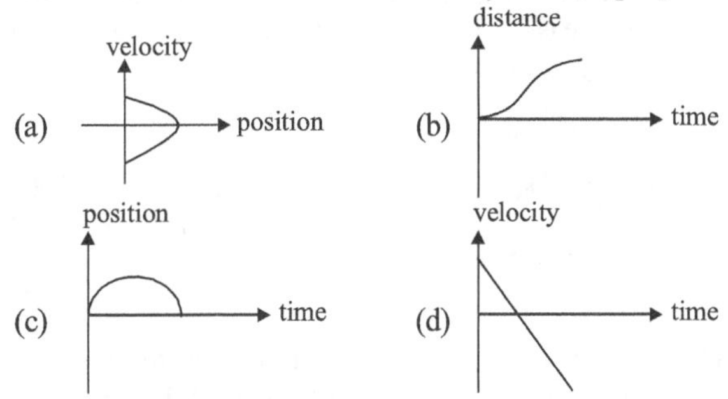

TOPIC-2 : Non-uniform Motion

8. An automobile, travelling at 40 km/h, can be stopped at a distance of 40 m by applying brakes. If the same automobile is travelling at 80 km/h, the minimum stopping distance, in metres, is (assume no skidding) **[Online April 15, 2018]**

(a) 75m (b) 160m (c) 100m (d) 150m

9. The velocity-time graphs of a car and a scooter are shown in the figure. (i) the difference between the distance travelled by the car and the scooter in 15 s and (ii) the time at which the car will catch up with the scooter are, respectively **[Online April 15, 2018]**

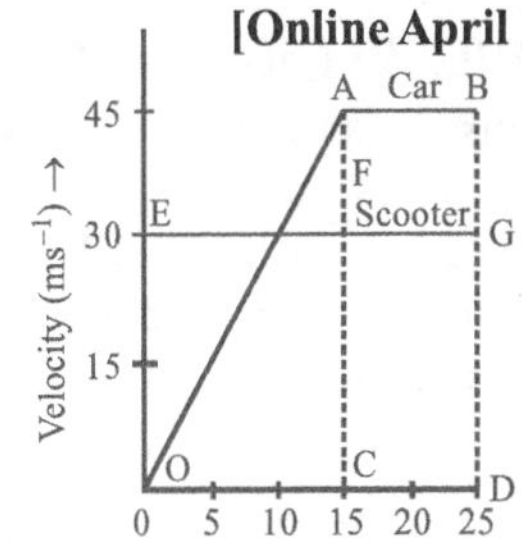

(a) 337.5m and 25s

(b) 225.5m and 10s

(c) 112.5m and 22.5s

(d) 11.2.5m and 15s

10. A man in a car at location Q on a straight highway is moving with speed v. He decides to reach a point P in a field at a distance d from highway (point M) as shown in the figure. Speed of the car in the field is half to that on the highway. What should be the distance RM, so that the time taken to reach P is minimum? **[Online April 15, 2018]**

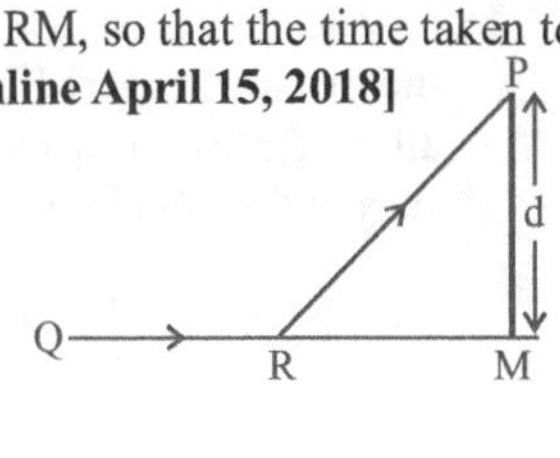

(a) $\frac{d}{\sqrt{3}}$ (b) $\frac{d}{2}$

(c) $\frac{d}{\sqrt{2}}$ (d) d

CHAPTER-3 : Motion in a Plane

TOPIC-1 : Vectors

11. Let $\vec{A} = (\hat{i} + \hat{j})$ and $\vec{B} = (\hat{i} - \hat{j})$. The magnitude of a coplanar vector $\vec{C}$ such that $\vec{A}.\vec{C} = \vec{B}.\vec{C} = \vec{A}.\vec{B}$ is given by **[Online April 16, 2018]**

(a) $\sqrt{\frac{5}{9}}$ (b) $\sqrt{\frac{10}{9}}$ (c) $\sqrt{\frac{20}{9}}$ (d) $\sqrt{\frac{9}{12}}$

CHAPTER-4 : Laws of Motion

TOPIC-3 : Friction

12. Two masses $m_1 = 5$ kg and $m_2 = 10$ kg, connected by an inextensible string over a frictionless pulley, are moving as shown in the figure. The coefficient of friction of horizontal surface is 0.15. The minimum weight m that should be put on top of m_2 to stop the motion is: **[2018]**

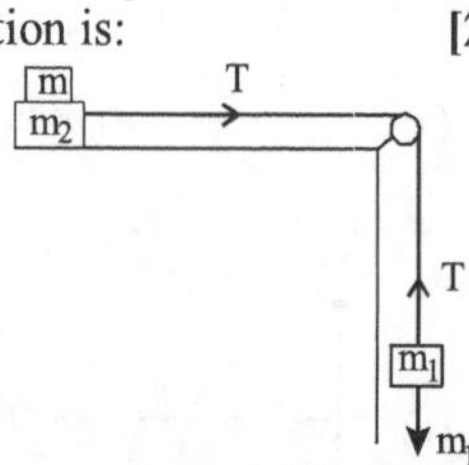

(a) 18.3 kg

(b) 27.3 kg

(c) 43.3 kg

(d) 10.3 kg

13. A given object takes *n* times more time to slide down a 45° rough inclined plane as it takes to slide down a perfectly smooth 45° incline. The coefficient of kinetic friction between the object and the incline is : **[Online April 15, 2018]**

(a) $\sqrt{1-\frac{1}{n^2}}$ (b) $1-\frac{1}{n^2}$ (c) $\frac{1}{2-n^2}$ (d) $\sqrt{\frac{1}{1-n^2}}$

14. A body of mass 2kg slides down with an acceleration of $3 m/s^2$ on a rough inclined plane having a slope of 30°. The external force required to take the same body up the plane with the same acceleration will be: ($g = 10 m/s^2$) **[Online April 15, 2018]**

(a) 4N (b) 14N (c) 6N (d) 20N

TOPIC-4 : Circular Motion, Banking of Road

15. A disc rotates about its axis of symmetry in a hoizontal plane at a steady rate of 3.5 revolutions per second. A coin placed at a distance of 1.25cm from the axis of rotation remains at rest on the disc. The coefficient of friction between the coin and the disc is ($g = 10 m/s^2$)

(a) 0.5 (b) 0.7 (c) 0.3 (d) 0.6

[Online April 15, 2018]

CHAPTER-5 : Work, Energy and Power

TOPIC-1 : Work

16. A body of mass starts moving from rest along x-axis so that its velocity varies as $v = a\sqrt{s}$ where a is a constant s and is the distance covered by the body. The total work done by all the forces acting on the body in the first second after the start of the motion is: **[Online April 16, 2018]**

(a) $\frac{1}{8}ma^4t^2$ (b) $4ma^4t^2$ (c) $8ma^4t^2$ (d) $\frac{1}{4}ma^4t^2$

TOPIC-2 : Energy

17. A particle is moving in a circular path of radius a under the action of an attractive potential $U = -\frac{k}{2r^2}$. Its total energy is: **[2018]**

(a) $-\frac{k}{4a^2}$ (b) $\frac{k}{2a^2}$ (c) zero (d) $-\frac{3}{2}\frac{k}{a^2}$

18. Two particles of the same mass m are moving in circular orbits because of force, given by $F(r) = \frac{-16}{r} - r^3$

The first particle is at a distance r = 1, and the second, at r = 4. The best estimate for the ratio of kinetic energies of the first and the second particle is closest to **[Online April 16, 2018]**

(a) 10^{-1} (b) 6×10^{-2}

(c) 6×10^{2} (d) 3×10^{-3}

TOPIC-4 : Collisions

19. In a collinear collision, a particle with an initial speed v_0 strikes a stationary particle of the same mass. If the final total kinetic energy is 50% greater than the original kinetic energy, the magnitude of the relative velocity between the two particles, after collision, is: **[2018]**

(a) $\frac{v_0}{4}$ (b) $\sqrt{2}v_0$

(c) $\frac{v_0}{2}$ (d) $\frac{v_0}{\sqrt{2}}$

20. The mass of a hydrogen molecule is 3.32×10^{-27} kg. If 10^{23} hydrogen molecules strike, per second, a fixed wall of area $2 cm^2$ at an angle of 45° to the normal, and rebound elastically with a speed of 10^3 m/s, then the pressure on the wall is nearly: **[2018]**

(a) $2.35 \times 10^3 N/m^2$ (b) $4.70 \times 10^3 N/m^2$

(c) $2.35 \times 10^2 N/m^2$ (d) $4.70 \times 10^2 N/m^2$

21. It is found that if a neutron suffers an elastic collinear collision with deuterium at rest, fractional loss of its energy is p_d; while for its similar collision with carbon nucleus at rest, fractional loss of energy is P_c. The values of P_d and P_c are respectively: **[2018]**

(a) (·89, ·28) (b) (·28, ·89)

(c) (0, 0) (d) (0, 1)

22. A proton of mass m collides elastically with a particle of unknown mass at rest. After the collision, the proton and the unknown particle are seen moving at an angle of 90° with respect to each other. The mass of unknown particle is: **[Online April 15, 2018]**

(a) $\frac{m}{\sqrt{3}}$ (b) $\frac{m}{2}$

(c) 2m (d) m

CHAPTER-6 : System of Particles and Rotational Motion

TOPIC-1 : Centre of Mass, Centre of Gravity & Principle of Moments

23. A force of 40 N acts on a point B at the end of an L-shaped object, as shown in the figure. The angle θ that will produce maximum moment of the force about point A is given by: **[Online April 15, 2018]**

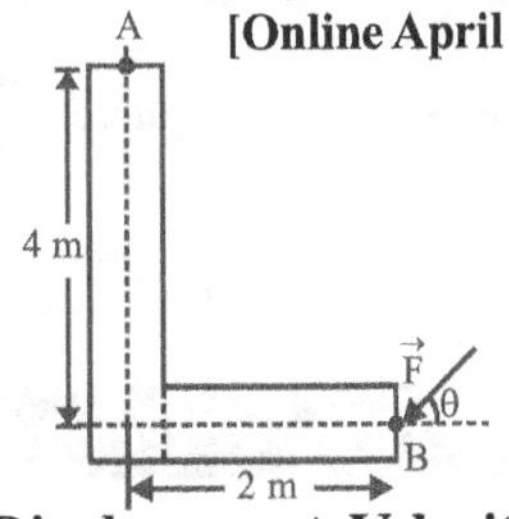

(a) $\tan\theta = \frac{1}{4}$

(b) $\tan\theta = 2$

(c) $\tan\theta = \frac{1}{2}$

(d) $\tan\theta = 4$

TOPIC-2 : Angular Displacement, Velocity and Acceleration

24. A particle is moving with a uniform speed in a circular orbit of radius R in a central force inversely proportional to the nth power of R. If the period of rotation of the particle is T, then: **[2018]**

(a) $T \propto R^{3/2}$ for any n. (b) $T \propto R^{n/2+1}$

(c) $T \propto R^{(n+1)/2}$ (d) $T \propto R^{n/2}$

TOPIC-3 : Torque, Couple and Angular Momentum

25.

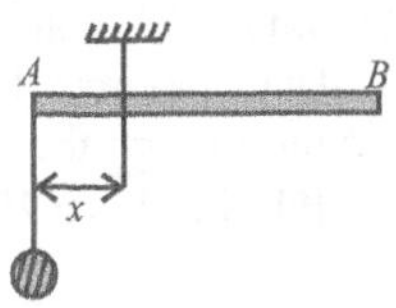

A uniform rod *AB* is suspended from a point *X*, at a variable distance from *x* from *A*, as shown. To make the rod horizontal, a mass *m* is suspended from its end *A*. A set of (*m*, *x*) values is recorded. The appropriate variable that give a straight line, when plotted, are: **[Online April 15, 2018]**

(a) $m, \frac{1}{x}$ (b) $m, \frac{1}{x^2}$ (c) m, x (d) m, x^2

26. A thin uniform bar of length L and mass 8m lies on a smooth horizontal table. Two point masses m and 2m moving in the same horizontal plane from opposite sides of the bar with speeds 2v and v respectively. The masses stick to the bar after collision at a distance $\frac{L}{3}$ and $\frac{L}{6}$ respectively from the centre of the bar. If the bar starts rotating about its center of mass as a result of collision, the angular speed of the bar will be: **[Online April 15, 2018]**

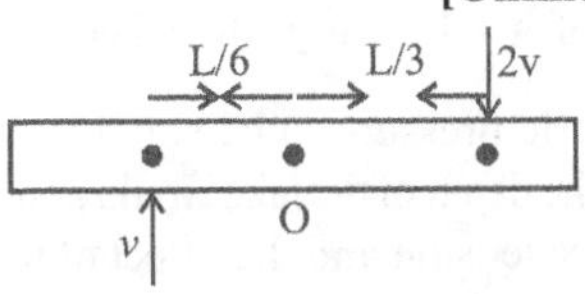

(a) $\frac{v}{6L}$ (b) $\frac{6v}{5L}$ (c) $\frac{3v}{5L}$ (d) $\frac{v}{5L}$

TOPIC-4 : Moment of Inertia and Rotational K.E.

27. Seven identical circular planar disks, each of mass M and radius R are welded symmetrically as shown. The moment of inertia of the arrangement about the axis normal to the plane and passing through the point P is: **[2018]**

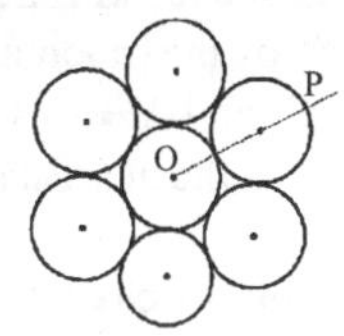

(a) $\frac{19}{2}MR^2$ (b) $\frac{55}{2}MR^2$ (c) $\frac{73}{2}MR^2$ (d) $\frac{181}{2}MR^2$

28. From a uniform circular disc of radius R and mass 9 M, a small disc of radius $\frac{R}{3}$ is removed as shown in the figure. The moment of inertia of the remaining disc about an axis perpendicular to the plane of the disc and passing, through centre of disc is : **[2018]**

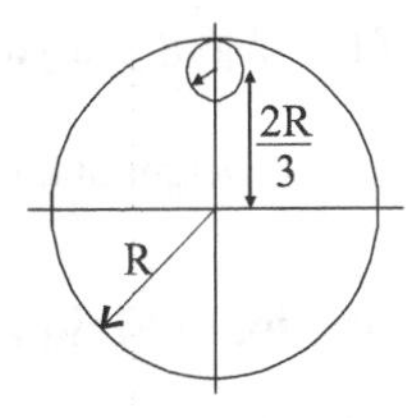

(a) $4MR^2$ (b) $\frac{40}{9}MR^2$ (c) $10\ MR^2$ (d) $\frac{37}{9}MR^2$

29. A thin circular disk is in the xy plane as shown in the figure. The ratio of its moment of inertia about z and z′ axes will be **[Online April 16, 2018]**

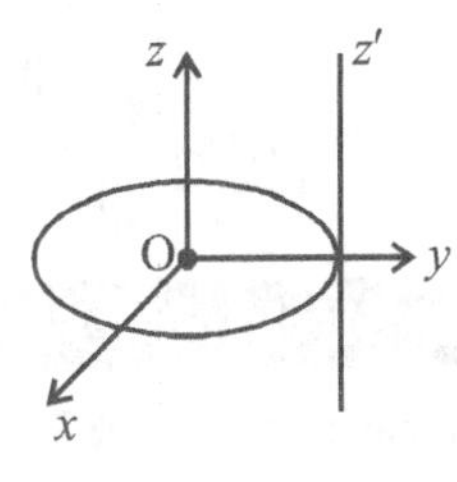

(a) 1 : 2 (b) 1 : 4 (c) 1 : 3 (d) 1 : 5

30. A thin rod MN, free to rotate in the vertical plane about the fixed end N, is held horizontal. When the end M is released the speed of this end, when the rod makes an angle α with the horizontal, will be proportional to: (see figure) **[Online April 15, 2018]**

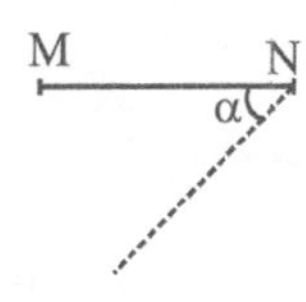

(a) $\sqrt{\cos\alpha}$ (b) $\cos\alpha$

(c) $\sin\alpha$ (d) $\sqrt{\sin\alpha}$

CHAPTER-7 : Gravitation

TOPIC-2 : Newton's Universal Law of Gravitation

31. Take the mean distance of the moon and the sun from the earth to be 0.4×10^6 km and 150×10^6 km respectively. Their masses are 8×10^{22} kg and 2×10^{30} kg respectively. The radius of the earth is 6400 km. Let ΔF_1 be the difference in the forces exerted by the moon at the nearest and farthest points on the earth and ΔF_2 be the difference in the force exerted by the sun at the nearest and farthest points on the earth. Then, the number closest to $\frac{\Delta F_1}{\Delta F_2}$ is: **[Online April 15, 2018]**

(a) 2 (b) 6 (c) 10^{-2} (d) 0.6

TOPIC-3 : Acceleration due to Gravity

32. Suppose that the angular velocity of rotation of earth is increased. Then, as a consequence. **[Online April 16, 2018]**

(a) There will be no change in weight anywhere on the earth
(b) Weight of the object, everywhere on the earth, wild decrease
(c) Weight of the object, everywhere on the earth, will increase
(d) Except at poles, weight of the object on the earth will decrease

TOPIC-4 : Gravitational Field and Potential nergy

33. A body of mass m is moving in a circular orbit of radius R about a planet of mass M. At some instant, it splits into two equal masses. The first mass moves in a circular orbit of radius $\frac{R}{2}$, and the other mass, in a circular orbit of radius $\frac{3R}{2}$. The difference between the final and initial total energies is: **[Online April 15, 2018]**

(a) $-\frac{GMm}{2R}$ (b) $+\frac{GMm}{6R}$ (c) $-\frac{GMm}{6R}$ (d) $\frac{GMm}{2R}$

CHAPTER-8 : Mechanical Properties of Solids

TOPIC-1 : Hooke's Law & Young's Modulus

34. As shown in the figure, forces of 10^5N each are applied in opposite directions, on the upper and lower faces of a cube of side 10cm, shifting the upper face parallel to itself by 0.5cm. If the side of another cube of the same material is, 20cm, then under similar conditions as above, the displacement will be: **[Online April 15, 2018]**

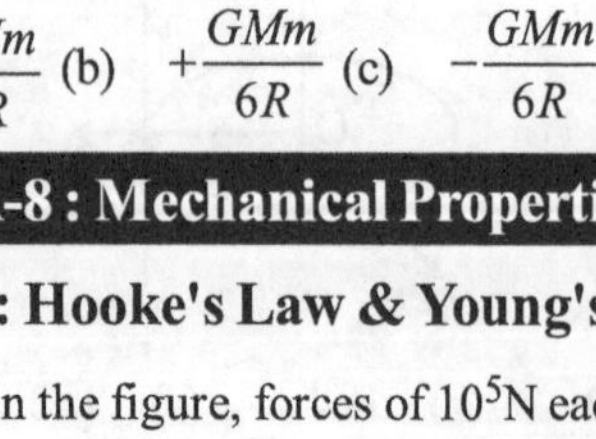

(a) 1.00cm (b) 0.25cm (c) 0.37cm (d) 0.75cm

TOPIC-2 : Bulk and Rigidity Modulus and Work Done in Stretching a Wire

35. A solid sphere of radius r made of a soft material of bulk modulus K is surrounded by a liquid in a cylindrical container. A massless piston of area a floats on the surface of the liquid, covering entire cross-section of cylindrical container. When a mass m is placed on the surface of the piston to compress the liquid, the fractional decrement in the radius of the sphere $\left(\frac{dr}{r}\right)$, is: **[2018]**

(a) $\frac{Ka}{mg}$ (b) $\frac{Ka}{3mg}$ (c) $\frac{mg}{3Ka}$ (d) $\frac{mg}{Ka}$

CHAPTER-9 : Mechanical Properties of Fluids

TOPIC-1 : Pressure, Density, Pascal's Law and Archimedes' Principle

36. A small soap bubble of radius 4cm is trapped inside another bubble of radius 6cm without any contact. Let P_2 be the pressure inside the inner bubble and P_0, the pressure outside the outer bubble. Radius of another bubble with pressure difference $P_2 - P_0$ between its inside and outside would be **[Online April 16, 2018]**

(a) 6cm (b) 12cm (c) 4.8cm (d) 2.4cm

37. A thin uniform tube is bent into a circle of radius r in the vertical plane. Equal volumes of two immiscible liquids, whose densities are ρ_1 and ρ_1 $(\rho_1 > \rho_2)$ fill half the circle. The angle θ between the radius vector passing through the common interface and the vertical is **[Online April 15, 2018]**

(a) $\theta = \tan^{-1}\left[\frac{\pi}{2}\left(\frac{\rho_1 - \rho_2}{\rho_1 + \rho_2}\right)\right]$

(b) $\theta = \tan^{-1}\frac{\pi}{2}\left(\frac{\rho_1 - \rho_2}{\rho_1 + \rho_2}\right)$

(c) $\theta = \tan^{-1}\pi\left(\frac{\rho_1}{\rho_2}\right)$

(d) None of above

TOPIC-2 : Fluid Flow, Reynold's Number and Bernoulli's Principle

38. When an air bubble of radius r rises from the bottom to the surface of a lake, its radius becomes $\frac{5r}{4}$. Taking the atmospheric pressure to be equal to 10m height of water column, the depth of the lake would approximately be (ignore the surface tension and the effect of temperature): **[Online April 15, 2018]**

(a) 10.5m (b) 8.7m (c) 11.2m (d) 9.5m

CHAPTER-10 : Thermal Properties of Matter

TOPIC-2 : Calorimetry and Heat Transfer

39. The value closest to the thermal velocity of a Helium atom at room temperature (300K) in ms^{-1} is: **[Online April 15, 2018]**
$[k_B = 1.4 \times 10^{-23} J/K; m_{He} = 7 \times 10^{-27} kg]$
(a) 1.3×10^4 (b) 1.3×10^5
(c) 1.3×10^2 (d) 1.3×10^3

TOPIC-3 : Newton's Law of Cooling

40. A body takes 10 minutes to cool from 60°C to 50°C. The temperature of surroundings is constant at 25°C. Then, the temperature of the body after next 10 minutes will be approximately **[Online April 15, 2018]**
(a) 43°C (b) 47°C (c) 41°C (d) 45°C

CHAPTER-11 : Thermodynamics

TOPIC-2 : Specific Heat Capacity and Thermodynamical Processes

41. One mole of an ideal monoatomic gas is taken along the path ABCA as shown in the PV diagram. The maximum temperature attained by the gas along the path BC is given by **[Online April 16, 2018]**
(a) $\frac{25}{8}\frac{P_0V_0}{R}$ (b) $\frac{25}{4}\frac{P_0V_0}{R}$
(c) $\frac{25}{16}\frac{P_0V_0}{R}$ (d) $\frac{5}{8}\frac{P_0V_0}{R}$

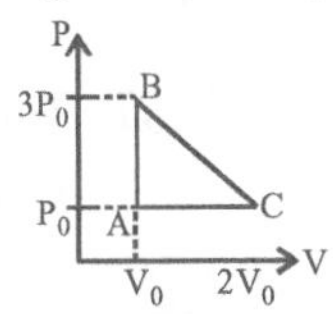

42. One mole of an ideal monoatomic gas is compressed isothermally in a rigid vessel to double its pressure at room temperature, 27°C. The work done on the gas will be: **[Online April 15, 2018]**
(a) 300R ln 6 (b) 300R
(c) 300R ln 7 (d) 300R ln 2

TOPIC-3 : Carnot Engine, Refrigerators and Second Law of Thermodynamics

43. A Carnot's engine works as a refrigerator between 250 K and 300 K. It receives 500 cal heat from the reservoir at the lower temperature. The amount of work done in each cycle to operate the refrigerator is: **[Online April 15, 2018]**
(a) 420 J (b) 2100 J (c) 772 J (d) 2520 J

44. Two Carnot engines A and B are operated in series. Engine A receives heat from a reservoir at 600K and rejects heat to a reservoir at temperature T. Engine B receives heat rejected by engine A and in turn rejects it to a reservoir at 100K. If the efficiencies of the two engines A and B are represented by η_A and η_B respectively, then what is the value of $\frac{\eta_A}{\eta_B}$
[Online April 15, 2018]
(a) $\frac{12}{7}$ (b) $\frac{12}{5}$ (c) $\frac{5}{12}$ (d) $\frac{7}{12}$

CHAPTER-12 : Kinetic Theory

TOPIC-3 : Degree of Freedom, Specific Heat Capacity, and Mean Free Path

45. Two moles of an ideal monoatomic gas occupies a volume V at 27°C. The gas expands adiabatically to a volume 2 V. Calculate (1) the final temperature of the gas and (2) change in its internal energy. **[2018]**
(a) (1) 189 K (2) 2.7 kJ
(b) (1) 195 K (2) –2.7 kJ
(c) (1) 189 K (2) –2.7 kJ
(d) (1) 195 K (2) 2.7 kJ

46. Two moles of helium are mixed with n with moles of hydrogen. If $\frac{C_P}{C_V} = \frac{3}{2}$ for the mixture, then the value of n is
[Online April 16, 2018]
(a) 3/2 (b) 2 (c) 1 (d) 3

CHAPTER-13 : Oscillations

TOPIC-1 : Displacement, Phase, Velocity and Acceleration in S.H.M.

47. Two simple harmonic motions, as shown, are at right angles. They are combined to form Lissajous figures.
$x(t) = A \sin (at + \delta)$
$y(t) = B \sin (bt)$
Identify the correct match below
[Online April 15, 2018]
(a) Parameters: $A = B, a = 2b; \delta = \frac{\pi}{2}$; Curve: Circle
(b) Parameters: $A = B, a = b; \delta = \frac{\pi}{2}$; Curve: Line
(c) Parameters: $A \neq B, a = b; \delta = \frac{\pi}{2}$; Curve: Ellipse
(d) Parameters: $A \neq B, a = b; \delta = 0$; Curve: Parabola

TOPIC-3 : Time Period, Frequency, Simple Pendulum and Spring Pendulum

48. A silver atom in a solid oscillates in simple harmonic motion in some direction with a frequency of 10^{12}/sec. What is the force constant of the bonds connecting one atom with the other? (Mole wt. of silver = 108 and Avagadro number = 6.02×10^{23} gm mole^{-1}) **[2018]**
(a) 6.4 N/m (b) 7.1 N/m (c) 2.2 N/m (d) 5.5 N/m

49. A particle executes simple harmonic motion and is located at x = a, b and c at times t_0, $2t_0$ and $3t_0$ respectively. The frequency of the oscillation is **[Online April 16, 2018]**
(a) $\frac{1}{2\pi t_0}\cos^{-1}\left(\frac{a+b}{2c}\right)$ (b) $\frac{1}{2\pi t_0}\cos^{-1}\left(\frac{a+b}{3c}\right)$
(c) $\frac{1}{2\pi t_0}\cos^{-1}\left(\frac{2a+3c}{b}\right)$ (d) $\frac{1}{2\pi t_0}\cos^{-1}\left(\frac{a+c}{2b}\right)$

TOPIC-4 : Damped, Forced Oscillations and Resonance

50. An oscillator of mass M is at rest in its equilibrium position in a potential $V = \frac{1}{2}k(x - X)^2$. A particle of mass m comes from right with speed u and collides completely inelastically with M and sticks to it. This process repeats every time the oscillator crosses its equilibrium position. The amplitude of oscillations after 13 collisions is: (M = 10, m = 5, u = 1, k = 1). **[Online April 16, 2018]**

(a) $\frac{1}{2}$ (b) $\frac{1}{\sqrt{3}}$

(c) $\frac{2}{3}$ (d) $\sqrt{\frac{3}{5}}$

CHAPTER-14 : Waves

TOPIC-2 : Vibration of String and Organ

51. A granite rod of 60 cm length is clamped at its middle point and is set into longitudinal vibrations. The density of granite is 2.7×10^3 kg/m^3 and its Young's modulus is 9.27×10^{10} Pa. What will be the fundamental frequency of the longitudinal vibrations? **[2018]**

(a) 5 kHz (b) 2.5 kHz (c) 10 kHz (d) 7.5 kHz

52. The end correction of a resonance column is 1cm. If the shortest length resonating with the tuning fork is 10cm, the next resonating length should be **[Online April 16, 2018]**

(a) 32cm (b) 40cm (c) 28cm (d) 36cm

TOPIC-3 : Beats, Interference and Superposition of Waves

53. A tuning fork vibrates with frequency 256 Hz and gives one beat per second with the third normal mode of vibration of an open pipe. What is the length of the pipe? (Speed of sound of air is 340 ms^{-1}) **[Online April 15, 2018]**

(a) 190 cm (b) 180 cm (c) 220 cm (d) 200 cm

54. 5 beats/ second are heard when a turning fork is sounded with a sonometer wire under tension, when the length of the sonometer wire is either 0.95m or 1m. The frequency of the fork will be: **[Online April 15, 2018]**

(a) 195Hz (b) 251Hz (c) 150Hz (d) 300Hz

TOPIC-4 : Musical Sound and Doppler's Effect

55. Two sitar strings, A and B, playing the note 'Dha' are slightly out of tune and produce beats and frequency 5 Hz. The tension of the string B is slightly increased and the beat frequency is found to decrease by 3 Hz. If the frequency of A is 425 Hz, the original frequency of B is **[Online April 16, 2018]**

(a) 430 Hz (b) 428 Hz (c) 422 Hz (d) 420 Hz

CHAPTER-15 : Electric Charges and Fields

TOPIC - 1: Electric Charges and Coulomb's Law

56. Two identical conducting spheres A and B, carry equal charge. They are separated by a distance much larger than their diameter, and the force between them is F. A third identical conducting sphere, C, is uncharged. Sphere C is first touched to A, then to B, and then removed. As a result, the force between A and B would be equal to **[Online April 16, 2018]**

(a) $\frac{3F}{4}$ (b) $\frac{F}{2}$ (c) F (d) $\frac{3F}{8}$

TOPIC - 2: Electric Field and Electric Field Lines

57. A body of mass M and charge q is connected to a spring of spring constant k. It is oscillating along x-direction about its equilibrium position, taken to be at $x = 0$, with an amplitude A. An electric field E is applied along the x-direction. Which of the following statements is correct? **[Online April 15, 2018]**

(a) The total energy of the system is $\frac{1}{2}m\omega^2 A^2 + \frac{1}{2}\frac{q^2E^2}{k}$

(b) The new equilibrium position is at a distance: $\frac{2qE}{k}$ from $x = 0$

(c) The new equilibrium position is at a distance: $\frac{qE}{2k}$ from x = 0

(d) The total energy of the system is $\frac{1}{2}m\omega^2 A^2 - \frac{1}{2}\frac{q^2E^2}{k}$

58. A solid ball of radius R has a charge density ρ given by $\rho = \rho_0\left(1 - \frac{r}{R}\right)$ for $0 \le r \le R$. The electric field outside the ball is: **[Online April 15, 2018]**

(a) $\frac{\rho_0 R^3}{\varepsilon_0 r^2}$ (b) $\frac{4\rho_0 R^3}{3\varepsilon_0 r^2}$ (c) $\frac{3\rho_0 R^3}{4\varepsilon_0 r^2}$ (d) $\frac{\rho_0 R^3}{12\varepsilon_0 r^2}$

TOPIC - 3 : Electric Dipole, Electric Flux and Gauss's Law

59. A charge Q is placed at a distance a/2 above the centre of the square surface of edge a as shown in the figure. The electric flux through the square surface is: **[Online April 15, 2018]**

(a) $\frac{Q}{3\varepsilon_0}$ (b) $\frac{Q}{6\varepsilon_0}$

(c) $\frac{Q}{2\varepsilon_0}$ (d) $\frac{Q}{\varepsilon_0}$

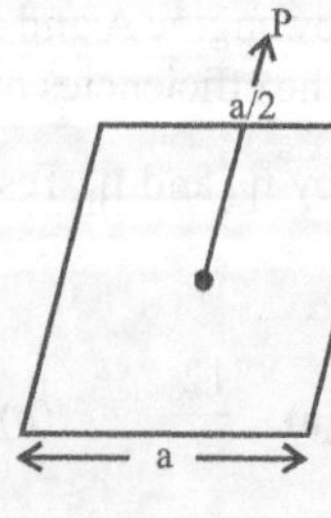

CHAPTER-16 : Electrostatic Potential and Capacitance

TOPIC - 1: Electrostatic Potential and Equipotential Surfacess

60. Three concentric metal shells A, B and C of respective radii *a*, *b* and *c* ($a < b < c$) have surface charge densities $+\sigma$, $-\sigma$ and $+\sigma$ respectively. The potential of shell B is: **[2018]**

(a) $\frac{\sigma}{\epsilon_0}\left[\frac{a^2-b^2}{a}+c\right]$ (b) $\frac{\sigma}{\epsilon_0}\left[\frac{a^2-b^2}{b}+c\right]$

(c) $\frac{\sigma}{\epsilon_0}\left[\frac{b^2-c^2}{b}+a\right]$ (d) $\frac{\sigma}{\epsilon_0}\left[\frac{b^2-c^2}{c}+a\right]$

TOPIC - 3: Capacitors, Grouping of Capacitor and Energy Stored in a Capacitor

61. A parallel plate capacitor of capacitance 90 pF is connected to a battery of emf 20V. If a dielectric material of dielectric constant $k = \frac{5}{3}$ is inserted between the plates, the magnitude of the induced charge will be: **[2018]**

(a) 1.2 n C (b) 0.3 n C (c) 2.4 n C (d) 0.9 n C

62. In the following circuit, the switch S is closed at t = 0. The charge on the capacitor C_1 as a function of time will be given by $\left(C_{eq} = \frac{C_1C_2}{C_1+C_2}\right)$. **[Online April 16, 2018]**

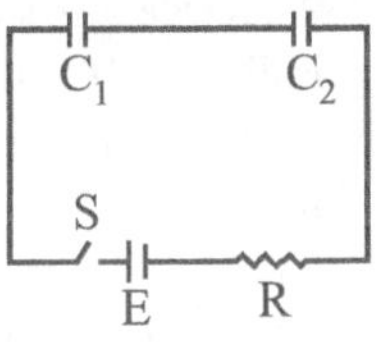

(a) $C_{eq}E[1-\exp(-t/RC_{eq})]$

(b) $C_1E[1-\exp(-tR/C_1)]$

(c) $C_2E[1-\exp(-t/RC_2)]$

(d) $C_{eq}E\exp(-t/RC_{eq})$

63. The equivalent capacitance between *A* and *B* in the circuit given below is:

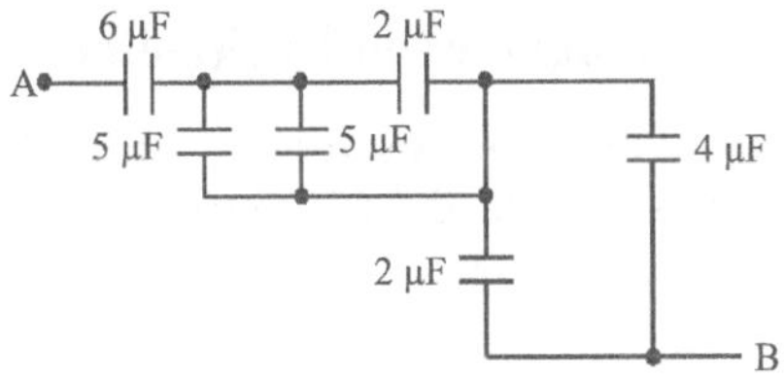

[Online April 15, 2018]

(a) 4.9 μF (b) 3.6 μF (c) 5.4 μF (d) 2.4 μF

64. A parallel plate capacitor with area 200cm^2 and separation between the plates 1.5cm, is connected across a battery of emf V. If the force of attraction between the plates is 25×10^{-6}N, the value of V is approximately: **[Online April 15, 2018]**

$$\left(\varepsilon_0 = 8.85 \times 10^{-12}\frac{C^2}{N.m^2}\right)$$

(a) 150V (b) 100V (c) 250V (d) 300V

65. A capacitor C_1 is charged up to a voltage V = 60V by connecting it to battery B through switch (1), Now C_1 is disconnected from battery and connected to a circuit consisting of two uncharged capacitors $C_2 = 3.0\mu F$ and $C_3 = 6.0\mu F$ through a switch (2) as shown in the figure. The sum of final charges on C_2 and C_3 is: **[Online April 15, 2018]**

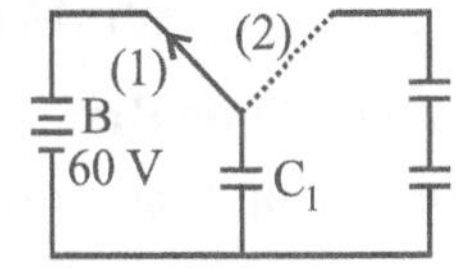

(a) 36μC (b) 20μC (c) 54μC (d) 40μC

CHAPTER-17 : Current Electricity

TOPIC - 1: Electric Current, Drift of Electrons, Ohm's Law, Resistance and Resistivity

66. A heating element has a resistance of 100Ω at room temperature. When it is connected to a supply of 220 V, a steady current of 2 A passes in it and temperature is 500°C more than room temperature. What is the temperature coefficient of resistance of the heating element? **[Online April 16, 2018]**

(a) $1 \times 10^{-4}\,°C^{-1}$ (b) $5 \times 10^{-4}\,°C^{-1}$

(c) $2 \times 10^{-4}\,°C^{-1}$ (d) $0.5 \times 10^{-4}\,°C^{-1}$

67. A copper rod of cross-sectional area A carries a uniform current I through it. At temperature T, if the volume charge density of the rod is ρ, how long will the charges take to travel a distance d ? **[Online April 15, 2018]**

(a) $\frac{2\rho dA}{IT}$ (b) $\frac{2\rho dA}{I}$ (c) $\frac{\rho dA}{I}$ (d) $\frac{\rho dA}{IT}$

TOPIC - 2: Combination of Resistances

68. In the given circuit all resistances are of value *R* ohm each. The equivalent resistance between *A* and *B* is : **[Online April 15, 2018]**

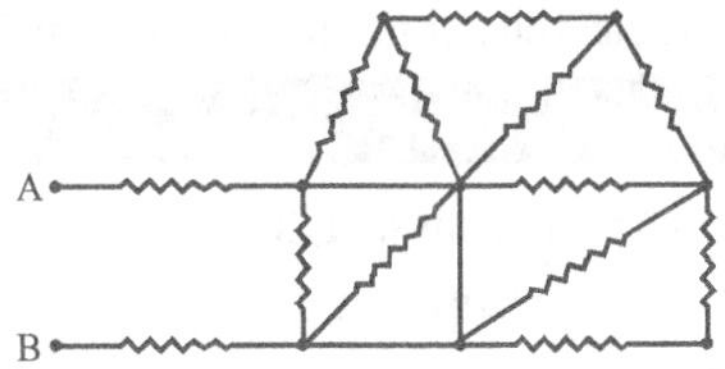

(a) 2*R* (b) $\frac{5R}{2}$ (c) $\frac{5R}{3}$ (d) 3*R*

TOPIC - 3: Kirchoff's Laws, Cells, Thermo e.m.f. Electrolysis

69. Two batteries with e.m.f. 12 V and 13 V are connected in parallel across a load resistor of 10 Ω. The internal resistances of the two batteries are 1 Ω and 2 Ω respectively. The voltage across the load lies between: **[2018]**

(a) 11.6 V and 11.7 V (b) 11.5 V and 11.6 V

(c) 11.4 V and 11.5 V (d) 11.7 V and 11.8 V

TOPIC - 4: Heating Effect of Current

70. A constant voltage is applied between two ends of a metallic wire. If the length is halved and the radius of the wire is doubled, the rate of heat developed in the wire will be: **[Online April 15, 2018]**

(a) Increased 8 times (b) Doubled
(c) Halved (d) Unchanged

TOPIC - 5: Wheatstone Bridge and Different Measuring Instruments

71. In a potentiometer experiment, it is found that no current passes through the galvanometer when the terminals of the cell are connected across 52 cm of the potentiometer wire. If the cell is shunted by a resistance of 5 Ω, a balance is found when the cell is connected across 40 cm of the wire. Find the internal resistance of the cell. **[2018]**

(a) 1 Ω (b) 1.5 Ω (c) 2 Ω (d) 2.5 Ω

72. On interchanging the resistances, the balance point of a meter bridge shifts to the left by 10 cm. The resistance of their series combination is 1kΩ. How much was the resistance on the left slot before interchanging the resistances? **[2018]**

(a) 990 Ω (b) 505 Ω (c) 550 Ω (d) 910 Ω

73. In a meter bridge, as shown in the figure, it is given that resistance Y=12.5 Ω and that the balance is obtained at a distance 39.5 cm from end *A* (by jockey J). After interchanging the resistances *X* and *Y*, a new balance point is found at a distance l_2 from end *A*. What are the values of *X* and l_2 ? **[Online April 15, 2018]**

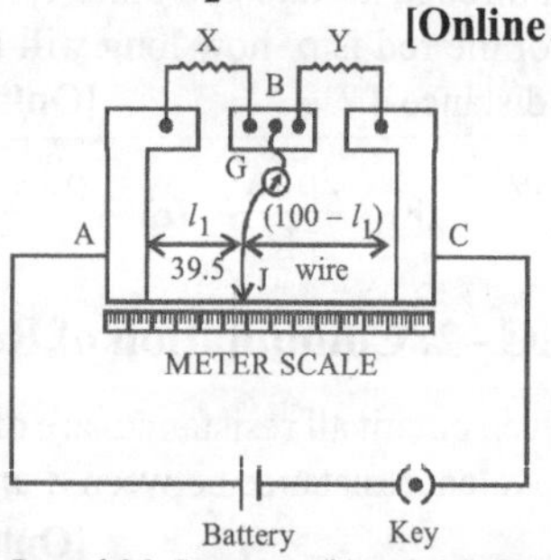

(a) 19.15 Ω and 39.5 cm (b) 8.16 Ω and 60.5 cm
(c) 19.15 Ω and 60.5 cm (d) 8.16 Ω and 39.5 cm

CHAPTER-18 : Moving Charges and Magnetism

TOPIC - 1: Motion of Charged Particle in Magnetic Field

74. An electron, a proton and an alpha particle having the same kinetic energy are moving in circular orbits of radii r_e, r_p, r_α respectively in a uniform magnetic field B. The relation between r_e, r_p, r_α is : **[2018]**

(a) $r_e > r_p = r_\alpha$ (b) $r_e < r_p = r_\alpha$
(c) $r_e < r_p < r_\alpha$ (d) $r_e < r_\alpha < r_p$

TOPIC - 2: Magnetic Field Lines, Biot-Savart's Law and Ampere's Circuital Law

75. The dipole moment of a circular loop carrying a current I, is m and the magnetic field at the centre of the loop is B_1. When the dipole moment is doubled by keeping the current constant, the magnetic field at the centre of the loop is B_2. The ratio $\frac{B_1}{B_2}$ is: **[2018]**

(a) 2 (b) $\sqrt{3}$ (c) $\sqrt{2}$ (d) $\frac{1}{\sqrt{2}}$

76. A Helmholtz coil has pair of loops, each with *N* turns and radius *R*. They are placed coaxially at distance *R* and the same current *I* flows through the loops in the same direction. The magnitude of magnetic field at *P*, midway between the centres *A* and *C*, is given by (Refer to figure): **[Online April 15, 2018]**

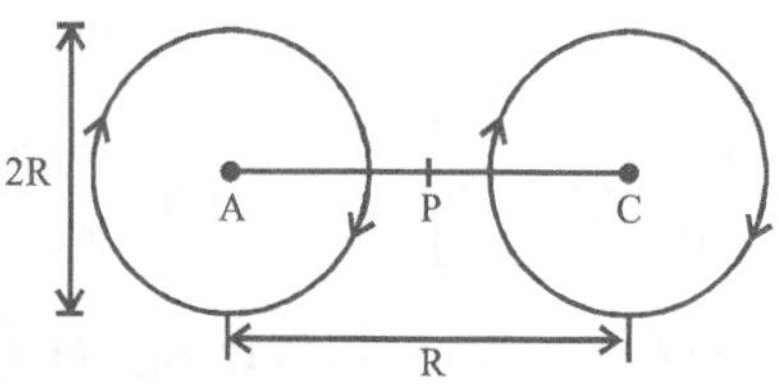

(a) $\frac{4N\mu_0 I}{5^{3/2}R}$ (b) $\frac{8N\mu_0 I}{5^{3/2}R}$ (c) $\frac{4N\mu_0 I}{5^{1/2}R}$ (d) $\frac{8N\mu_0 I}{5^{1/2}R}$

77. A current of 1A is flowing on the sides of an equilateral triangle of side 4.5×10^{-2}m. The magnetic field at the centre of the triangle will be: **[Online April 15, 2018]**

(a) 4×10^{-5}Wb/m^2 (b) Zero
(c) 2×10^{-5}Wb/m^2 (d) 8×10^{-5}Wb/m^2

TOPIC - 3: Force and Torque on Current Carrying Conductor

78. A charge q is spread uniformly over an insulated loop of radius r . If it is rotated with an angular velocity ω with respect to normal axis then the magnetic moment of the loop is **[Online April 16, 2018]**

(a) $\frac{1}{2}q\omega r^2$ (b) $\frac{4}{3}q\omega r^2$ (c) $\frac{3}{2}q\omega r^2$ (d) $q\omega r^2$

TOPIC - 4: Galvanometer and its Conversion into Ammeter and Voltmeter

79. In a circuit for finding the resistance of a galvanometer by half deflection method, a 6 V battery and a high resistance of 11kΩ are used. The figure of merit of the galvanometer 60μA/division. In the absence of shunt resistance, the galvanometer produces a deflection of θ = 9 divisions when current flows in the circuit. The value of the shunt resistance that can cause the deflection of θ/2 , is closest to **[Online April 16, 2018]**

(a) 55Ω (b) 110Ω (c) 220Ω (d) 550Ω

80. A galvanometer with its coil resistance 25Ω requires a current of 1mA for its full deflection. In order to construct an ammeter to read up to a current of 2A, the approximate value of the shunt resistance should be **[Online April 16, 2018]**

(a) 2.5×10^{-2}Ω (b) 1.25×10^{-3}Ω
(c) 2.5×10^{-3}Ω (d) 1.25×10^{-2}Ω

CHAPTER-19 : Magnetism and Matter

TOPIC - 2: The Earth Magnetism, Magnetic Materials and their properties

81. The B-H curve for a ferromagnet is shown in the figure. The ferromagnet is placed inside a long solenoid with 1000 turns/cm.. The current that should be passed in the solenoid to demagnetise the ferromagnet completely is: **[Online April 15, 2018]**

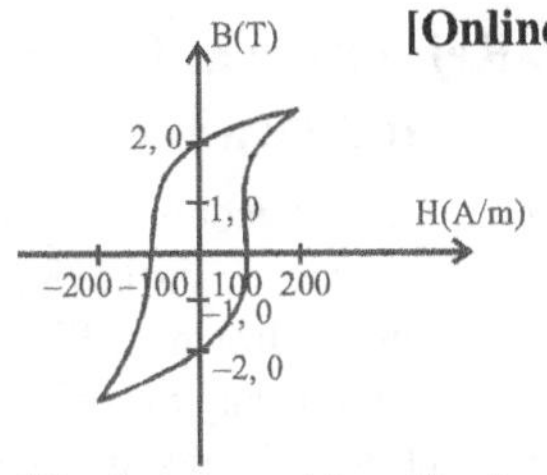

(a) 2 mA (b) 1 mA (c) 40 μA (d) 20 μA

CHAPTER-20 : Electromagnetic Induction

TOPIC - 2: Motional and Static EMI and Application of EMI

82. A coil of cross-sectional area A having n turns is placed in a uniform magnetic field B. When it is rotated with an angular velocity ω, the maximum e.m.f. induced in the coil will be **[Online April 16, 2018]**

(a) nBAω (b) $\frac{3}{2}$nBAω (c) 3nBAω (d) $\frac{1}{2}$nBAω

83. An ideal capacitor of capacitance 0.2 μF is charged to a potential difference of 10V. The charging battery is then disconnected. The capacitor is then connected to an ideal inductor of self inductance 0.5mH. The current at a time when the potential difference across the capacitor is 5V, is: **[Online April 15, 2018]**

(a) 0.17A (b) 0.15A (c) 0.34A (d) 0.25A

84. A copper rod of mass m slides under gravity on two smooth parallel rails, with separation 1 and set at an angle of θ with the horizontal. At the bottom, rails are joined by a resistance R. There is a uniform magnetic field B normal to the plane of the rails, as shown in the figure. The terminal speed of the copper rod is: **[Online April 15, 2018]**

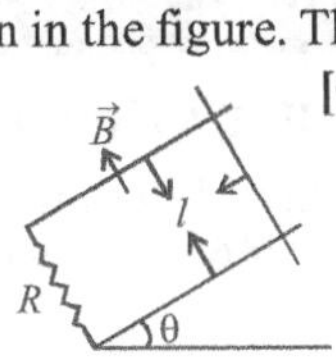

(a) $\frac{mgR\cos\theta}{B^2l^2}$ (b) $\frac{mgR\sin\theta}{B^2l^2}$

(c) $\frac{mgR\tan\theta}{B^2l^2}$ (d) $\frac{mgR\cot\theta}{B^2l^2}$

85. At the centre of a fixed large circular coil of radius R, a much smaller circular coil of radius r is placed. The two coils are concentric and are in the same plane. The larger coil carries a current I. The smaller coil is set to rotate with a constant angular velocity ω about an axis along their common diameter. Calculate the emf induced in the smaller coil after a time t of its start of rotation. **[Online April 15, 2018]**

(a) $\frac{\mu_0 I}{2R}\omega r^2\sin\omega t$ (b) $\frac{\mu_0 I}{4R}\omega\pi r^2\sin\omega t$

(c) $\frac{\mu_0 I}{2R}\omega\pi r^2\sin\omega t$ (d) $\frac{\mu_0 I}{4R}\omega r^2\sin\omega t$

CHAPTER-21 : Alternating Current

TOPIC - 2: AC Circuit, LCR Circuit, Quality and Power Factor

86. In an a.c. circuit, the instantaneous e.m.f. and current are given by

$e = 100\sin 30t$

$i = 20\sin\left(30t - \frac{\pi}{4}\right)$

In one cycle of a.c., the average power consumed by the circuit and the wattless current are, respectively: **[2018]**

(a) 50W, 10A (b) $\frac{1000}{\sqrt{2}}$ W, 10A

(c) $\frac{50}{\sqrt{2}}$ W, 0 (d) 50W, 0

87. For an RLC circuit driven with voltage of amplitude v_m and frequency $\omega_0 = \frac{1}{\sqrt{LC}}$ the current exhibits resonance. The quality factor, Q is given by: **[2018]**

(a) $\frac{\omega_0 L}{R}$ (b) $\frac{\omega_0 R}{L}$ (c) $\frac{R}{(\omega_0 C)}$ (d) $\frac{CR}{\omega_0}$

TOPIC - 3: Transformers and LC Oscillations

88. A power transmission line feeds input power at 2300 V to a step down transformer with its primary windings having 4000 turns, giving the output power at 230 V. If the current in the primary of the transformer is 5 A, and its efficiency is 90%, the output current would be: **[Online April 16, 2018]**

(a) 20 A (b) 40 A (c) 45 A (d) 25 A

CHAPTER-22 : Electromagnetic Waves

TOPIC-1 : Electromagnetic Waves, Conduction and Displacement Current

89. An EM wave from air enters a medium. The electric fields are $\vec{E}_1 = E_{01}\hat{x}\cos\left[2\pi\nu\left(\frac{z}{c} - t\right)\right]$ in air and

$\vec{E}_2 = E_{02}\hat{x}\cos[k(2z - ct)]$ in medium, where the wave number k and frequency ν refer to their values in air. The medium is nonmagnetic. If ϵ_{r_1} and ϵ_{r_2} refer to relative permittivities of air and medium respectively, which of the following options is correct? **[2018]**

(a) $\frac{\epsilon_{r_1}}{\epsilon_{r_2}} = 4$ (b) $\frac{\epsilon_{r_1}}{\epsilon_{r_2}} = 2$

(c) $\frac{\epsilon_{r_1}}{\epsilon_{r_2}} = \frac{1}{4}$ (d) $\frac{\epsilon_{r_1}}{\epsilon_{r_2}} = \frac{1}{2}$

90. A plane electromagnetic wave of wavelength λ has an intensity I. It is propagating along the positive Y– direction. The allowed expressions for the electric and magnetic fields are given by **[Online April 16, 2018]**

(a) $\vec{E}=\sqrt{\frac{I}{\varepsilon_0 C}}\cos\left[\frac{2\pi}{\lambda}(y-ct)\right]\hat{i};\vec{B}=\frac{1}{c}E\hat{k}$

(b) $\vec{E}=\sqrt{\frac{I}{\varepsilon_0 C}}\cos\left[\frac{2\pi}{\lambda}(y-ct)\right]\hat{k};\vec{B}=-\frac{1}{c}E\hat{i}$

(c) $\vec{E}=\sqrt{\frac{2I}{\varepsilon_0 C}}\cos\left[\frac{2\pi}{\lambda}(y-ct)\right]\hat{k};\vec{B}=+\frac{1}{c}E\hat{i}$

(d) $\vec{E}=\sqrt{\frac{2I}{\varepsilon_0 C}}\cos\left[\frac{2\pi}{\lambda}(y+ct)\right]\hat{k};\vec{B}=\frac{1}{c}E\hat{i}$

91. A monochromatic beam of light has a frequency $\nu=\frac{3}{2\pi}\times10^{12}$ Hz and is propagating along the direction $\frac{\hat{i}+\hat{j}}{\sqrt{2}}$. It is polarized along the $\hat{k}$ direction. The acceptable form for the magnetic field is: **[Online April 15, 2018]**

(a) $k\frac{E_0}{C}\left(\frac{\hat{i}-\hat{j}}{\sqrt{2}}\right)\cos\left[10^4\left(\frac{\hat{i}-\hat{j}}{\sqrt{2}}\right).\vec{r}-(3\times10^{12})t\right]$

(b) $\frac{E_0}{C}\left(\frac{\hat{i}-\hat{j}}{\sqrt{2}}\right)\cos\left[10^4\left(\frac{\hat{i}+\hat{j}}{\sqrt{2}}\right).\vec{r}-(3\times10^{12})t\right]$

(c) $\frac{E_0}{C}\hat{k}\cos\left[10^4\left(\frac{\hat{i}+\hat{j}}{\sqrt{2}}\right).\vec{r}+(3\times10^{12})t\right]$

(d) $\frac{E_0}{C}\frac{(\hat{i}+\hat{j}+\hat{k})}{\sqrt{3}}\cos\left[10^4\left(\frac{\hat{i}+\hat{j}}{\sqrt{2}}\right).\vec{r}+(3\times10^{12})t\right]$

92. A plane polarized monochromatic EM wave is travelling a vacuum along z direction such that at $t=t_1$ it is found that the electric field is zero at a spatial point z_1. The next zero that occurs in its neighbourhood is at z_2. The frequency of the electromagnetic wave is: **[Online April 15, 2018]**

(a) $\frac{3\times10^8}{|z_2-z_1|}$ (b) $\frac{6\times10^8}{|z_2-z_1|}$

(c) $\frac{1.5\times10^8}{|z_2-z_1|}$ (d) $\frac{1}{t_1+\frac{|z_2-z_1|}{3\times10_8}}$

CHAPTER-23 : Ray Optics and Optical Instruments

TOPIC - 1: Plane Mirror, Spherical Mirror and Reflection of Light

93. A particle is oscillating on the X-axis with an amplitude 2 cm about the point x_0 = 10 cm with a frequency ω. A concave mirror of focal length 5 cm is placed at the origin (see figure)

Identify the correct statements: **[Online April 15, 2018]**

(A) The image executes periodic motion

(B) The image executes non-periodic motion

(C) The turning points of the image are asymmetric w.r.t the image of the point at x = 10 cm

(D) The distance between the turning points of the oscillation of the image is $\frac{100}{21}$

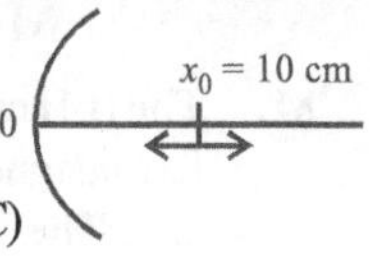

(a) (B), (D) (b) (B), (C)

(c) (A), (C), (D) (d) (A), (D)

TOPIC - 3: Refraction at Curved Surface Lenses and Power of Lens

94. A planoconvex lens becomes an optical system of 28 cm focal length when its plane surface is silvered and illuminated from left to right as shown in Fig-A. If the same lens is instead silvered on the curved surface and illuminated from other side as in Fig. B, it acts like an optical system of focal length 10 cm. The refractive index of the material of lens if: **[Online April 15, 2018]**

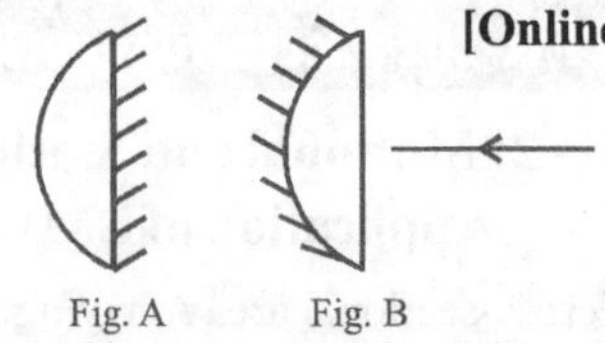

Fig. A Fig. B

(a) 1.50 (b) 1.55 (c) 1.75 (d) 1.51

95. A convergent doublet of separated lenses, corrected for spherical aberration, has resultant focal length of 10cm. The separation between the two lenses is 2cm. The focal lengths of the component lenses **[Online April 15, 2018]**

(a) 18cm, 20cm (b) 10cm, 12cm

(c) 12cm, 14cm (d) 16cm, 18cm

TOPIC - 4: Prism and Dispersion of Light

96. A ray of light is incident at an angle of 60° on one face of a prism of angle 30°. The emergent ray of light makes an angle of 30° with incident ray. The angle made by the emergent ray with second face of prism will be: **[Online April 16, 2018]**

(a) 30° (b) 90° (c) 0° (d) 45°

CHAPTER-24 : Wave Optics

TOPIC - 2: Young's Double Slit Experiment

97. The angular width of the central maximum in a single slit diffraction pattern is 60°. The width of the slit is 1 μm. The slit is illuminated by monochromatic plane waves. If another slit of same width is made near it, Young's fringes can be observed on a screen placed at a distance 50 cm from the slits. If the observed fringe width is 1 cm, what is slit separation distance?

(i.e. distance between the centres of each slit.) **[2018]**

(a) 25 μm (b) 50 μm (c) 75 μm (d) 100 μm

98. Light of wavelength 550 nm falls normally on a slit of width 22.0×10^{-5}cm. The angular position of the second minima from the central maximum will be (in radians) **[Online April 15, 2018]**

(a) $\frac{\pi}{8}$ (b) $\frac{\pi}{12}$ (c) $\frac{\pi}{4}$ (d) $\frac{\pi}{6}$

TOPIC - 3: Diffraction, Polarisation of Light and Resolving Power

99. Unpolarized light of intensity I passes through an ideal polarizer A. Another indentical polarizer B is placed behind A. The intensity of light beyond B is found to be $\frac{I}{2}$. Now another identical polarizer C is placed between A and B. The intensity beyond B is now found to be $\frac{I}{8}$. The angle between polarizer A and C is: **[2018]**

(a) 0° (b) 30° (c) 45° (d) 60°

100. Unpolarized light of intensity I is incident on a system of two polarizers, A followed by B. The intensity of emergent light is I/2. If a third polarizer C is placed between A and B, the intensity of emergent light is reduced to I/3 . The angle between the polarizers A and C is θ. Then **[Online April 16, 2018]**

(a) $\cos\theta = \left(\frac{2}{3}\right)^{1/4}$ (b) $\cos\theta = \left(\frac{1}{3}\right)^{1/4}$

(c) $\cos\theta = \left(\frac{1}{3}\right)^{1/2}$ (d) $\cos\theta = \left(\frac{2}{3}\right)^{1/2}$

101. A plane polarized light is incident on a polariser with its pass axis making angle θ with x-axis, as shown in the figure. At four different values of θ, $\theta = 8°, 38°, 188°$ and $218°$, the observed intensities are same. What is the angle between the direction of polarization and x-axis **[Online April 15, 2018]**

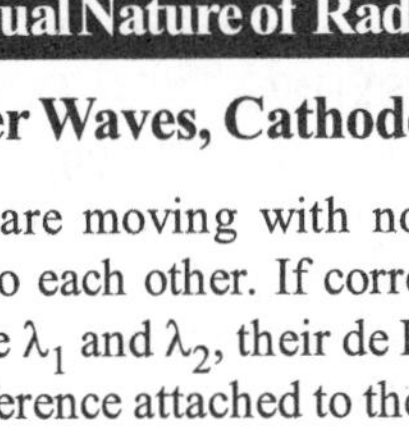

(a) 203° (b) 45° (c) 98° (d) 128°

CHAPTER-25 : Dual Nature of Radiation and Matter

TOPIC - 1: Matter Waves, Cathode and Positive Rays

102. Two electrons are moving with non-relativistic speeds perpendicular to each other. If corresponding de Broglie wavelengths are λ_1 and λ_2, their de Broglie wavelength in the frame of reference attached to their centre of mass is: **[Online April 15, 2018]**

(a) $\lambda_{CM} = \lambda_1 = \lambda_2$ (b) $\frac{1}{\lambda_1} = \frac{1}{\lambda_1} + \frac{1}{\lambda_2}$

(c) $\lambda_{CM} = \frac{2\lambda_1\lambda_2}{\sqrt{\lambda_1^2 + \lambda_2^2}}$ (d) $\lambda_{CM} = \left(\frac{\lambda_1 + \lambda_2}{2}\right)$

103. If the de Broglie wavelengths associated with a proton and an α-particle are equal, then the ratio of velocities of the proton and the α-particle will be: **[Online April 15, 2018]**

(a) 1 : 4 (b) 1 : 2 (c) 4 : 1 (d) 2 : 1

TOPIC - 2: Photon, Photoelectric Effect X-rays and Davisson-Germer Experiment

104. Both the nucleus and the atom of some element are in their respective first excited states. They get de-excited by emitting photons of wavelengths λ_N, λ_A respectively. The ratio $\frac{\lambda_N}{\lambda_A}$ is closest to **[Online April 16, 2018]**

(a) 10^{-6} (b) 10 (c) 10^{-1} (d) 10^{-10}

CHAPTER-26 : Atoms

TOPIC - 2 : Bohr's Model and the Spectra of the Hydrogen Atom

105. An electron from various excited states of hydrogen atom emit radiation to come to the ground state. Let λ_n, λ_g be the de Broglie wavelength of the electron in the nth state and the ground state respectively. Let Λ_n be the wavelength of the emitted photon in the transition from the nth state to the ground state. For large n, (A, B are constants) **[2018]**

(a) $\Lambda_n \approx A + \frac{B}{\lambda_n^2}$ (b) $\Lambda_n \approx A + B\lambda_n$

(c) $\Lambda_n^2 \approx A + B\lambda_n^2$ (d) $\Lambda_n^2 \approx \lambda$

106. If the series limit frequency of the Lyman series is v_l, then the series limit frequency of the P-fund series is : **[2018]**

(a) $25\,v_L$ (b) $16\,v_L$ (c) $v_L/16$ (d) $v_L/25$

107. The de-Broglie wavelength (λ_B) associated with the electron orbiting in the second excited state of hydrogen atom is related to that in the ground state (λ_G) by **[Online April 16, 2018]**

(a) $\lambda_B = \lambda_{G/3}$ (b) $\lambda_B = \lambda_{G/2}$

(c) $\lambda_B = 2\lambda_G$ (d) $\lambda_B = 3\lambda_G$

108. The energy required to remove the electron from a singly ionized Helium atom is 2.2 times the energy required to remove an electron from Helium atom. The total energy required to ionize the Helium atom completely is: **[Online April 15, 2018]**

(a) 20 eV (b) 79 eV (c) 109 eV (d) 34 eV

109. Muon (μ^{-1}) is negatively charged ($|q| = |e|$) with a mass $m_\mu = 200m_e$, where m_e is the mass of the electron and e is the electronic charge. If μ^{-1} is bound to a proton to form a hydrogen like atom, identify the correct statements **[Online April 15, 2018]**

(A) Radius of the muonic orbit is 200 times smaller than that of the electron

(B) the speed of the μ^{-1} in the nth orbit is $\frac{1}{200}$ times that of the election in the nth orbit

(C) The lonization energy of muonic atom is 200 times more than that of an hydrogen atom

(D) The momentum of the muon in the nth orbit is 200 times more than that of the electron

(a) (A), (B), (D) (b) (B), (D)

(c) (C), (D) (d) (A), (C), (D)

CHAPTER-27 : Nuclei

TOPIC - 1: Composition and Size of the Nuclei

110. An unstable heavy nucleus at rest breaks into two nuclei which move away with velocities in the ratio of 8:27. The ratio of the radii of the nuclei (assumed to be spherical) is: **[Online April 15, 2018]**

(a) 8:27 (b) 2:3 (c) 3:2 (d) 4:9

TOPIC - 3: Radioactivity

111. At some instant, a radioactive sample S_1 having an activity 5μCi has twice the number of nuclei as another sample S_2 which has an activity of 10μCi. The half lives of S_1 and S_2 are **[Online April 16, 2018]**

(a) 10 years and 20 years, respectively
(b) 5 years and 20 years, respectively
(c) 20 years and 10 years, respectively
(d) 20 years and 5 years, respectively

112. A solution containing active cobalt $^{60}_{27}Co$ having activity of 0.8 μCi and decay constant λ is injected in an animal's body. If 1cm^3 of blood is drawn from the animal's body after 10 hrs of injection, the activity found was 300 decays per minute. What is the volume of blood that is flowing in the body? (1Ci = 3.7 × 10^{10} decay per second and at t = 10 hrs $e^{-\lambda t}$ = 0.84) **[Online April 15, 2018]**

(a) 6 litres (b) 7 litres (c) 4 litres (d) 5 litres

CHAPTER-28 : Semiconductor Electronics : Materials, Devices and Simple Circuits

TOPIC - 1: Solids, Semiconductors and P-N Junction Diode

113. The reading of the ammeter for a silicon diode in the given circuit is : **[2018]**

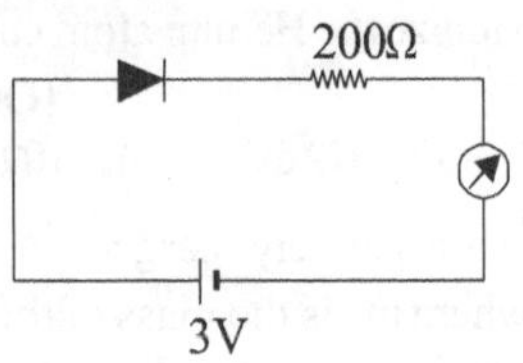

(a) 0 (b) 15 mA
(c) 11.5 mA (d) 13.5 mA

114. In the given circuit, the current through zener diode is: **[Online April 16, 2018]**

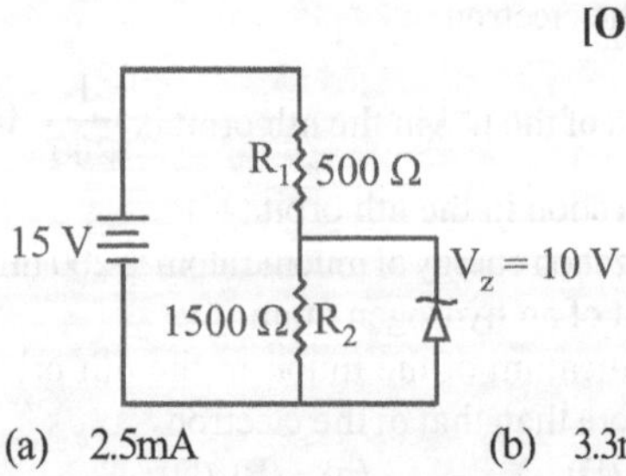

(a) 2.5mA (b) 3.3mA
(c) 5.5mA (d) 6.7mA

TOPIC - 2: Junction Transistor

115. In a common emitter configuration with suitable bias, it is given than R_L is the load resistance and R_{BE} is small signal dynamic resistance (input side). Then, voltage gain, current gain and power gain are given, respectively, by:
(β is current gain, I_B, I_C, I_E are respectively base, collector and emitter currents:) **[Online April 15, 2018]**

(a) $\beta\frac{R_L}{R_{BE}}, \frac{\Delta I_E}{\Delta I_B}, \beta^2\frac{R_L}{R_{BE}}$ (b) $\beta^2\frac{R_L}{R_{BE}}, \frac{\Delta I_C}{\Delta I_B}, \beta\frac{R_L}{R_{BE}}$

(c) $\beta^2\frac{R_L}{R_{BE}}, \frac{\Delta I_C}{\Delta I_E}, \beta^2\frac{R_L}{R_{BE}}$ (d) $\beta\frac{R_L}{R_{BE}}, \frac{\Delta I_C}{\Delta I_B}, \beta^2\frac{R_L}{R_{BE}}$

TOPIC - 3: Digital Electronics and Logic Gates

116. Truth table for the given circuit will be **[Online April 15, 2018]**

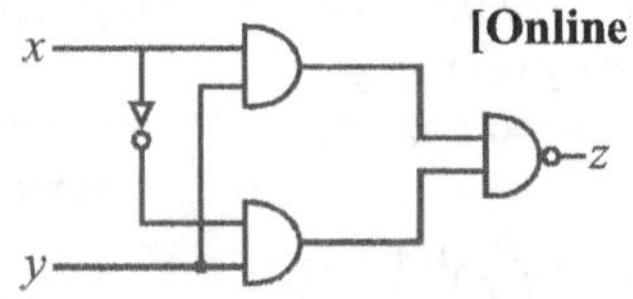

(a)

x	y	z
0	0	1
0	1	1
1	0	1
1	1	0

(b)

x	y	z
0	0	0
0	1	0
1	0	0
1	1	1

(c)

x	y	z
0	0	1
0	1	1
1	0	1
1	1	1

(d)

x	y	z
0	0	0
0	1	1
1	0	1
1	1	1

CHAPTER-29 : Communication Systems

TOPIC-1 : Communication Systems

117. A telephonic communication service is working at carrier frequency of 10 GHz. Only10% of it is utilized for transmission. How many telephonic channels can be transmitted simultaneously if each channel requires a bandwidth of 5 kHz? **[2018]**

(a) 2×10^3 (b) 2×10^4 (c) 2×10^5 (d) 2×10^6

118. A carrier wave of peak voltage 14 V is used for transmitting a message signal. The peak voltage of modulating signal given to achieve a modulation index of 80% will be: **[2018]**

(a) 11.2V (b) 7V (c) 22.4V (d) 28V

119. The number of amplitude modulated broadcast stations that can be accommodated in a 300 kHz band width for the highest modulating frequency 15 kHz will be: **[Online April 15, 2018]**

(a) 20 (b) 10 (c) 8 (d) 15

120. The carrier frequency of a transmitter is provided by a tank circuit of a coil of inductance 49μH and a capactiance of 2.5nF . It is modulated by an audio signal of 12kHz. The frequency range occupied by the side bands is: **[Online April 15, 2018]**

(a) 18kHz–30kHz (b) 63kHz–75kHz
(c) 442kHz–466kHz (d) 13482kHz–13494kHz

Hints and Solutions

CHAPTER-1 : Physical World, Units and Measurements

TOPIC-2 : Dimensions of Physical Quantities

1. **(b)** Plank length is a unit of length, $l_p = 1.616229 \times 10^{-35}$ m

$$l_p = \sqrt{\frac{hG}{c^3}}$$

TOPIC-3 : Errors in Measurements

2. **(c)** Density $(d) = \frac{\text{Mass (M)}}{\text{Volume (V)}} = \frac{M}{L^3}$

$\therefore$ Error in density, $\frac{\Delta d}{d} = \frac{\Delta M}{M} + \frac{3\Delta L}{L}$

$= 1.5\% + 3(1\%) = 4.5\%$

3. **(d)** Maximum percentage error in A

$= 3(\%\text{ error in P}) + 2(\%\text{ error in Q})$

$+ \frac{1}{2}(\%\text{ error in R}) + 1(\%\text{ error in S})$

$= 3 \times 0.5 + 2 \times 1 + \frac{1}{2} \times 3 + 1 \times 1.5$

$= 1.5 + 2 + 1.5 + 1.5 = 6.5\%$

4. **(c)** From Kepler's law, time period of a satellite,

$T = 2\pi\sqrt{\frac{r^3}{Gm}} \qquad T^2 = \frac{4\pi^2}{GM} r^3$

Relative uncertainty in the mass of the earth

$\left|\frac{\Delta M}{M}\right| = 2\frac{\Delta T}{T} = 2 \times 10^{-2}$ ($\because$ 4π & G constant and relative uncertainty in radius $\frac{\Delta r}{r}$ negligible)

5. **(c)** Relative error in Surface area, $\frac{\Delta s}{s} = 2 \times \frac{\Delta r}{r} = \alpha$ and relative error in volume, $\frac{\Delta v}{v} = 3 \times \frac{\Delta r}{r}$

$\therefore$ Relative error in volume w.r.t. relative error in area,

$\frac{\Delta v}{v} = \frac{3}{2}\alpha$

6. **(d)** Least count $= \frac{\text{Value of 1 part on main scale}}{\text{Number of parts on vernier scale}}$

$= \frac{0.25}{5 \times 100}$ cm $= 5 \times 10^{-4}$ cm

Reading $= 4 \times 0.05$ cm $+ 30 \times 5 \times 10^{-4}$ cm

$= (0.2 + 0.0150)$ cm $= 0.2150$ cm (Thickness of wire)

CHAPTER-2 : Motion in a Straight Line

TOPIC-1 : Distance, Displacement & Uniform Motion

7. **(b)** Graphs in option (c) position-time and option (a) velocity-position are corresponding to velocity-time graph option (d) and its distance-time graph is as given below. Hence distance-time graph option (b) is incorrect.

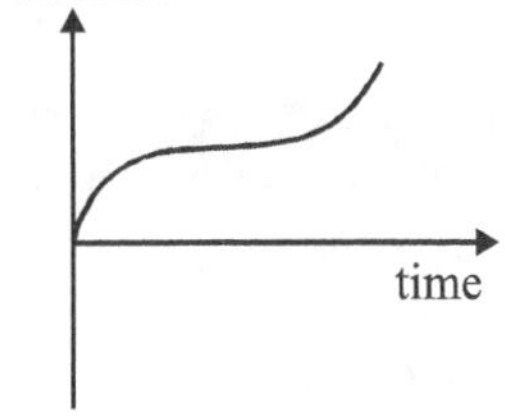

TOPIC-2 : Non-uniform Motion

8. **(b)** According to question, $u_1 = 40$ km/h, $v_1 = 0$ and $s_1 = 40$ m

using $v^2 - u^2 = 2as$; $0^2 - 40^2 = 2a \times 40$ ...(i)

Again, $0^2 - 80^2 = 2as$ ...(ii)

From eqn. (i) and (ii)

Stopping distance, $s = 160$ m

9. **(c)** Using equation, $a = \frac{v-u}{t}$ and $S = ut + \frac{1}{2}at^2$

Distance travelled by car in 15 sec $= \frac{1}{2}\frac{(45)}{15}(15)^2$

$= \frac{675}{2}$ m

Distance traveled by scooter in 15 seconds $= 30 \times 15 = 450$ ($\because$ distance = speed × time)

Difference between distance travelled by car and scooter in 15 sec, $450 - 337.5 = 112.5$ m

Let car catches scooter in time t;

$\frac{675}{2} + 45(t - 15) = 30t$

$337.5 + 45t - 675 = 30t \Rightarrow 15t = 337.5$

$\Rightarrow t = 22.5$ sec

10. **(a)** Let the car turn of the highway at a distance 'x' from the point M. So, RM = x

And if speed of car in field is v, then time taken by the car to cover the distance $QR = QM - x$ on the highway,

$t_1 = \frac{QM - x}{2v}$ .....(i)

Time taken to travel the distance 'RP' in the field

$$t_2 = \frac{\sqrt{d^2+x^2}}{v} \quad ..... (ii)$$

Total time elapsed to move the car from Q to P

$$t = t_1 + t_2 = \frac{QM - x}{2v} + \frac{\sqrt{d^2+x^2}}{v}$$

For 't' to be minimum $\frac{dt}{dx} = 0$

$$\frac{1}{v}\left[-\frac{1}{2} + \frac{x}{\sqrt{d^2+x^2}}\right] = 0$$

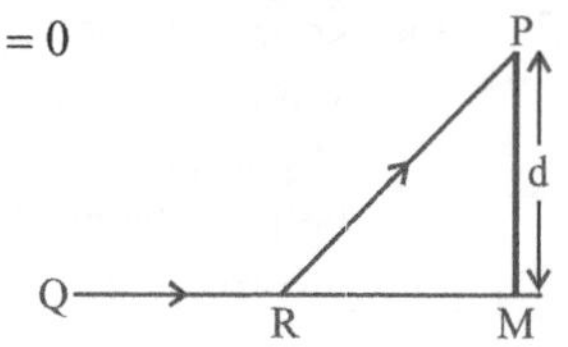

or $x = \frac{d}{\sqrt{2^2-1}} = \frac{d}{\sqrt{3}}$

CHAPTER-3 : Motion in a Plane

TOPIC-1 : Vectors

11. **(a)** If $\vec{C} = a\hat{i} + b\hat{j}$ then $\vec{A}.\vec{C} = \vec{A}.\vec{B}$

$a + b = 1 \quad ..... (i)$

$\vec{B}.\vec{C} = \vec{A}.\vec{B}$

$2a - b = 1 \quad ..... (ii)$

Solving equation (i) and (ii) we get

$a = \frac{1}{3}, b = \frac{2}{3}$

$\therefore$ Magnitude of coplanar vector, $|\vec{C}| = \sqrt{\frac{1}{9} + \frac{4}{9}} = \sqrt{\frac{5}{9}}$

CHAPTER-4 : Laws of Motion

TOPIC-3 : Friction

12 **(b)** Given : $m_1 = 5$kg; $m_2 = 10$kg; $\mu = 0.15$

FBD for m_1, $m_1 g - T = m_1 a$

$\Rightarrow 50 - T = 5 \times a$

and, $T - 0.15\,(m + 10)\,g = (10 + m)a$

For rest $a = 0$

or, $50 = 0.15\,(m + 10)\,10$

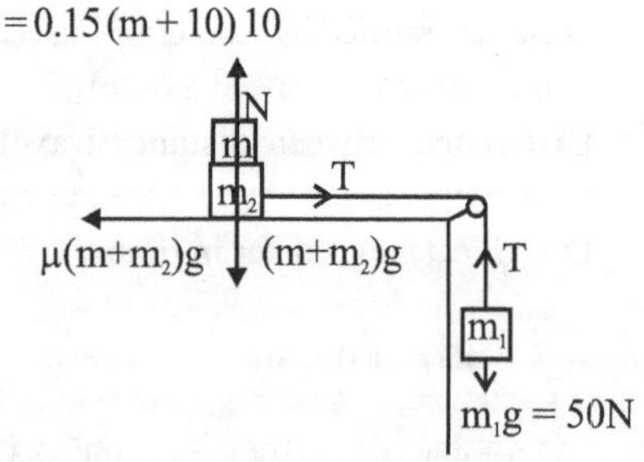

$\Rightarrow \quad 5 = \frac{3}{20}(m + 10)$

$\frac{100}{3} = m + 10 \quad \therefore \; m = 23.3$kg ; close to option (b)

13. **(b)** The coefficients of kinetic friction between the object and the incline

$\mu = \tan\theta\left(1 - \frac{1}{n^2}\right) \Rightarrow \mu = 1 - \frac{1}{n^2} \quad (\because \; \theta = 45°)$

14. **(d)** Equation of motion when the mass slides down

$Mg \sin\theta - f = Ma$

$\Rightarrow \; 10 - f = 6 \; (M = 2$ kg, $a = 3$ m/s^2, $\theta = 30°$ given)

$\therefore \; f = 4$N

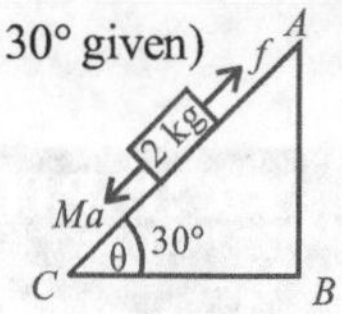

Equation of motion when the block is pushed up

Let the external force required to take the block up the plane with same acceleration be F

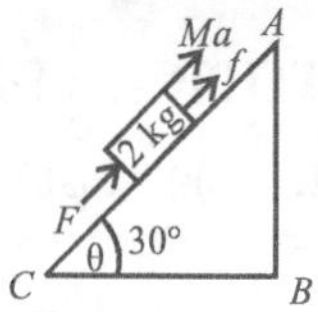

$F - Mg \sin\theta - f = Ma$

$\Rightarrow \; F - 10 - 4 = 6$

$F = 20$ N

TOPIC-4 : Circular Motion, Banking of Road

15. **(d)** Using, $\mu mg = \frac{mv^2}{r} = mr\omega^2$

$\omega = 2\pi n = 2\pi \times 3.5 = 7\pi$ rad/sec

Radius, $r = 1.25$ cm $= 1.25 \times 10^{-2}$ m

Coefficient of friction, $\mu = ?$

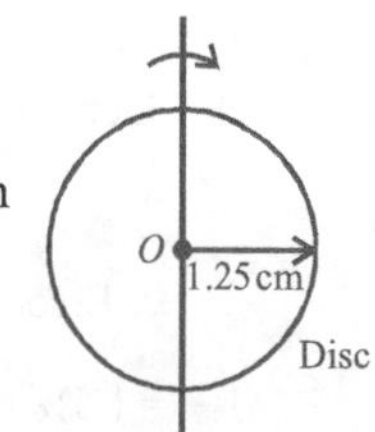

$\mu mg = \frac{m(r\omega)^2}{r} \quad (\because \; v = r\omega)$

$\mu mg = mr\omega^2$

$$\Rightarrow \quad \mu = \frac{r\omega^2}{g} = \frac{1.25 \times 10^{-2} \times \left(7 \times \frac{22}{7}\right)^2}{10}$$

$$= \frac{1.25 \times 10^{-2} \times 22^2}{10} = 0.6$$

CHAPTER-5 : Work, Energy and Power

TOPIC-1 : Work

16. **(a)** From question, $v = a\sqrt{s} = \frac{ds}{dt}$

or, $\quad 2\sqrt{s} = at \Rightarrow S = \frac{a^2t^2}{4}$

$F = m \times \frac{a^2}{2}$

Work done $= \frac{ma^2}{2} \times \frac{a^2t^2}{4} = \frac{1}{8}ma^4t^2$

TOPIC-2 : Energy

17. **(c)** $F = -\frac{\partial u}{\partial r}\hat{r} = \frac{K}{r^3}\hat{r}$

Since particle is moving in circular path

$F = \frac{mv^2}{r} = \frac{K}{r^3} \Rightarrow mv^2 = \frac{K}{r^2}$

$\therefore$ K.E. $= \frac{1}{2}mv^2 = \frac{K}{2r^2}$

Total energy = P.E. + K.E.

$= -\frac{K}{2r^2} + \frac{K}{2r^2} =$ Zero $\quad (\because$ P.E. $= -\frac{K}{2r^2}$ given)

18. **(b)** As the particles moving in circular orbits, So

$$\frac{mv^2}{r}=\frac{16}{r}+r^2$$

Kinetic energy, $KE_0=\frac{1}{2}mv^2=\frac{1}{2}[16+r^4]$

For first particle, $r=1,\ K_1=\frac{1}{2}m(16+1)$

Similarly, for second particle, $r=4,\ K_2=\frac{1}{2}m(16+256)$

$$\therefore\ \frac{K_1}{K_2}=\frac{\frac{16+1}{2}}{\frac{16+256}{2}}=\frac{17}{272}\simeq 6\times10^{-2}$$

TOPIC-4 : Collisions

19. **(b)**

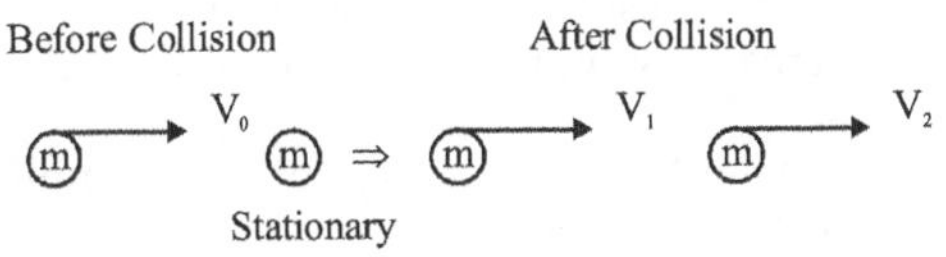

$$\frac{1}{2}mv_1^2+\frac{1}{2}mv_2^2=\frac{3}{2}\left(\frac{1}{2}mv_0^2\right)$$

$$\Rightarrow\ v_1^2+v_2^2=\frac{3}{2}v_0^2 \quad ....(i)$$

From momentum conservation

$mv_0=m(v_1+v_2)$ ....(ii)

Squarring both sides,

$(v_1+v_2)^2=v_0{}^2$

$\Rightarrow\ v_1{}^2+v_2{}^2+2v_1v_2=v_0{}^2$

$$2v_1v_2=-\frac{v_0^2}{2}$$

$$(v_1-v_2)^2=v_1^2+v_2^2-2v_1v_2=\frac{3}{2}v_0^2+\frac{v_0^2}{2}$$

Solving we get relative velocity between the two particles

$v_1-v_2=\sqrt{2}v_0$

20. **(a)** Change in momentum

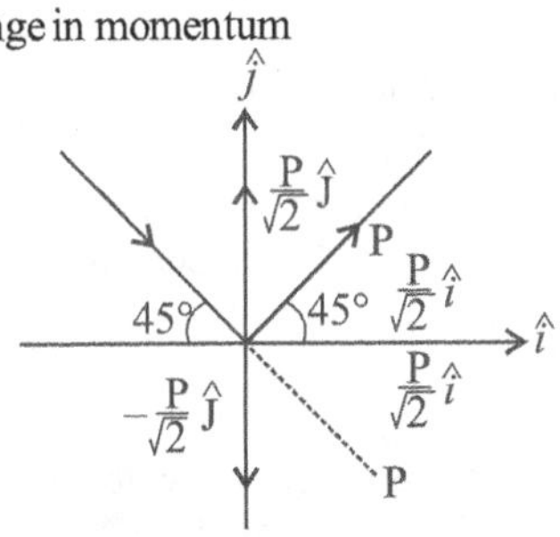

$$\Delta P=\frac{P}{\sqrt{2}}\hat{j}+\frac{P}{\sqrt{2}}\hat{j}+\frac{P}{\sqrt{2}}\hat{i}-\frac{P}{\sqrt{2}}\hat{i}$$

$$\Delta P=\frac{2P}{\sqrt{2}}\hat{j}=I_H\ \text{molecule}$$

$$\Rightarrow\ I_{wall}=-\frac{2P}{\sqrt{2}}\hat{j}$$

Pressure, P

$$=\frac{F}{A}=\frac{\sqrt{2}P}{A}n \quad (\because n=\text{no. of particles})$$

$$=\frac{\sqrt{2}\times3.32\times10^{-27}\times10^3\times10^{23}}{2\times10^{-4}}=2.35\times10^3 N/m^2$$

21. **(a)** For collision of neutron with deuterium:

Applying conservation of momentum :

$mv+0=mv_1+2mv_2$ .....(i)

$v_2-v_1=v$ .....(ii)

$\because$ Collision is elastic, e = 1

From eqn (i) and eqn (ii) $v_1=-\frac{v}{3}$

$$P_d=\frac{\frac{1}{2}mv^2-\frac{1}{2}mv_1^2}{\frac{1}{2}mv^2}=\frac{8}{9}=0.89$$

Now, For collision of neutron with carbon nucleus

Applying Conservation of momentum

$mv+0=mv_1+12mv_2$ ....(iii)

$v=v_2-v_1$ ....(iv)

From eqn (iii) and eqn (iv)

$$v_1=-\frac{11}{13}v$$

$$P_c=\frac{\frac{1}{2}mv^2-\frac{1}{2}m\left(\frac{11}{13}v\right)^2}{\frac{1}{2}mv^2}=\frac{48}{169}\approx0.28$$

22. **(d)** Apply principle of conservation of momentum along *x*-direction,

$mu=mv_1\cos45°+Mv_2\cos45°$

$$mu=\frac{1}{\sqrt{2}}(mv_1+Mv_2) \quad ..... (i)$$

Along *y*-direction,

$o=mv_1\sin45°-Mv_2\sin45°$

$$o=(mv_1-Mv_2)\frac{1}{\sqrt{2}} \quad ..... (ii)$$

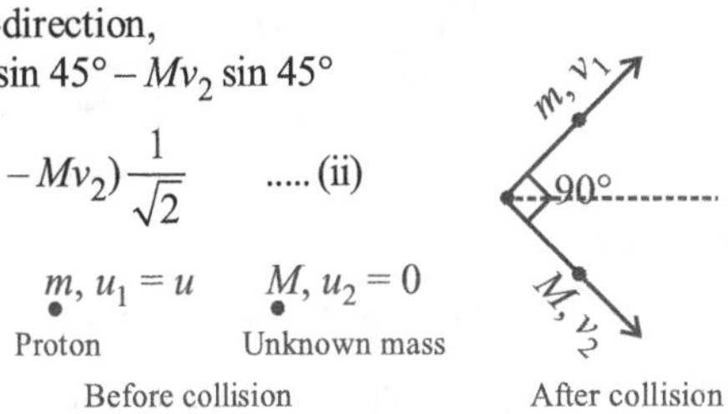

$$\text{Coefficient of restution } e=1=\frac{v_2-v_1\cos90}{u\cos45}$$

($\because$ Collision is elastic)

$$\Rightarrow\ \frac{v_2}{\frac{u}{\sqrt{2}}}=1$$

$\Rightarrow u=\sqrt{2}v_2$ ..... (iii)

Solving eqs (i), (ii), & (iii), we get mass of unknown particle, $M=m$

CHAPTER-6 : System of Particles and Rotational Motion

TOPIC-1 : Centre of Mass, Centre of Gravity & Principle of Moments

23. (c) To produce maximum moment of force line of action of force must be perpendicular to line AB.

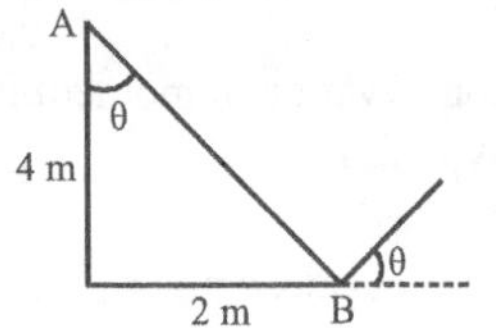

$\therefore \tan\theta = \frac{2}{4} = \frac{1}{2}$

TOPIC-2 : Angular Displacement, Velocity and Acceleration

24. (c) $m\omega^2 R = \text{Force} \propto \frac{1}{R^n}$ $\left(\text{Force} = \frac{mv^2}{R}\right)$

$\Rightarrow \omega^2 \propto \frac{1}{R^{n+1}} \Rightarrow \omega \propto \frac{1}{R^{\frac{n+1}{2}}}$

Time period $T = \frac{2\pi}{\omega}$

Time period, $T \propto R^{\frac{n+1}{2}}$

TOPIC-3 : Torque, Couple and Angular Momentum

25. (a) Balancing torque w.r.t. point of suspension

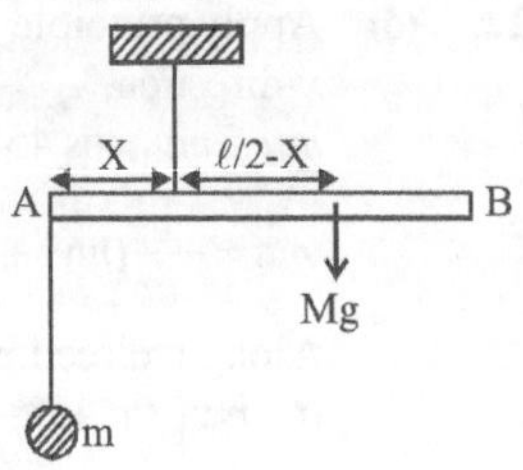

$mg\,x = Mg\left(\frac{\ell}{2} - x\right)$

$\Rightarrow mx = M\frac{\ell}{2} - Mx$

$m = \left(M\frac{\ell}{2}\right)\frac{1}{x} - M$

$y = \alpha\frac{1}{x} - C$ Straight line equation.

26. (a)

TOPIC-4 : Moment of Inertia and Rotational K.E.

27. (d) Using parallel axes theorem, moment of inertia about 'O'

$I_o = I_{cm} + md^2$

$= \frac{7MR^2}{2} + 6(M \times (2R)^2) = \frac{55MR^2}{2}$

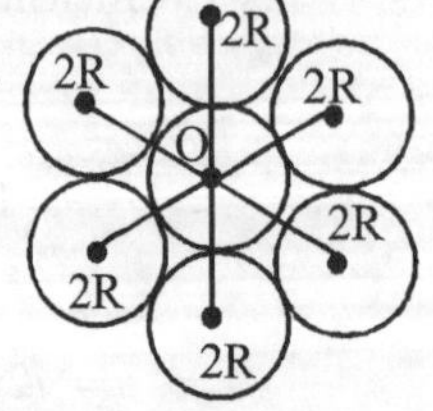

Again, moment of inertia about point P, $I_p = I_o + md^2$

$= \frac{55MR^2}{2} + 7M(3R)^2 = \frac{181}{2}MR^2$

28. (a) Let σ be the mass per unit area.

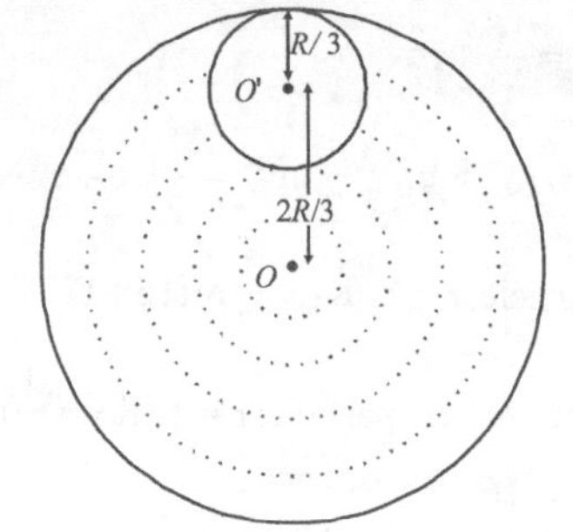

The total mass of the disc $= \sigma \times \pi R^2 = 9M$

The mass of the circular disc cut

$= \sigma \times \pi\left(\frac{R}{3}\right)^2 = \sigma \times \frac{\pi R^2}{9} = M$

Let us consider the above system as a complete disc of mass $9M$ and a negative mass M super imposed on it.

Moment of inertia (I_1) of the complete disc $= \frac{1}{2}9MR^2$ about an axis passing through O and perpendicular to the plane of the disc.

M.I. of the cut out portion about an axis passing through O' and perpendicular to the plane of disc

$= \frac{1}{2} \times M \times \left(\frac{R}{3}\right)^2$

$\therefore$ *M.I.* (I_2) of the cut out portion about an axis passing through O and perpendicular to the plane of disc

$= \left[\frac{1}{2} \times M \times \left(\frac{R}{3}\right)^2 + M \times \left(\frac{2R}{3}\right)^2\right]$

[Using perpendicular axis theorem]

$\therefore$ The total *M.I.* of the system about an axis passing through O and perpendicular to the plane of the disc is

$I = I_1 + I_2$

$= \frac{1}{2}9MR^2 - \left[\frac{1}{2} \times M \times \left(\frac{R}{3}\right)^2 + M \times \left(\frac{2R}{3}\right)^2\right]$

$= \frac{9MR^2}{2} - \frac{9MR^2}{18} = \frac{(9-1)MR^2}{2} = 4MR^2$

29. (c) As we know, moment of inertia of a disc about an axis passing through C.G. and perpendicular to its plane,

$I_z = \frac{mR^2}{2}$

Moment of inertia of a disc about a tangential axis perpendicular to its own plane,

$I_z' = \frac{3}{2}mR^2$

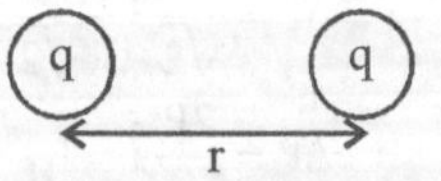

$\therefore \quad I_z / I_z' = \frac{mR^2}{2} \Big/ \frac{3mR^2}{2} = 1/3$

30. (a) When the rod makes an angle α

Displacement of centre of mass $= \frac{l}{2}\cos\alpha$

$$mg\frac{l}{2}\cos\alpha = \frac{l}{2}I\omega^2$$

$$mg\frac{l}{2}\cos\alpha = \frac{ml^2}{6}\omega^2$$ ($\because$ M.I. of thin uniform rod about an axis passing through its centre of mass and perpendicular to the rod $I = \frac{ml^2}{12}$)

$$\Rightarrow \quad \omega = \sqrt{\frac{3g\cos\alpha}{l}}$$

Speed of end $= \omega \times l = \sqrt{3g\cos\alpha l}$

i.e., Speed of end, $\omega \propto \sqrt{\cos\alpha}$

CHAPTER-7 : Gravitation

TOPIC-2 : Newton's Universal Law of Gravitation

31. (a) As we know, Gravitational force of attraction,

$$F = \frac{GMm}{R^2}$$

$$F_1 = \frac{GM_e m}{r_1^2} \text{ and } F_2 = \frac{GM_e M_s}{r_2^2}$$

$$\Delta F_1 = \frac{2GM_e m}{r_1^3}\Delta r_1 \text{ and } \Delta F_2 = \frac{GM_e M_s}{r_2^3}\Delta r_2$$

$$\frac{\Delta F_1}{\Delta F_2} = \frac{m\Delta r_1}{r_1^3}\frac{r_2^3}{M_s \Delta r_2} = \left(\frac{m}{M_s}\right)\left(\frac{r_2^3}{r_1^3}\right)\left(\frac{\Delta r_1}{\Delta r_2}\right)$$

Using $\Delta r_1 = \Delta r_2 = 2R_{earth}$; $m = 8\times10^{22}$ kg;
$M_s = 2\times10^{30}$ kg
$r_1 = 0.4\times10^6$ km and $r_2 = 150\times10^6$ km

$$\frac{\Delta F_1}{\Delta F_2} = \left(\frac{8\times10^{22}}{2\times10^{30}}\right)\left(\frac{150\times10^6}{0.4\times10^6}\right)^3 \times 1 \cong 2$$

TOPIC-3 : Acceleration due to Gravity

32. (d) With rotation of earth or latitude, acceleration due to gravity vary as $g' = g - \omega^2 R\cos^2\phi$
Where ϕ is latitude, there will be no change in gravity at poles as $\phi = 90°$
At all other points as ω increases g' will decreases hence, weight, W = mg decreases.

TOPIC-4 : Gravitational Field and Potential nergy

33. (c) Initial gravitational potential energy, $E_i = -\frac{GMm}{2R}$
Final gravitational potential energy,

$$E_f = -\frac{GMm/2}{2\left(\frac{R}{2}\right)} - \frac{GMm/2}{2\left(\frac{3R}{2}\right)} = -\frac{GMm}{2R} - \frac{GMm}{6R}$$

$$= -\frac{4GMm}{6R} = -\frac{2GMm}{3R}$$

$\therefore$ Difference between initial and final energy,

$$E_f - E_i = \frac{GMm}{R}\left(-\frac{2}{3}+\frac{1}{2}\right) = -\frac{GMm}{6R}$$

CHAPTER-8 : Mechanical Properties of Solids

TOPIC-1 : Hooke's Law & Young's Modulus

34. (b) For same material the ratio of stress to strain is same
For first cube

$$\text{Stress}_1 = \frac{\text{force}_1}{\text{area}_1} = \frac{10^5}{(0.1^2)}$$

$$\text{Strain}_1 = \frac{\text{change in length}_1}{\text{original length}_1} = \frac{0.5\times10^{-2}}{0.1}$$

For second block,

$$\text{stress}_2 = \frac{\text{force}_2}{\text{area}_2} = \frac{10^5}{(0.2^2)}$$

$$\text{strain}_2 = \frac{\text{change in length}_2}{\text{original length}_2} = \frac{x}{0.2}$$

x is the displacement for second block.

For same material, $\frac{\text{stress}_1}{\text{strain}_1} = \frac{\text{stress}_2}{\text{strain}_2}$

or, $$\frac{\frac{10.5}{(0.1)^2}}{\frac{0.5\times10^{-2}}{0.1}} = \frac{\frac{10^5}{(0.2)^2}}{\frac{x}{0.2}}$$

Solving we get, $x = 0.25$ cm

TOPIC-2 : Bulk and Rigidity Modulus and Work Done in Stretching a Wire

35. (c) Bulk modulus, $K = \frac{\text{volumetric stress}}{\text{volumetric strain}}$

$$K = \frac{mg}{a\left(\frac{dV}{V}\right)} \Rightarrow \frac{dV}{V} = \frac{mg}{Ka} \quad ....(i)$$

volume of sphere, $V = \frac{4}{3}\pi R^3$

Fractional change in volume $\frac{dV}{V} = \frac{3dr}{r}$ ...(ii)

Using eq. (i) & (ii) $\frac{3dr}{r} = \frac{mg}{Ka}$

$\therefore \quad \frac{dr}{r} = \frac{mg}{3Ka}$ (fractional decrement in radius)

CHAPTER-9 : Mechanical Properties of Fluids

TOPIC-1 : Pressure, Density, Pascal's Law and Archimedes' Principle

36. (d) Clearly from figure,

$$P_2 = P_0 + \frac{4T}{6} + \frac{4t}{4} \text{ or, } P_2 - P_0 = \frac{4T}{6} + \frac{4T}{4} \quad .....(i)$$

Let r be the radius of bubble with pressure difference $P_2 - P_0$ so,

$$P_2 - P_0 = \frac{4T}{r} \quad .....(ii)$$

From eq^n (i) and (ii),

$$\frac{4T}{r} = \frac{4T}{6} + \frac{4T}{4}$$

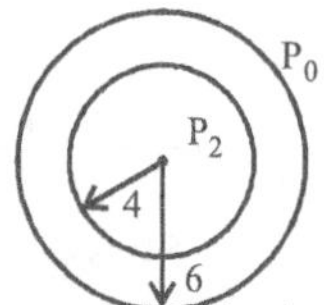

$$\Rightarrow \frac{1}{r} = \frac{1}{6} + \frac{1}{4} \Rightarrow r = 2.4 \text{ cm}$$

37. (d) Pressure at interface A must be same from both the sides to be in equilibrium.

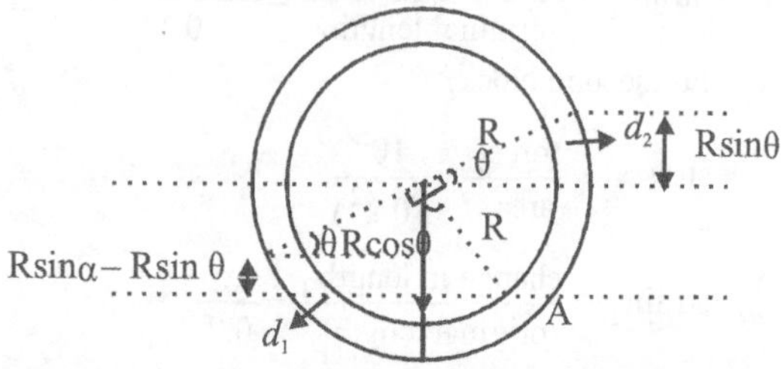

$$\therefore \quad (R\cos\theta + R\sin\theta)\rho_2 g = (R\cos\theta - R\sin\theta)\rho_1 g$$

$$\Rightarrow \frac{d_1}{d_2} = \frac{\cos\theta + \sin\theta}{\cos\theta - \sin\theta} = \frac{1+\tan\theta}{1-\tan\theta}$$

$$\Rightarrow \rho_1 - \rho_1 \tan\theta = \rho_2 + \rho_2 \tan\theta$$

$$\Rightarrow (\rho_1 + \rho_2)\tan\theta = \rho_1 - \rho_2$$

$$\therefore \quad \theta = \tan^{-1}\left(\frac{\rho_1 - \rho_2}{\rho_1 + \rho_2}\right)$$

TOPIC-2 : Fluid Flow, Reynold's Number and Bernoulli's Principle

38. (d) Using $P_1V_1 = P_2V_2$

$$(P_1)\frac{4}{3}\pi r^3 = (P_2)\frac{4}{3}\pi\frac{125r^3}{64}$$

$$\frac{\rho g(10) + \rho g h}{\rho g(10)} = \frac{125}{64}$$

$640 + 64h = 1250$

On solving we get $h = 9.5$ m

CHAPTER-10 : Thermal Properties of Matter

TOPIC-2 : Calorimetry and Heat Transfer

39. (d) $v = \sqrt{3k_BT/m_{He}} = \sqrt{\dfrac{3\times1.4\times10^{-23}\times300}{7\times10^{-27}}}$

$= 1.34 \times 10^3$ m/s

TOPIC-3 : Newton's Law of Cooling

40. (a) According to Newton's law of cooling,

$$\left(\frac{\theta_1 - \theta_2}{t}\right) = K\left(\frac{\theta_1 + \theta_2}{2} - \theta_0\right)$$

$$\left(\frac{60-50}{10}\right) = K\left(\frac{60+50}{2} - 25\right) \quad .....(i)$$

$$\text{and, } \left(\frac{50-\theta}{10}\right) = K\left(\frac{50+\theta}{2} - 25\right) \quad .....(ii)$$

Dividing eq. (i) by (ii),

$$\frac{10}{(50-\theta)} = \frac{60}{\theta} \Rightarrow \theta = 42.85°C \cong 43°C$$

CHAPTER-11 : Thermodynamics

TOPIC-2 : Specific Heat Capacity and Thermodynamical Processes

41. (a) Equation of the BC

$$P = P_0 - \frac{2P_0}{V_0}(V - 2V_0)$$

using $PV = nRT$

$$\text{Temperature, } T = \frac{P_0V - \dfrac{2P_0V^2}{V_0} + 4P_0V}{1\times R}$$

($\because$ n = 1 mole given)

$$T = \frac{P_0}{F}\left[5V - \frac{2V^2}{V_0}\right]$$

$$\frac{dT}{dV} = 0 \Rightarrow 5 - \frac{4V}{V_0} = 0 \Rightarrow V = \frac{5}{4}V_0$$

$$T = \frac{P_0}{R}\left[5\times\frac{5V_0}{4} - \frac{2}{V_0}\times\frac{25}{16}V_0^2\right] = \frac{25}{8}\frac{P_0V_0}{R}$$

42. (d) Work done on gas $= nRT\ \ell n\left(\frac{p_f}{p_i}\right) = R(300)\ \ell n(2) =$

$300\ R\ln 2 \quad \left(\because \frac{P_f}{P_i} = 2 \text{ given}\right)$

TOPIC-3 : Carnot Engine, Refrigerators and Second Law of Thermodynamics

43. (a) Given: Temperature of cold body, T_2 = 250 K temperature of hot body; T_1 = 300 K

Heat received, Q_2 = 500 cal work done, W = ?

$$\text{Efficiency} = 1 - \frac{T_2}{T_1} = \frac{W}{Q_2 + W} \Rightarrow 1 - \frac{250}{300} = \frac{W}{Q_2 + W}$$

$$W = \frac{Q_2}{5} = \frac{500\times4.2}{5}J = 420\text{ J}$$

44. (d) Efficiency of engine A, $n_A = \frac{T_1 - T_2}{T_1}$

and $n_B = \frac{T_2 - T_3}{T_2}$; $T_2 = \frac{T_1 + T_3}{2} = 350\ K$

or $\frac{n_A}{n_B} = \frac{\frac{600-350}{600}}{\frac{350-100}{350}} = \frac{7}{12}$

CHAPTER-12 : Kinetic Theory

TOPIC-3 : Degree of Freedom, Specific Heat Capacity, and Mean Free Path

45. (c) In an adiabatic process

$TV^{\gamma-1} = \text{Constant}$ or, $T_1V_1^{\gamma-1} = T_2V_2^{\gamma-1}$

For monoatomic gas $\gamma = \frac{5}{3}$

$(300)V^{2/3} = T_2(2V)^{2/3} \Rightarrow T_2 = \frac{300}{(2)^{2/3}}$

$T_2 = 189$ K (final temperature)

Change in internal energy $\Delta U = n\frac{f}{2}R\ \Delta T$

$= 2\left(\frac{3}{2}\right)\left(\frac{25}{3}\right)(-111) = -2.7\text{kJ}$

46. (b) Using formula,

$$\gamma_{mixture} = \left(\frac{C_p}{C_v}\right)_{mix} = \frac{\frac{n_1\gamma_1}{\gamma_1 - 1} + \frac{n_2\gamma_2}{\gamma_2 - 1}}{\frac{n_1}{\gamma_1 - 1} + \frac{n_2}{\gamma_2 - 1}}$$

Putting the value of $n_1 = 2$, $n_2 = n$, $\left(\frac{C_p}{C_v}\right)_{mix} = \frac{3}{2}$

$\gamma_1 = \frac{5}{3}, \gamma_2 = \frac{7}{5}$ and solving we get, $n = 2$

CHAPTER-13 : Oscillations

TOPIC-1 : Displacement, Phase, Velocity and Acceleration in S.H.M.

47. (c) From the two mutually perpendicular S.H.M.'s, the general equation of Lissajous figure,

$$\frac{x^2}{A^2} + \frac{y^2}{B^2} - \frac{2xy}{AB}\cos\delta = \sin^2\delta$$

$x = A\sin(at + \delta)$

$y = B\sin(bt + r)$

Clearly $A \neq B$ hence ellipse.

TOPIC-3 : Time Period, Frequency, Simple Pendulum and Spring Pendulum

48. (b) As we know, frequency in SHM

$f = \frac{1}{2\pi}\sqrt{\frac{k}{m}} = 10^{12}$ where m = mass of one atom

Mass of one atom of silver, $= \frac{108}{(6.02\times10^{23})} \times 10^{-3}$ kg

$\frac{1}{2\pi}\sqrt{\frac{k}{108\times10^{-3}} \times 6.02\times10^{23}} = 10^{12}$

Solving we get, spring constant, K = 7.1N/m

49. (d) Using $y = A\sin\omega t$

$a = A\sin\omega t_0$

$b = A\sin 2\omega t_0$

$c = A\sin 3\omega t_0$

$a + c = A[\sin\omega t_0 + A\sin 3\omega t_0] = 2A\sin 2\omega t_0\cos\omega t_0$

$\frac{a+c}{b} = 2\cos\omega t_0$

$\Rightarrow \omega = \frac{1}{t_0}\cos^{-1}\left(\frac{a+c}{2b}\right) \Rightarrow f = \frac{1}{2\pi t_0}\cos^{-1}\left(\frac{a+c}{2b}\right)$

TOPIC-4 : Damped, Forced Oscillations and Resonance

50. (b) In first collision mu momentum will be imparted to system, in second collision when momentum of (M + m) is in opposite direction mu momentum of particle will make its momentum zero.

On 13th collision, $\boxed{m} \rightarrow \boxed{M+12}$; $\boxed{M+13m} \rightarrow V$

$mu = (M + 13m)v \Rightarrow v = \frac{mu}{M+13m} = \frac{u}{15}$

$v = \omega A \Rightarrow \frac{u}{15} = \sqrt{\frac{K}{M-13m}} \times A$

Putting value of M, m, u and K we get amplitude

$A = \frac{1}{15}\sqrt{\frac{75}{1}} = \frac{1}{\sqrt{3}}$

CHAPTER-14 : Waves

TOPIC-2 : Vibration of String and Organ

51. (a) In solids, Velocity of wave $V = \sqrt{\frac{Y}{\rho}} = \sqrt{\frac{9.27\times10^{10}}{2.7\times10^3}}$

$v = 5.85 \times 10^3$ m/sec

Since rod is clamped at middle fundamental wave shape is as follow

$\frac{\lambda}{2} = L \Rightarrow \lambda = 2L$

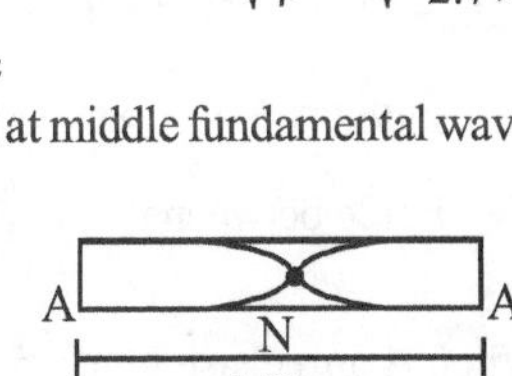

$\lambda = 1.2\text{m}$ ($\because$ L = 60 cm = 0.6m (given))

Using $v = f\lambda$

$$\Rightarrow f = \frac{v}{\lambda} = \frac{5.85\times10^3}{1.2}$$

$= 4.88 \times 10^3$ Hz $\simeq 5$ KHz

52. (a) For first resonance, $\frac{\lambda}{4} = \ell_1 + e = 11$ cm

($\because$ end correction e = 1 cm given)

For second resonance, $\frac{3\lambda}{4} = \ell_2 + e$

$\Rightarrow \ell_2 = 3\times11-1 = 32$ cm

TOPIC-3 : Beats, Interference and Superposition of Waves

53. (d) According to question, tuning fork gives 1 beat/second with (N) 3rd normal mode. Therefore, organ pipe will have frequency (256 ± 1) Hz. In open organ pipe,

frequency $n = \frac{NV}{2\ell}$

or, $255 = \frac{3\times340}{2\times\ell} \Rightarrow \ell = 2\text{m} = 200$ cm

54. (a) Probable frequencies of tuning fork be $n \pm 5$

Frequency of sonometer wire, $n \propto \frac{1}{l}$

$\therefore \frac{n+5}{n-5} = \frac{100}{95} \Rightarrow 95(n+5) = 100(n-5)$

or, $95n + 475 = 100n - 500$

or, $5n = 975$

or, $n = \frac{975}{5} = 195$ Hz

TOPIC-4 : Musical Sound and Doppler's Effect

55. (d) $n_A = 425$ Hz, $n_B = ?$

Beat frequency x = 5 Hz which is decreasing ($5 \to 3$) after increasing the tension of the string B.

Also tension of string B increasing so

$n_B\uparrow$ ($\because n \propto \sqrt{T}$)

Hence $n_A - n_B\uparrow = x\downarrow \longrightarrow$ correct

$n_B\uparrow - n_A = x\downarrow \longrightarrow$ incorrect

$\therefore n_B = n_A - x = 425 - 5 = 420$ Hz

CHAPTER-15 : Electric Charges and Fields

TOPIC - 1: Electric Charges and Coulomb's Law

56. (d) Spheres A and B carry equal charge say 'q'

$\therefore$ Force between them, $F = \frac{kqq}{r^2}$

When A and C are touched, charge on both $q_A = q_C = \frac{q}{2}$

Then when B and C are touched, charge on B

$$q_B = \frac{\frac{q}{2}+q}{2} = \frac{3q}{4}$$

Now, the force between charge q_A and q_B

$$F' = \frac{kq_Aq_B}{r^2} = \frac{k\times\frac{q}{2}\times\frac{3q}{4}}{r^2} = \frac{3}{8}\frac{kq^2}{r^2} = \frac{3}{8}F$$

TOPIC - 2: Electric Field and Electric Field Lines

57. (a) Equilibrium position will shift to point where resultant force = 0

$kx_{eq} = qE \Rightarrow x_{eq} = \frac{qE}{k}$

Total energy $= \frac{1}{2}m\omega^2A^2 + \frac{1}{2}kx_{eq}^2$

Total energy $= \frac{1}{2}m\omega^2A^2 + \frac{1}{2}\frac{q^2E^2}{k}$

58. (d) Charge density, $\rho = \rho_0\left(1-\frac{r}{R}\right)$

$dq = \rho dv$

$q_{in} = \int dq = \rho dv$

$= \rho_0\left(1-\frac{r}{R}\right)4\pi r^2 dr$ ($\because dv = 4\pi r^2 dr$)

$= 4\pi\rho_0\int_0^R\left(1-\frac{r}{R}\right)r^2dr$

$= 4\pi\rho_0\int_0^R r^2dr - \frac{r^2}{R}dr$

$= 4\pi\rho_0\left[\left[\frac{r^3}{3}\right]_0^R - \left[\frac{r^4}{4R}\right]_0^R\right] = 4\pi\rho_0\left[\frac{R^3}{3} - \frac{R^4}{4R}\right]$

$= 4\pi\rho_0\left[\frac{R^3}{3} - \frac{R^3}{4}\right] = 4\pi\rho_0\left[\frac{R^3}{12}\right]$

$q = \frac{\pi\rho_0R^3}{3}$

$E.4\pi r^2 = \left(\frac{\pi\rho_0R^3}{3\epsilon_0}\right)$

$\therefore$ Electric field outside the ball, $E = \frac{\rho_0R^3}{12\epsilon_0 r^2}$

TOPIC - 3 : Electric Dipole, Electric Flux and Gauss's Law

59. (b) When cube is of side a and point charge Q is at the center of the cube then the total electric flux due to this charge will pass evenly through the six faces of the cube. So, the electric flux through one face will be equal to 1/6 of the total electric flux due to this charge.

Flux through 6 faces $= \frac{Q}{\epsilon_0}$

$\therefore$ Flux through 1 face, $= \frac{Q}{6\epsilon_0}$

CHAPTER-16 : Electrostatic Potential and Capacitance

TOPIC - 1: Electrostatic Potential and Equipotential Surfacess

60. (b) Potential outside the shell, $V_{outside} = \frac{KQ}{r}$

where r is distance of point from the centre of shell

Potential inside the shell,

$V_{inside} = \frac{KQ}{R}$

where 'R" is radius of the shell

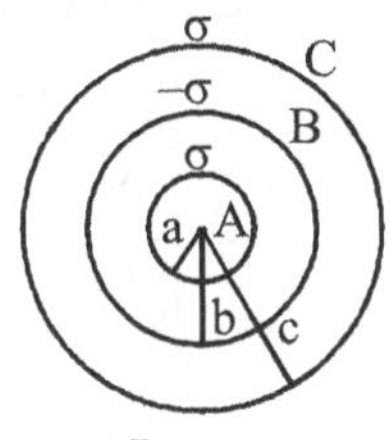

$$V_B = \frac{Kq_A}{r_b} + \frac{Kq_B}{r_b} + \frac{Kq_C}{r_c}$$

$$V_B = \frac{1}{4\pi \in_0}\left[\frac{\sigma 4\pi a^2}{b} - \frac{\sigma 4\pi b^2}{b} + \frac{\sigma 4\pi c^2}{c}\right]$$

$$V_B = \frac{\sigma}{\in_0}\left[\frac{a^2 - b^2}{b} + c\right]$$

TOPIC - 3: Capacitors, Grouping of Capacitor and Energy Stored in a Capacitor

61. (a) Charge on Capacitor, $Q_i = CV$

After inserting dielectric of dielectric constant = K

$Q_f = (kC)\,V$

Induced charges on dielectric

$$Q_{ind} = Q_f - Q_i = KCV - CV$$

$$= (K-1)CV = \left(\frac{5}{3} - 1\right) \times 90\text{pF} \times 2\text{V} = 1.2\text{nC}$$

62. (a) During charging charge on the capacitor increases with time. Charge on the capacitor C_1 as a function of time,

$Q = Q_0(1 - e^{-t/RC})$

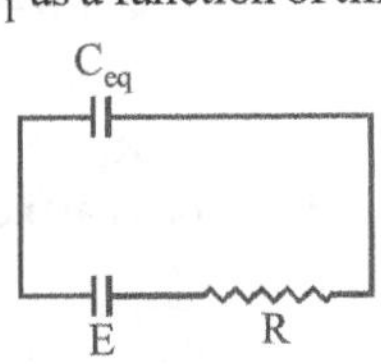

$$Q = C_{eq}E\left[1 - e^{-t/RC_{eq}}\right]$$

$(\because\ Q_0 = C_{eq}E)$

Both capacitor will have charge as they are connected in series

63. (d) The simplified circuit of the circuit given in question as follows:

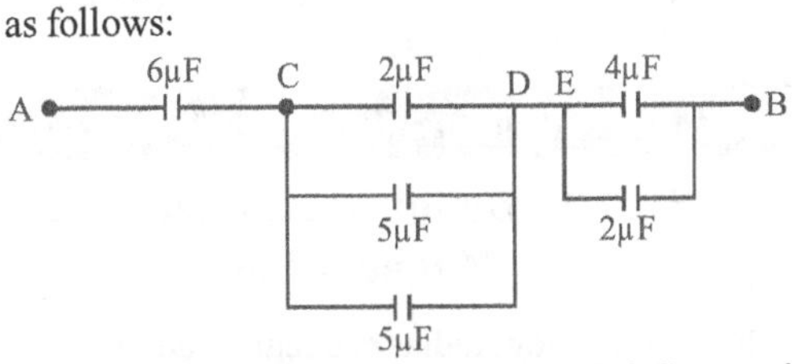

The equivalent capacitance between C & D capacitors of 2μF, 5μF and 5 μF are in parallel.

$\therefore\ C_{CD} = 2 + 5 + 5 = 12\ \mu F$ ($\because$ In parallel grouping $C_{eq} = C_1 + C_2 + ... + C_n$)

Similarly equivalent capacitance between E & B $C_{EB} = 4 + 2 = 6\mu F$

Now equivalent capacitance between A & B

$$\frac{1}{C_{eq}} = \frac{1}{6} + \frac{1}{12} + \frac{1}{6} = \frac{5}{12}$$

$\Rightarrow C_{eq} = \frac{12}{5} = 2.4\ \mu F$ ($\because$ In series grouping, $\frac{1}{C_{eq}} = \frac{1}{C_1} + \frac{1}{C_2} + ... + \frac{1}{C_n}$)

64. (c) Given area of Parallel plate capacitor, $A = 200\ cm^2$

Separation between the plates, $d = 1.5$ cm

Force of attraction between the plates, $F = 25 \times 10^{-6}$N

$F = QE$

$F = \frac{Q^2}{2A \in_0}$ (E due to parallel plate $= \frac{\sigma}{2\in_0} = \frac{Q}{A2\in_0}$)

But $Q = CV = \frac{\in_0 A(V)}{d}$

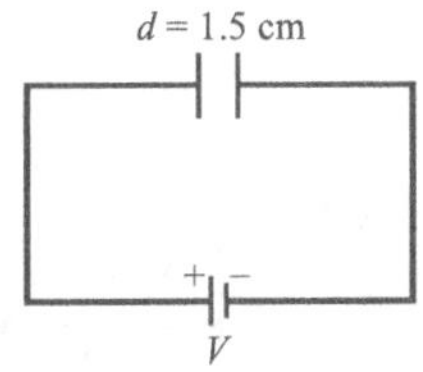

$$\therefore\quad F = \frac{(\in_0 AV)^2}{d^2 \times 2A\in_0}$$

$$= \frac{(\in_0 A)^2 \times V^2}{d^2 \times 2 \times (A\in_0)} = \frac{(\in_0 A) \times V^2}{d^2 \times 2}$$

or, $$25 \times 10^{-6} = \frac{(8.85 \times 10^{-12}) \times (200 \times 10^{-4}) \times V^2}{2.25 \times 10^{-4} \times 2}$$

$$\Rightarrow\quad V = \sqrt{\frac{25 \times 10^{-6} \times 2.25 \times 10^{-4} \times 2}{8.85 \times 10^{-12} \times 200 \times 10^{-4}}} \approx 250\text{ V}$$

65. (a) The sum of final charges on C_2 and C_3 is 36 μC.

CHAPTER-17 : Current Electricity

TOPIC - 1: Electric Current, Drift of Electrons, Ohm's Law, Resistance and Resistivity

66. (c) Resistance after temperature increases by 500°C i.e.,

$$R_t = \frac{V}{I} = \frac{220}{2} = 110\Omega$$

$R_0 = 100$ (given) temperature coefficient of resistance, $\alpha = ?$

using $R_t = R_0(1 + \alpha t)$

$110 = 100(1 + \alpha 500)$

$$\alpha = \frac{10}{100 \times 500}$$

or, $\alpha = 2 \times 10^{-4}\,°C^{-1}$

67. (c) Charge density $\rho = \frac{\text{charge}}{\text{volume}} = \frac{q}{Ad} \Rightarrow q = \rho Ad$

Also, $q = IT \Rightarrow T = \frac{q}{I} = \frac{\rho Ad}{I}$

TOPIC - 2: Combination of Resistances

68. (a) $R_{series} = R_1 + R_2 + ... + R_n$

$$\frac{1}{R_{parallel}} = \frac{1}{R_1} + \frac{1}{R_2} + ... + \frac{1}{R_n}$$

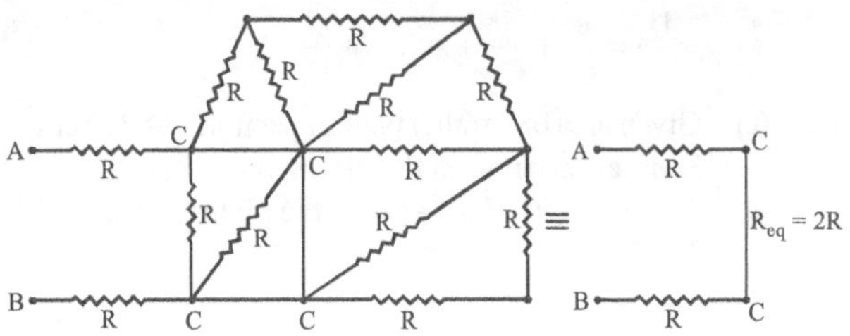

TOPIC - 3: Kirchoff 's Laws, Cells, Thermo e.m.f. Electrolysis

69. (b)

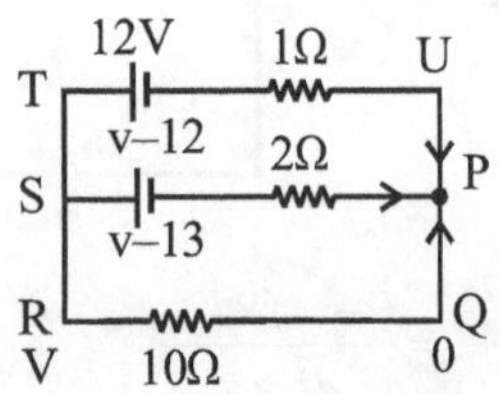

Using Kirchhoff's law at P we get

$$\frac{V-12}{1} + \frac{V-13}{2} + \frac{V-0}{10} = 0$$

[Let potential at P, Q, U = 0 and at R = V

$$\Rightarrow \frac{V}{1} + \frac{V}{2} + \frac{V}{10} = \frac{12}{1} + \frac{13}{2} + \frac{0}{10}$$

$$\Rightarrow \frac{10+5+1}{10}V = \frac{24+13}{2} \Rightarrow V\left(\frac{16}{10}\right) = \frac{37}{2}$$

$$\Rightarrow V = \frac{37 \times 10}{16 \times 2} = \frac{370}{32} = 11.56 \text{ volt}$$

TOPIC - 4: Heating Effect of Current

70. (a) Rate of heat i.e., Power developed in the wire $= P = \dfrac{V^2}{R}$

Resistance of the wire of length, L $R_1 = \dfrac{\rho L}{A} = \dfrac{\rho L}{\pi r^2}$

$\therefore$ Power, $P_1 = \dfrac{V^2}{R_1}$

Resistance of the wire when length is halved i.e., $L/2$

$$R_2 = \frac{\rho \frac{L}{2}}{\pi(2r)^2} = \frac{\rho L}{\pi 8r^2} = \frac{R_1}{8}$$

$\therefore$ Power, $P_2 = \dfrac{V}{\frac{R_1}{8}} = \dfrac{8V}{R_1}$

or, $P_2 = 8P_1$ i.e., power increased 8 times of previous or original wire.

TOPIC - 5: Wheatstone Bridge and Different Measuring Instruments

71. (b) Using formula, internal resistance,

$$r = \left(\frac{l_1 - l_2}{l_2}\right)s = \left(\frac{52-40}{40}\right) \times 5 = 1.5\Omega$$

72. (c) $R_1 + R_2 = 1000$

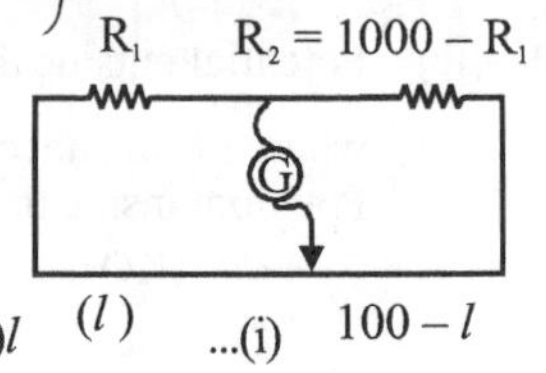

$\Rightarrow R_2 = 1000 - R_1$

On balancing condition

$R_1(100 - l) = (1000 - R_1)l$ ...(i)

On Interchanging resistance balance point shifts left by 10 cm

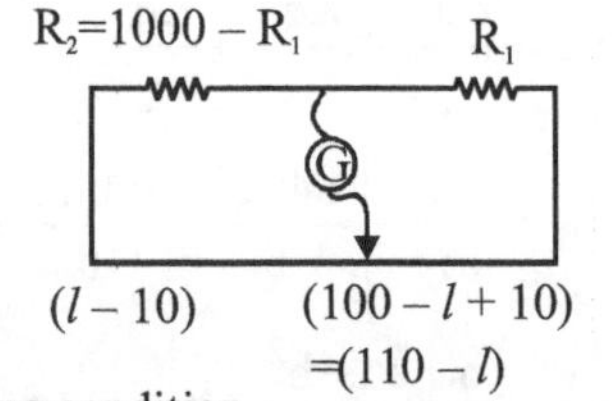

On balancing condition

$(1000 - R_1)(110 - l) = R_1(l - 10)$

or, $R_1(l - 10) = (1000 - R_1)(110 - l)$ ...(ii)

Dividing eqn (i) by (ii)

$$\frac{100-l}{l-10} = \frac{l}{110-l}$$

$\Rightarrow (100 - l)(110 - l) = l(l - 10)$

$\Rightarrow 11000 - 100l - 110l + l^2 = l^2 - 10l$

$\Rightarrow 11000 = 200l$

or, $l = 55$

Putting the value of 'l' in eqn (i)

$R_1(100 - 55) = (1000 - R_1)55$

$\Rightarrow R_1(45) = (1000 - R_1)55$

$\Rightarrow R_1(9) = (1000 - R_1)11$

$\Rightarrow 20R_1 = 11000$

$\therefore R_1 = 550\,\Omega$

73. (b) For a balanced meter bridge,

$$\frac{X}{39.5} = \frac{Y}{(100-39.5)} \Rightarrow Y = 39.5 = X \times (100 - 39.5)$$

or, $X = \dfrac{12.5 \times 39.5}{60.5} = 8.16\Omega$

When X and Y are interchanged l_1 and $(100 - l_1)$ will also interchange so, $l_2 = 60.5$ cm

CHAPTER-18 : Moving Charges and Magnetism

TOPIC - 1: Motion of Charged Particle in Magnetic Field

74. (b) As we know, radius of circular path in magnetic field

$$r = \frac{\sqrt{2Km}}{qB}$$

For electron, $r_e = \dfrac{\sqrt{2Km_e}}{eB}$ ....(i)

For proton, $r_p = \frac{\sqrt{2Km_p}}{eB}$ ....(ii)

For α particle,

$$r_\alpha = \frac{\sqrt{2Km_a}}{q_\alpha B} = \frac{\sqrt{2K4m_p}}{2eB} = \frac{\sqrt{2Km_p}}{eB} \text{ ...(iii)}$$

$\therefore \quad r_e < r_p = r_\alpha \quad (\because m_e < m_p)$

TOPIC - 2: Magnetic Field Lines, Biot-Savart's Law and Ampere's Circuital Law

75. (c) Magnetic field at the centre of loop, $B_1 = \frac{\mu_0 I}{2R}$

Dipole moment of circular loop is m = IA

$m_1 = I.A = I.\pi R^2$ {R = Radius of the loop}

If moment is doubled (keeping current constant)

R becomes $\sqrt{2}R$

$$m_2 = I.\pi\left(\sqrt{2}R\right)^2 = 2.I\pi R^2 = 2m_1$$

$$B_2 = \frac{\mu_0 I}{2\left(\sqrt{2}R\right)}$$

$$\therefore \frac{B_1}{B_2} = \frac{\frac{\mu_0 I}{2R}}{\frac{\mu_0 I}{2\left(\sqrt{2}R\right)}} = \sqrt{2}$$

76. (b) Point *P* is situated at the mid-point of the line joining the centres of the circular wires which have same radii (R). The magnetic fields ($\vec{B}$) at P due to the currents in the wires are in same direction.

Magnitude of magnetic field at point, *P*

$$B = 2\left\{\frac{\mu_0 NIR^2}{2\left(R^2 + \frac{R^2}{4}\right)^{3/2}}\right\} = \frac{\mu_0 NIR^2}{\frac{5^{3/2}}{8}} = \frac{8\mu_0 NI}{5^{3/2} R}$$

77. (a) Here, side of the triangle, $l = 4.5 \times 10^{-2}$ m, current, I = 1A magnetic field at the centre of the triangle '*O*' *B* = ?

From figure, $\tan 60° = \sqrt{3} = \frac{1}{2d}$

$$\Rightarrow d = \frac{l}{2\sqrt{3}} = \left(\frac{4.5 \times 10^{-2}}{2\sqrt{3}}\right) \text{m}$$

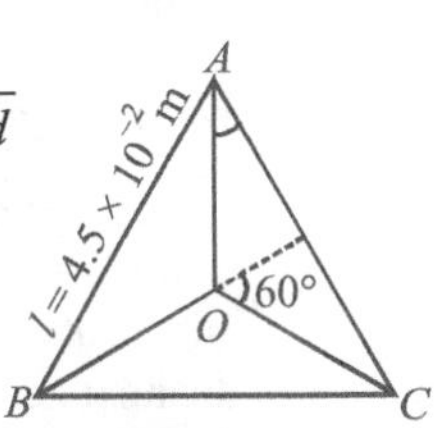

Magnetic field, $B = \frac{\mu_0 i}{4\pi d}(\cos\theta_1 + \cos\theta_2)$

Putting value of $\mu = 4\pi \times 10^{-7}$ and θ_1 and θ_2 we will get $B = 4 \times 10^{-5}$ Wb/m^2

TOPIC - 3: Force and Torque on Current Carrying Conductor

78. (a) Magnetic moment, $\mu = IA = \frac{qv}{2\pi r}(\pi r^2)$

or, $\mu = \frac{qr\omega}{2\pi r}(\pi r^2) = \frac{1}{2}qr^2\omega$

TOPIC - 4: Galvanometer and its Conversion into Ammeter and Voltmeter

79. (b) Figure of merit of a galvanometer is the correct required to produce a deflection of one division in the galvanometer i.e., figure of merit $= \frac{I}{\theta}$

$$I = \frac{\varepsilon}{R+G} \qquad G = \frac{1}{9}K\Omega$$

$$\frac{1}{2} = \frac{\varepsilon}{R + \frac{GS}{G+S}} \times \frac{S}{S+G} \Rightarrow \frac{1}{2} = \frac{\varepsilon S}{R(S+G)+GS}$$

$$S = \frac{RG \times \frac{1}{2}}{\varepsilon - \frac{(R+G)I}{2}}$$

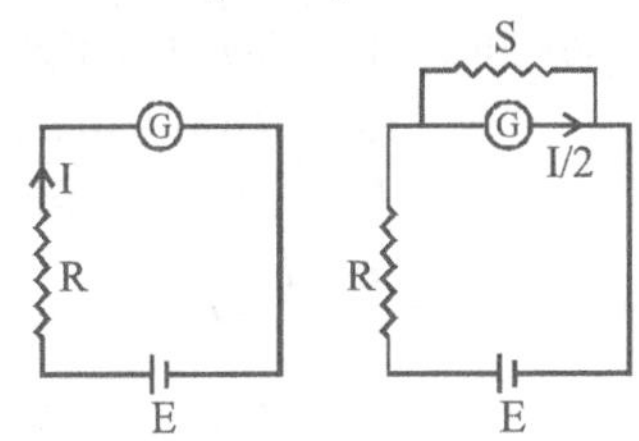

$$S = \frac{11 \times 10^3 \times \frac{1}{2} \times 10^2 \times 270 \times 10^{-6}}{6 - \left(\frac{6}{2}\right)} = 110\Omega$$

80. (d) According to question, current through galvanometer, $I_g = 1$ mA

Current through shunt $(I - I_g) = 2$ A

Galvanometer resistance $R_g = 25\Omega$

Resistance of shunt, S = ?

$I_0R_0 = (I - I_g)S$

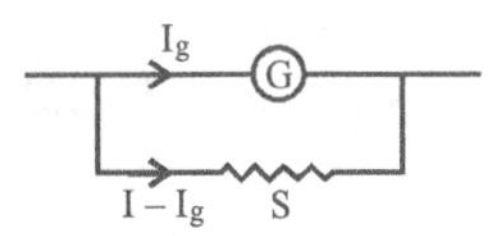

$$\Rightarrow S = \frac{10^{-3} \times 25}{2}$$

$S \simeq 1.25 \times 10^{-2}\Omega$

CHAPTER-19 : Magnetism and Matter

TOPIC - 2: The Earth Magnetism, Magnetic Materials and their properties

81. (b) Given Number of turns,

n = 1000 turns/cm = 1000 × 100 turns/m

Coercivity of ferromagnet, H = 100 A/m

Current to demagnetise the ferromagnet, I = ?

Using, H = nI

or, $100 = 10^5 \times I$

$$\therefore \quad I = \frac{100}{10^5} = 1 \text{ mA}$$

CHAPTER-20 : Electromagnetic Induction

TOPIC - 2: Motional and Static EMI and Application of EMI

82. **(a)** Induced emf in a coil, $e = -\frac{d\phi}{dt} = NBA \sin \omega t$

Also, $e = e_0 \sin \omega t$

$\therefore$ Maximum emf induced, $e_0 = nBA\omega$

83. **(a)** Given: Capacitance, $C = 0.2\,\mu F = 0.2 \times 10^{-6}$ F

Inductance $L = 0.5$ mH $= 0.5 \times 10^{-3}$ H

Current I = ?

Using energy conservation

$$\frac{1}{2}CV^2 = \frac{1}{2}CV_1^2 + \frac{1}{2}LI^2$$

$$\frac{1}{2} \times 0.2 \times 10^{-6} \times 10^2 + 0$$

$$= \frac{1}{2} \times 0.2 \times 10^{-6} \times 5^2 + \frac{1}{2} \times 0.5 \times 10^{-3} I^2$$

$$\therefore \quad I = \sqrt{3} \times 10^{-1}\,A = 0.17\,A$$

84. **(b)** From Faraday's law of electomagnetic induction,

$$e = \frac{d\phi}{dt} = \frac{d(BA)}{lt} = \frac{d(Bll)}{dt}$$

$$= \frac{Bdl \times l}{dt} = BVl$$

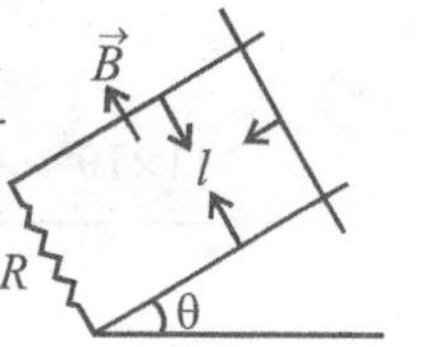

Also, $F = ilB = \left(\frac{BV}{R}\right)(l^2 B) = \frac{B^2 l^2 V}{R}$

At equilibrium

$$mg \sin\theta = \frac{B^2 lV}{R} \Rightarrow V = \frac{mgR\sin\theta}{B^2 l^2}$$

85. **(c)** According to Faraday's law of electromagnetic induction,

$$e = -\frac{d\phi}{dt} \text{ and } \phi = BA\cos\omega t = B\pi r^2 \cos\omega t$$

$$\Rightarrow \quad e = -\frac{d}{dt}(\pi r^2 B\cos\omega t) = \pi r^2 B \sin\omega t(\omega)$$

$$\therefore \quad e = \frac{\mu_0 I}{2R}\pi\omega r^2 \sin\omega t \quad \left(\because B = \frac{\mu_0 I}{2R}\right)$$

CHAPTER-21 : Alternating Current

TOPIC - 2: AC Circuit, LCR Circuit, Quality and Power Factor

86. **(b)** As we know, average power $P_{avg} = V_{rms} I_{rms} \cos\theta$

$$= \left(\frac{V_0}{\sqrt{2}}\right)\left(\frac{I_0}{\sqrt{2}}\right)\cos\theta = \left(\frac{100}{\sqrt{2}}\right)\left(\frac{20}{\sqrt{2}}\right)\cos 45^\circ \quad (\because \theta = 45^\circ)$$

$$P_{avg} = \frac{1000}{\sqrt{2}} \text{ watt}$$

Wattless current $I = I_{rms} \sin\theta$

$$= \frac{I_0}{\sqrt{2}}\sin\theta = \frac{20}{\sqrt{2}}\sin 45^\circ = 10A$$

87. **(a)** Quality factor $Q = \frac{\omega_0}{2\Delta\omega} = \frac{\omega_0 L}{R}$

TOPIC - 3: Transformers and LC Oscillations

88. **(c)** Given : $V_P = 2300$ V, $V_s = 230$ V, $I_P = 5$ A, $n = 90\% = 0.9$

Efficiency $n = 0.9 = \frac{P_s}{P_P} \Rightarrow P_s = 0.9\,P_p$

$V_s I_s = 0.9 \times V_P I_P \quad (\because P = VI)$

$$I_s = \frac{0.9 \times 2300 \times 5}{230} = 45\,A$$

CHAPTER-22 : Electromagnetic Waves

TOPIC-1 : Electromagnetic Waves, Conduction and Displacement Current

89. **(c)** Velocity of EM wave is given by $v = \frac{1}{\sqrt{\mu \in}}$

Velocity in air $= \frac{\omega}{k} = C$

Velocity in medium $= \frac{C}{2}$

Here, $\mu_1 = \mu_2 = 1$ as medium is non-magnetic

$$\therefore \quad \frac{\frac{1}{\sqrt{\in_{r_1}}}}{\frac{1}{\sqrt{\in_{r_2}}}} = \frac{C}{\left(\frac{C}{2}\right)} = 2 \quad \Rightarrow \quad \frac{\in_{r_1}}{\in_{r_2}} = \frac{1}{4}$$

90. **(c)** If E_0 is magnitude of electric field then

$$\frac{1}{2}\varepsilon_0 E^2 \times C = 1 \Rightarrow E_0 = \sqrt{\frac{2I}{C\varepsilon_0}}$$

$$E_0 = \frac{E_0}{C}$$

Direction of $\vec{E} \times \vec{B}$ will be along $+\hat{j}$.

91. **(a)** $\hat{E} \times \hat{B}$ should give the direction of wave propagation

$$\Rightarrow \quad \hat{K} \times \hat{B} \,||\, \frac{\hat{i} \times \hat{j}}{\sqrt{2}} \Rightarrow \hat{K} \times \left(\frac{\hat{i} + \hat{j}}{\sqrt{2}}\right) = \frac{\hat{j} - (-\hat{i})}{\sqrt{2}} = \frac{\hat{i} + \hat{j}}{\sqrt{2}} \,||\, \frac{\hat{i} + \hat{j}}{\sqrt{2}}$$

Option-1, option-2 and option-4 does not satisfy.

Wave propagation vector $\hat{K}$ should along $\frac{\hat{i} + \hat{j}}{\sqrt{2}}$ so correct option is 3.

92. **(a)** Using $E = E_0 - e^{i}(kz - \omega t)$

Given, at $t = t_1, z = z_1, E = 0$

the next zero that occurs in it's neighborhood is at z_2, the frequency of the electromagnetic wave at t_2

$$e^{i(kz_1 - \omega t_1)} = e^{i(kz_2 - \omega t_2)}$$

$$kz_1 - \omega t_1 = kz_2 - \omega t_2$$

$$(t_2 - t_1)\omega = k(z - z_1)$$

where $k = \frac{2\pi}{\lambda} = 2\pi v$

$$(t_2 - t_1) = \frac{2\pi}{\lambda \times 2\pi v}(z_2 - z_1) = \frac{1}{x \times v}(z_2 - z_1)$$

$$\Rightarrow \quad \lambda \times v = \frac{(z_2 - z_1)}{(t_2 - t_1)} = C$$

$$(t_2 - t_1) = \frac{(z_2 - z_1)}{C}$$

Frequency is $f \propto \frac{1}{t}$ then $\frac{1}{(t_2 - t_1)} = \frac{C}{(z_2 - z_1)}$

$\therefore$ Frequency, $f = \frac{3 \times 10^8}{(z_2 - z_1)}$

CHAPTER-23 : Ray Optics and Optical Instruments

TOPIC - 1: Plane Mirror, Spherical Mirror and Reflection of Light

93. **(c)** When object is at 8 cm

Image $V_1 = \frac{f \times u}{u - f} = \frac{5 \times 8}{8 - 5} = -\frac{40}{3}$ cm

When object is at 12 cm

Image $V_2 = \frac{f \times u}{u - f} = \frac{5 \times 12}{12 - 5} = -\frac{60}{7}$ cm

Separation $= |V_1 - V_2| = \frac{40}{3} - \frac{60}{7} = \frac{100}{21}$ cm

So A, C and D are correct statements.

TOPIC - 3: Refraction at Curved Surface Lenses and Power of Lens

94. **(a)** **Case-1**

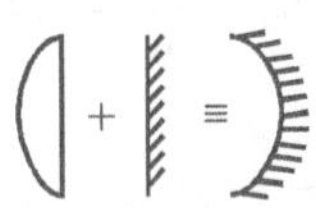

$\frac{1}{f_1} = \left(\frac{\mu - 1}{R}\right)$ f = –28

$P = 2P_1 + P_2 \Rightarrow \frac{1}{28} = 2\left(\frac{\mu - 1}{R}\right)$ ($\because$ Power, $P = \frac{1}{f}$ & $f_{\text{plane mirror}} = \infty$)

Case-2

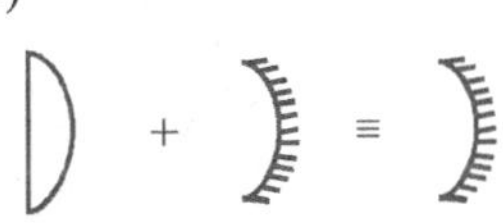

$\frac{1}{f_1} = \left(\frac{\mu - 1}{R}\right)$ $f_2 = -\frac{R}{2}$ $f = -10$ cm

$$P = 2P_1 + P_2 \Rightarrow \frac{1}{10} = 2\left(\frac{\mu - 1}{2}\right) + \frac{2}{R}$$

or, $\frac{1}{10} = \frac{1}{28} + \frac{2}{R} \Rightarrow \frac{2}{R} = \frac{1}{10} - \frac{2}{28} = \frac{18}{280}$

or, $R = \frac{280}{9}$ cm

or, $\frac{1}{28} = 2\left(\frac{\mu - 1}{280}\right)9 \Rightarrow \mu - 1 = \frac{5}{9}$

$\therefore \quad \mu = 1 + \frac{5}{9} = \frac{14}{9} = 1.55$

95. **(a)** For minimum spherical aberration separation,
$d = f_1 - f_2 = 2$ cm
Resultant focal length = F = 10 cm

Using $\frac{1}{F} = \frac{1}{f_1} + \frac{1}{f_2} - \frac{d}{f_1 f_2}$ and solving, we get f_1, f_2 18 cm and 20 cm respectively.

TOPIC - 4: Prism and Dispersion of Light

96. **(c)** Angle of prism, A = 30°, i = 60°,
angle of deviation, δ = 30°

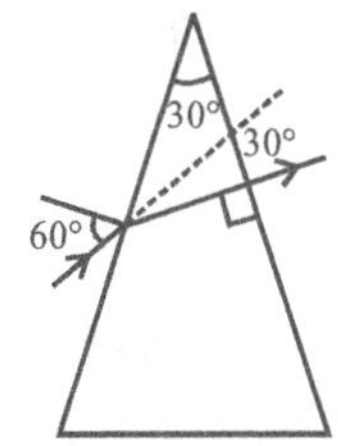

Using formula, δ = i + e – A

⇒ e = δ + A – i

= 30° + 30° – 60° = 0°

$\therefore$ Emergent ray will be perpendicular to the face
So it will make angle 90° with the force through which it emerges.

CHAPTER-24 : Wave Optics

TOPIC - 2: Young's Double Slit Experiment

97. **(a)** Angular width of central maxima $= \frac{2\lambda}{d}$

or, $\lambda = \frac{d}{2}$; Fringe width, $\beta = \frac{\lambda \times D}{d'}$

$$10^{-2} = \frac{d}{2} \times \frac{50 \times 10^{-2}}{d'} = \frac{10^{-6} \times 50 \times 10^{-2}}{2 \times d'}$$

Therefore, slit separation distance, d' = 25μm

98. **(a)** If angular position of 2nd maxima from central maxima is θ then

$$\sin\theta = \frac{(2n - 1)\lambda}{2a} = \frac{3\lambda}{20} = \frac{3 \times 550 \times 10^{-9}}{2 \times 22 \times 10^{-7}}$$

$\therefore \quad \theta \simeq \frac{\pi}{8}$ rad

TOPIC - 3: Diffraction, Polarisation of Light and Resolving Power

99. **(c)** Axis of transmission of A & B are parallel.

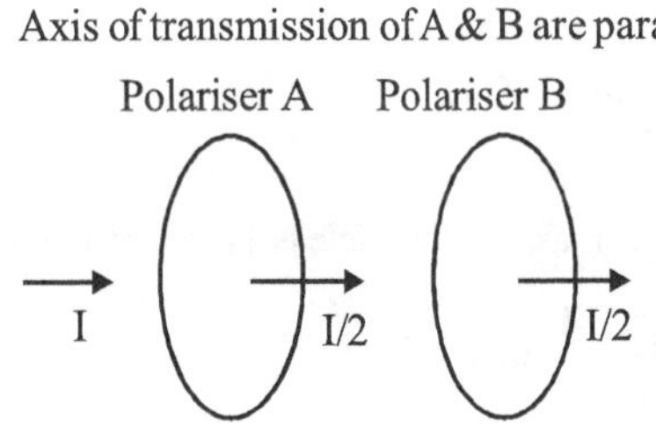

After introducing polariser C between A and B,

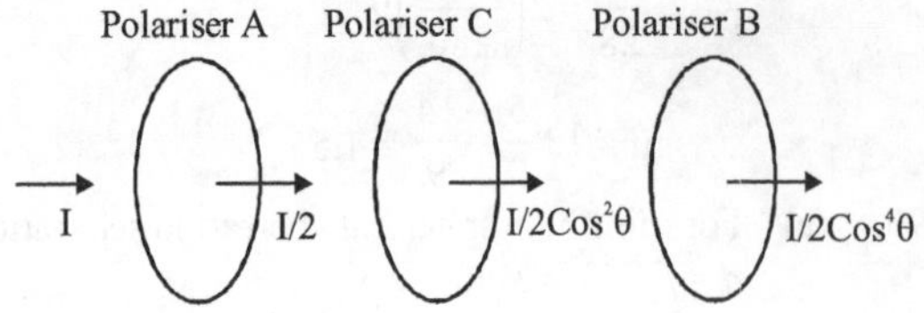

$$\frac{I}{2}\cos^4\theta = \frac{I}{8} \Rightarrow \cos^4\theta = \frac{1}{4}$$

$$\Rightarrow \cos\theta = \frac{1}{\sqrt{2}} \text{ or, } \theta = 45°$$

100. (a) Polariser A and B have same alignment of transmission axis.
Lets assume polariser c is introduced at θ angle

$$\frac{1}{2}\cos^2\theta \times \cos^2\theta = \frac{1}{3}$$

or, $\cos^4\theta = \frac{2}{3} \Rightarrow \cos\theta = \left(\frac{2}{3}\right)^{1/4}$

101. (a)

CHAPTER-25 : Dual Nature of Radiation and Matter

TOPIC - 1: Matter Waves, Cathode and Positive Rays

102. (c) Momentum (p) of each electron $\frac{h}{\lambda_1}\hat{i}$ and $\frac{h}{\lambda_2}\hat{j}$

Velocity of centre of mass

$$V_{cm} = \frac{h}{2m\lambda_1}\hat{i} + \frac{h}{2m\lambda_2}\hat{j} \quad (\because p = mv)$$

Velocity of 1st particle about centre of mass

$$V_{1cm} = \frac{h}{2m\lambda_1}\hat{i} - \frac{h}{2m\lambda_2}\hat{j}$$

$$\lambda_{cm} = \frac{h}{\sqrt{\frac{h^2}{4\lambda_1^2} + \frac{h^2}{4\lambda_2^2}}} = \frac{2\lambda_1\lambda_2}{\sqrt{\lambda_1^2 + \lambda_2^2}} \quad \left(\because \lambda = \frac{h}{p}\right)$$

103. (c) According to question, $\lambda_p = \lambda_\alpha$

Using, $\lambda = \frac{h}{p} = \frac{h}{mv}$

So, $\frac{h}{m_p \times v_p} = \frac{h}{m_\alpha \times v_\alpha}$

$$\Rightarrow \frac{v_p}{v_\alpha} = \frac{m_\alpha}{m_p} = \frac{4m_p}{m_p}$$

($\because$ mass of α-particle is 4 times of mass of proton)

So, $\frac{v_p}{v_\alpha} = \frac{4}{1}$; i.e., 4 : 1

TOPIC - 2: Photon, Photoelectric Effect X-rays and Davisson-Germer Experiment

104. (a) Energy $E = \frac{hc}{\lambda}$;

$$= \frac{\lambda_N}{\lambda_a} = \frac{E_a}{E_N}$$

where E_a and E_N are energies of photons from atom and nucleus respectively. E_N is of the order of MeV = 10^6 eV and E_a in few eV.

So $\frac{\lambda_N}{\lambda_a} = 10^{-6}$

CHAPTER-26 : Atoms

TOPIC - 2 : Bohr's Model and the Spectra of the Hydrogen Atom

105. (a) Wavelength of emitted photon from n^{th} state to the ground state, $\frac{1}{\Lambda_n} = RZ^2\left(\frac{1}{1^2} - \frac{1}{n^2}\right)$

$$\Lambda_n = \frac{1}{RZ^2}\left(1 - \frac{1}{n^2}\right)^{-1}$$

Since n is very large, using binomial theorem

$$\Lambda_n = \frac{1}{RZ^2}\left(1 + \frac{1}{n^2}\right)$$

$$\Lambda_n = \frac{1}{RZ^2} + \frac{1}{RZ^2}\left(\frac{1}{n^2}\right)$$

As we know, $\lambda_n = \frac{2\pi r}{n} = 2\pi\left(\frac{n^2h^2}{4\pi^2 mZe^2}\right)\frac{1}{n} \propto n$

$$\Lambda_n \approx A + \frac{B}{\lambda_n^2}$$

106. (d) $h\nu_L = E_\infty - E_1$ ...(i)

$h\nu_f = E_\infty - E_5$ ...(ii)

$$E \propto \frac{z^2}{n^2} \Rightarrow \frac{E_5}{E_1} = \left(\frac{1}{5}\right)^2 = \frac{1}{25}$$

Eqn (i) / (ii) $\Rightarrow \frac{h\nu_L}{h\nu_f} = \frac{E_1}{E_5}$

$$\Rightarrow \frac{\nu_L}{\nu_f} = \frac{25}{1} \Rightarrow \nu_f = \frac{\nu_L}{25}$$

107. (d) de-Broglie wavelength, $\lambda = \frac{h}{P}$

$$\frac{\lambda_B}{\lambda_G} = \frac{P_a}{P_B} = \frac{mv_G}{mv_B}$$

Speed of electron $V \propto \frac{z}{n}$

so $\frac{\lambda_B}{\lambda_G} = \frac{n_B}{n_G} = \frac{3}{1} \Rightarrow \lambda_B = 3\lambda_G$

108. (b) Energy required to remove e^- from singly ionized helium atom $= \frac{(13.6)Z^2}{1^2} = 54.4\,eV \quad (\because Z = 2)$

Energy required to remove e^- from helium atom = x eV

According to question, 54.4 eV = 2.2x ⇒ x = 24.73 eV

Therefore, energy required to ionize helium atom = (54.4 + 24.73) eV = 79.12 eV

109. (d) (A) Radius of muon $= \frac{\text{Radius of hydrogen}}{200}$

Radius of H atom $= r = \frac{\epsilon_0 n^2 h^2}{\pi m e^2}$

Radius of muon $= r_\mu = \frac{\epsilon_0 n^2 h^2}{\pi \times 200\, m e^2}$

$r_\mu = \frac{r}{200}$

(B) Velocity relation given is wrong

(C) Ionization energy in e^-H atom

$E = \frac{+me^4}{8\epsilon_0^2 n^2 h^2}$

$E_\mu = \frac{200me^4}{8\epsilon_0^2 n^2 h^2} = 200E$

(D) Momentum of H-atom

$mvr = \frac{nh}{2\pi}$

Hence (A), (C), (D) are correct.

CHAPTER-27 : Nuclei

TOPIC - 1: Composition and Size of the Nuclei

110. (c) Let heavy nucleus breaks into two nuclei of mass m_1 and m_2 and move away with velocities V_1 and V_2 respectively.

According to question, $\frac{V_1}{V_2} = \frac{8}{27}$

$m_1V_1 = m_2V_2$ (Law of momentum conservation)

$\Rightarrow \frac{m_1}{m_2} = \frac{V_2}{V_1} = \frac{27}{8}$

$\frac{\rho \times \frac{4}{3}\pi R_1^3}{\rho \times \frac{4}{3}\pi R_2^3} \quad \left(\because \text{density } \rho = \frac{\text{mass}}{\text{volume}}\right)$

$\Rightarrow \left(\frac{R_1}{R_2}\right) = \left(\frac{27}{8}\right)^{\frac{1}{3}} = \left(\frac{3}{2}\right)^{3\times\frac{1}{3}}$

$\therefore \frac{R_1}{R_2} = \frac{3}{2}$

TOPIC - 3: Radioactivity

111. (b) Given : $N_1 = 2N_2$

Activity of radioactive substance = λN

Half life period $t = \frac{\ln 2}{\lambda}$ or, $\lambda = \frac{\ln 2}{T}$

$\lambda_1 N_1 = \frac{\ln 2}{t_1} \times N_1 = 5\,\mu c_i \quad \text{..... (i)}$

$\lambda_2 N_2 = \frac{\ln 2}{t_2} \times N_2 = 10\,\mu c_i \quad \text{..... (ii)}$

Dividing equation (ii) by (i)

$\frac{t_2}{t_1} \times \frac{N_1}{N_2} = \frac{1}{2}$

$\frac{t_2}{t_1} = \frac{1}{4} \Rightarrow t_1 = 4t_2$

i.e., Half life of S_1 is four times of sample S_2.

Hence 5 years and 20 years.

112. (d) Let initial activity = No = 0.8 μ ci

$0.8 \times 3.7 \times 10^4$ dps

Activity in 1 cm^3 of blood at t = 10 hr,

$n = \frac{300}{60}$ dps = 5 dps

N = Activity of whole blood at time t = 10 hr.

Total volume of the blood in the person, $V = \frac{N}{n}$

$= \frac{N_0 e - \lambda t}{n} = \frac{0.8 \times 3.7 \times 10^4 \times 0.7927}{5} \cong 5$ litres

CHAPTER-28 : Semiconductor Electronics : Materials, Devices and Simple Circuits

TOPIC - 1: Solids, Semiconductors and P-N Junction Diode

113. (c) Clearly from fig. given in question, Silicon diode is in forward bias.

∴ Potential barrier across diode

$\Delta V = 0.7$ volts

Current, $I = \frac{V - \Delta V}{R} = \frac{3 - 0.7}{200} = \frac{2.3}{200} = 11.5$mA

114. (b)

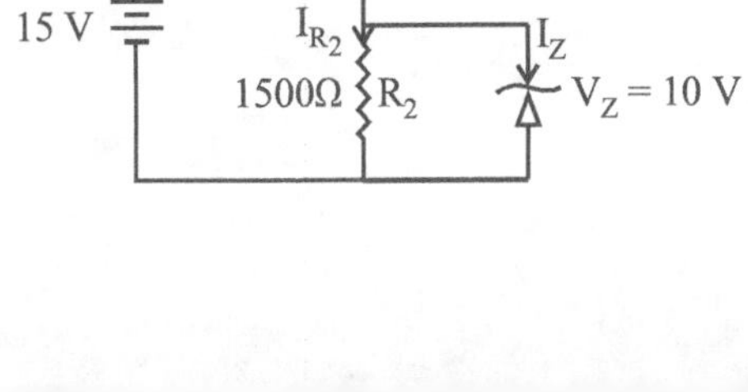

The voltage drop across R_2 is $V_{R_2} = V_Z = 10V$

The current through R_2 is

$$I_{R_2} = \frac{V_{R_2}}{R_2} = \frac{10\,V}{1500\Omega} = 0.667 \times 10^{-2} A$$

$= 6.67 \times 10^{-3} A = 6.67\,mA$

The voltage drop across R_1 is

$V_{R_1} = 15V - V_{R_2} = 15V - 10V = 5V$

The current through R_1 is

$$I_{R_1} = \frac{V_{R_1}}{R_1} = \frac{5\,V}{500\Omega} = 10^{-2} A = 10 \times 10^{-3} A = 10\,mA$$

The current through the zener diode is

$I_Z = I_{R_1} - I_{R_2} = (10 - 6.67)mA = 3.3mA$

TOPIC - 2: Junction Transistor

115. (d) Curent gain $\beta = \frac{\Delta I_C}{I_B}$

Voltage gain A_v = Current gain × Resistance gain = $\beta \frac{R_L}{R_{BE}}$

Power gain A_p = (Current gain)^2 × Resistance gain

$= \beta^2 \frac{R_L}{R_{BE}}$

TOPIC - 3: Digital Electronics and Logic Gates

116. (c) Truth table of the circuit is as follows

x	y	$\overline{x}$	$a = x.y$	$b = \overline{x}.y$	$z = \overline{a.b}$
0	0	1	0	0	1
0	1	1	0	1	1
1	0	0	0	0	1
1	1	0	1	0	1

CHAPTER-29 : Communication Systems

TOPIC-1 : Communication Systems

117. (c) If n = no. of channels

10% of 10 GHz = n × 5 KHz

or, $\frac{10}{100} \times 10 \times 10^9 = n \times 5 \times 10^3 \Rightarrow n = 2 \times 10^5$

118. (a) Given : modulation index m = 80% = 0.8

$E_c = 14\,V, E_m = ?$

using, $m = \frac{E_m}{E_c} \Rightarrow E_m = m \times E_c = 0.8 \times 14 = 11.2V$

119. (b) Given, modulating frequency f_m = 15 KHz

∴ Bandwidth of one channel = $2f_m$ = 30 kHz

∴ No of channels accommodate = $\frac{300kHz}{30kHz} = 10$

120. (c) Given : Inductance, $L = 49\,\mu H = 49 \times 10^{-6}$ H, capacitance $C = 2.5\,nF = 2.5 \times 10^{-9}$ F

Using $\omega = \frac{1}{\sqrt{LC}}$

$$= \frac{1}{\sqrt{49 \times 10^{-6} \times \frac{2.5}{10} \times 10^{-9}}} = \frac{1}{7 \times 5 \times 10^{-8}} = \frac{10^8}{7 \times 5}$$

or, $\frac{10^8}{7 \times 5} = 2\pi \times f = 2 \times \frac{22}{7} \times f \quad (\because \omega = 2\pi f)$

or, $f = \frac{10^7}{22} = \frac{10^4}{22} kHz = 454.54 kHz$

Therefore frequency range 454.54 ± 12kHz

i.e., 442 kHz – 466 kHz

PHYSICS

Chapter 1 Physical World, Units and Measurements

TOPIC-1 : Unit of Physical Quantities

1. A metal sample carrying a current along X-axis with density J_x is subjected to a magnetic field B_z (along z-axis). The electric field E_y developed along Y-axis is directly proportional to J_x as well as B_z. The constant of proportionality has SI unit. **[Online April 25, 2013]**

(a) $\frac{m^2}{A}$ (b) $\frac{m^3}{As}$ (c) $\frac{m^2}{As}$ (d) $\frac{As}{m^3}$

TOPIC-2 : Dimensions of Physical Quantities

2. Time (T), velocity (C) and angular momentum (h) are chosen as fundamental quantities instead of mass, length and time. In terms of these, the dimensions of mass would be : **[Online April 8, 2017]**

(a) $[M]=[T^{-1}C^{-2}h]$ (b) $[M]=[T^{-1}C^{2}h]$
(c) $[M]=[T^{-1}C^{-2}h^{-1}]$ (d) $[M]=[TC^{-2}h]$

3. A, B, C and D are four different physical quantities having different dimensions. None of them is dimensionless. But we know that the equation AD = C ln (BD) holds true. Then which of the combination is not a meaningful quantity? **[Online April 10, 2016]**

(a) $\frac{C}{BD}-\frac{AD^2}{C}$ (b) $A^2-B^2C^2$
(c) $\frac{A}{B}-C$ (d) $\frac{(A-C)}{D}$

4. In the following 'I' refers to current and other symbols have their usual meaning, Choose the option that corresponds to the dimensions of electrical conductivity : **[Online April 9, 2016]**

(a) $M^{-1}L^{-3}T^3I$ (b) $M^{-1}L^{-3}T^3I^2$
(c) $M^{-1}L^3T^3I$ (d) $ML^{-3}T^{-3}I^2$

5. If electronic charge e, electron mass m, speed of light in vacuum c and Planck's constant h are taken as fundamental quantities, the permeability of vacuum μ_0 can be expressed in units of : **[Online April 11, 2015]**

(a) $\left(\frac{h}{me^2}\right)$ (b) $\left(\frac{hc}{me^2}\right)$ (c) $\left(\frac{h}{ce^2}\right)$ (d) $\left(\frac{mc^2}{he^2}\right)$

6. If the capacitance of a nanocapacitor is measured in terms of a unit '*u*' made by combining the electric charge '*e*', Bohr radius 'a_0', Planck's constant 'h' and speed of light '*c*' then: **[Online April 10, 2015]**

(a) $u=\frac{e^2h}{a_0}$ (b) $u=\frac{hc}{e^2a_0}$
(c) $u=\frac{e^2c}{ha_0}$ (d) $u=\frac{e^2a_0}{hc}$

7. From the following combinations of physical constants (expressed through their usual symbols) the only combination, that would have the same value in different systems of units, is: **[Online April 12, 2014]**

(a) $\frac{ch}{2\pi\varepsilon_0^2}$

(b) $\frac{e^2}{2\pi\varepsilon_0 Gm_e^2}$ (m_e = mass of electron)

(c) $\frac{\mu_0\varepsilon_0}{c^2}\frac{G}{he^2}$

(d) $\frac{2\pi\sqrt{\mu_0\varepsilon_0}}{ce^2}\frac{h}{G}$

8. In terms of resistance R and time T, the dimensions of ratio $\frac{\mu}{\varepsilon}$ of the permeability μ and permittivity ε is: **[Online April 11, 2014]**

(a) $[RT^{-2}]$ (b) $[R^2T^{-1}]$ (c) $[R^2]$ (d) $[R^2T^2]$

9. Let $[\epsilon_0]$ denote the dimensional formula of the permittivity of vacuum. If M = mass, L = length, T = time and A = electric current, then: **[2013]**

(a) $\epsilon_0=[M^{-1}L^{-3}T^2A]$ (b) $\epsilon_0=[M^{-1}L^{-3}T^4A^2]$
(c) $\epsilon_0=[M^1L^2T^1A^2]$ (d) $\epsilon_0=[M^1L^2T^1A]$

10. If the time period *t* of the oscillation of a drop of liquid of density *d*, radius *r*, vibrating under surface tension *s* is given by the formula $t=\sqrt{r^{2b}s^c d^{a/2}}$. It is observed that the time period is directly proportional to $\sqrt{\frac{d}{s}}$. The value of *b* should therefore be : **[Online April 23, 2013]**

(a) $\frac{3}{4}$ (b) $\sqrt{3}$ (c) $\frac{3}{2}$ (d) $\frac{2}{3}$

11. The dimensions of angular momentum, latent heat and capacitance are, respectively. **[Online April 22, 2013]**
(a) $ML^2T^1A^2$, L^2T^{-2}, $M^{-1}L^{-2}T^2$
(b) ML^2T^{-2}, L^2T^2, $M^{-1}L^{-2}T^4A^2$
(c) ML^2T^{-1}, L^2T^{-2}, ML^2TA^2
(d) ML^2T^{-1}, L^2T^{-2}, $M^{-1}L^{-2}T^4A^2$

12. Given that K = energy, V = velocity, T = time. If they are chosen as the fundamental units, then what is dimensional formula for surface tension? **[Online May 7, 2012]**
(a) $[KV^{-2}T^{-2}]$ (b) $[K^2V^2T^{-2}]$
(c) $[K^2V^{-2}T^{-2}]$ (d) $[KV^2T^2]$

13. The dimensions of magnetic field in M, L, T and C (coulomb) is given as **[2008]**
(a) $[MLT^{-1}C^{-1}]$ (b) $[MT^2C^{-2}]$
(c) $[MT^{-1}C^{-1}]$ (d) $[MT^{-2}C^{-1}]$

14. Which of the following units denotes the dimension $\frac{ML^2}{Q^2}$, where Q denotes the electric charge? **[2006]**
(a) Wb/m^2 (b) Henry (H)
(c) H/m^2 (d) Weber (Wb)

15. Out of the following pair, which one does NOT have identical dimensions? **[2005]**
(a) Impulse and momentum
(b) Angular momentum and planck's constant
(c) Work and torque
(d) Moment of inertia and moment of a force

16. Which one of the following represents the correct dimensions of the coefficient of viscosity? **[2004]**
(a) $[ML^{-1}T^{-1}]$ (b) $[MLT^{-1}]$
(c) $[ML^{-1}T^{-2}]$ (d) $[ML^{-2}T^{-2}]$

17. Dimensions of $\frac{1}{\mu_0\varepsilon_0}$, where symbols have their usual meaning, are **[2003]**
(a) $[L^{-1}T]$ (b) $[L^{-2}T^2]$
(c) $[L^2T^{-2}]$ (d) $[LT^{-1}]$

18. The physical quantities not having same dimensions are **[2003]**
(a) torque and work
(b) momentum and planck's constant
(c) stress and young's modulus
(d) speed and $(\mu_0\varepsilon_0)^{-1/2}$

19. Identify the pair whose dimensions are equal **[2002]**
(a) torque and work (b) stress and energy
(c) force and stress (d) force and work

TOPIC-3 : Errors in Measurements

20. The following observations were taken for determining surface tensiton T of water by capillary method :
Diameter of capilary, $D = 1.25 \times 10^{-2}$ m
rise of water, $h = 1.45 \times 10^{-2}$ m
Using $g = 9.80$ m/s^2 and the simplified relation $T = \frac{rhg}{2} \times 10^3$ N/m, the possible error in surface tension is closest to : **[2017]**
(a) 2.4% (b) 10% (c) 0.15% (d) 1.5%

21. A physical quantity P is described by the relation
$P = a^{1/2} b^2 c^3 d^{-4}$
If the relative errors in the measurement of a, b, c and d respectively, are 2%, 1%, 3% and 5%, then the relative error in P will be : **[Online April 9, 2017]**
(a) 8% (b) 12% (c) 32% (d) 25%

22. A screw gauge with a pitch of 0.5 mm and a circular scale with 50 divisions is used to measure the thickness of a thin sheet of Aluminium. Before starting the measurement, it is found that wen the two jaws of the screw gauge are brought in contact, the 45th division coincides with the main scale line and the zero of the main scale is barely visible. What is the thickness of the sheet if the main scale reading is 0.5 mm and the 25th division coincides with the main scale line? **[2016]**
(a) 0.70 mm (b) 0.50 mm (c) 0.75 mm (d) 0.80 mm

23. A student measures the time period of 100 oscillations of a simple pendulum four times. The data set is 90 s, 91 s, 95 s, and 92 s. If the minimum division in the measuring clock is 1 s, then the reported mean time should be: **[2016]**
(a) 92 ± 1.8 s (b) 92 ± 3s
(c) 92 ± 1.5 s (d) 92 ± 5.0 s

24. The period of oscillation of a simple pendulum is $T = 2\pi\sqrt{\frac{L}{g}}$. Measured value of L is 20.0 cm known to 1 mm accuracy and time for 100 oscillations of the pendulum is found to be 90 s using a wrist watch of 1s resolution. The accuracy in the determination of g is : **[2015]**
(a) 1% (b) 5% (c) 2% (d) 3%

25. Diameter of a steel ball is measured using a Vernier callipers which has divisions of 0.1 cm on its main scale (MS) and 10 divisions of its vernier scale (VS) match 9 divisions on the main scale. Three such measurements for a ball are given as: **[Online April 10, 2015]**

S.No.	MS(cm)	VS divisions
1.	0.5	8
2.	0.5	4
3.	0.5	6

If the zero error is – 0.03 cm, then mean corrected diameter is:
(a) 0.52 cm (b) 0.59 cm (c) 0.56 cm (d) 0.53 cm

26. The current voltage relation of a diode is given by $I = \left(e^{1000V/T} - 1\right)$ mA, where the applied voltage V is in volts and the temperature T is in degree kelvin. If a student makes an error measuring ±0.01 V while measuring the current of 5 mA at 300 K, what will be the error in the value of current in mA? **[2014]**
(a) 0.2 mA (b) 0.02 mA (c) 0.5 mA (d) 0.05 mA

27. A student measured the length of a rod and wrote it as 3.50 cm. Which instrument did he use to measure it? [2014]
(a) A meter scale.
(b) A vernier calliper where the 10 divisions in vernier scale matches with 9 division in main scale and main scale has 10 divisions in 1 cm.
(c) A screw gauge having 100 divisions in the circular scale and pitch as 1 mm.
(d) A screw gauge having 50 divisions in the circular scale and pitch as 1 mm.

28. Match List - I (Event) with List-II (Order of the time interval for happening of the event) and select the correct option from the options given below the lists: [Online April 19, 2014]

	List - I		List - II
(1)	Rotation period of earth	(i)	10^5 s
(2)	Revolution period of earth	(ii)	10^7 s
(3)	Period of light wave	(iii)	10^{-15} s
(4)	Period of sound wave	(iv)	10^{-3} s

(a) (1)-(i), (2)-(ii), (3)-(iii), (4)-(iv)
(b) (1)-(ii), (2)-(i), (3)-(iv), (4)-(iii)
(c) (1)-(i), (2)-(ii), (3)-(iv), (4)-(iii)
(d) (1)-(ii), (2)-(i), (3)-(iii), (4)-(iv)

29. In the experiment of calibration of voltmeter, a standard cell of e.m.f. 1.1 volt is balanced against 440 cm of potential wire. The potential difference across the ends of resistance is found to balance against 220 cm of the wire. The corresponding reading of voltmeter is 0.5 volt. The error in the reading of volmeter will be: [Online April 12, 2014]
(a) -0.15 volt (b) 0.15 volt
(c) 0.5 volt (d) -0.05 volt

30. An experiment is performed to obtain the value of acceleration due to gravity g by using a simple pendulum of length L. In this experiment time for 100 oscillations is measured by using a watch of 1 second least count and the value is 90.0 seconds. The length L is measured by using a meter scale of least count 1 mm and the value is 20.0 cm. The error in the determination of g would be: [Online April 9, 2014]
(a) 1.7% (b) 2.7% (c) 4.4% (d) 2.27%

31. Resistance of a given wire is obtained by measuring the current flowing in it and the voltage difference applied across it. If the percentage errors in the measurement of the current and the voltage difference are 3% each, then error in the value of resistance of the wire is [2012]
(a) 6% (b) zero (c) 1% (d) 3%

32. A spectrometer gives the following reading when used to measure the angle of a prism.
Main scale reading : 58.5 degree
Vernier scale reading : 09 divisions
Given that 1 division on main scale corresponds to 0.5 degree. Total divisions on the Vernier scale is 30 and match with 29 divisions of the main scale. The angle of the prism from the above data is [2012]
(a) 58.59 degree (b) 58.77 degree
(c) 58.65 degree (d) 59 degree

33. N divisions on the main scale of a vernier calliper coincide with $(N+1)$ divisions of the vernier scale. If each division of main scale is 'a' units, then the least count of the instrument is [Online May 19, 2012]
(a) a (b) $\frac{a}{N}$
(c) $\frac{N}{N+1}\times a$ (d) $\frac{a}{N+1}$

34. A student measured the diameter of a wire using a screw gauge with the least count 0.001 cm and listed the measurements. The measured value should be recorded as [Online May 12, 2012]
(a) 5.3200 cm (b) 5.3 cm
(c) 5.32 cm (d) 5.320 cm

35. A screw gauge gives the following reading when used to measure the diameter of a wire.
Main scale reading : 0 mm
Circular scale reading : 52 divisions
Given that 1mm on main scale corresponds to 100 divisions of the circular scale. The diameter of wire from the above data is
(a) 0.052 cm (b) 0.026 cm [2011]
(c) 0.005 cm (d) 0.52 cm

36. The respective number of significant figures for the numbers 23.023, 0.0003 and 2.1×10^{-3} are [2010]
(a) 5, 1, 2 (b) 5, 1, 5 (c) 5, 5, 2 (d) 4, 4, 2

37. In an experiment the angles are required to be measured using an instrument, 29 divisions of the main scale exactly coincide with the 30 divisions of the vernier scale. If the smallest division of the main scale is half- a degree (= 0.5°), then the least count of the instrument is: [2009]
(a) half minute (b) one degree
(c) half degree (d) one minute

38. A body of mass m = 3.513 kg is moving along the x-axis with a speed of 5.00 ms^{-1}. The magnitude of its momentum is recorded as [2008]
(a) 17.6 kg ms^{-1} (b) 17.565 kg ms^{-1}
(c) 17.56 kg ms^{-1} (d) 17.57 kg ms^{-1}

39. Two full turns of the circular scale of a screw gauge cover a distance of 1mm on its main scale. The total number of divisions on the circular scale is 50. Further, it is found that the screw gauge has a zero error of – 0.03 mm. While measuring the diameter of a thin wire, a student notes the main scale reading of 3 mm and the number of circular scale divisions in line with the main scale as 35. The diameter of the wire is [2008]
(a) 3.32 mm (b) 3.73 mm (c) 3.67 mm (d) 3.38 mm

Hints & Solutions

TOPIC-1 : Unit of Physical Quantities

1. (b) According to question

$E_y \propto J_x B_Z$

$\therefore$ Constant of proportionality

$$K = \frac{E_y}{B_Z J_x} = \frac{C}{J_x} = \frac{m^3}{As}$$

$\left[\text{As } \frac{E}{B} = C \text{ (speed of light) and } J = \frac{I}{\text{Area}}\right]$

TOPIC-2 : Dimensions of Physical Quantities

2. (a) Let mass, related as $M \propto T^x C^y h^z$

$M^1L^0T^0 = (T^1)^x (L^1T^{-1})^y (M^1L^2T^{-1})^z$

$M^1L^0T^0 = M^z L^{y+2z} + T^{x-y-z}$

$z = 1$

$y + 2z = 0$ $\qquad x - y - z = 0$

$y = -2$ $\qquad x + 2 - 1 = 0$

$x = -1$

$M = [T^{-1}C^{-2}h^1]$

3. (d) Dimension of A $\neq$ dimension of (C)

Hence A – C is not possible.

4. (b) We know that resistivity

$$\rho = \frac{RA}{\ell}$$

$$\text{Conductivity} = \frac{1}{\text{resistivity}} = \frac{\ell}{RA}$$

$$= \frac{\ell I}{VA} \quad (\because V = RI)$$

$$= \frac{[L][I]}{\left[\frac{[ML^2T^{-2}]}{[I][T]}\right] \times [L^2]} \qquad \because V = \frac{W}{q} = \frac{W}{it}$$

$$= [M^{-1}L^{-3}T^3][I^2] = [M^{-1}L^{-3}T^3I^2]$$

5. (c) Let μ_0 related with e, m, c and h as follows.

$\mu_0 = ke^a m^b c^c h^d$

$[MLT^{-2}A^{-2}] = [AT]^a [M]^b [LT^{-1}]^c [ML^2T^{-1}]^d$

$= [M^{b+d}\ L^{c+2d}\ T^{a-c-d}\ A^a]$

On comparing both sides we get

$a = -2$ ...(i)

$b + d = 1$ ...(ii)

$c + 2d = 1$ ...(iii)

$a - c - d = -2$ ...(iv)

By equation (i), (ii), (iii) & (iv) we get,

$a = -2,\ b = 0,\ c = -1,\ d = 1$

$$\therefore [\mu_0] = \left[\frac{h}{ce^2}\right]$$

6. (d) Let unit 'u' related with e, a_0, h and c as follows.

$[u] = [e]^a [a_0]^b [h]^c [C]^d$

Using dimensional method,

$[M^{-1}L^{-2}T^{+4}A^{+2}] = [A^1T^1]^a [L]^b [ML2T^{-1}]^c [LT^{-1}]^d$

$[M^{-1}L^{-2}T^{+4}A^{+2}] = [M^c L^{b+2c+d} T^{a-c-d} A^a]$

$a = 2,\ b = 1,\ c = -1,\ d = -1$

$$\therefore \quad u = \frac{e^2 a_0}{hc}$$

7. (b) The dimensional formulae of

$e = [M^0L^0T^1A^1]$

$\varepsilon_0 = [M^{-1}L^{3}T^4A^2]$

$G = [M^{-1}L^3T^{-2}]$

and $m_e = [M^1L^0T^0]$

Now, $\dfrac{e^2}{2\pi\varepsilon_0 Gm_e^2}$

$$= \frac{[M^0L^0T^1A^1]^2}{2\pi[M^{-1}L^{-3}T^4A^2][M^{-1}L^3T^{-2}][M^1L^0T^0]^2}$$

$$= \frac{[T^2A^2]}{2\pi[M^{-1-1+2}L^{-3+3}T^{4-2}A^2]}$$

$$= \frac{[T^2A^2]}{2\pi[M^0L^0T^2A^2]} = \frac{1}{2\pi}$$

$\because \dfrac{1}{2\pi}$ is dimensionless thus the combination $\dfrac{e^2}{2\pi\varepsilon_0 Gm_e^2}$ would have the same value in different systems of units.

8. (c) Dimensions of $\mu = [MLT^{-2}A^{-2}]$

Dimensions of $\in = [M^{-1}L^{-3}T^4A^2]$

Dimensions of $R = [ML^2T^{-3}A^{-2}]$

$$\therefore \frac{\text{Dimensions of } \mu}{\text{Dimensions of } \in} = \frac{[MLT^{-2}A^{-2}]}{[M^{-1}L^{-3}T^4A^2]}$$

$$= [M^2L^4T^{-6}A^{-4}] = [R^2]$$

9. (b) As we know,

$$F = \frac{1}{4\pi\varepsilon_0}\frac{q_1q_2}{R^2} \Rightarrow \varepsilon_0 = \frac{q_1q_2}{4\pi FR^2}$$

Hence, $\varepsilon_0 = \frac{C^2}{N.m^2} = \frac{[AT]^2}{MLT^{-2}.L^2} = [M^{-1}L^{-3}T^4A^2]$

10. (c)

11. (d) Angular momentum $= m \times v \times r = ML^2T^{-1}$

Latent heat $L = \frac{Q}{m} = \frac{ML^2T^{-2}}{M} = L^2T^{-2}$

Capacitance $C = \frac{\text{Charge}}{\text{P.d.}} = M^{-1}L^{-2}T^4A^2$

12. (a) Surface tension, $T = \frac{F}{\ell} = \frac{F}{\ell}.\frac{\ell}{\ell}.\frac{T^2}{T^2}$

(As, $F.\ell = K$ (energy); $\frac{T^2}{\ell^2} = V^{-2}$)

Therefore, surface tension $= [KV^{-2}T^{-2}]$

13. (c) We know that $F = q\,v\,B$

$\therefore\ B = \frac{F}{qv} = \frac{MLT^{-2}}{C \times LT^{-1}} = MT^{-1}C^{-1}$

14. (b) Mutual inductance $= \frac{\phi}{I} = \frac{BA}{I}$

$[\text{Henry}] = \frac{[MT^{-1}Q^{-1}L^2]}{[QT^{-1}]} = ML^2Q^{-2}$

15. (d) Moment of Inertia, $I = Mr^2$

$[I] = [ML^2]$

Moment of force, $\vec{\tau} = \vec{r} \times \vec{F}$

$[\vec{\tau}] = [L][MLT^{-2}] = [ML^2T^{-2}]$

16. (a) From Stokes law,

$F = 6\pi\eta r v \Rightarrow \eta = \frac{F}{6\pi r v}$

$\therefore \eta = \frac{[MLT^{-2}]}{[L][LT^{-1}]} \Rightarrow \eta = [ML^{-1}T^{-1}]$

17. (c) We know that the velocity of light in vacuum is given by

$c = \frac{1}{\sqrt{\mu_o\varepsilon_o}} \qquad \therefore \frac{1}{\mu_o\varepsilon_o} = c^2 = L^2T^{-2}$

18. (b) Momentum $= mv = [MLT^{-1}]$
Planck's constant,

$h = \frac{E}{\nu} = \frac{[ML^2T^{-2}]}{[T^{-1}]} = [ML^2T^{-1}]$

19. (a) $W = \vec{F}\cdot\vec{s} = Fs\cos\theta$

$= [MLT^{-2}][L] = [ML^2T^{-2}]$;

$\vec{\tau} = \vec{r} \times \vec{F} \Rightarrow \tau = rF\sin\theta$

$= [L][MLT^{-2}] = [ML^2T^{-2}]$

TOPIC-3 : Errors in Measurements

20. (d) Surface tension, $T = \frac{rhg}{2} \times 10^3$

Relative error in surface tension, $\frac{\Delta T}{T} = \frac{\Delta r}{r} + \frac{\Delta h}{h} + 0$

($\because$ g, 2 and 10^3 are constant)

Percentage error

$$100 \times \frac{\Delta T}{T} = \left(\frac{10^{-2} \times 0.01}{1.25 \times 10^{-2}} + \frac{10^{-2} \times 0.01}{1.45 \times 10^{-2}}\right)100$$

$= (0.8 + 0.689)$
$= (1.489) = 1.489\% \cong 1.5\%$

21. (c) Given, $P = a^{1/2}b^2c^2d^{-4}$,
Maximum relative error,

$\frac{\Delta P}{P} = \frac{1}{2}\frac{\Delta a}{a} + 2\frac{\Delta b}{b} + 3\frac{\Delta c}{c} + 4\frac{\Delta d}{d}$

$= \frac{1}{2} \times 2 + 2 \times 1 + 3 \times 3 + 4 \times 5 = 32\%$

22. (d) L.C. $= \frac{0.5}{50} = 0.01$ mm

Zero error $= 5 \times 0.01 = 0.05$ mm (Negative)
Reading $= (0.5 + 25 \times 0.01) + 0.05 = 0.80$ mm

23. (c) $\Delta T = \frac{|\Delta T_1| + |\Delta T_2| + |\Delta T_3| + |\Delta T_4|}{4}$

$= \frac{2 + 1 + 3 + 0}{4} = 1.5$

As the resolution of measuring clock is 1.5 therefore the mean time should be 92 ± 1.5

24. (d) As, $g = 4\pi^2\frac{l}{T^2}$

So, $\frac{\Delta g}{g} \times 100 = \frac{\Delta l}{l} \times 100 + 2\frac{\Delta T}{T} \times 100$

$= \frac{0.1}{20} \times 100 + 2 \times \frac{1}{90} \times 100 = 2.72 \simeq 3\%$

25. (b) Least count $= \frac{0.1}{10} = 0.01$ cm

$d_1 = 0.5 + 8 \times 0.01 + 0.03 = 0.61$ cm
$d_2 = 0.5 + 4 \times 0.01 + 0.03 = 0.57$ cm
$d_3 = 0.5 + 6 \times 0.01 + 0.03 = 0.59$ cm

Mean diameter $= \frac{0.61 + 0.57 + 0.59}{3}$

$= 0.59$ cm

26. (a) The current voltage relation of diode is

$I = (e^{1000\,V/T} - 1)$ mA (given)

When, $I = 5mA$, $e^{1000\,V/T} = 6mA$

Also, $dI = (e^{1000\,V/T}) \times \frac{1000}{T}$ (By exponential function)

$= (6\,mA) \times \frac{1000}{300} \times (0.01) = 0.2$ mA

27. (b) Measured length of rod = 3.50 cm
For vernier scale with 1 Main Scale Division = 1 mm
9 Main Scale Division = 10 Vernier Scale Division,
Least count = 1 MSD – 1 VSD = 0.1 mm

28. (a) Rotation period of earth is about 24 hrs $\simeq 10^5$ s
Revolution period of earth is about 365 days $\simeq 10^7$ s
Speed of light wave $C = 3 \times 10^8$ m/s
Wavelength of visible light of spectrum
$\lambda = 4000 - 7800$ Å

$$C = f\lambda \left(\text{and } T = \frac{1}{f}\right)$$

Therefore period of light wave is 10^{-15} s (approx)

29. (d) In a voltmeter

$V \propto l$
$V = kl$
Now, it is given E = 1.1 volt for $l_1 = 440$ cm
and V = 0.5 volt for $l_2 = 220$ cm
Let the error in reading of voltmeter be ΔV then,
$1.1 = 400$ K and $(0.5 - \Delta V) = 220$ K.

$$\Rightarrow \frac{1.1}{440} = \frac{0.5 - \Delta V}{220}$$

$$\therefore \Delta V = -0.05 \text{ volt}$$

30. (b) According to the question.

$$t = (90 \pm 1) \text{ or, } \frac{\Delta t}{t} = \frac{1}{90}$$

$$l = (20 \pm 0.1) \text{ or, } \frac{\Delta l}{l} = \frac{0.1}{20}$$

$$\frac{\Delta g}{g}\% = ?$$

As we know,

$$t = 2\pi\sqrt{\frac{l}{g}}$$

$$\Rightarrow g = \frac{4\pi^2 l}{t^2}$$

$$\text{or, } \frac{\Delta g}{g} = \pm\left(\frac{\Delta l}{l} + 2\frac{\Delta t}{t}\right)$$

$$= \left(\frac{0.1}{20} + 2 \times \frac{1}{90}\right)$$

$$= 0.027$$

$$\therefore \frac{\Delta g}{g}\% = 2.7\%$$

31. (a) $R = \frac{V}{I} \Rightarrow R \pm \Delta R = \frac{V \pm \Delta V}{I \pm \Delta I}$

$$R\left(1 \pm \frac{\Delta R}{R}\right) = \frac{V}{I}\left(\frac{1 \pm \Delta V/V}{1 \pm \dfrac{\Delta I}{I}}\right)$$

$$\left(\frac{\Delta R}{R}\right) = \left(\frac{\Delta V}{V}\right) + \left(\frac{\Delta I}{I}\right) = (3+3)\% = 6\%$$

32. (c) ∵ Reading of Vernier = Main scale reading + Vernier scale reading × least count.
Main scale reading = 58.5
Vernier scale reading = 09 division
least count of Vernier = 0.5°/30

$$\text{Thus, } R = 58.5° + 9 \times \frac{0.5°}{30}$$

R = 58.65°

33. (d) No of divisions on main scale = N
No of divisions on vernier scale = $N + 1$
size of main scale division = a
Let size of vernier scale division be b
then we have

$$aN = b(N+1) \Rightarrow b = \frac{aN}{N+1}$$

$$\text{Least count is } a - b = a - \frac{aN}{N+1}$$

$$= a\left[\frac{N+1-N}{N+1}\right] = \frac{a}{N+1}$$

34. (d) The least count (L.C.) of a screw guage is the smallest length which can be measured accurately with it.

As least count is 0.001 cm = $\frac{1}{1000}$ cm

Hence measured value should be recorded upto 3 decimal places i.e., 5.320 cm

35. (a) L.C. = $\frac{1}{100}$ mm
Diameter of wire = $MSR + CSR \times L.C.$

$$= 0 + \frac{1}{100} \times 52 = 0.52 \text{ mm} = 0.052 \text{ cm}$$

36. (a) Number of significant figures in 23.023 = 5
Number of significant figures in 0.0003 = 1
Number of significant figures in $2.1 \times 10^{-3} = 2$
So, the radiation belongs to X-rays part of the spectrum.

37. (d) 30 Divisions of vernier scale coincide with 29 divisions of main scales

$$\text{Therefore 1 V.S.D} = \frac{29}{30} \text{ MSD}$$

Least count = 1 MSD – 1VSD

$$= 1 \text{ MSD} - \frac{29}{30} \text{ MSD}$$

$$= \frac{1}{30} \text{ MSD}$$

$$= \frac{1}{30} \times 0.5° = 1 \text{ minute.}$$

38. (a) Momentum, $p = m \times v$
$= (3.513) \times (5.00) = 17.565$ kg m/s
= 17.6 (Rounding off to get three significant figures)

39. (d) Least count of screw gauge

$$= \frac{0.5}{50} \text{ mm} = 0.01 \text{mm}$$

∴ Reading = [Main scale reading + circular scale reading × L.C] – (zero error)
$= [3 + 35 \times 0.01] - (-0.03) = 3.38$ mm

Chapter 2 Motion in a Straight Line

TOPIC-1 : Distance, Displacement & Uniform Motion

1. A car covers the first half of the distance between two places at 40 km/h and other half at 60 km/h. The average speed of the car is **[Online May 7, 2012]**
(a) 40 km/h (b) 45 km/h (c) 48 km/h (d) 60 km/h

2. The velocity of a particle is $v = v_0 + gt + ft^2$. If its position is $x = 0$ at $t = 0$, then its displacement after unit time ($t = 1$) is **[2007]**
(a) $v_0 + g/2 + f$ (b) $v_0 + 2g + 3f$
(c) $v_0 + g/2 + f/3$ (d) $v_0 + g + f$

3. A particle located at $x = 0$ at time $t = 0$, starts moving along with the positive x-direction with a velocity 'v' that varies as $v = \alpha\sqrt{x}$. The displacement of the particle varies with time as **[2006]**
(a) t^2 (b) t (c) $t^{1/2}$ (d) t^3

TOPIC-2 : Non-uniform Motion

4. Which graph corresponds to an object moving with a constant negative acceleration and a positive velocity ? **[Online April 8, 2017]**

(a)
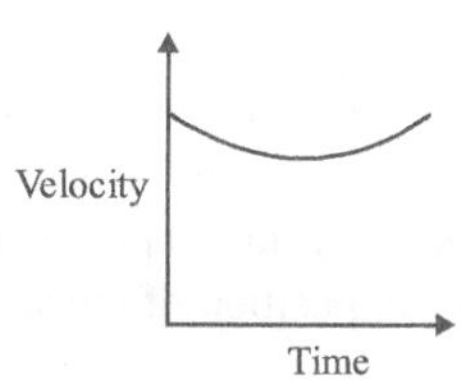

(b)
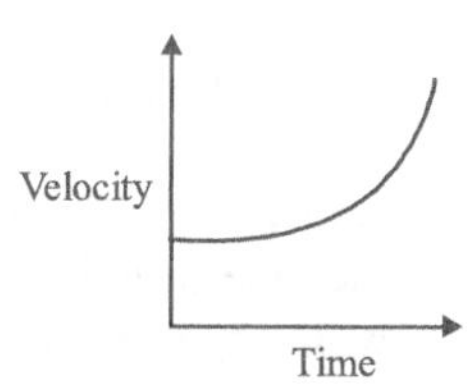

(c)
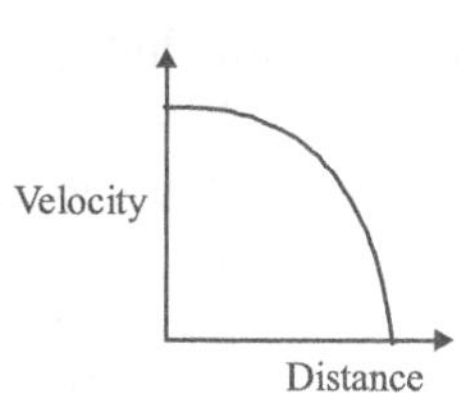

(d)
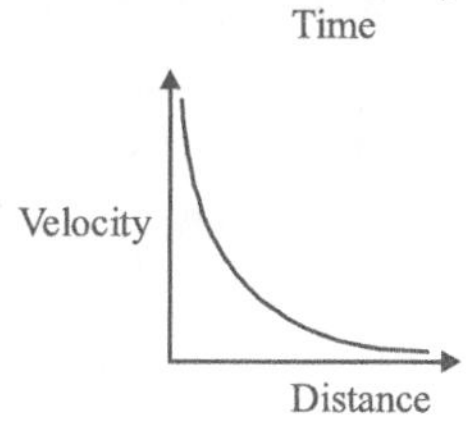

5. The distance travelled by a body moving along a line in time t is proportional to t^3.
The acceleration-time (a, t) graph for the motion of the body will be **[Online May 12, 2012]**

(a)
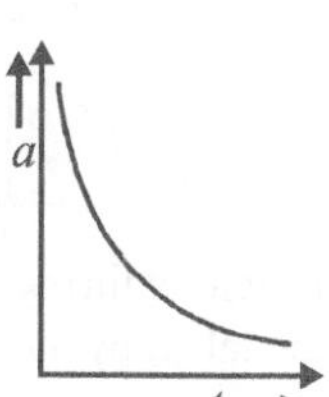

(b)
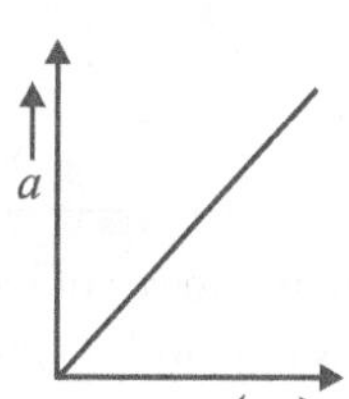

(c)
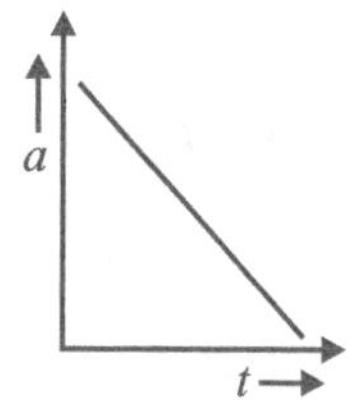

(d)
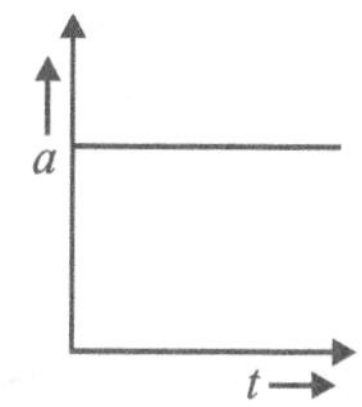

6. The graph of an object's motion (along the x-axis) is shown in the figure. The instantaneous velocity of the object at points A and B are v_A and v_B respectively. Then **[Online May 7, 2012]**

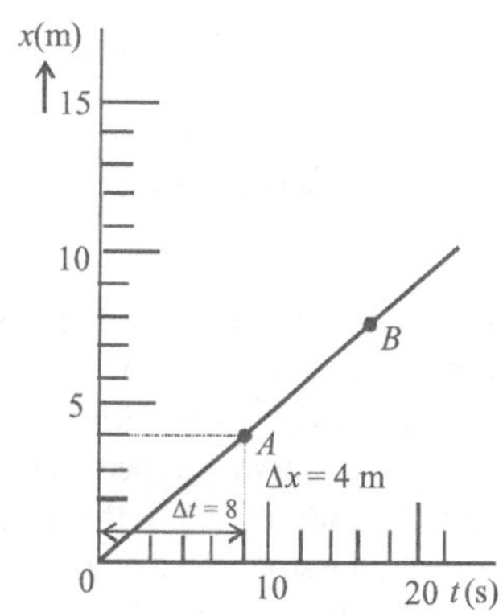

(a) $v_A = v_B = 0.5$ m/s (b) $v_A = 0.5$ m/s $< v_B$
(c) $v_A = 0.5$ m/s $> v_B$ (d) $v_A = v_B = 2$ m/s

7. An object, moving with a speed of 6.25 m/s, is decelerated at a rate given by
$\frac{dv}{dt} = -2.5\sqrt{v}$ where v is the instantaneous speed. The time taken by the object, to come to rest, would be: **[2011]**
(a) 2 s (b) 4 s (c) 8 s (d) 1 s

8. A body is at rest at $x = 0$. At $t = 0$, it starts moving in the positive x-direction with a constant acceleration. At the same instant another body passes through $x = 0$ moving in the positive x-direction with a constant speed. The position of the first body is given by $x_1(t)$ after time 't'; and that of the second body by $x_2(t)$ after the same time interval. Which of the following graphs correctly describes $(x_1 - x_2)$ as a function of time 't'? **[2008]**

(a)
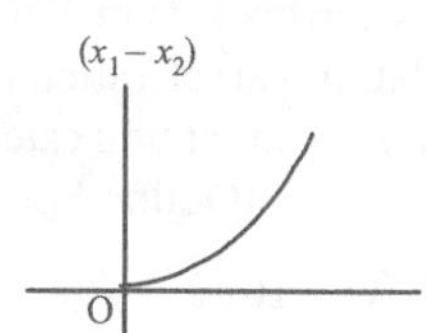

(b)
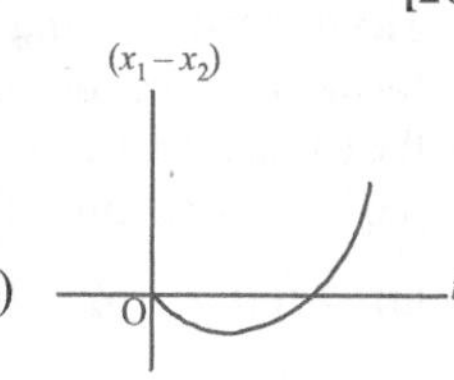

(c) 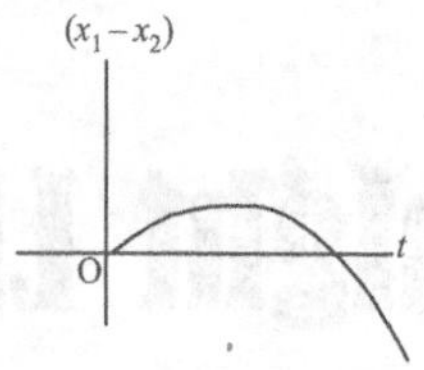

(d) 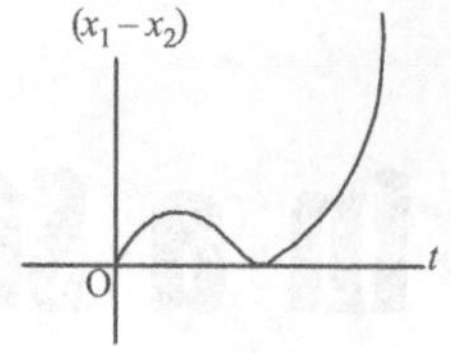

9. A car, starting from rest, accelerates at the rate f through a distance S, then continues at constant speed for time t and then decelerates at the rate $\frac{f}{2}$ to come to rest. If the total distance traversed is 15 S, then **[2005]**

(a) $S=\frac{1}{6}ft^2$ (b) $S=ft$

(c) $S=\frac{1}{4}ft^2$ (d) $S=\frac{1}{72}ft^2$

10. A particle is moving eastwards with a velocity of 5 ms^{-1}. In 10 seconds the velocity changes to 5 ms^{-1} northwards. The average acceleration in this time is **[2005]**

(a) $\frac{1}{2}ms^{-2}$ towards north

(b) $\frac{1}{\sqrt{2}}ms^{-2}$ towards north - east

(c) $\frac{1}{\sqrt{2}}ms^{-2}$ towards north - west

(d) zero

11. The relation between time t and distance x is $t = ax^2 + bx$ where a and b are constants. The acceleration is **[2005]**

(a) $2bv^3$ (b) $-2abv^2$ (c) $2av^2$ (d) $-2av^3$

12. An automobile travelling with a speed of 60 km/h, can brake to stop within a distance of 20m. If the car is going twice as fast i.e., 120 km/h, the stopping distance will be **[2004]**

(a) 60m (b) 40m (c) 20m (d) 80m

13. A car, moving with a speed of 50 km/hr, can be stopped by brakes after at least 6 m. If the same car is moving at a speed of 100 km/hr, the minimum stopping distance is **[2003]**

(a) 12m (b) 18m (c) 24m (d) 6m

14. If a body looses half of its velocity on penetrating 3 cm in a wooden block, then how much will it penetrate more before coming to rest? **[2002]**

(a) 1 cm (b) 2 cm (c) 3 cm (d) 4 cm.

15. Speeds of two identical cars are u and $4u$ at the specific instant. The ratio of the respective distances in which the two cars are stopped from that instant is **[2002]**

(a) 1 : 1 (b) 1 : 4 (c) 1 : 8 (d) 1 : 16

TOPIC-3 : Relative Velocity

16. A car is standing 200 m behind a bus, which is also at rest. The two start moving at the same instant but with different forward accelerations. The bus has acceleration 2 m/s^2 and the car has acceleration 4 m/s^2. The car will catch up with the bus after a time of : **[Online April 9, 2017]**

(a) $\sqrt{110}$ s (b) $\sqrt{120}$ s (c) $10\sqrt{2}$ s (d) 15 s

17. A person climbs up a stalled escalator in 60 s. If standing on the same but escalator running with constant velocity he takes 40 s. How much time is taken by the person to walk up the moving escalator? **[Online April 12, 2014]**

(a) 37 s (b) 27 s (c) 24 s (d) 45 s

18. A goods train accelerating uniformly on a straight railway track, approaches an electric pole standing on the side of track. Its engine passes the pole with velocity u and the guard's room passes with velocity v. The middle wagon of the train passes the pole with a velocity. **[Online May 19, 2012]**

(a) $\frac{u+v}{2}$ (b) $\frac{1}{2}\sqrt{u^2+v^2}$

(c) $\sqrt{uv}$ (d) $\sqrt{\left(\frac{u^2+v^2}{2}\right)}$

TOPIC-4 : Motion Under Gravity

19. A body is thrown vertically upwards. Which one of the following graphs correctly represent the velocity vs time? **[2017]**

(a) 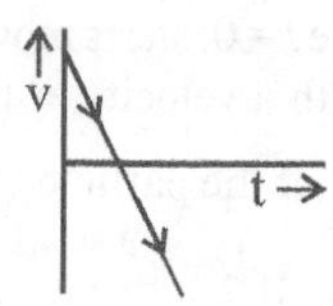

(b) 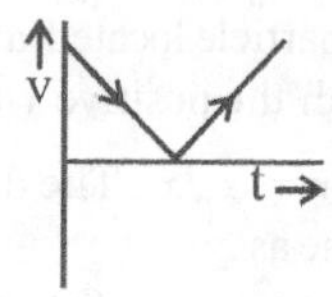

(c) 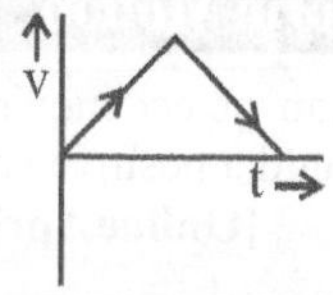

(d) 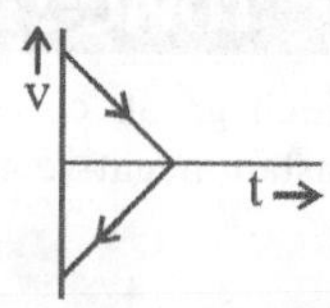

20. Two stones are thrown up simultaneously from the edge of a cliff 240 m high with initial speed of 10 m/s and 40 m/s respectively. Which of the following graph best represents the time variation of relative position of the second stone with respect to the first ?

(Assume stones do not rebound after hitting the ground and neglect air resistance, take g = 10 m/ s^2) **[2015]**

(*The figures are schematic and not drawn to scale*)

(a) 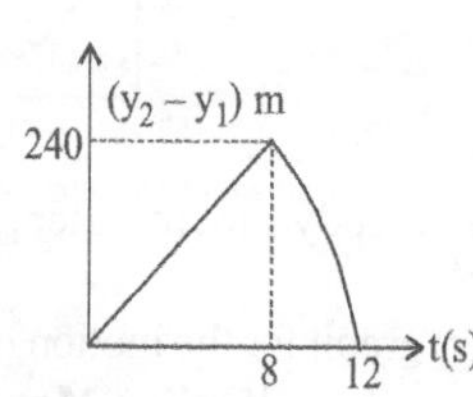

(b) 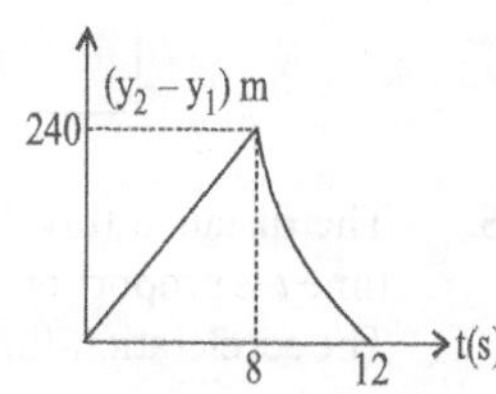

(c) 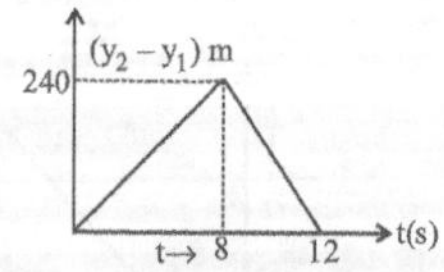

(d) 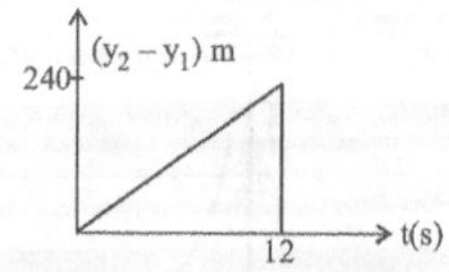

21. From a tower of height H, a particle is thrown vertically upwards with a speed u. The time taken by the particle, to hit the ground, is n times that taken by it to reach the highest point of its path. The relation between H, u and n is: **[2014]**

(a) $2gH = n^2u^2$ (b) $gH = (n-2)^2 u^2 d$
(c) $2gH = nu^2(n-2)$ (d) $gH = (n-2)u^2$

22. Consider a rubber ball freely falling from a height $h = 4.9$ m onto a horizontal elastic plate. Assume that the duration of collision is negligible and the collision with the plate is totally elastic.
Then the velocity as a function of time and the height as a function of time will be: **[2009]**

(a) 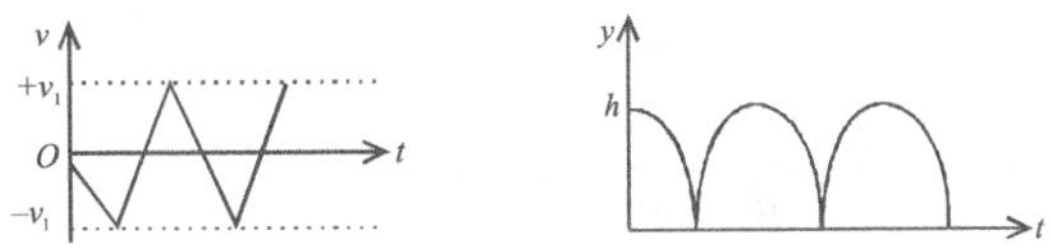

(b) 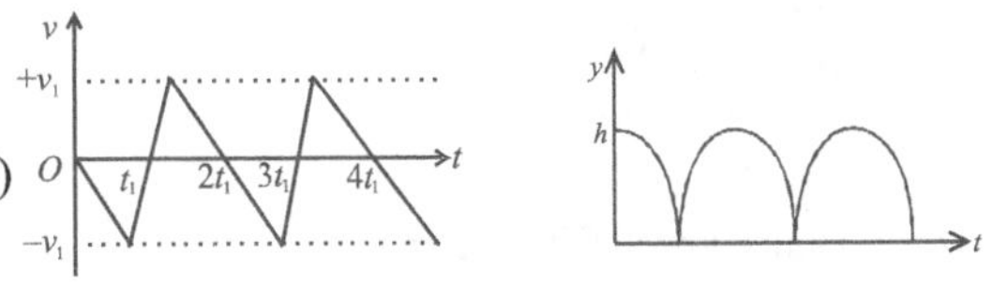

(c) 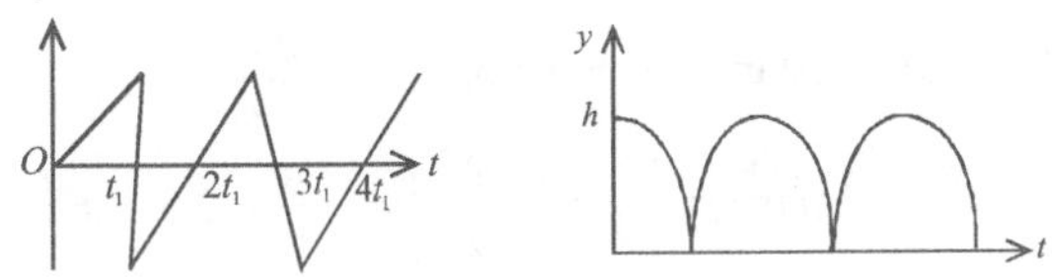

(d) 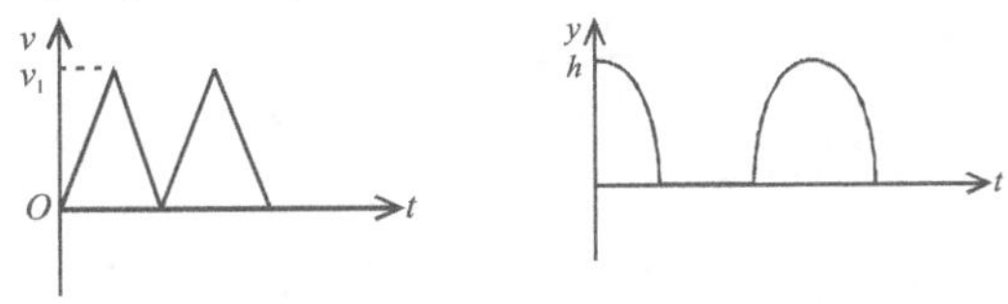

23. A parachutist after bailing out falls 50 m without friction. When parachute opens, it decelerates at 2 m/s^2. He reaches the ground with a speed of 3 m/s. At what height, did he bail out? **[2005]**

(a) 182m (b) 91m (c) 111m (d) 293m

24. A ball is released from the top of a tower of height h meters. It takes T seconds to reach the ground. What is the position of the ball at $\frac{T}{3}$ second **[2004]**

(a) $\frac{8h}{9}$ meters from the ground

(b) $\frac{7h}{9}$ meters from the ground

(c) $\frac{h}{9}$ meters from the ground

(d) $\frac{17h}{18}$ meters from the ground

25. From a building two balls A and B are thrown such that A is thrown upwards and B downwards (both vertically). If v_A and v_B are their respective velocities on reaching the ground, then **[2002]**

(a) $v_B > v_A$
(b) $v_A = v_B$
(c) $v_A > v_B$
(d) their velocities depend on their masses.

Hints & Solutions

TOPIC-1 : Distance, Displacement & Uniform motion

1. (c) Average speed $= \frac{\text{Total distance travelled}}{\text{Total time taken}} = \frac{x}{T}$

$$= \frac{x}{\frac{x}{2\times 40}+\frac{x}{2\times 60}} = 48 \text{ km/h}$$

2. (c) We know that, $v = \frac{dx}{dt} \Rightarrow dx = v\,dt$

Integrating, $\int_0^x dx = \int_0^t v\,dt$

or $x = \int_0^t (v_0 + gt + ft^2)\,dt$

$$= \left[v_0 t + \frac{gt^2}{2} + \frac{ft^3}{3}\right]_0^t$$

or, $x = v_0 t + \frac{gt^2}{2} + \frac{ft^3}{3}$

At $t = 1$, $x = v_0 + \frac{g}{2} + \frac{f}{3}$.

3. (a) $v = \alpha\sqrt{x}$, $\frac{dx}{dt} = \alpha\sqrt{x} \Rightarrow \frac{dx}{\sqrt{x}} = \alpha\,dt$

$$\int_0^x \frac{dx}{\sqrt{x}} = \alpha\int_0^t dt$$

$$\left[\frac{2\sqrt{x}}{1}\right]_0^x = \alpha[t]_0^t$$

$$\Rightarrow 2\sqrt{x} = \alpha t \Rightarrow x = \frac{\alpha^2}{4}t^2$$

TOPIC-2 : Non-uniform motion

4. (c) According to question, object is moving with constant negative acceleration i.e., a = – constant (C)

$$\frac{vdv}{dx} = -C$$

$$vdv = -Cdx$$

$$\frac{v^2}{2} = -Cx + k$$

$$x = -\frac{v^2}{2C} + \frac{k}{C}$$

Hence, graph (3) represents correctly.

5. (b) Distance along a line i.e., displacement (s) $= t^3$ ($\because s \propto t^3$ given)

By double differentiation of displacement, we get acceleration.

$$V = \frac{ds}{dt} = \frac{dt^3}{dt} = 3t^2 \text{ and}$$

$$a = \frac{dv}{dt} = \frac{d3t^2}{dt} = 6t$$

$a = 6t$ or $a \propto t$

Hence graph (b) is correct.

6. (a) Instantaneous velocity $v = \frac{\Delta x}{\Delta t}$

From graph, $v_A = \frac{\Delta x_A}{\Delta t_A} = \frac{4m}{8s} = 0.5$ m/s

and $v_B = \frac{\Delta x_B}{\Delta t_B} = \frac{8m}{16s} = 0.5$ m/s

i.e., $v_A = v_B = 0.5$ m/s

7. (a) $\frac{dv}{dt} = -2.5\sqrt{v}$

$$\Rightarrow \frac{dv}{\sqrt{v}} = -2.5\,dt$$

Integrating,

$$\int_{6.25}^{0} v^{-1/2} dv = -2.5\int_0^t dt$$

$$\Rightarrow \left[\frac{v^{+1/2}}{(1/2)}\right]_{6.25}^{0} = -2.5[t]_0^t$$

$\Rightarrow -2(6.25)^{1/2} = -2.5t$

$\Rightarrow t = 2$ sec

8. (b) **For the body starting from rest**

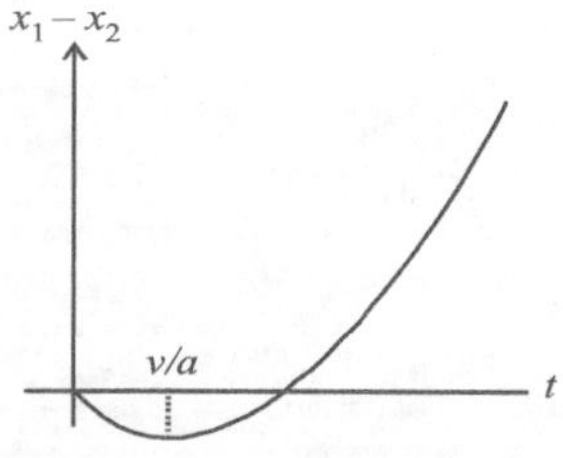

$$x_1 = 0 + \frac{1}{2}at^2$$

$$\Rightarrow x_1 = \frac{1}{2}at^2$$

For the body moving with constant speed

$x_2 = vt$

$\therefore\ x_1 - x_2 = \frac{1}{2}at^2 - vt$

at $t = 0$, $x_1 - x_2 = 0$

For $t < \frac{v}{a}$; the slope is negative

For $t = \frac{v}{a}$; the slope is zero

For $t > \frac{v}{a}$; the slope is positive

These characteristics are represented by graph (b).

9. **(d)** Distance from A to $B = S = \frac{1}{2} f t_1^2$

Distance from B to $C = (f t_1) t$

Distance from C to $D = \frac{u^2}{2a} = \frac{(f t_1)^2}{2(f/2)} = f t_1^2 = 2S$

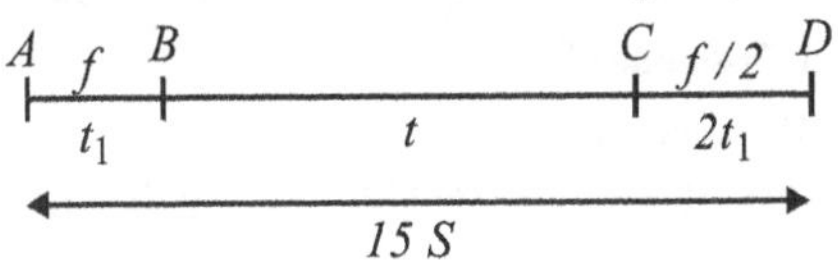

$\Rightarrow \quad S + f t_1 t + 2S = 15S$

$\Rightarrow \quad f t_1 t = 12S$ .... (i)

$\frac{1}{2} f t_1^2 = S$ .... (ii)

Dividing (i) by (ii), we get $t_1 = \frac{t}{6}$

$\Rightarrow \quad S = \frac{1}{2} f \left(\frac{t}{6}\right)^2 = \frac{f t^2}{72}$

10. **(c)** Average acceleration

$= \frac{\text{change in velocity}}{\text{time interval}} = \frac{\Delta \vec{v}}{t}$

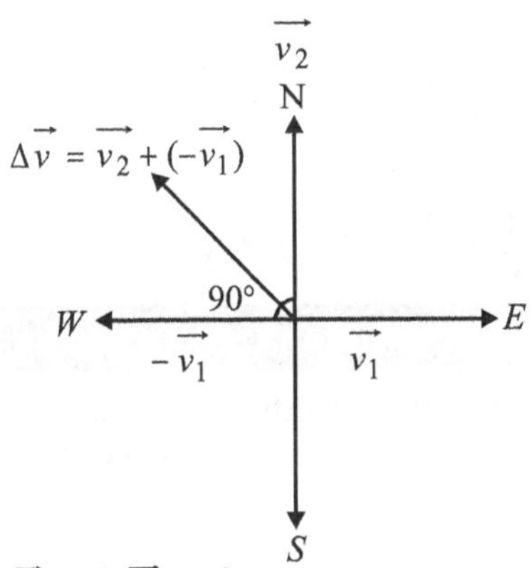

$\vec{v_1} = 5\hat{i}, \vec{v_2} = 5\hat{j}$

$\Delta \vec{v} = (\vec{v}_2 - \vec{v}_1)$

$= \sqrt{v_1^2 + v_2^2 + 2 v_1 v_2 \cos 90}$

$= \sqrt{5^2 + 5^2 + 0}$

[As $|v_1| = |v_2| = 5$ m/s]

$= 5\sqrt{2}$ m/s

Avg. acc. $= \frac{\Delta \vec{v}}{t} = \frac{5\sqrt{2}}{10} = \frac{1}{\sqrt{2}}$ m/s^2

$\tan \theta = \frac{5}{-5} = -1$

which means θ is in the second quadrant. (towards north -west)

11. **(d)** $t = ax^2 + bx$; Diff. with respect to time (t)

$\frac{d}{dt}(t) = a\frac{d}{dt}(x^2) + b\frac{dx}{dt} = a.2x\frac{dx}{dt} + \text{b.v.}$

$1 = 2axv + bv = v(2ax + b)(v = \text{velocity})$

$2ax + b = \frac{1}{v}.$

Again differentiating,

$2a\frac{dx}{dt} + 0 = -\frac{1}{v^2}\frac{dv}{dt}$

$\Rightarrow \quad \frac{dv}{dt} = f = -2av^3 \left(\because \frac{dx}{dt} = v\right)$

12. **(d)** Speed, $u = 60 \times \frac{5}{18}$ m/s $= \frac{50}{3}$ m/s

$d = 20\text{m}, u' = 120 \times \frac{5}{18} = \frac{100}{3}$ m/s

Let declaration be a then $(0)^2 - u^2 = -2ad$

or $\quad u^2 = 2ad$ ...(1)

and $(0)^2 - u'^2 = -2ad'$

or $\quad u'^2 = 2ad'$ ...(2)

(2) divided by (1) gives,

$4 = \frac{d'}{d} \Rightarrow d' = 4 \times 20 = 80\text{m}$

13. **(c)** **Case-1 :** $u = 50 \times \frac{5}{18}$ m/s,

$v = 0, s = 6\text{m}, a = a$

$v^2 - u^2 = 2as$

$\Rightarrow 0^2 - \left(50 \times \frac{5}{18}\right)^2 = 2 \times a \times 6$

$\Rightarrow -\left(50 \times \frac{5}{18}\right)^2 = 2 \times a \times 6$ ....(i)

Case-2 : $u = 100$ km/hr $= 100 \times \frac{5}{18}$ m/sec

$v = 0, s = s, a = a \quad \therefore v^2 - u^2 = 2as$

$\Rightarrow 0^2 - \left(100 \times \frac{5}{18}\right)^2 = 2as$

$\Rightarrow -\left(100 \times \frac{5}{18}\right)^2 = 2as$ ...(ii)

Dividing (i) and (ii) we get

$\frac{100 \times 100}{50 \times 50} = \frac{2 \times a \times s}{2 \times a \times 6} \Rightarrow s = 24\text{m}$

14. (a) Activity *A* to *B*

$u_1 = u\,;\, v_1 = \dfrac{u}{2}, s_1 = 0.03$ m, $a_1 = ?$

$v_1^2 - u_1^2 = 2a_1 s_1$ ...(i)

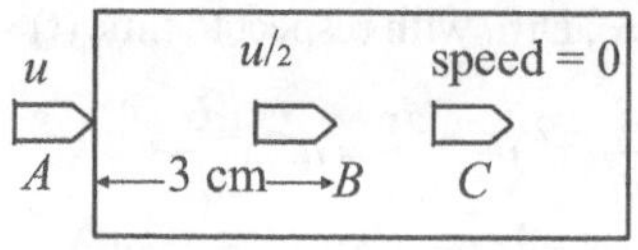

$\therefore \left(\dfrac{u}{2}\right)^2 - u^2 = 2 \times a \times 0.03$

$\Rightarrow \dfrac{u^2}{4} - u^2 = 0.06a \Rightarrow -\dfrac{3}{4}u^2 = 0.06a$

$\Rightarrow a = \dfrac{-3}{4 \times 0.06}u^2$

Activity *B* to *C*: Assuming the same retardation

$u_2 = u/2\,;\, v_2 = 0\,;\, s_2 = ?\,;\, a_2 = \dfrac{-3}{4 \times 0.06}u^2$

$v_2^2 - u_2^2 = 2a_2 \times s_2$ ...(ii)

$\therefore 0 - \dfrac{u^2}{4} = 2\left(\dfrac{-3\ u^2}{4 \times 0.06}\right) \times s_2$

$\Rightarrow s_2 = \dfrac{1}{100} m = 1\,cm$

Alternatively, dividing (i) and (ii),

$\dfrac{v_1^2 - u_1^2}{v_2^2 - u_2^2} = \dfrac{2a \times s_1}{2a \times s_2}$

$\Rightarrow \dfrac{\left(\dfrac{u}{2}\right)^2 - u^2}{0 - \left(\dfrac{u}{2}\right)^2} = \dfrac{0.03}{s_2} \Rightarrow s_2 = 1\ cm.$

15. (d) For car 1

$u_1 = u,\, v_1 = 0,\, a_1 = -a,\, s_1 = s_1$

$\therefore \quad v_1^2 - u_1^2 = 2a_1 s_1 \Rightarrow -u^2 = -2as_1$

$\Rightarrow u^2 = 2as_1$ ...(i)

For car 2

$u_2 = 4u,\, v_1 = 0,\, a_2 = -a,\, s_2 = s_2$

$\therefore \quad v_2^2 - u_2^2 = 2a_2 s_2 \Rightarrow -(4u)^2 = 2(-a)\,s_2$

$\Rightarrow 16\,u^2 = 2as_2$ ...(ii)

Dividing (i) and (ii),

$\dfrac{u^2}{16u^2} = \dfrac{2as_1}{2as_2} \Rightarrow \dfrac{1}{16} = \dfrac{s_1}{s_2}$

TOPIC-3 : Relative Velocity

16. (c)

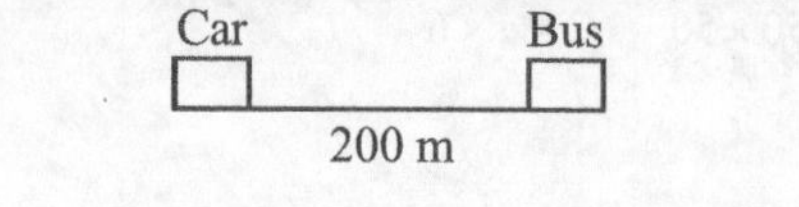

Given, $u_C = u_B = 0,\, a_C = 4\ m/s^2,\, a_B = 2\ m/s^2$

hence relative acceleration, $a_{CB} = 2\ m/sec^2$

Now, we know, $s = ut + \dfrac{1}{2}at^2$

$200 = \dfrac{1}{2} \times 2t^2 \quad \because u = 0$

Hence, the car will catch up with the bus after time

$t = 10\sqrt{2}$ second

17. (c) Person's speed walking only is $\dfrac{1}{60} \dfrac{\text{"escalator"}}{\text{second}}$

Standing the escalator without walking the speed is

$\dfrac{1}{40} \dfrac{\text{"escalator"}}{\text{second}}$

Walking with the escalator going, the speed add.

So, the person's speed is $\dfrac{1}{60} + \dfrac{1}{40} = \dfrac{15}{120} \dfrac{\text{"escalator"}}{\text{second}}$

So, the time to go up the escalator $t = \dfrac{120}{5} = 24$ second.

18. (d) Let '*S*' be the distance between two ends '*a*' be the constant acceleration

As we know $v^2 - u^2 = 2aS$

or, $aS = \dfrac{v^2 - u^2}{2}$

Let *v* be velocity at mid point.

Therefore, $v_c^2 - u^2 = 2a\dfrac{S}{2}$

$v_c^2 = u^2 + aS$

$v_c^2 = u^2 + \dfrac{v^2 - u^2}{2}$

$v_c = \sqrt{\dfrac{u^2 + v^2}{2}}$

TOPIC-4 : Motion Under Gravity

19. (a) For a body thrown vertically upwards acceleration remains constant ($a = -g$) and velocity at anytime *t* is given by $V = u - gt$

During rise velocity decreases linearly and during fall velocity increases linearly and direction is opposite to each other.

Hence graph (1) correctly depicts velocity versus time.

20. (b) $y_1 = 10t - 5t^2\,;\, y_2 = 40t - 5t^2$

for $y_1 = -240$m, $t = 8$s

$\therefore \quad y_2 - y_1 = 30t$ for $t \leq 8$s.

for $t > 8$s,

$y_2 - y_1 = 240 - 40t - \dfrac{1}{2}gt^2$

21. (c) Speed on reaching ground

$v = \sqrt{u^2 + 2gh}$

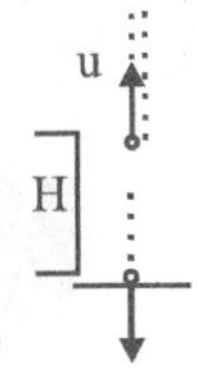

Now, $v = u + at$

$\Rightarrow \sqrt{u^2 + 2gh} = -u + gt$

Time taken to reach highest point is $t = \frac{u}{g}$,

$\Rightarrow t = \frac{u + \sqrt{u^2 + 2gH}}{g} = \frac{nu}{g}$ (from question)

$\Rightarrow 2gH = n(n-2)u^2$

22. **(b)** For downward motion $v = -gt$
The velocity of the rubber ball increases in downward direction and we get a straight line between v and t with a negative slope.

Also applying $y - y_0 = ut + \frac{1}{2}at^2$

We get $y - h = -\frac{1}{2}gt^2 \Rightarrow y = h - \frac{1}{2}gt^2$

The graph between y and t is a parabola with $y = h$ at $t = 0$. As time increases y decreases.

For upward motion.

The ball suffer elastic collision with the horizontal elastic plate therefore the direction of velocity is reversed and the magnitude remains the same.
Here $v = u - gt$ where u is the velocity just after collision.
As t increases, v decreases. We get a straight line between v and t with negative slope.

Also $y = ut - \frac{1}{2}gt^2$

All these characteristics are represented by graph (b).

23. **(d)** Initial velocity of parachute after bailing out,

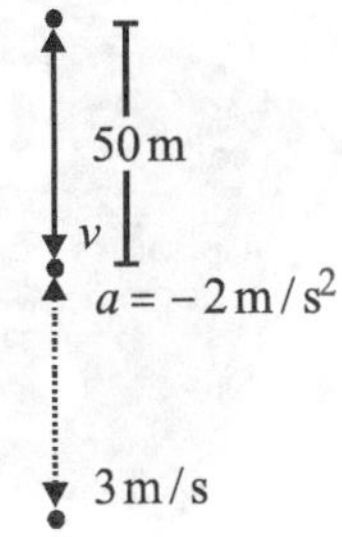

$u = \sqrt{2gh}$

$u = \sqrt{2 \times 9.8 \times 50} = 14\sqrt{5}$

The velocity at ground,
$v = 3 m/s$

$S = \frac{v^2 - u^2}{2 \times 2} = \frac{3^2 - 980}{4} \approx 243$ m

Initially he has fallen 50 m.
$\therefore$ Total height from where he bailed out $= 243 + 50 = 293$ m

24. **(a)** We have $s = ut + \frac{1}{2}gt^2$,

or $h = \frac{1}{2}gT^2$ $\quad (\because u = 0)$

now for $T/3$ second, vertical distance moved is given by

$h' = \frac{1}{2}g\left(\frac{T}{3}\right)^2 \Rightarrow h' = \frac{1}{2} \times \frac{gT^2}{9} = \frac{h}{9}$

$\therefore$ position of ball from ground $= h - \frac{h}{9} = \frac{8h}{9}$

25. **(b)** Ball A is thrown upwards from the building. During its downward journey when it comes back to the point of throw, its speed is equal to the speed of throw. So, for the journey of both the balls from point A to B.

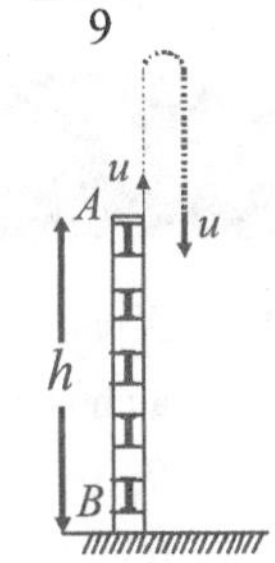

We can apply $v^2 - u^2 = 2gh$.
As u, g, h are same for both the balls, $v_A = v_B$

Chapter 3

Motion in a Plane

TOPIC-1 : Vectors

1. A vector $\vec{A}$ is rotated by a small angle $\Delta\theta$ radian ($\Delta\theta << 1$) to get a new vector $\vec{B}$ In that case $|\vec{B}-\vec{A}|$ is : **[Online April 11, 2015]**

(a) $|\vec{A}|\Delta\theta$ (b) $|\vec{B}|\Delta\theta-|\vec{A}|$

(c) $|\vec{A}|\left(1-\frac{\Delta\theta^2}{2}\right)$ (d) 0

2. If $\vec{A}\times\vec{B}=\vec{B}\times\vec{A}$, then the angle between A and B is **[2004]**

(a) $\frac{\pi}{2}$ (b) $\frac{\pi}{3}$ (c) π (d) $\frac{\pi}{4}$

TOPIC-2 : Motion in a Plane with Constant Acceleration

3. A particle is moving with velocity $\vec{v}=k(y\hat{i}+x\hat{j})$, where k is a constant. The general equation for its path is **[2010]**

(a) $y=x^2+$ constant (b) $y^2=x+$ constant

(c) $xy=$ constant (d) $y^2=x^2+$ constant

4. A particle has an initial velocity of $3\hat{i}+4\hat{j}$ and an acceleration of $0.4\hat{i}+0.3\hat{j}$. Its speed after 10 s is : **[2009]**

(a) $7\sqrt{2}$ units (b) 7 units

(c) 8.5 units (d) 10 units

5. The co-ordinates of a moving particle at any time 't' are given by $x=\alpha t^3$ and $y=\beta t^3$. The speed of the particle at time 't' is given by **[2003]**

(a) $3t\sqrt{\alpha^2+\beta^2}$ (b) $3t^2\sqrt{\alpha^2+\beta^2}$

(c) $t^2\sqrt{\alpha^2+\beta^2}$ (d) $\sqrt{\alpha^2+\beta^2}$

TOPIC-3 : Projectile Motion

6. The initial speed of a bullet fired from a rifle is 630 m/s. The rifle is fired at the centre of a target 700 m away at the same level as the target. How far above the centre of the target ? **[Online April 11, 2014]**

(a) 1.0m (b) 4.2m (c) 6.1m (d) 9.8m

7. The position of a projectile launched from the origin at $t=0$ is given by $\vec{r}=(40\hat{i}+50\hat{j})$ m at $t=2$s. If the projectile was launched at an angle θ from the horizontal, then θ is (take g = 10 ms^{-2}) **[Online April 9, 2014]**

(a) $\tan^{-1}\frac{2}{3}$ (b) $\tan^{-1}\frac{3}{2}$ (c) $\tan^{-1}\frac{7}{4}$ (d) $\tan^{-1}\frac{4}{5}$

8. A projectile is given an initial velocity of $(\hat{i}+2\hat{j})$ m/s, where $\hat{i}$ is along the ground and $\hat{j}$ is along the vertical. If g = 10 m/s^2, the equation of its trajectory is : **[2013]**

(a) $y=x-5x^2$ (b) $y=2x-5x^2$

(c) $4y=2x-5x^2$ (d) $4y=2x-25x^2$

9. The maximum range of a bullet fired from a toy pistol mounted on a car at rest is R_0= 40 m. What will be the acute angle of inclination of the pistol for maximum range when the car is moving in the direction of firing with uniform velocity v = 20 m/s, on a horizontal surface ? (g = 10 m/s^2) **[Online April 25, 2013]**

(a) 30° (b) 60° (c) 75° (d) 45°

10. A ball projected from ground at an angle of 45° just clears a wall in front. If point of projection is 4 m from the foot of wall and ball strikes the ground at a distance of 6 m on the other side of the wall, the height of the wall is : **[Online April 22, 2013]**

(a) 4.4m (b) 2.4m (c) 3.6m (d) 1.6m

11. A boy can throw a stone up to a maximum height of 10 m. The maximum horizontal distance that the boy can throw the same stone up to will be **[2012]**

(a) $20\sqrt{2}$ m (b) 10m

(c) $10\sqrt{2}$ m (d) 20m

12. A water fountain on the ground sprinkles water all around it. If the speed of water coming out of the fountain is v, the total area around the fountain that gets wet is : **[2011]**

(a) $\pi\frac{v^4}{g^2}$ (b) $\frac{\pi}{2}\frac{v^4}{g^2}$ (c) $\pi\frac{v^2}{g^2}$ (d) $\pi\frac{v^2}{g}$

13. A projectile can have the same range 'R' for two angles of projection. If 'T_1' and 'T_2' to be time of flights in the two cases, then the product of the two time of flights is directly proportional to. **[2004]**

(a) R (b) $\frac{1}{R}$ (c) $\frac{1}{R^2}$ (d) R^2

14. A ball is thrown from a point with a speed 'v_0' at an elevation angle of θ. From the same point and at the same instant, a person starts running with a constant speed $\frac{'v_0'}{2}$ to catch the ball. Will the person be able to catch the ball? If yes, what should be the angle of projection θ ? **[2004]**

(a) No (b) Yes, 30° (c) Yes, 60° (d) Yes, 45°

15. A boy playing on the roof of a 10 m high building throws a ball with a speed of 10m/s at an angle of 30° with the horizontal. How far from the throwing point will the ball be at the height of 10 m from the ground ? **[2003]**

$[g = 10\text{m/s}^2,\ \sin 30^o = \frac{1}{2},\ \cos 30^o = \frac{\sqrt{3}}{2}]$

(a) 5.20m (b) 4.33m (c) 2.60m (d) 8.66m

TOPIC-4 : Relative Velocity in Two Dimensions & Uniform Circular Motion

16. If a body moving in circular path maintains constant speed of 10 ms^{-1}, then which of the following correctly describes relation between acceleration and radius ?

[Online April 10, 2015]

(a) 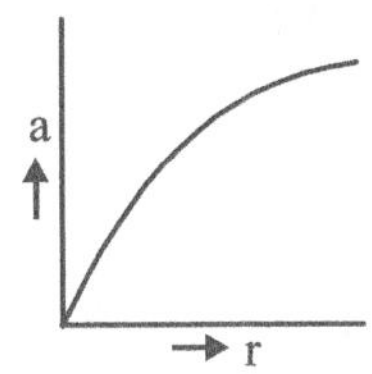

(b) 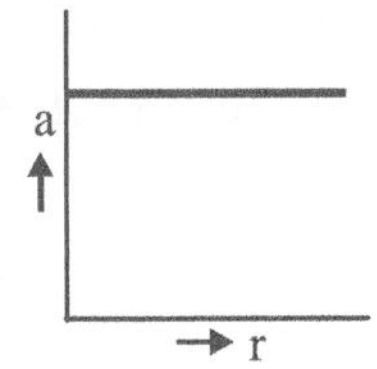

(c) 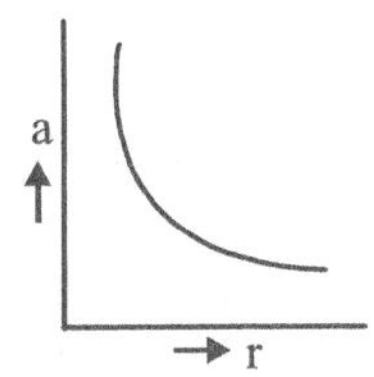

(d) 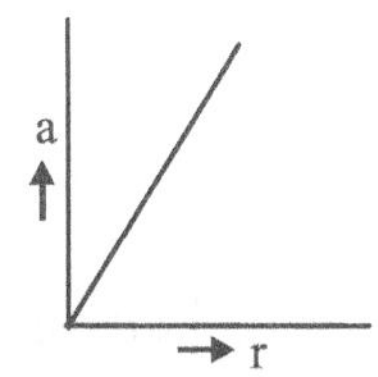

Hints & Solutions

TOPIC-1 : Vectors

1. (a) Arc length = radius × angle

So, $|\vec{B}-\vec{A}|=|\vec{A}|\Delta\theta$

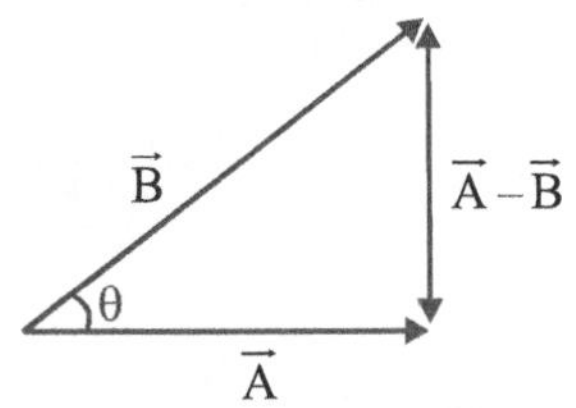

2. (c) $\vec{A}\times\vec{B}-\vec{B}\times\vec{A}=0 \Rightarrow \vec{A}\times\vec{B}+\vec{A}\times\vec{B}=0$

$\therefore \vec{A}\times\vec{B}=0$

Angle between them is 0, π, or 2 π

from the given options, $\theta=\pi$

TOPIC-2 : Motion in a Plane with Constant Acceleration

3. (d) $\vec{v}=k(y\hat{i}+x\hat{j})$

x-component of $v=ky$

$$\Rightarrow \frac{dx}{dt}=ky \quad ...(1)$$

y-component of $v=kx$

$$\Rightarrow \frac{dy}{dt}=kx \quad ...(2)$$

From (1) and (2), $\frac{dy}{dx}=\frac{x}{y}$

$\Rightarrow ydy=xdx \Rightarrow y^2=x^2+\text{constant}$

4. (a) Given $\vec{u}=3\hat{i}+4\hat{j}$, $\vec{a}=0.4\hat{i}+0.3\hat{j}$, $t=10$ s

$\vec{v}=\vec{u}+\vec{a}t=3\hat{i}+4\hat{j}+(0.4\hat{i}+0.3\hat{j})\times 10$

$=7\hat{i}+7\hat{j}$

$\therefore |\vec{v}|=\sqrt{7^2+7^2}=7\sqrt{2}$ units

5. (b) $x=\alpha t^3$ and $y=\beta t^3$

$v_x=\frac{dx}{dt}=3\alpha t^2$ and $v_y=\frac{dy}{dt}=3\beta t^2$

$\therefore v=\sqrt{v_x^2+v_y^2}=\sqrt{9\alpha^2t^4+9\beta^2t^4}$

$=3t^2\sqrt{\alpha^2+\beta^2}$

TOPIC-3 : Projectile Motion

6. (c) Let 't' be the time taken by the bullet to hit the target.

$\therefore$ 700 m = 630 ms^{-1} t

$$\Rightarrow t=\frac{700\text{m}}{630\text{ms}^{-1}}=\frac{10}{9}\text{sec}$$

For vertical motion,

Here, $u=0$

$$\therefore h=\frac{1}{2}gt^2$$

$$=\frac{1}{2}\times 10\times\left(\frac{10}{9}\right)^2$$

$$=\frac{500}{81}\text{m}=6.1\text{ m}$$

Therefore, the rifle must be aimed 6.1 m above the centre of the target to hit the target.

7. (c) From question,

Horizontal velocity (initial),

$$u_x=\frac{40}{2}=20\text{m/s}$$

Vertical velocity (initial), $50=u_y t+\frac{1}{2}gt^2$

$$\Rightarrow u_y\times 2+\frac{1}{2}(-10)\times 4$$

or, $50=2u_y-20$

or, $u_y=\frac{70}{2}=35\text{m/s}$

$$\therefore \tan\theta=\frac{u_y}{u_x}=\frac{35}{20}=\frac{7}{4}$$

$$\Rightarrow \text{Angle } \theta=\tan^{-1}\frac{7}{4}$$

8. (b) From equation, $\vec{v}=\hat{i}+2\hat{j}$

$\Rightarrow x=t$ ...(i)

$y=2t-\frac{1}{2}(10t^2)$ ...(ii)

From (i) and (ii), $y=2x-5x^2$

9. (b)

10. (b) 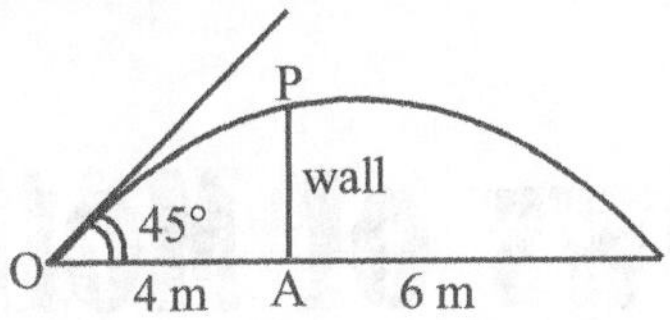

As ball is projected at an angle 45° to the horizontal therefore Range = 4H

or $10 = 4H \Rightarrow H = \frac{10}{4} = 2.5\,m$

($\because$ Range = 4 m + 6 m = 10m)

Maximum height, $H = \frac{u^2 \sin^2\theta}{2g}$

$$\therefore\ u^2 = \frac{H \times 2g}{\sin^2\theta} = \frac{2.5 \times 2 \times 10}{\left(\frac{1}{\sqrt{2}}\right)^2} = 100$$

or, $u = \sqrt{100} = 10\ ms^{-1}$

Height of wall PA

$$= OA\tan\theta - \frac{1}{2}\frac{g(OA)^2}{u^2\cos^2\theta}$$

$$= 4 - \frac{1}{2} \times \frac{10 \times 16}{10 \times 10 \times \frac{1}{\sqrt{2}} \times \frac{1}{\sqrt{2}}} = 2.4\,m$$

11. (d) $R = \frac{u^2\sin^2\theta}{g}$, $H = \frac{u^2\sin^2\theta}{2g}$

H_{max} at $2\theta = 90°$

$$H_{max} = \frac{u^2}{2g}$$

$$\frac{u^2}{2g} = 10 \Rightarrow u^2 = 10g \times 2$$

$$R = \frac{u^2\sin 2\theta}{g} \Rightarrow R_{max} = \frac{u^2}{g}$$

$$R_{max} = \frac{10 \times g \times 2}{g} = 20 \text{ metre}$$

12. (a) Total area around fountain

$A = \pi R_{max}^2$

Where $R_{max} = \frac{v^2 \sin 2\theta}{g} = \frac{v^2 \sin 90°}{g} = \frac{v^2}{g}$

$$\therefore\ A = \pi\frac{v^4}{g^2}$$

13. (a) The angle for which the ranges are same is complementary.

Let one angle be θ, then other is $90° - \theta$

$$T_1 = \frac{2u\sin\theta}{g}, T_2 = \frac{2u\cos\theta}{g}$$

$$T_1T_2 = \frac{4u^2\sin\theta\cos\theta}{g} = 2R$$

$$(\because R = \frac{u^2\sin^2\theta}{g})$$

Hence it is proportional to R.

14. (c) Yes, the person can catch the ball when horizontal velocity is equal to the horizontal component of ball's velocity, the motion of ball will be only in vertical direction with respect to person for that,

$$\frac{v_o}{2} = v_o\cos\theta \text{ or } \theta = 60°$$

15. (d) From the figure it is clear that range is required

$$R = \frac{u^2\sin 2\theta}{g} = \frac{(10)^2\sin(2 \times 30°)}{10} = 5\sqrt{3}$$

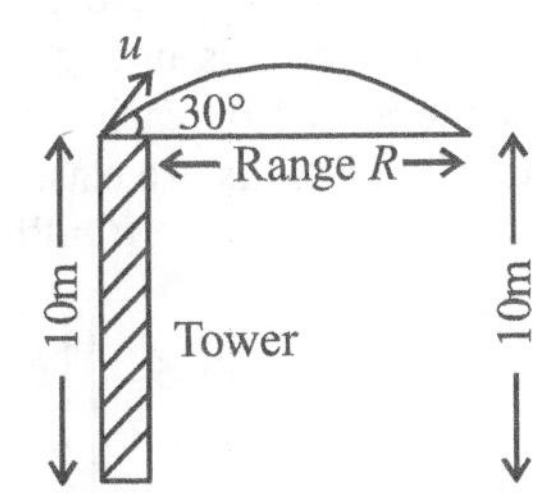

TOPIC-4 : Relative Velocity in Two Dimensions & Uniform Circular Motion

16. (c) Speed, V = constant (from question)

Centripetal acceleration,

$$a = \frac{V^2}{r}$$

ra = constant

Hence graph (c) correctly describes relation between acceleration and radius.

Chapter 4

Laws of Motion

TOPIC-1 : Ist, IInd & IIIrd Laws of Motion

1. A particle of mass m is acted upon by a force F given by the empirical law $F = \frac{R}{t^2} v(t)$. If this law is to be tested experimentally by observing the motion starting from rest, the best way is to plot : **[Online April 10, 2016]**

(a) $\log v(t)$ against $\frac{1}{t}$ (b) $v(t)$ against t^2

(c) $\log v(t)$ against $\frac{1}{t^2}$ (d) $\log v(t)$ against t

2. A large number (n) of identical beads, each of mass m and radius r are strung on a thin smooth rigid horizontal rod of length L (L >> r) and are at rest at random positions. The rod is mounted between two rigid supports (see figure). If one of the beads is now given a speed v, the average force experienced by each support after a long time is (assume all collisions are elastic) : **[Online April 11, 2015]**

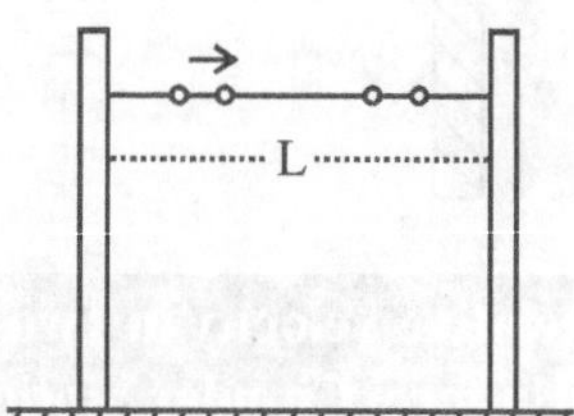

(a) $\frac{mv^2}{2(L-nr)}$ (b) $\frac{mv^2}{L-2nr}$

(c) $\frac{mv^2}{L-nr}$ (d) zero

3. A body of mass 5 kg under the action of constant force $\vec{F} = F_x\hat{i} + F_y\hat{j}$ has velocity at t = 0 s as $\vec{v} = (6\hat{i} - 2\hat{j})$ m/s and at t = 10s as $\vec{v} = +6\hat{j}$ m/s. The force $\vec{F}$ is: **[Online April 11, 2014]**

(a) $(-3\hat{j} + 4\hat{j})$N (b) $\left(-\frac{3}{5}\hat{i} + \frac{4}{5}\hat{j}\right)$N

(c) $(3\hat{i} - 4\hat{j})$N (d) $\left(\frac{3}{5}\hat{i} - \frac{4}{5}\hat{j}\right)$N

4. A particle of mass m is at rest at the origin at time $t = 0$. It is subjected to a force $F(t) = F_0 e^{-bt}$ in the x direction. Its speed $v(t)$ is depicted by which of the following curves? **[2012]**

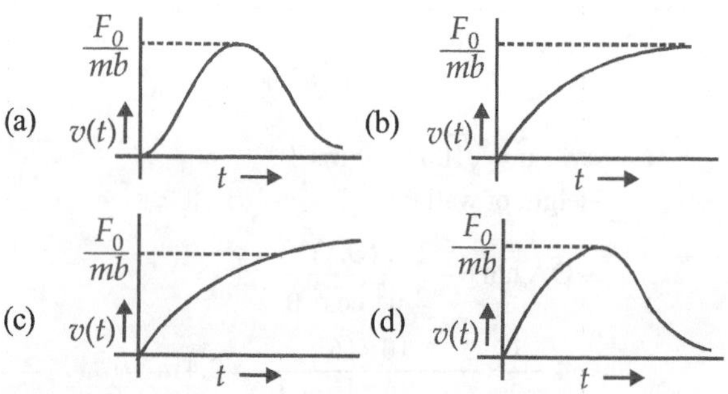

5. This question has Statement 1 and Statement 2. Of the four choices given after the Statements, choose the one that best describes the two Statements.
Statement 1: If you push on a cart being pulled by a horse so that it does not move, the cart pushes you back with an equal and opposite force.
Statement 2: The cart does not move because the force described in statement 1 cancel each other. **[Online May 26, 2012]**

(a) Statement 1 is true, Statement 2 is true, Statement 2 is the correct explanation of Statement 1.
(b) Statement 1 is false, Statement 2 is true.
(c) Statement 1 is true, Statement 2 is false.
(d) Statement 1 is true, Statement 2 is true, Statement 2 is not the correct explanation of Statement 1.

6. Two fixed frictionless inclined planes making an angle 30° and 60° with the vertical are shown in the figure. Two blocks A and B are placed on the two planes. What is the relative vertical acceleration of A with respect to B ? **[2010]**

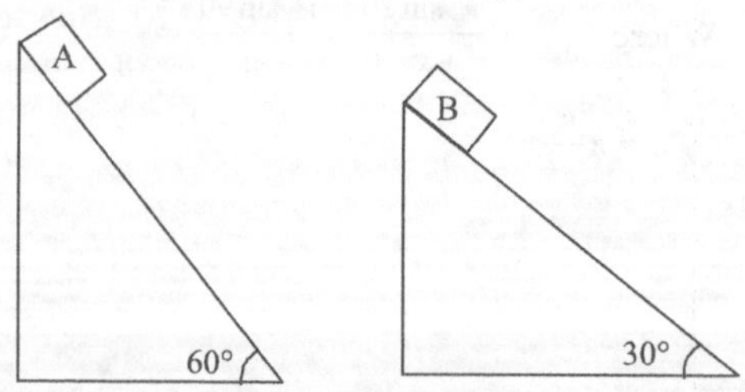

(a) 4.9 ms^{-2} in horizontal direction
(b) 9.8 ms^{-2} in vertical direction
(c) Zero
(d) 4.9 ms^{-2} in vertical direction

7. A ball of mass 0.2 kg is thrown vertically upwards by applying a force by hand. If the hand moves 0.2 m while applying the force and the ball goes upto 2 m height further, find the magnitude of the force. (Consider g = 10 m/s^2). **[2006]**
(a) 4 N (b) 16 N (c) 20 N (d) 22 N

8. A player caught a cricket ball of mass 150 g moving at a rate of 20 m/s. If the catching process is completed in 0.1s, the force of the blow exerted by the ball on the hand of the player is equal to **[2006]**
(a) 150 N (b) 3 N (c) 30 N (d) 300 N

9. A particle of mass 0.3 kg subject to a force $F = -kx$ with $k = 15$ N/m. What will be its initial acceleration if it is released from a point 20 cm away from the origin ? **[2005]**
(a) 15 m/s^2 (b) 3 m/s^2 (c) 10 m/s^2 (d) 5 m/s^2

10. A block is kept on a frictionless inclined surface with angle of inclination 'α'. The incline is given an acceleration 'a' to keep the block stationary. Then a is equal to **[2005]**

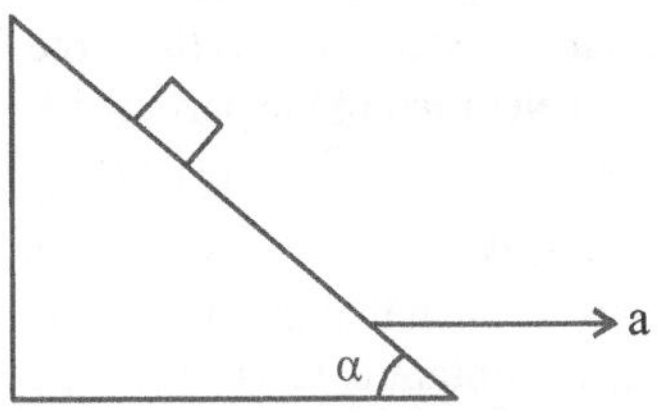

(a) g cosec α (b) g / tan α
(c) g tan α (d) g

11. A rocket with a lift-off mass 3.5×10^4 kg is blasted upwards with an initial acceleration of 10m/s^2. Then the initial thrust of the blast is **[2003]**
(a) 3.5×10^5 N (b) 7.0×10^5 N
(c) 14.0×10^5 N (d) 1.75×10^5 N

12. Three forces start acting simultaneously on a particle moving with velocity, $\vec{v}$. These forces are represented in magnitude and direction by the three sides of a triangle ABC. The particle will now move with velocity **[2003]**

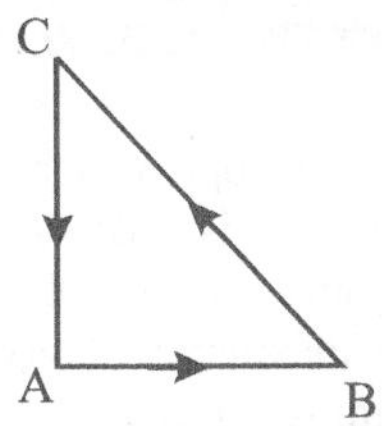

(a) less than $\vec{v}$
(b) greater than $\vec{v}$
(c) $|\vec{v}|$ in the direction of the largest force BC
(d) $\vec{v}$, remaining unchanged

13. A solid sphere, a hollow sphere and a ring are released from top of an inclined plane (frictionless) so that they slide down the plane. Then maximum acceleration down the plane is for (no rolling) **[2002]**
(a) solid sphere (b) hollow sphere
(c) ring (d) all same

TOPIC-2 : Motion of Connected Bodies, Pulley & Equilibrium of Forces

14. A mass 'm' is supported by a massless string wound around a uniform hollow cylinder of mass m and radius R. If the string does not slip on the cylinder, with what acceleration will the mass fall or release? **[2014]**

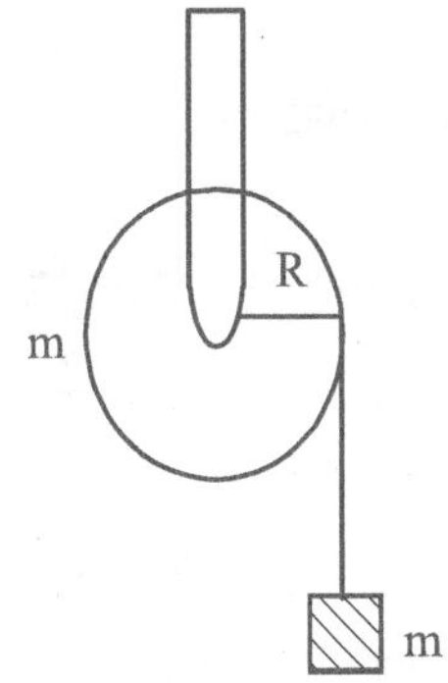

(a) $\frac{2g}{3}$ (b) $\frac{g}{2}$ (c) $\frac{5g}{6}$ (d) g

15. Two blocks of mass M_1 = 20 kg and M_2 = 12 kg are connected by a metal rod of mass 8 kg. The system is pulled vertically up by applying a force of 480 N as shown. The tension at the mid-point of the rod is : **[Online April 22, 2013]**

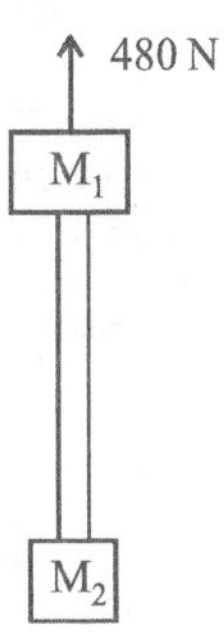

(a) 144N (b) 96N (c) 240N (d) 192N

16. A uniform sphere of weight W and radius 5 cm is being held by a string as shown in the figure. The tension in the string will be : **[Online April 9, 2013]**

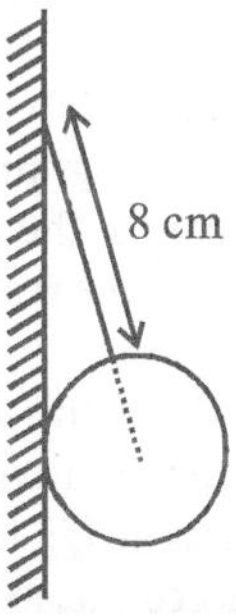

(a) $12\frac{W}{5}$ (b) $5\frac{W}{12}$ (c) $13\frac{W}{5}$ (d) $13\frac{W}{12}$

17. A spring is compressed between two blocks of masses m_1 and m_2 placed on a horizontal frictionless surface as shown in the figure. When the blocks are released, they have initial velocity of v_1 and v_2 as shown. The blocks travel distances x_1 and x_2 respectively before coming to rest. The ratio $\left(\frac{x_1}{x_2}\right)$ is **[Online May 12, 2012]**

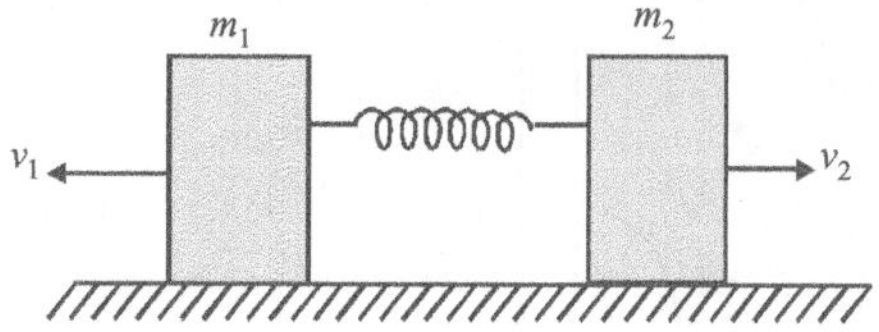

(a) $\frac{m_2}{m_1}$ (b) $\frac{m_1}{m_2}$

(c) $\sqrt{\frac{m_2}{m_1}}$ (d) $\sqrt{\frac{m_1}{m_2}}$

18. A block of mass m is connected to another block of mass M by a spring (massless) of spring constant k. The block are kept on a smooth horizontal plane. Initially the blocks are at rest and the spring is unstretched. Then a constant force F starts acting on the block of mass M to pull it. Find the force of the block of mass m. **[2007]**

(a) $\frac{MF}{(m+M)}$ (b) $\frac{mF}{M}$

(c) $\frac{(M+m)F}{m}$ (d) $\frac{mF}{(m+M)}$

19. Two masses $m_1 = 5\text{g}$ and $m_2 = 4.8$ kg tied to a string are hanging over a light frictionless pulley. What is the acceleration of the masses when left free to move ? $(g = 9.8\text{m/s}^2)$ **[2004]**

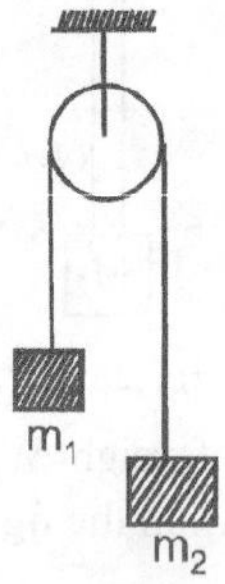

(a) $5\ \text{m/s}^2$ (b) $9.8\ \text{m/s}^2$

(c) $0.2\ \text{m/s}^2$ (d) $4.8\ \text{m/s}^2$

20. A spring balance is attached to the ceiling of a lift. A man hangs his bag on the spring and the spring reads 49 N, when the lift is stationary. If the lift moves downward with an acceleration of $5\ \text{m/s}^2$, the reading of the spring balance will be **[2003]**

(a) 24 N (b) 74 N (c) 15 N (d) 49 N

21. A block of mass M is pulled along a horizontal frictionless surface by a rope of mass m. If a force P is applied at the free end of the rope, the force exerted by the rope on the block is **[2003]**

(a) $\frac{Pm}{M+m}$ (b) $\frac{Pm}{M-m}$ (c) P (d) $\frac{PM}{M+m}$

22. A light spring balance hangs from the hook of the other light spring balance and a block of mass M kg hangs from the former one. Then the true statement about the scale reading is **[2003]**

(a) both the scales read M kg each

(b) the scale of the lower one reads M kg and of the upper one zero

(c) the reading of the two scales can be anything but the sum of the reading will be M kg

(d) both the scales read $M/2$ kg each

23. A lift is moving down with acceleration a. A man in the lift drops a ball inside the lift. The acceleration of the ball as observed by the man in the lift and a man standing stationary on the ground are respectively **[2002]**

(a) g, g (b) $g-a, g-a$

(c) $g-a, g$ (d) a, g

24. When forces F_1, F_2, F_3 are acting on a particle of mass m such that F_2 and F_3 are mutually perpendicular, then the particle remains stationary. If the force F_1 is now removed then the acceleration of the particle is **[2002]**

(a) F_1/m (b) F_2F_3/mF_1

(c) $(F_2 - F_3)/m$ (d) F_2/m.

25. Two forces are such that the sum of their magnitudes is 18 N and their resultant is 12 N which is perpendicular to the smaller force. Then the magnitudes of the forces are **[2002]**

(a) 12 N, 6 N (b) 13 N, 5 N

(c) 10 N, 8 N (d) 16N, 2N.

26. A light string passing over a smooth light pulley connects two blocks of masses m_1 and m_2 (vertically). If the acceleration of the system is $g/8$, then the ratio of the masses is **[2002]**

(a) 8 : 1 (b) 9 : 7 (c) 4 : 3 (d) 5 : 3

27. Three identical blocks of masses $m = 2$ kg are drawn by a force $F = 10.2$ N with an acceleration of $0.6\ \text{ms}^{-2}$ on a frictionless surface, then what is the tension (in N) in the string between the blocks B and C? **[2002]**

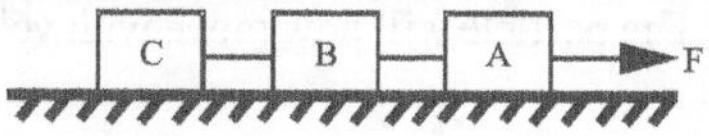

(a) 9.2 (b) 3.4 (c) 4 (d) 9.8

28. One end of a massless rope, which passes over a massless and frictionless pulley P is tied to a hook C while the other end is free. Maximum tension that the rope can bear is 360 N. With what value of maximum safe acceleration (in ms^{-2}) can a man of 60 kg climb on the rope? **[2002]**

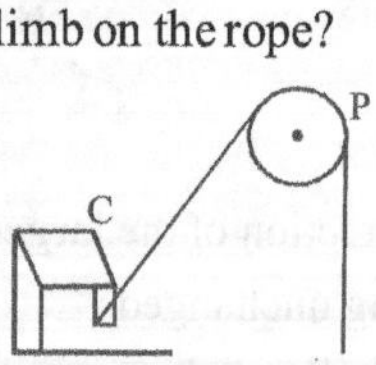

(a) 16 (b) 6 (c) 4 (d) 8

TOPIC-3 : Friction

29. A rocket is fired vertically from the earth with an acceleration of 2g, where g is the gravitational acceleration. On an inclined

plane inside the rocket, making an angle θ with the horizontal, a point object of mass m is kept. The minimum coefficient of friction μ_{min} between the mass and the inclined surface such that the mass does not move is : **[Online April 9, 2016]**

(a) tan2θ (b) tanθ
(c) 3 tanθ (d) 2 tan θ

30. Given in the figure are two blocks A and B of weight 20 N and 100 N, respectively. These are being pressed against a wall by a force F as shown. If the coefficient of friction between the blocks is 0.1 and between block B and the wall is 0.15, the frictional force applied by the wall on block B is: **[2015]**

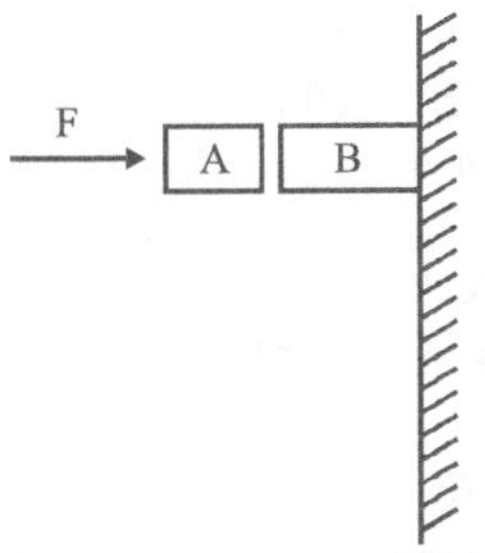

(a) 120N (b) 150N (c) 100N (d) 80N

31. A block of mass m = 10 kg rests on a horizontal table. The coefficient of friction between the block and the table is 0.05. When hit by a bullet of mass 50 g moving with speed v, that gets embedded in it, the block moves and comes to stop after moving a distance of 2 m on the table. If a freely falling object were to acquire speed $\frac{v}{10}$ after being dropped from height H, then neglecting energy losses and taking g = 10 ms^{-2}, the value of H is close to: **[Online April 10, 2015]**

(a) 0.05 km (b) 0.02 km
(c) 0.03 km (d) 0.04 km

32. A block of mass m is placed on a surface with a vertical cross section given by $y = \frac{x^3}{6}$. If the coefficient of friction is 0.5, the maximum height above the ground at which the block can be placed without slipping is: **[2014]**

(a) $\frac{1}{6}$m (b) $\frac{2}{3}$m (c) $\frac{1}{3}$m (d) $\frac{1}{2}$m

33. Consider a cylinder of mass M resting on a rough horizontal rug that is pulled out from under it with acceleration 'a' perpendicular to the axis of the cylinder. What is $F_{friction}$ at point P? It is assumed that the cylinder does not slip. **[Online April 19, 2014]**

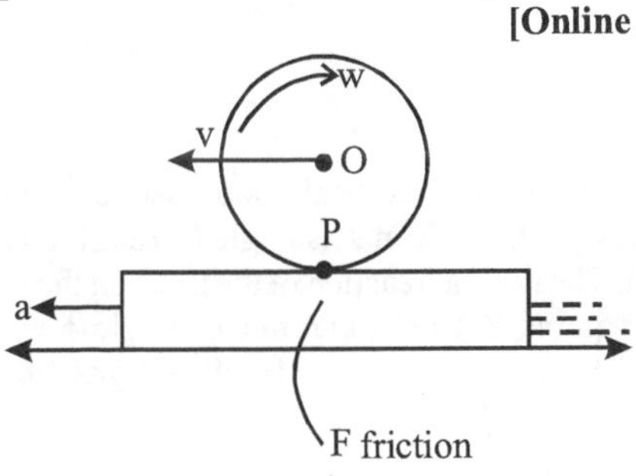

(a) Mg (b) Ma (c) $\frac{Ma}{2}$ (d) $\frac{Ma}{3}$

34. A heavy box is to dragged along a rough horizontal floor. To do so, person A pushes it at an angle 30° from the horizontal and requires a minimum force F_A, while person B pulls the box at an angle 60° from the horizontal and needs minimum force F_B. If the coefficient of friction between the box and the floor is $\frac{\sqrt{3}}{5}$, the ratio $\frac{F_A}{F_B}$ is **[Online April 19, 2014]**

(a) $\sqrt{3}$ (b) $\frac{5}{\sqrt{3}}$ (c) $\sqrt{\frac{3}{2}}$ (d) $\frac{2}{\sqrt{3}}$

35. A small ball of mass m starts at a point A with speed v_o and moves along a frictionless track AB as shown. The track BC has coefficient of friction μ. The ball comes to stop at C after travelling a distance L which is: **[Online April 11, 2014]**

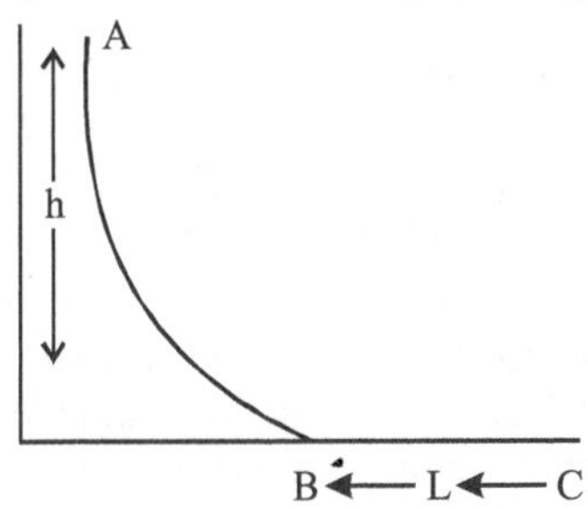

(a) $\frac{2h}{\mu}+\frac{v_o^2}{2\mu g}$ (b) $\frac{h}{\mu}+\frac{v_o^2}{2\mu g}$

(c) $\frac{h}{2\mu}+\frac{v_o^2}{\mu g}$ (d) $\frac{h}{2\mu}+\frac{v_o^2}{2\mu g}$

36. A block A of mass 4 kg is placed on another block B of mass 5 kg, and the block B rests on a smooth horizontal table. If the minimum force that can be applied on A so that both the blocks move together is 12 N, the maximum force that can be applied to B for the blocks to move together will be: **[Online April 9, 2014]**

(a) 30 N (b) 25 N (c) 27 N (d) 48 N

37. A block is placed on a rough horizontal plane. A time dependent horizontal force F = kt acts on the block, where k is a positive constant. The acceleration - time graph of the block is : **[Online April 25, 2013]**

(a)
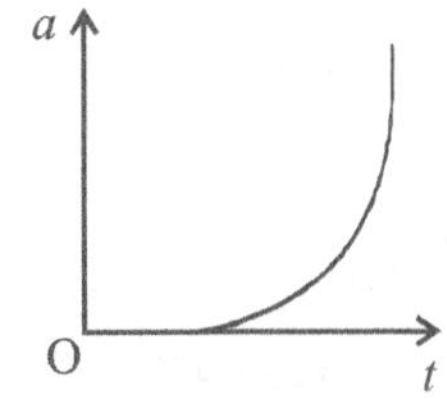

(b)
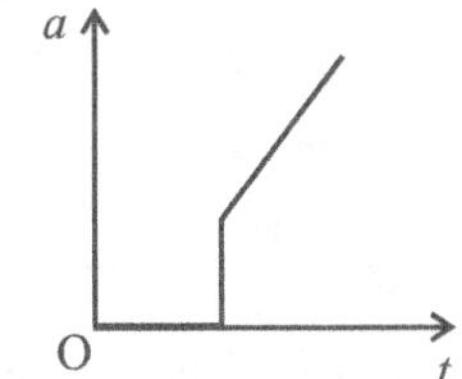

(c)
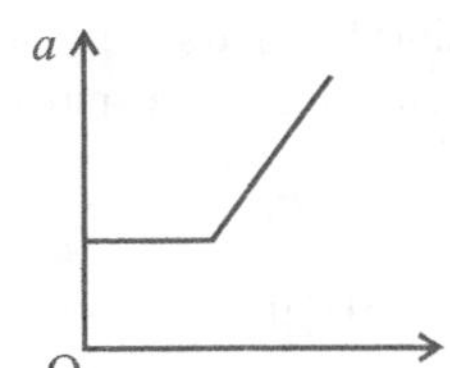

(d)
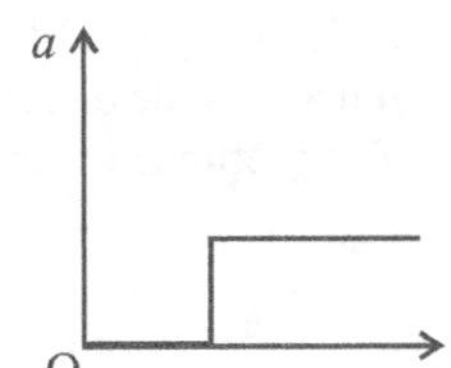

38. A body starts from rest on a long inclined plane of slope 45°. The coefficient of friction between the body and the plane varies as $\mu = 0.3\,x$, where x is distance travelled down the plane. The body will have maximum speed (for $g = 10\ \text{m/s}^2$) when $x =$ **[Online April 22, 2013]**

(a) 9.8m (b) 27m (c) 12m (d) 3.33m

39. A block of weight W rests on a horizontal floor with coefficient of static friction μ. It is desired to make the block move by applying minimum amount of force. The angle θ from the horizontal at which the force should be applied and magnitude of the force F are respectively. **[Online May 19, 2012]**

(a) $\theta = \tan^{-1}(\mu), F = \dfrac{\mu W}{\sqrt{1+\mu^2}}$

(b) $\theta = \tan^{-1}\left(\dfrac{1}{\mu}\right), F = \dfrac{\mu W}{\sqrt{1+\mu^2}}$

(c) $\theta = 0, F = \mu W$

(d) $\theta = \tan^{-1}\left(\dfrac{\mu}{1+\mu}\right), F = \dfrac{\mu W}{1+\mu}$

40. An insect crawls up a hemispherical surface very slowly. The coefficient of friction between the insect and the surface is 1/3. If the line joining the centre of the hemispherical surface to the insect makes an angle α with the vertical, the maximum possible value of α so that the insect does not slip is given by **[Online May 12, 2012]**

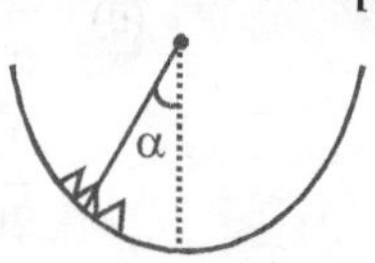

(a) $\cot\alpha = 3$ (b) $\sec\alpha = 3$
(c) $\operatorname{cosec}\alpha = 3$ (d) $\cos\alpha = 3$

41. The minimum force required to start pushing a body up rough (frictional coefficient μ) inclined plane is F_1 while the minimum force needed to prevent it from sliding down is F_2. If the inclined plane makes an angle θ from the horizontal such that $\tan\theta = 2\mu$ then the ratio $\dfrac{F_1}{F_2}$ is

(a) 1 (b) 2 **[2011 RS]**
(c) 3 (d) 4

42. If a spring of stiffness 'k' is cut into parts 'A' and 'B' of length $\ell_A : \ell_B = 2:3$, then the stiffness of spring 'A' is given by **[2011 RS]**

(a) $\dfrac{3k}{5}$ (b) $\dfrac{2k}{5}$ (c) k (d) $\dfrac{5k}{2}$

43. A smooth block is released at rest on a 45° incline and then slides a distance 'd'. The time taken to slide is 'n' times as much to slide on rough incline than on a smooth incline. The coefficient of friction is **[2005]**

(a) $\mu_k = \sqrt{1-\dfrac{1}{n^2}}$ (b) $\mu_k = 1-\dfrac{1}{n^2}$

(c) $\mu_s = \sqrt{1-\dfrac{1}{n^2}}$ (d) $\mu_s = 1-\dfrac{1}{n^2}$

44. The upper half of an inclined plane with inclination ϕ is perfectly smooth while the lower half is rough. A body starting from rest at the top will again come to rest at the bottom if the coefficient of friction for the lower half is given by **[2005]**

(a) $2\cos\phi$ (b) $2\sin\phi$ (c) $\tan\phi$ (d) $2\tan\phi$

45. Consider a car moving on a straight road with a speed of 100 m/s . The distance at which car can be stopped is $[\mu_k = 0.5]$ **[2005]**

(a) 1000 m (b) 800 m (c) 400 m (d) 100 m

46. A block rests on a rough inclined plane making an angle of 30° with the horizontal. The coefficient of static friction between the block and the plane is 0.8. If the frictional force on the block is 10 N, the mass of the block (in kg) is (take $g = 10\ \text{m/s}^2$) **[2004]**

(a) 1.6 (b) 4.0 (c) 2.0 (d) 2.5

47. A horizontal force of 10 N is necessary to just hold a block stationary against a wall. The coefficient of friction between the block and the wall is 0.2. The weight of the block is

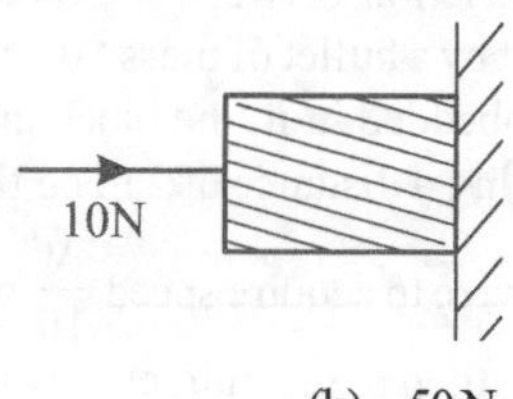

(a) 20 N (b) 50 N **[2003]**
(c) 100 N (d) 2 N

48. A marble block of mass 2 kg lying on ice when given a velocity of 6 m/s is stopped by friction in 10 s. Then the coefficient of friction is **[2003]**

(a) 0.02 (b) 0.03 (c) 0.04 (d) 0.06

TOPIC-4 : Circular Motion, Banking of Road

49. A conical pendulum of length 1 m makes an angle $\theta = 45°$ w.r.t. Z-axis and moves in a circle in the XY plane. The radius of the circle is 0.4 m and its centre is vertically below O. The speed of the pendulum, in its circular path, will be :(Take $g = 10\ \text{ms}^{-2}$) **[Online April 9, 2017]**

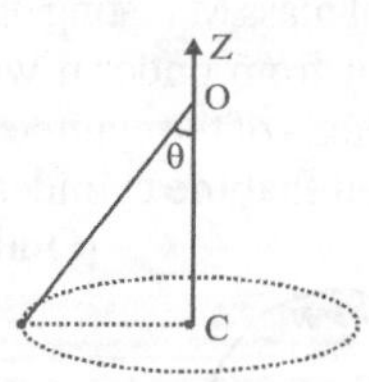

(a) 0.4 m/s

(b) 4 m/s

(c) 0.2 m/s

(d) 2 m/s

50. A particle is released on a vertical smooth semicircular track from point X so that OX makes angle θ from the vertical (see figure). The normal reaction of the track on the particle vanishes at point Y where OY makes angle ϕ with the horizontal. Then: **[Online April 19, 2014]**

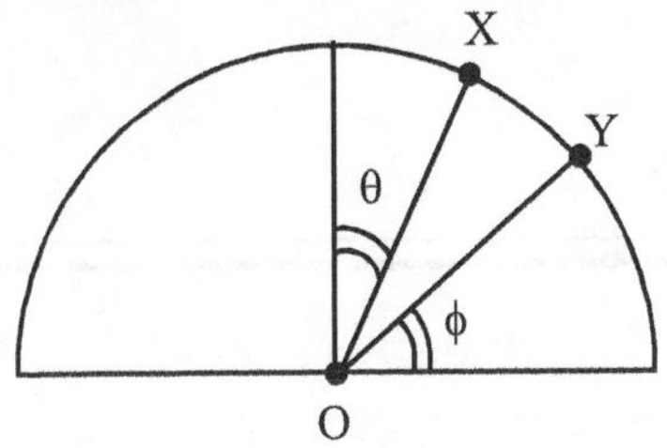

(a) $\sin\phi = \cos\phi$ (b) $\sin\phi = \frac{1}{2}\cos\theta$

(c) $\sin\phi = \frac{2}{3}\cos\theta$ (d) $\sin\phi = \frac{3}{4}\cos\theta$

51. A body of mass '*m*' is tied to one end of a spring and whirled round in a horizontal plane with a constant angular velocity. The elongation in the spring is 1 cm. If the angular velocity is doubled, the elongation in the spring is 5 cm. The original length of the spring is : **[Online April 23, 2013]**

(a) 15 cm (b) 12 cm (c) 16 cm (d) 10 cm

52. A point P moves in counter-clockwise direction on a circular path as shown in the figure. The movement of 'P' is such that it sweeps out a length $s = t^3 + 5$, where s is in metres and t is in seconds. The radius of the path is 20 m. The acceleration of 'P' when $t = 2$ s is nearly. **[2010]**

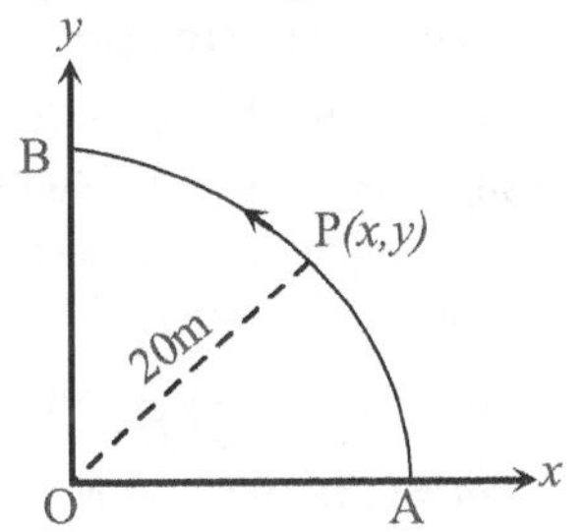

(a) $13 m/s^2$ (b) $12 m/s^2$ (c) $7.2 ms^2$ (d) $14 m/s^2$

53. For a particle in uniform circular motion, the acceleration $\vec{a}$ at a point P(R,θ) on the circle of radius R is (Here θ is measured from the x-axis) **[2010]**

(a) $-\frac{v^2}{R}\cos\theta\,\hat{i} + \frac{v^2}{R}\sin\theta\,\hat{j}$

(b) $-\frac{v^2}{R}\sin\theta\,\hat{i} + \frac{v^2}{R}\cos\theta\,\hat{j}$

(c) $-\frac{v^2}{R}\cos\theta\,\hat{i} - \frac{v^2}{R}\sin\theta\,\hat{j}$

(d) $\frac{v^2}{R}\hat{i} + \frac{v^2}{R}\hat{j}$

54. An annular ring with inner and outer radii R_1 and R_2 is rolling without slipping with a uniform angular speed. The ratio of the forces experienced by the two particles situated on the inner and outer parts of the ring, $\frac{F_1}{F_2}$ is` **[2005]**

(a) $\left(\frac{R_1}{R_2}\right)^2$ (b) $\frac{R_2}{R_1}$ `(c) $\frac{R_1}{R_2}$ (d) 1

55. Which of the following statements is **FALSE** for a particle moving in a circle with a constant angular speed ? **[2004]**

(a) The acceleration vector points to the centre of the circle
(b) The acceleration vector is tangent to the circle
(c) The velocity vector is tangent to the circle
(d) The velocity and acceleration vectors are perpendicular to each other.

56. The minimum velocity (in ms^{-1}) with which a car driver must traverse a flat curve of radius 150 m and coefficient of friction 0.6 to avoid skidding is **[2002]**

(a) 60 (b) 30 (c) 15 (d) 25

Hints & Solutions

TOPIC-1 : Ist, IInd & IIIrd Laws of Motion

1. **(a)** From $F=\frac{R}{t^2}v(t) \Rightarrow m\frac{dv}{dt}=\frac{R}{t^2}v(t)$

Integrating both sides $\int\frac{dv}{dt}=\int\frac{Rdt}{mt^2}$

In $v=-\frac{R}{mt}$

$\therefore \ln v \propto \frac{1}{t}$

2. **(b)** Space between the supports for motion of beads is L–2nr

Average force experienced by each support,

$$F=\frac{2mV}{\frac{2(L-2nr)}{V}}=\frac{mV^2}{L-2nr}$$

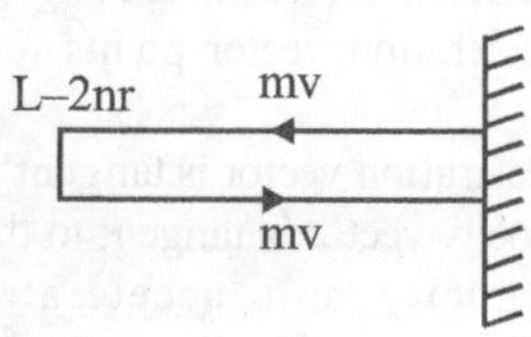

3. **(a)** From question,

Mass of body, $m = 5$ kg

Velocity at $t = 0$,

$u = (6\hat{i} - 2\hat{j})$ m/s

Velocity at $t = 10$ s,

$v = +6\,\hat{j}$ m/s

Force, $F = ?$

Acceleration, $a=\frac{v-u}{t}$

$=\frac{6\hat{j}-(6\hat{i}-2\hat{j})}{10}=\frac{-3\hat{i}+4\hat{j}}{5}$ m/s^2

Force, $F = ma$

$=5\times\frac{(-3\hat{i}+4\hat{j})}{5}=(-3\hat{i}+4\hat{j})N$

4. **(c)** Given that $F(t) = F_0e^{-bt}$

$\Rightarrow\ m\frac{dv}{dt}=F_0e^{-bt}$

$\frac{dv}{dt}=\frac{F_0}{m}e^{-bt}$

$\int_0^v dv=\frac{F_0}{m}\int_0^t e^{-bt}dt$

$v=\frac{F_0}{m}\left[\frac{e^{-bt}}{-b}\right]_0^t=\frac{F_0}{mb}\left[-\left(e^{-bt}-e^{-0}\right)\right]$

$\Rightarrow\ v=\frac{F_0}{mb}\left[1-e^{-bt}\right]$

5. **(a)** According to newton third law of motion i.e. every action is associated with equal and opposite reaction.

6. **(d)** $mg\sin\theta = ma$

$\therefore a = g\sin\theta$

where a is along the inclined plane

$\therefore$ vertical component of acceleration is $g\sin^2\theta$

$\therefore$ relative vertical acceleration of A with respect to B is

$g(\sin^2 60-\sin^2 30]=\frac{g}{2}=4.9$ m/s^2

in vertical direction

7. **(d)** Let the velocity of the ball just when it leaves the hand is u then applying,

$v^2 - u^2 = 2as$ for upward journey

$\Rightarrow -u^2 = 2(-10)\times 2 \Rightarrow u^2 = 40$

Again applying $v^2 - u^2 = 2as$ for the upward journey of the ball, when the ball is in the hands of the thrower,

$v^2 - u^2 = 2as$

$\Rightarrow 40 - 0 = 2\ (a)\ 0.2 \Rightarrow a = 100$ m/s^2

$\therefore F = ma = 0.2\times 100 = 20\ N$

$\Rightarrow N - mg = 20 \Rightarrow N = 20 + 2 = 22N$

8. **(c)** $F=\frac{m(v-u)}{t}=\frac{0.15(0-20)}{0.1}=30\,N$

9. **(c)** Mass $(m) = 0.3$ kg $\Rightarrow F = m.a = -15$ x

$a=-\frac{15}{0.3}x=\frac{-150}{3}x=-50x$

$a=-50\times 0.2=10\,\text{m/s}^2$

10. **(c)** From free body diagram,

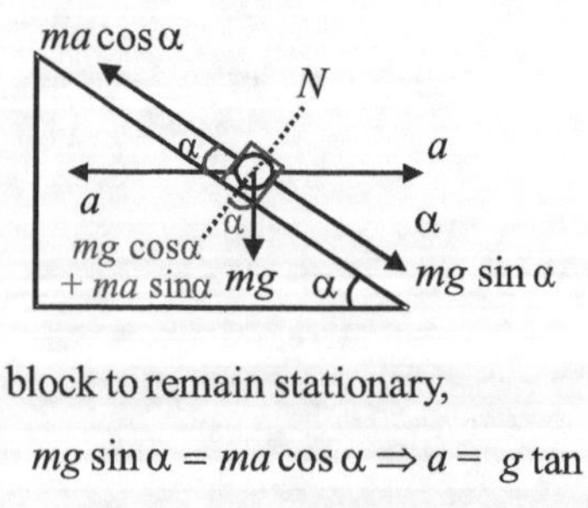

For block to remain stationary,

$mg\sin\alpha = ma\cos\alpha \Rightarrow a = g\tan\alpha$

11. (b) As shown in the figure $F - mg = ma$

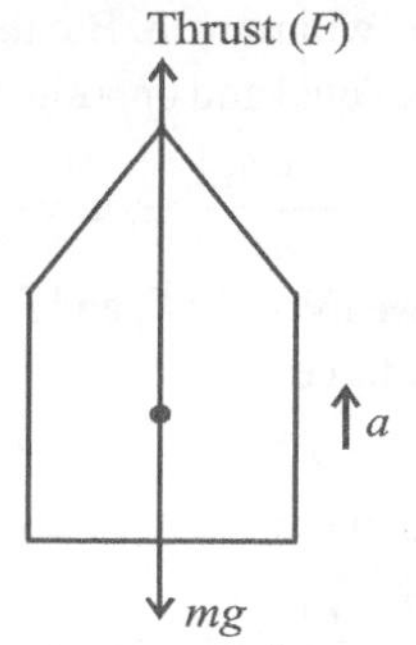

$\therefore\ F = m(g + a) = 3.5 \times 10^4 (10+10)$
$= 7 \times 10^5 N$

12. (d) As shown in the figure, the three forces are represented by the sides of a triangle taken in the same order. Therefore the resultant force is zero. $\vec{F}_{net} = m\vec{a}$. Therefore, acceleration is also zero i.e., velocity remains unchanged.

13. (d) This is a case of sliding (the plane being frictionless) and therefore the acceleration of all the bodies is same ($g \sin \theta$).

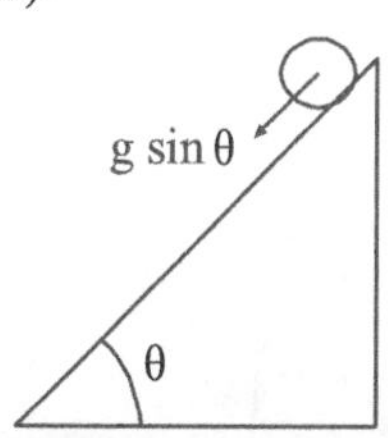

TOPIC-2 : Motion of Connected Bodies, Pulley & Equilibrium of Forces

14. (b) From figure,

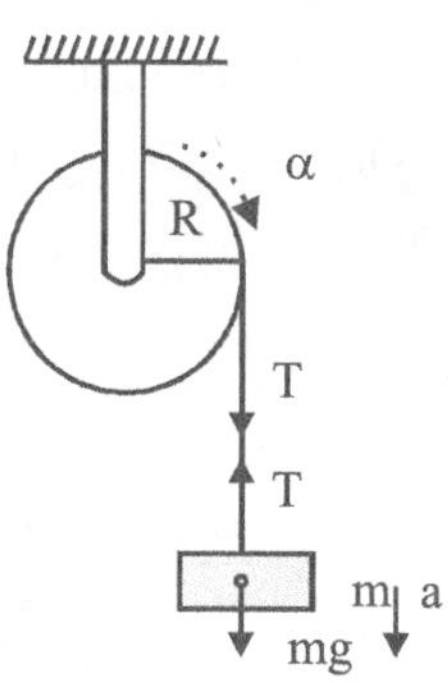

Acceleration $a = R\alpha$ ...(i)
and $mg - T = ma$ ...(ii)
From equation (i) and (ii)

$$T \times R = mR^2\alpha = mR^2\left(\frac{a}{R}\right)$$

or $T = ma$
$\Rightarrow\ mg - ma = ma$
$$\Rightarrow\ a = \frac{g}{2}$$

15. (d) Acceleration produced in upward direction

$$a = \frac{F}{M_1 + M_2 + \text{Mass of metal rod}}$$

$$= \frac{480}{20+12+8} = 12\ ms^{-2}$$

Tension at the mid point

$$T = \left(M_2 + \frac{\text{Mass of rod}}{2}\right)a$$

$$= (12+4) \times 12 = 192\ N$$

16. (d)

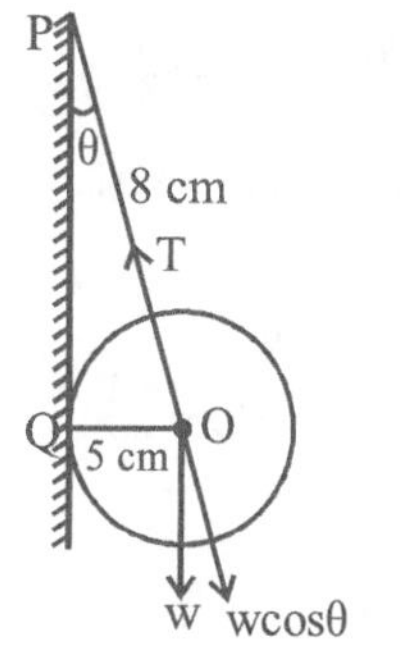

$$PQ = \sqrt{OP^2 + OQ^2}$$

$$= \sqrt{13^2 + 5^2} = 12$$

Tension in the string

$$T = w \cos\theta = \frac{13}{12} W$$

17. (a)

18. (d) Writing free body-diagrams for m & M,

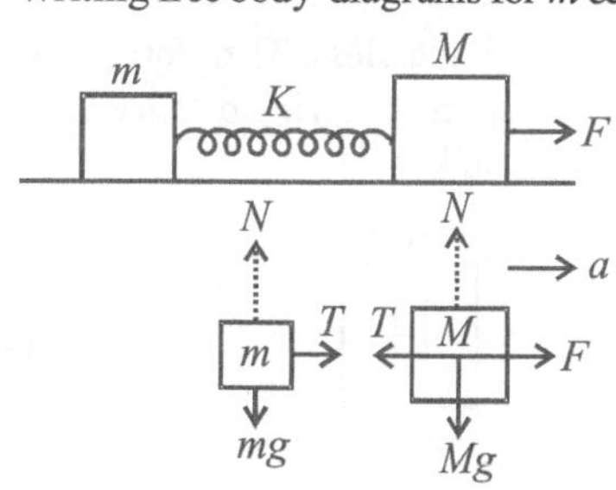

we get $T = ma$ and $F - T = Ma$
where T is force due to spring
$\Rightarrow\ F - ma = Ma$ or, $F = Ma + ma$

$$\therefore\ a = \frac{F}{M+m}.$$

Now, force acting on the block of mass m is

$$ma = m\left(\frac{F}{M+m}\right) = \frac{mF}{m+M}.$$

19. (c) Acceleration $a = \left(\dfrac{m_1 - m_2}{m_1 + m_2}\right) g$

$$= \frac{(5-4.8) \times 9.8}{(5+4.8)} m/s^2 = 0.2\ m/s^2$$

20. **(a)** For the bag accelerating down

$mg - T = ma$

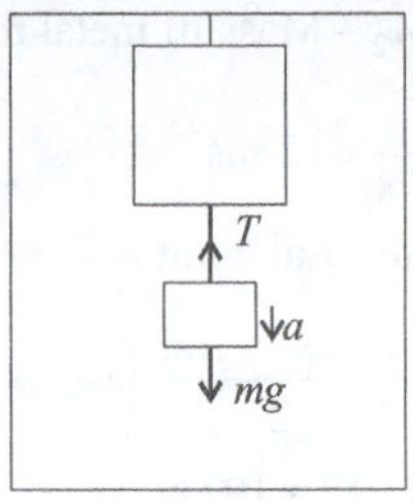

$\therefore\ T = m(g-a) = \frac{49}{10}(10-5) = 24.5\text{ N}$

21. **(d)** Taking the rope and the block as a system

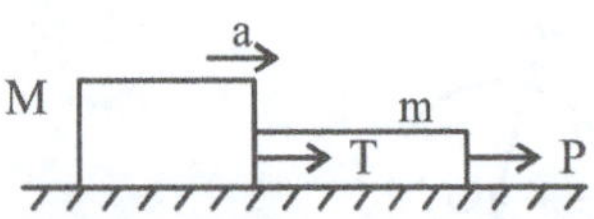

we get $P = (m+M)\,a$

$\therefore\ a = \frac{P}{m+M}$

Taking the block as a system,

we get $T = Ma$

$\therefore\ T = \frac{MP}{m+M}$

22. **(a)** The Earth pulls the block by a force Mg. The block in turn exerts a force Mg on the spring of spring balance S_1 which therefore shows a reading of M kgf.

The spring S_1 is massless. Therefore, it exerts a force of Mg on the spring of spring balance S_2 which shows the reading of M kgf.

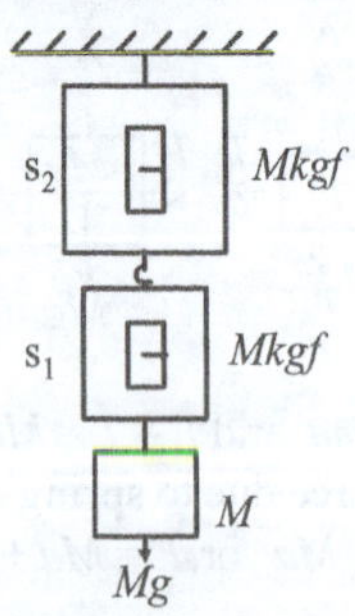

23. **(c)**
- For the man standing in the left, the acceleration of the ball

  $\vec{a}_{bm} = \vec{a}_b - \vec{a}_m \Rightarrow a_{bm} = g - a$

  Where 'a' is the acceleration of the mass (because the acceleration of the lift is 'a')
- For the man standing on the ground, the acceleration of the ball

  $\vec{a}_{bm} = \vec{a}_b - \vec{a}_m \Rightarrow a_{bm} = g - 0 = g$

24. **(a)** When F_1, F_2 and F_3 are acting on a particle then the particle remains stationary. This means that the resultant of F_1, F_2 and F_3 is zero. When F_1 is removed, F_2 and F_3 will remain. But the resultant of F_2 and F_3 should be equal and opposite to F_1. i.e. $|F_2 + F_3| = |F_1|$

$\therefore\quad a = \frac{|F_2 + F_3|}{m} \Rightarrow a = \frac{F_1}{m}$

25. **(b)** Let the two forces be F_1 and F_2 and let $F_2 < F_1$. R is the resultant force.

Given $F_1 + F_2 = 18$ ...(i)

From the figure $F_2^2 + R^2 = F_1^2$

$F_1^2 - F_2^2 = R^2$

$\therefore\quad F_1^2 - F_2^2 = 144$ ...(ii)

Only option (b) follows equation (i) and (ii).

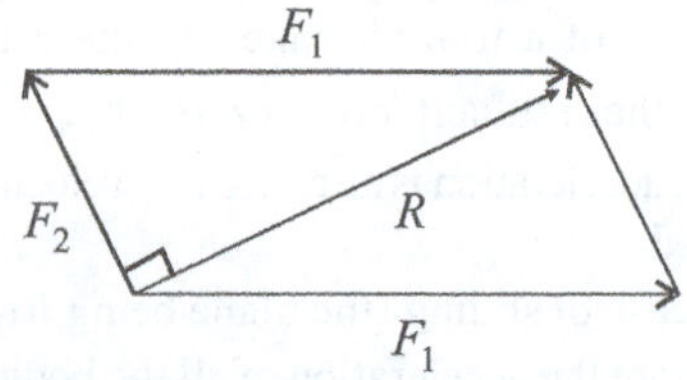

26. **(b)** **For mass m_1**

$m_1g - T = m_1a$

For mass m_2

$T - m_2g = m_2a$

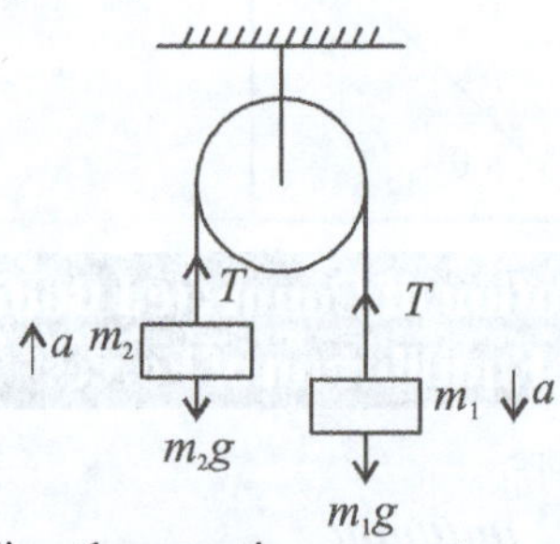

Adding the equations we get

$a = \frac{(m_1 - m_2)g}{m_1 + m_2}$

Here $a = \frac{g}{8}$

$\therefore\ \frac{1}{8} = \frac{\frac{m_1}{m_2} - 1}{\frac{m_1}{m_2} + 1} \Rightarrow \frac{m_1}{m_2} + 1 = 8\frac{m_1}{m_2} - 8 \Rightarrow \frac{m_1}{m_2} = \frac{9}{7}$

27. **(b)** $F = (m+m+m) \times a$

$\therefore\ a = \frac{10.2}{6}\text{ m/s}^2$

$\therefore\ T_2 = ma = 2 \times \frac{10.2}{6} = 3.4\text{N}$

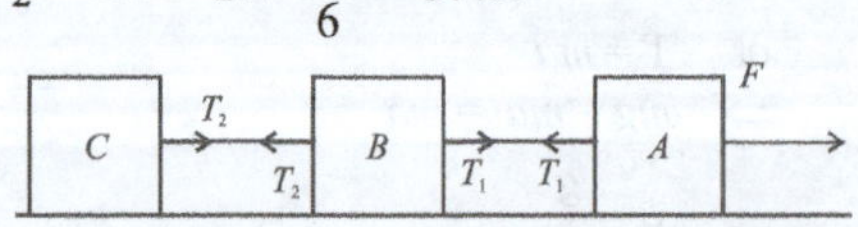

28. (c) $mg - T = ma$

$$\therefore \quad a = g - \frac{T}{m} = 10 - \frac{360}{60} = 4 m/s^2$$

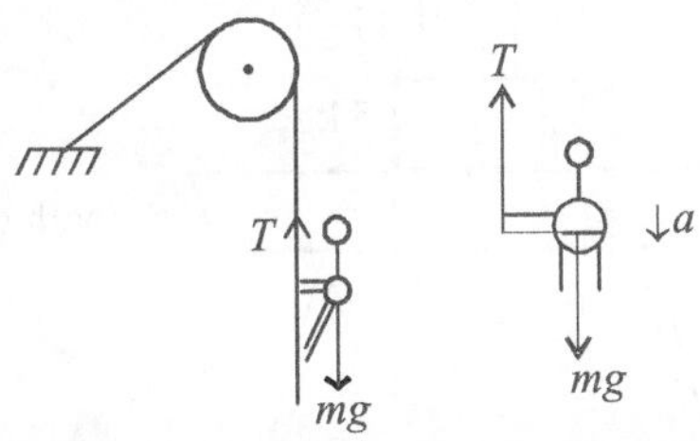

TOPIC-3 : Friction

29. (b) Let μ be the minimum coefficient of friction

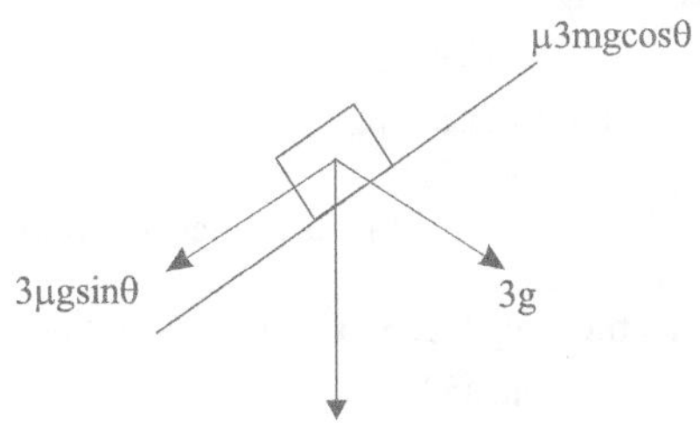

At equilibrium, mass does not move so,
$3mg\sin\theta = \mu 3mg\cos\theta$

$\therefore \mu_{min} = \tan\theta$

30. (a)

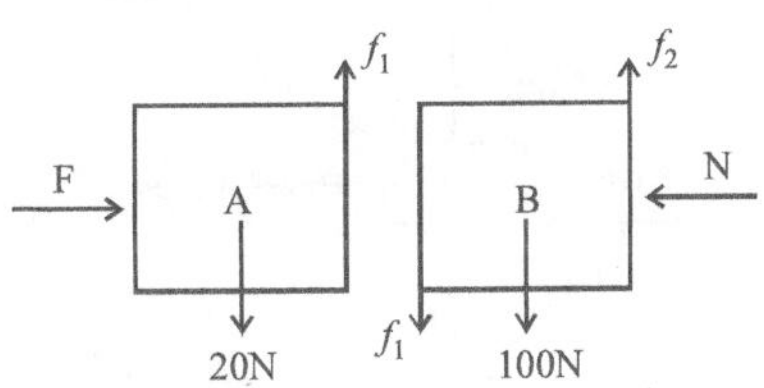

Assuming both the blocks are stationary
N = F
$f_1 = 20$ N
$f_2 = 100 + 20 = 120$N

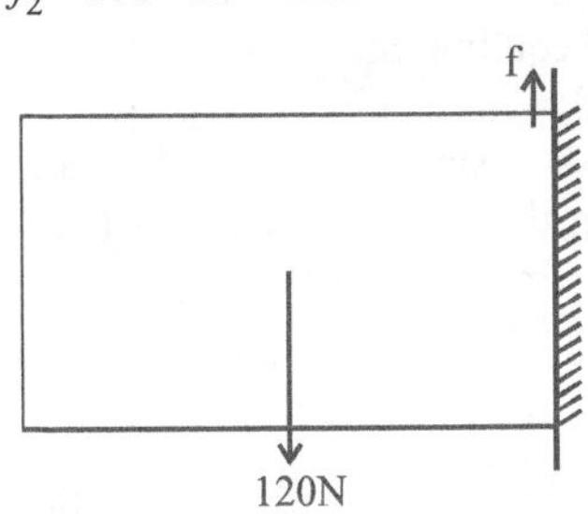

Considering the two blocks as one system and due to equilibrium f = 120N

31. (d) $f = \mu(M + m)g$

$$a = \frac{f}{M+m} = \frac{\mu(M+m)g}{(M+m)} = \mu g$$

$= 0.05 \times 10 = 0.5 \text{ ms}^{-2}$

$$V_0 = \frac{\text{Initial momentum}}{(M+m)} = \frac{0.05V}{10.05}$$

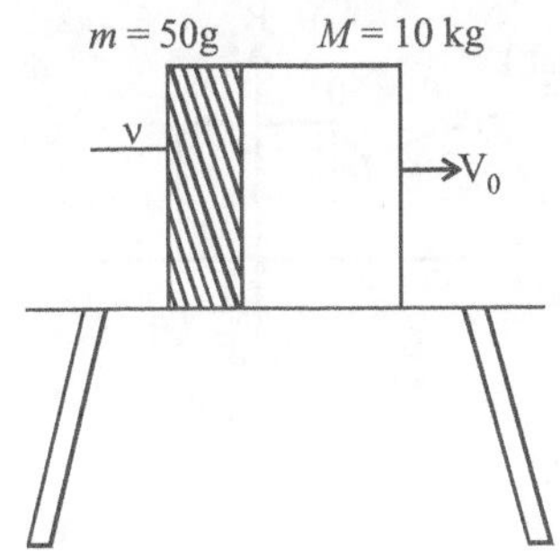

$v^2 - u^2 = 2as$
$0 - u^2 = 2as$
$u^2 = 2as$

$$\left(\frac{0.05v}{10.05}\right)^2 = 2 \times 0.5 \times 2$$

Solving we get $v = 201\sqrt{2}$
Object falling from height H.

$$\frac{V}{10} = \sqrt{2gH}$$

$$\frac{201\sqrt{2}}{10} = \sqrt{2 \times 10 \times H}$$

$H = 40$ m $= 0.04$ km

32. (a) At limiting equilibrium,
$\mu = \tan\theta$

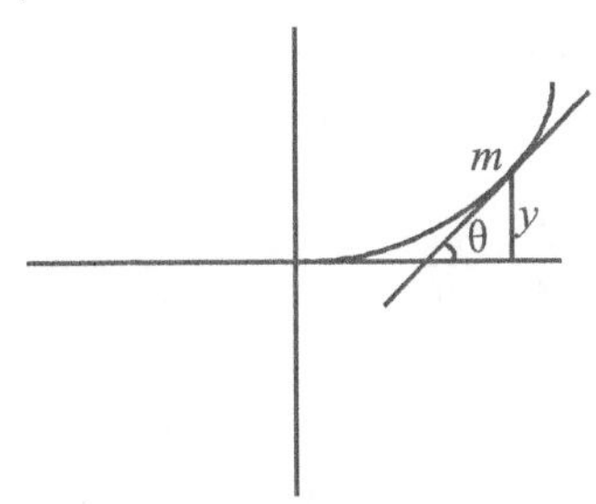

$\tan\theta = \mu = \frac{dy}{dx} = \frac{x^2}{2}$ (from question)

$\because$ Coefficient of friction $\mu = 0.5$

$\therefore \quad 0.5 = \frac{x^2}{2}$

$\Rightarrow \quad x = \pm 1$

Now, $y = \frac{x^3}{6} = \frac{1}{6} m$

33. (d) Force of friction at point P,

$$F_{friction} = \frac{1}{3} Ma\sin\theta$$

$= \frac{1}{3} Ma\sin 90°$ [here θ = 90°]

$= \frac{Ma}{3}$

34. (d)

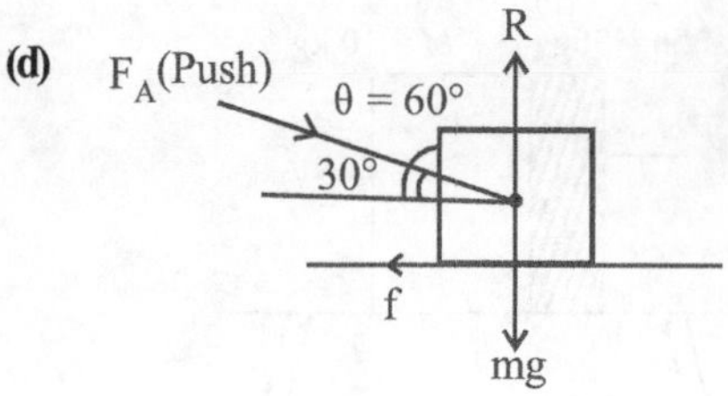

$$F_A = \frac{\mu mg}{\sin\theta - \mu\cos\theta}$$

Similarly,

$$F_B = \frac{\mu mg}{\sin\theta + \mu\cos\theta}$$

$$\therefore \quad \frac{F_A}{F_B} = \frac{\dfrac{\mu mg}{\sin\theta - \mu\cos\theta}}{\dfrac{\mu mg}{\sin\theta + \mu\cos\theta}}$$

$$= \frac{\dfrac{\mu mg}{\sin 60° - \dfrac{\sqrt{3}}{5}\cos 60°}}{\dfrac{\mu mg}{\sin 30° + \dfrac{\sqrt{3}}{5}\cos 30°}} \qquad \left[\mu = \frac{\sqrt{3}}{5}\text{ given}\right]$$

$$= \frac{\sin 30° + \dfrac{\sqrt{3}}{5}\cos 30°}{\sin 60° - \dfrac{\sqrt{3}}{5}\cos 60°}$$

$$= \frac{\dfrac{1}{2} + \dfrac{\sqrt{3}}{5}\times\dfrac{\sqrt{3}}{2}}{\dfrac{\sqrt{3}}{2} - \dfrac{\sqrt{3}}{5}\times\dfrac{1}{2}}$$

$$= \frac{\dfrac{1}{2}\left(1+\dfrac{3}{5}\right)}{\dfrac{\sqrt{3}}{5}\left(1-\dfrac{1}{5}\right)} = \frac{\dfrac{1}{2}\times\dfrac{8}{5}}{\dfrac{\sqrt{3}\times 4}{10}}$$

$$= \frac{\dfrac{8}{10}}{\dfrac{\sqrt{3}\times 4}{10}} = \frac{8}{\sqrt{3}\times 4} = \frac{2}{\sqrt{3}}$$

35. (b) Initial speed at point A, $u = v_0$

Speed at point B, $v = ?$

$$v^2 - u^2 = 2gh$$

$$v^2 = v_0^2 + 2gh$$

Let ball travels distance 'S' before coming to rest

$$S = \frac{v^2}{2\mu g} = \frac{v_0^2 + 2gh}{2\mu g}$$

$$= \frac{v_0^2}{2\mu g} + \frac{2gh}{2\mu g} = \frac{h}{\mu} + \frac{v_0^2}{2\mu g}$$

36. (c) Minimum force on A

= frictional force between the surfaces

$= 12\,N$

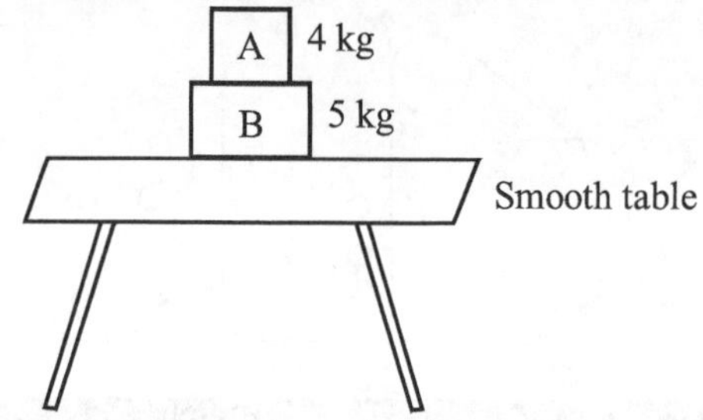

Therefore maximum acceleration

$$a_{max} = \frac{12\text{N}}{4\text{kg}} = 3\text{m/s}^2$$

Hence maximum force,

F_{max} = total mass × a_{max}

$= 9 \times 3 = 27$ N

37. (b) Graph (b) correctly dipicts the acceleration-time graph of the block.

38. (d) When the body has maximum speed then

$\mu = 0.3x = \tan 45°$

$\therefore x = 3.33$ m

39. (a) Let the force F is applied at an angle θ with the horizontal.

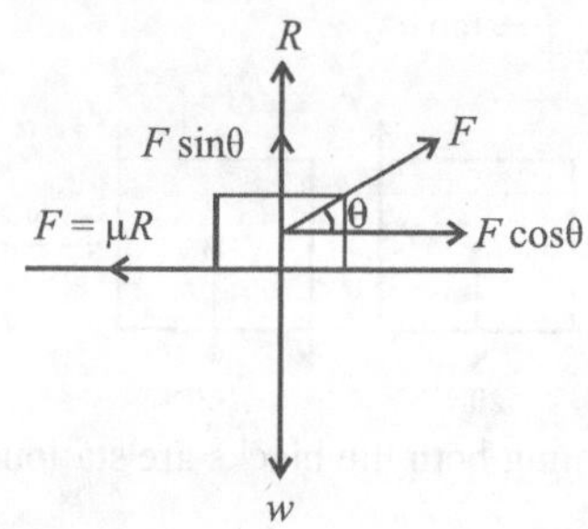

For horizontal equilibrium,

$F\cos\theta = \mu R$ ...(i)

For vertical equilibrium,

$R + F\sin\theta = mg$

or, $R = mg - F\sin\theta$ ...(ii)

Substituting this value of R in eq. (i), we get

$F\cos\theta = \mu(mg - F\sin\theta)$

$= \mu mg - \mu F\sin\theta$

or, $F(\cos\theta + \mu\sin\theta) = \mu mg$

or, $F = \dfrac{\mu mg}{\cos\theta + \mu\sin\theta}$ ...(iii)

For F to be minimum, the denominator ($\cos\theta + \mu\sin\theta$) should be maximum.

$\therefore \dfrac{d}{d\theta}(\cos\theta + \mu\sin\theta) = 0$

or, $-\sin\theta + \mu\cos\theta = 0$

or, $\tan\theta = \mu$

or, $\theta = \tan^{-1}(\mu)$

Then, $\sin\theta = \dfrac{\mu}{\sqrt{1+\mu^2}}$ and

$$\cos\theta = \frac{1}{\sqrt{1+\mu^2}}$$

Hence, F_{min}

$$= \frac{\mu w}{\frac{1}{\sqrt{1+\mu^2}} + \frac{\mu^2}{\sqrt{1+\mu^2}}} = \frac{\mu w}{\sqrt{1+\mu^2}}$$

40. **(a)**

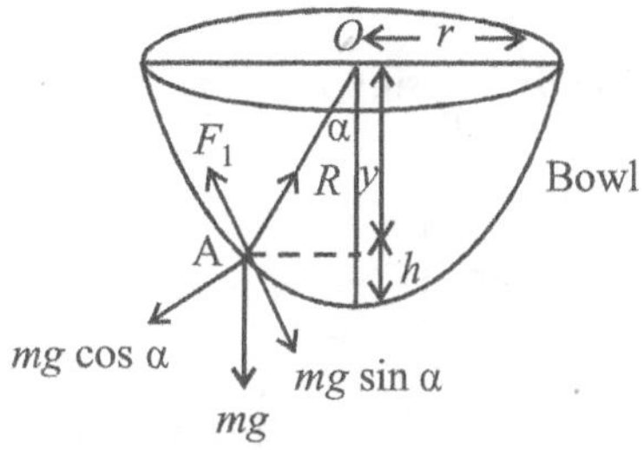

The insect crawls up the bowl upto a certain height h only till the component of its weight along the bowl is balanced by limiting frictional force.

For limiting condition at point A

$R = mg\cos\alpha$ ...(i)

$F_1 = mg\sin\alpha$ ...(ii)

Dividing eq. (ii) by (i)

$$\tan\alpha = \frac{1}{\cot\alpha} = \frac{F_1}{R} = \mu\left[As\ F_1 = \mu R\right]$$

$$\Rightarrow \quad \tan\alpha = \mu = \frac{1}{3}\left[\because \mu = \frac{1}{3}(\text{Given})\right]$$

$\therefore \quad \cot\alpha = 3$

41. **(c)**

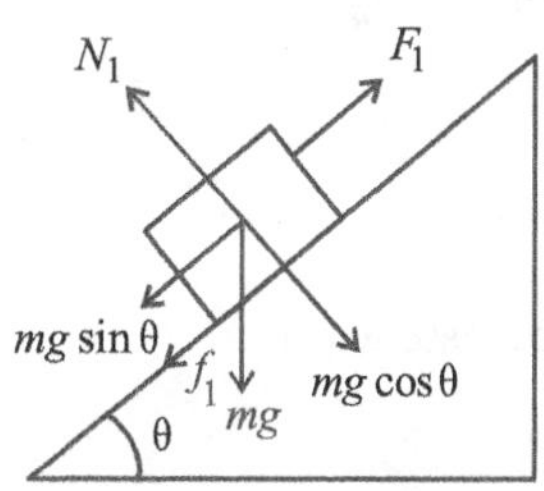

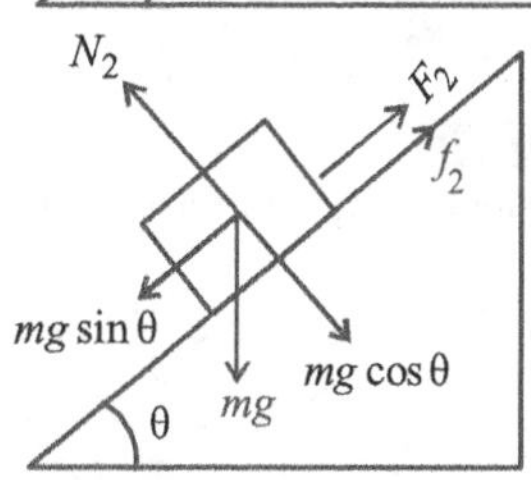

For the upward motion of the body

$mg\sin\theta + f_1 = F_1$

or, $F_1 = mg\sin\theta + \mu mg\cos\theta$

For the downward motion of the body,

$mg\sin\theta - f_2 = F_2$

or $F_2 = mg\sin\theta - \mu mg\cos\theta$

$$\therefore \quad \frac{F_1}{F_2} = \frac{\sin\theta + \mu\cos\theta}{\sin\theta - \mu\cos\theta}$$

$$\Rightarrow \quad \frac{\tan\theta+\mu}{\tan\theta-\mu} = \frac{2\mu+\mu}{2\mu-\mu} = \frac{3\mu}{\mu} = 3$$

42. **(d)** Here, $\ell_A = \frac{2\ell}{5}$, $\ell_B = \left(\frac{3\ell}{5}\right)$

$k\ell = k_A\ell_A = k_B\ell_B$

$k\ell = k_A\left(\frac{2\ell}{5}\right)$

$k_A = \frac{5k}{2}$

43. **(b)**

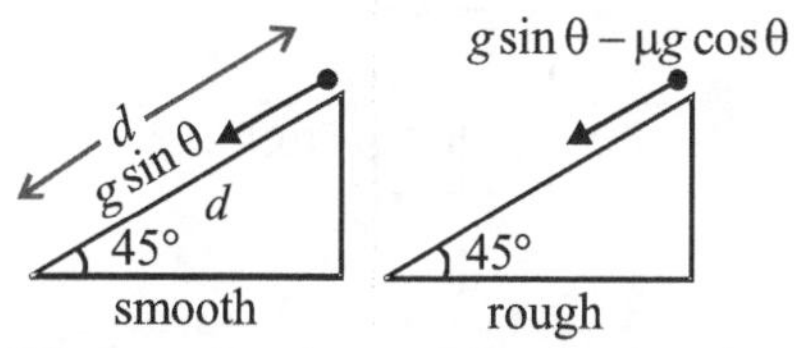

When surface is smooth

When surface is rough

$d = \frac{1}{2}(g\sin\theta)t_1^2$,

$d = \frac{1}{2}(g\sin\theta - \mu g\cos\theta)t_2^2$

$$t_1 = \sqrt{\frac{2d}{g\sin\theta}},\ t_2 = \sqrt{\frac{2d}{g\sin\theta - \mu g\cos\theta}}$$

According to question, $t_2 = nt_1$

$$n\sqrt{\frac{2d}{g\sin\theta}} = \sqrt{\frac{2d}{g\sin\theta - \mu g\cos\theta}}$$

μ, as applicable here, is coefficient of kinetic friction as the block moves over the inclined plane.

$$n = \frac{1}{\sqrt{1-\mu_k}}\ \left(\because \cos 45° = \sin 45° = \frac{1}{\sqrt{2}}\right)$$

$$n^2 = \frac{1}{1-\mu_k} \text{ or } 1-\mu_k = \frac{1}{n^2}$$

$$\text{or } \mu_k = 1 - \frac{1}{n^2}$$

44. **(d)** Acceleration of block while sliding down upper half $= g\sin\phi$;

retardation of block while sliding down lower half

$= -(g\sin\phi - \mu g\cos\phi)$

For the block to come to rest at the bottom, acceleration in I half = retardation in II half.

$g\sin\phi = -(g\sin\phi - \mu g\cos\phi)$

$\Rightarrow \mu = 2\tan\phi$

45. **(a)** $v^2 - u^2 = 2as$ or $0^2 - u^2 = 2(-\mu_k g)s$

$$-100^2 = 2\times -\frac{1}{2}\times 10\times s$$

$$s = 1000 \text{ m}$$

46. **(c)**

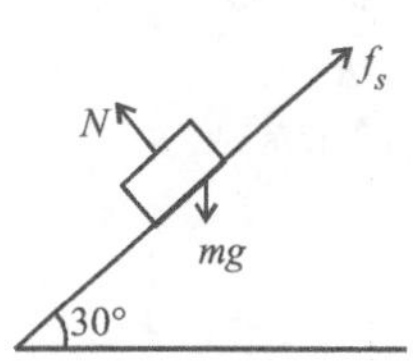

mg sinθ = f_s(for body to be at rest)

$\Rightarrow m \times 10 \times \sin 30° = 10$

$\Rightarrow m \times 5 = 10 \Rightarrow m = 2.0$ kg

47. **(d)** For the block to remain stationary with the wall

$f = W$

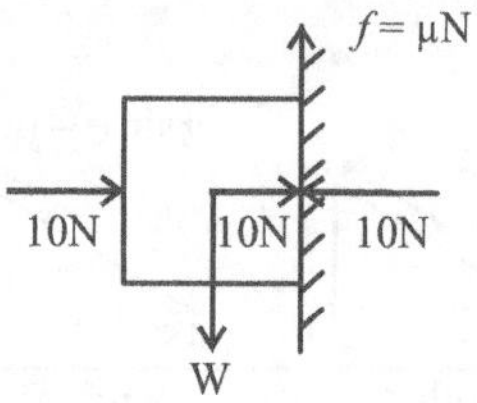

$\mu N = W$

$0.2 \times 10 = W \Rightarrow W = 2N$

48. **(d)** $u = 6$ m/s, $v = 0$, $t = 10s$, $a = ?$

$v = u + at \Rightarrow 0 = 6 + a \times 10$

$\Rightarrow \quad a = \frac{-6}{10} = -0.6 \text{m/s}^2$

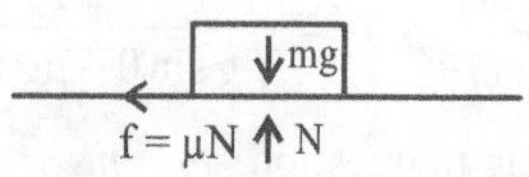

The retardation is due to the frictional force

$\therefore \quad f = ma \Rightarrow \mu N = ma \Rightarrow \mu mg = ma$

$\Rightarrow \mu = \frac{a}{g} = \frac{0.6}{10} = 0.06$

TOPIC-4 : Circular Motion, Banking of Road

49. **(d)** Given, θ = 45°, r = 0.4 m, g = 10 m/s²

$T \sin\theta = \frac{mv^2}{r}$ ...... (i)

$T \cos\theta = mg$ ...... (ii)

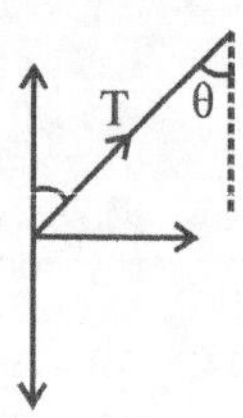

From equation (i) & (ii) we have,

$\tan\theta = \frac{v^2}{rg}$

$v^2 = rg \quad \because \theta = 45°$

Hence, speed of the pendulum in its circular path,

$v = \sqrt{rg} = \sqrt{0.4 \times 10} = 2$ m/s

50. **(c)**

51. **(a)**

52. **(d)** $s = t^3 + 5$

$\Rightarrow$ velocity, $v = \frac{ds}{dt} = 3t^2$

Tangential acceleration $a_t = \frac{dv}{dt} = 6t$

Radial acceleration $a_c = \frac{v^2}{R} = \frac{9t^4}{R}$

At $t = 2s$, $a_t = 6 \times 2 = 12$ m/s²

$a_c = \frac{9 \times 16}{20} = 7.2$ m/s²

$\therefore$ Resultant acceleration

$= \sqrt{a_t^2 + a_c^2}$

$= \sqrt{(12)^2 + (7.2)^2} = \sqrt{144 + 51.84}$

$= \sqrt{195.84} = 14$ m/s²

53. **(c)** Clearly $\vec{a} = a_c \cos\theta(-\hat{i}) + a_c \sin\theta(-\hat{j})$

$= \frac{-v^2}{R}\cos\theta\,\hat{i} - \frac{v^2}{R}\sin\theta\,\hat{j}$

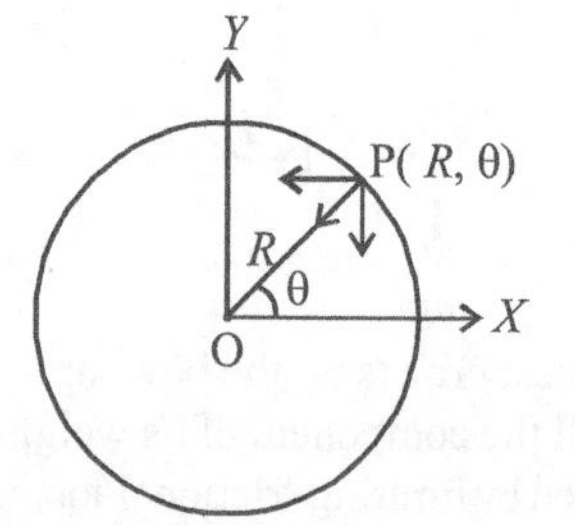

54. **(c)**

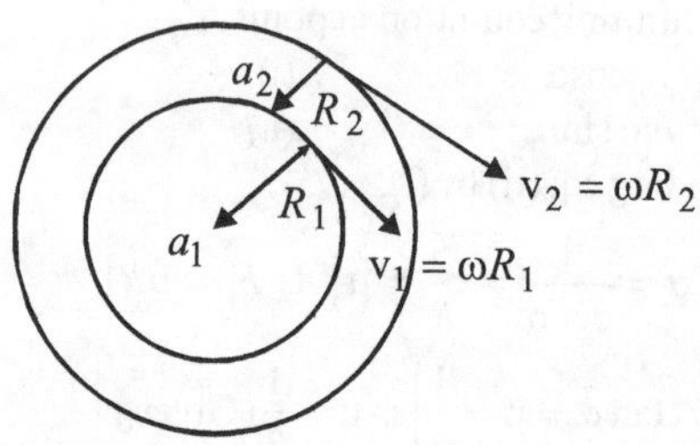

$a_1 = \frac{v_1^2}{R_1} = \frac{\omega^2 R_1^2}{R_1} = \omega^2 R_1$

$a_2 = \frac{v_2^2}{R_2} = \omega^2 R_2$

Taking particle masses equal

$\frac{F_1}{F_2} = \frac{ma_1}{ma_2} = \frac{a_1}{a_2} = \frac{R_1}{R_2}$

ALTERNATE SOLUTION

The force experienced by any particle is only along radial direction.

Force experienced by the particle, $F = m\omega^2 R$

$\therefore \frac{F_1}{F_2} = \frac{R_1}{R_2}$

55. **(b)** Only option (b) is false since acceleration vector is always radial (i.e. towards the center) for uniform circular motion.

56. **(b)** For negotiating a circular curve on a levelled road, the maximum velocity of the car is $v_{max} = \sqrt{\mu rg}$

Here $\mu = 0.6$, $r = 150$ m, $g = 9.8$

$\therefore v_{max} = \sqrt{0.6 \times 150 \times 9.8} \simeq 30 \text{m/s}$

Chapter 5

Work, Energy and Power

TOPIC-1 : Work

1. A time dependent force F = 6t acts on a particle of mass 1 kg. If the particle starts from rest, the work done by the force during the first 1 second will be **[2017]**
(a) 9 J (b) 18 J (c) 4.5 J (d) 22 J

2. Velocity–time graph for a body of mass 10 kg is shown in figure. Work–done on the body in first two seconds of the motion is : **[Online April 10, 2016]**

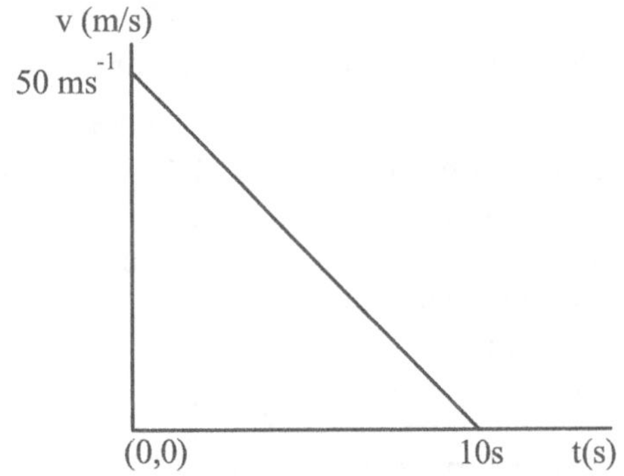

(a) −9300 J (b) 12000 J (c) −4500 J (d) −12000 J

3. When a rubber-band is stretched by a distance x, it exerts restoring force of magnitude $F = ax + bx^2$ where a and b are constants. The work done in stretching the unstretched rubber-band by L is: **[2014]**
(a) $aL^2 + bL^3$ (b) $\frac{1}{2}(aL^2 + bL^3)$
(c) $\frac{aL^2}{2} + \frac{bL^3}{3}$ (d) $\frac{1}{2}\left(\frac{aL^2}{2} + \frac{bL^3}{3}\right)$

4. A uniform chain of length 2 m is kept on a table such that a length of 60 cm hangs freely from the edge of the table. The total mass of the chain is 4 kg. What is the work done in pulling the entire chain on the table ? **[2004]**
(a) 12 J (b) 3.6 J (c) 7.2 J (d) 1200 J

5. A force $\vec{F} = (5\vec{i} + 3\vec{j} + 2\vec{k})N$ is applied over a particle which displaces it from its origin to the point $\vec{r} = (2\vec{i} - \vec{j})m$. The work done on the particle in joules is **[2004]**
(a) +10 (b) +7 (c) −7 (d) +13

6. A spring of spring constant 5×10^3 N/m is stretched initially by 5cm from the unstretched position. Then the work required to stretch it further by another 5 cm is **[2003]**
(a) 12.50 N-m (b) 18.75 N-m
(c) 25.00 N-m (d) 6.25 N-m

7. A spring of force constant 800 N/m has an extension of 5 cm. The work done in extending it from 5 cm to 15 cm is **[2002]**
(a) 16 J (b) 8 J (c) 32 J (d) 24 J

TOPIC-2 : Energy

8. A body of mass $m = 10^{-2}$ kg is moving in a medium and experiences a frictional force $F = -kv^2$. Its intial speed is $v_0 = 10$ ms^{-1}. If, after 10 s, its energy is $\frac{1}{8}mv_0^2$, the value of k will be: **[2017]**
(a) 10^{-4} kg m^{-1} (b) 10^{-1} kg m^{-1} s^{-1}
(c) 10^{-3} kg m^{-1} (d) 10^{-3} kg s^{-1}

9. An object is dropped from a height h from the ground. Every time it hits the ground it looses 50% of its kinetic energy. The total distance covered as $t \to \infty$ is : **[Online April 8, 2017]**
(a) 3h (b) ∞ (c) $\frac{5}{3}$h (d) $\frac{8}{3}$h

10. A point particle of mass m, moves long the uniformly rough track PQR as shown in the figure. The coefficient of friction, between the particle and the rough track equals μ. The particle is released, from rest from the point P and it comes to rest at a point R. The energies, lost by the ball, over the parts, PQ and QR, of the track, are equal to each other, and no energy is lost when particle changes direction from PQ to QR.
The value of the coefficient of friction μ and the distance x (= QR), are, respectively close to : **[2016]**

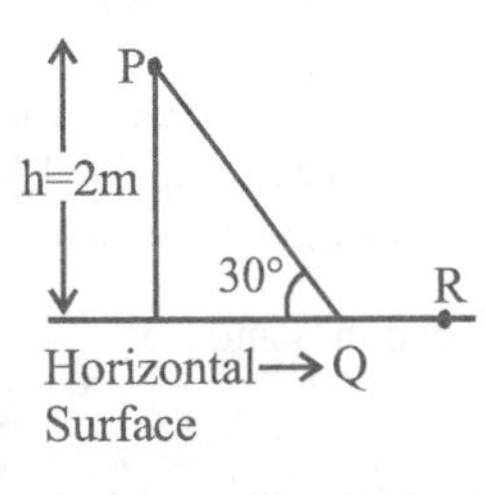

(a) 0.29 and 3.5 m (b) 0.29 and 6.5 m
(c) 0.2 and 6.5 m (d) 0.2 and 3.5 m

11. A person trying to lose weight by burning fat lifts a mass of 10 kg upto a height of 1 m 1000 times. Assume that the potential energy lost each time he lowers the mass is dissipated. How much fat will he use up considering the work done only when the weight is lifted up? Fat supplies 3.8×10^7 J of energy per kg which is converted to mechanical energy with a 20% efficiency rate. Take g = 9.8 ms^{-2} : **[2016]**

(a) 9.89×10^{-3} kg (b) 12.89×10^{-3} kg
(c) 2.45×10^{-3} kg (d) 6.45×10^{-3} kg

12. A particle is moving in a circle of radius r under the action of a force F = αr^2 which is directed towards centre of the circle. Total mechanical energy (kinetic energy + potential energy) of the particle is (take potential energy = 0 for r = 0) : **[Online April 11, 2015]**

(a) $\frac{1}{2}\alpha r^3$ (b) $\frac{5}{6}\alpha r^3$ (c) $\frac{4}{3}\alpha r^3$ (d) αr^3

13. A block of mass m = 0.1 kg is connected to a spring of unknown spring constant k. It is compressed to a distance x from its equilibrium position and released from rest. After approaching half the distance $\left(\frac{x}{2}\right)$ from equilibrium position, it hits another block and comes to rest momentarily, while the other block moves with a velocity 3 ms^{-1}.
The total initial energy of the spring is : **[Online April 10, 2015]**

(a) 0.3 J (b) 0.6 J (c) 0.8 J (d) 1.5 J

14. A bullet looses $\left(\frac{1}{n}\right)^{th}$ of its velocity passing through one plank. The number of such planks that are required to stop the bullet can be: **[Online April 19, 2014]**

(a) $\frac{n^2}{2n-1}$ (b) $\frac{2n^2}{n-1}$ (c) infinite (d) n

15. A spring of unstretched length l has a mass m with one end fixed to a rigid support. Assuming spring to be made of a uniform wire, the kinetic energy possessed by it if its free end is pulled with uniform velocity v is: **[Online April 12, 2014]**

(a) $\frac{1}{2}mv^2$ (b) mv^2 (c) $\frac{1}{3}mv^2$ (d) $\frac{1}{6}mv^2$

16. Two springs of force constants 300 N/m (Spring A) and 400 N/m (Spring B) are joined together in series. The combination is compressed by 8.75 cm. The ratio of energy stored in A and B is $\frac{E_A}{E_B}$. Then $\frac{E_A}{E_B}$ is equal to : **[Online April 9, 2013]**

(a) $\frac{4}{3}$ (b) $\frac{16}{9}$ (c) $\frac{3}{4}$ (d) $\frac{9}{16}$

17. The force $\vec{F} = F\hat{i}$ on a particle of mass 2 kg, moving along the x-axis is given in the figure as a function of its position x. The particle is moving with a velocity of 5 m/s along the x-axis at x = 0. What is the kinetic energy of the particle at x = 8 m? **[Online May 26, 2012]**

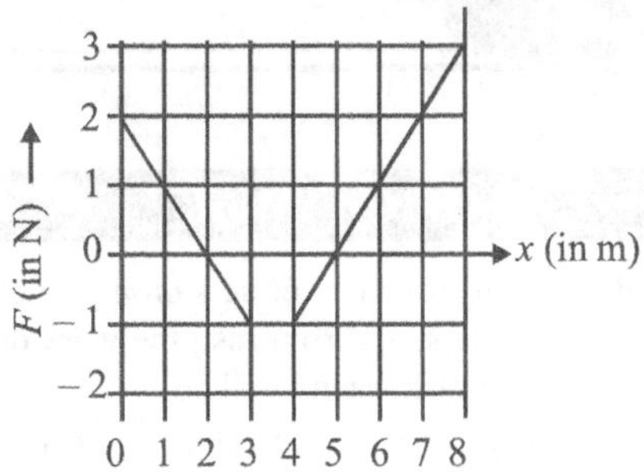

(a) 34 J (b) 34.5 J (c) 4.5 J (d) 29.4 J

18. A particle gets displaced by $\Delta\vec{r} = (2\hat{i} + 3\hat{j} + 4\hat{k})$ m under the action of a force $\vec{F} = (7\hat{i} + 4\hat{j} + 3\hat{k})$. The change in its kinetic energy is **[Online May 7, 2012]**

(a) 38 J (b) 70 J (c) 52.5 J (d) 126 J

19. At time t = 0 a particle starts moving along the x-axis. If its kinetic energy increases uniformly with time 't', the net force acting on it must be proportional to **[2011 RS]**

(a) constant (b) t
(c) $\frac{1}{\sqrt{t}}$ (d) $\sqrt{t}$

20. The potential energy function for the force between two atoms in a diatomic molecule is approximately given by $U(x) = \frac{a}{x^{12}} - \frac{b}{x^6}$, where a and b are constants and x is the distance between the atoms. If the dissociation energy of the molecule is

$D = \left[U(x = \infty) - U_{\text{at equilibrium}}\right]$, D is **[2010]**

(a) $\frac{b^2}{2a}$ (b) $\frac{b^2}{12a}$ (c) $\frac{b^2}{4a}$ (d) $\frac{b^2}{6a}$

21. An athlete in the olympic games covers a distance of 100 m in 10 s. His kinetic energy can be estimated to be in the range **[2008]**

(a) 200 J - 500 J (b) 2×10^5 J - 3×10^5 J
(c) 20,000 J - 50,000 J (d) 2,000 J - 5,000 J

22. A 2 kg block slides on a horizontal floor with a speed of 4m/s. It strikes a uncompressed spring, and compresses it till the block is motionless. The kinetic friction force is 15N and spring constant is 10,000 N/m. The spring compresses by **[2007]**

(a) 8.5 cm (b) 5.5 cm
(c) 2.5 cm (d) 11.0 cm

23. A particle is projected at 60° to the horizontal with a kinetic energy K. The kinetic energy at the highest point is [2007]
(a) $K/2$ (b) K
(c) Zero (d) $K/4$

24. A particle of mass 100g is thrown vertically upwards with a speed of 5 m/s. The work done by the force of gravity during the time the particle goes up is [2006]
(a) –0.5 J (b) –1.25 J
(c) 1.25 J (d) 0.5 J

25. The potential energy of a 1 kg particle free to move along the x-axis is given by $V(x) = \left(\frac{x^4}{4} - \frac{x^2}{2}\right) J$.
The total mechanical energy of the particle is 2 J. Then, the maximum speed (in m/s) is [2006]
(a) $\frac{3}{\sqrt{2}}$ (b) $\sqrt{2}$ (c) $\frac{1}{\sqrt{2}}$ (d) 2

26. A mass of M kg is suspended by a weightless string. The horizontal force that is required to displace it until the string makes an angle of 45° with the initial vertical direction is [2006]
(a) $Mg(\sqrt{2}+1)$ (b) $Mg\sqrt{2}$
(c) $\frac{Mg}{\sqrt{2}}$ (d) $Mg(\sqrt{2}-1)$

27. A spherical ball of mass 20 kg is stationary at the top of a hill of height 100 m. It rolls down a smooth surface to the ground, then climbs up another hill of height 30 m and finally rolls down to a horizontal base at a height of 20 m above the ground. The velocity attained by the ball is [2005]
(a) 20 m/s (b) 40 m/s
(c) $10\sqrt{30}$ m/s (d) 10 m/s

28. A particle moves in a straight line with retardation proportional to its displacement. Its loss of kinetic energy for any displacement x is proportional to [2004]
(a) x (b) e^x (c) x^2 (d) $\log_e x$

29. A particle is acted upon by a force of constant magnitude which is always perpendicular to the velocity of the particle, the motion of the particles takes place in a plane. It follows that [2004]
(a) its kinetic energy is constant
(b) its acceleration is constant
(c) its velocity is constant
(d) it moves in a straight line

30. A wire suspended vertically from one of its ends is stretched by attaching a weight of 200N to the lower end. The weight stretches the wire by 1 mm. Then the elastic energy stored in the wire is [2003]
(a) 0.2 J (b) 10 J (c) 20 J (d) 0.1 J

31. A ball whose kinetic energy is E, is projected at an angle of 45° to the horizontal. The kinetic energy of the ball at the highest point of its flight will be [2002]
(a) E (b) $E/\sqrt{2}$ (c) $E/2$ (d) zero.

TOPIC-3 : Power

32. A particle of mass M is moving in a circle of fixed radius R in such a way that its centripetal acceleration at time t is given by n^2Rt^2 where n is a constant. The power delivered to the particle by the force acting on it, is : [Online April 10, 2016]
(a) $\frac{1}{2}Mn^2R^2t^2$ (b) Mn^2R^2t
(c) MnR^2t^2 (d) MnR^2t

33. A car of weight W is on an inclined road that rises by 100 m over a distance of 1 Km and applies a constant frictional force $\frac{W}{20}$ on the car. While moving uphill on the road at a speed of 10 ms^{-1}, the car needs power P. If it needs power $\frac{P}{2}$ while moving downhill at speed v then value of v is: [Online April 9, 2016]
(a) 20 ms^{-1} (b) 5 ms^{-1} (c) 15 ms^{-1} (d) 10 ms^{-1}

34. A wind-powered generator converts wind energy into electrical energy. Assume that the generator converts a fixed fraction of the wind energy intercepted by its blades into electrical energy. For wind speed v, the electrical power output will be most likely proportional to [Online April 25, 2013]
(a) v^4 (b) v^2 (c) v (d) v

35. A 70 kg man leaps vertically into the air from a crouching position. To take the leap the man pushes the ground with a constant force F to raise himself. The center of gravity rises by 0.5 m before he leaps. After the leap the c.g. rises by another 1 m. The maximum power delivered by the muscles is : (Take g = 10 ms^{-2}) [Online April 23, 2013]
(a) 6.26×10^3 Watts at the start
(b) 6.26×10^3 Watts at take off
(c) 6.26×10^4 Watts at the start
(d) 6.26×10^4 Watts at take off

36. A body of mass 'm', accelerates uniformly from rest to 'v_1' in time 't_1'. The instantaneous power delivered to the body as a function of time 't' is [2004]
(a) $\frac{mv_1t^2}{t_1}$ (b) $\frac{mv_1^2t}{t_1^2}$ (c) $\frac{mv_1t}{t_1}$ (d) $\frac{mv_1^2t}{t_1}$

37. A body is moved along a straight line by a machine delivering a constant power. The distance moved by the body in time 't' is proportional to [2003]
(a) $t^{3/4}$ (b) $t^{3/2}$ (c) $t^{1/4}$ (d) $t^{1/2}$

TOPIC-4 : Collisions

38. Two particles A and B of equal mass M are moving with the same speed v as shown in the figure. They collide completely inelastically and move as a single particle C. The angle θ that the path of C makes with the X-axis is given by: **[Online April 9, 2017]**

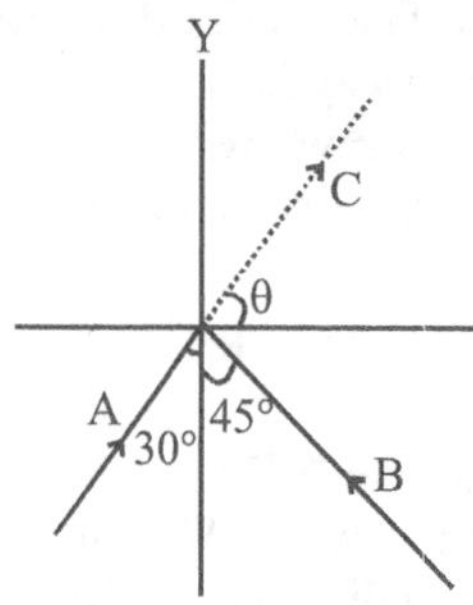

(a) $\tan\theta = \dfrac{\sqrt{3}+\sqrt{2}}{1-\sqrt{2}}$

(b) $\tan\theta = \dfrac{\sqrt{3}-\sqrt{2}}{1-\sqrt{2}}$

(c) $\tan\theta = \dfrac{1-\sqrt{2}}{\sqrt{2}(1+\sqrt{3})}$

(d) $\tan\theta = \dfrac{1-\sqrt{3}}{1+\sqrt{2}}$

39. A neutron moving with a speed 'v' makes a head on collision with a stationary hydrogen atom in ground state. The minimum kinetic energy of the neutron for which inelastic collision will take place is : **[Online April 10, 2016]**

(a) 20.4 eV (b) 10.2 eV (c) 12.1 eV (d) 16.8 eV

40. A particle of mass m moving in the x direction with speed $2v$ is hit by another particle of mass $2m$ moving in the y direction with speed v. If the collision is perfectly inelastic, the percentage loss in the energy during the collision is close to : **[2015]**

(a) 56% (b) 62% (c) 44% (d) 50%

41. A bullet of mass 4 g is fired horizontally with a speed of 300 m/s into 0.8 kg block of wood at rest on a table. If the coefficient of friction between the block and the table is 0.3, how far will the block slide approximately? **[Online April 12, 2014]**

(a) 0.19m (b) 0.379m (c) 0.569m (d) 0.758m

42. Three masses m, 2m and 3m are moving in x-y plane with speed 3u, 2u and u respectively as shown in figure. The three masses collide at the same point at P and stick together. The velocity of resulting mass will be: **[Online April 12, 2014]**

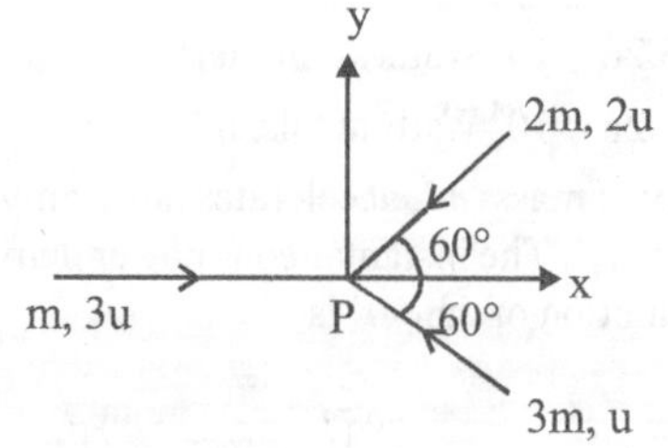

(a) $\frac{u}{12}\left(\hat{i}+\sqrt{3}\hat{j}\right)$ (b) $\frac{u}{12}\left(\hat{i}-\sqrt{3}\hat{j}\right)$

(c) $\frac{u}{12}\left(-\hat{i}+\sqrt{3}\hat{j}\right)$ (d) $\frac{u}{12}\left(-\hat{i}-\sqrt{3}\hat{j}\right)$

43. This question has statement I and statement II. Of the four choices given after the statements, choose the one that best describes the two statements.

Statement - I: A point particle of mass m moving with speed υ collides with stationary point particle of mass M. If the maximum energy loss possible is given as $f\left(\frac{1}{2}mv^2\right)$ then

$$f=\left(\frac{m}{M+m}\right).$$

Statement - II: Maximum energy loss occurs when the particles get stuck together as a result of the collision. **[2013]**

(a) Statement - I is true, Statment - II is true, Statement - II is the correct explanation of Statement - I.

(b) Statement-I is true, Statment - II is true, Statement - II is not the correct explanation of Statement - II.

(c) Statement - I is true, Statment - II is false.

(d) Statement - I is false, Statment - II is true.

44. A projectile of mass M is fired so that the horizontal range is 4 km. At the highest point the projectile explodes in two parts of masses $M/4$ and $3M/4$ respectively and the heavier part starts falling down vertically with zero initial speed. The horizontal range (distance from point of firing) of the lighter part is : **[Online April 23, 2013]**

(a) 16 km (b) 1 km (c) 10 km (d) 2 km

45. A moving particle of mass m, makes a head on elastic collision with another particle of mass $2m$, which is initially at rest. The percentage loss in energy of the colliding particle on collision, is close to **[Online May 19, 2012]**

(a) 33% (b) 67% (c) 90% (d) 10%

46. Two bodies A and B of mass m and $2m$ respectively are placed on a smooth floor. They are connected by a spring of negligible mass. A third body C of mass m is placed on the floor. The body C moves with a velocity v_0 along the line joining A and B and collides elastically with A. At a certain time after the collision it is found that the instantaneous velocities of A and B are same and the compression of the spring is x_0. The spring constant k will be **[Online May 12, 2012]**

(a) $m\dfrac{v_0^2}{x_0^2}$ (b) $m\dfrac{v_0}{2x_0}$

(c) $2m\dfrac{v_0}{x_0}$ (d) $\dfrac{2}{3}m\left(\dfrac{v_0}{x_0}\right)^2$

47. A projectile moving vertically upwards with a velocity of 200 ms^{-1} breaks into two equal parts at a height of 490 m. One part starts moving vertically upwards with a velocity of 400 ms^{-1}. How much time it will take, after the break up with the other part to hit the ground? **[Online May 12, 2012]**

(a) $2\sqrt{10}$ s (b) 5 s (c) 10 s (d) $\sqrt{10}$ s

48. **Statement -1:** Two particles moving in the same direction do not lose all their energy in a completely inelastic collision.

Statement -2 : Principle of conservation of momentum holds true for all kinds of collisions. **[2010]**

(a) Statement -1 is true, Statement -2 is true ; Statement -2 is the correct explanation of Statement -1.

(b) Statement -1 is true, Statement -2 is true; Statement -2 is **not** the correct explanation of Statement -1

(c) Statement -1 is false, Statement -2 is true.

(d) Statement -1 is true, Statement -2 is false.

49. A block of mass 0.50 kg is moving with a speed of 2.00 ms^{-1} on a smooth surface. It strikes another mass of 1.00 kg and then they move together as a single body. The energy loss during the collision is **[2008]**

(a) 0.16 J (b) 1.00 J (c) 0.67 J (d) 0.34 J

50. A bomb of mass 16kg at rest explodes into two pieces of masses 4 kg and 12 kg. The velolcity of the 12 kg mass is 4 ms^{-1}. The kinetic energy of the other mass is **[2006]**

(a) 144 J (b) 288 J (c) 192 J (d) 96 J

51. The block of mass M moving on the frictionless horizontal surface collides with the spring of spring constant k and compresses it by length L. The maximum momentum of the block after collision is **[2005]**

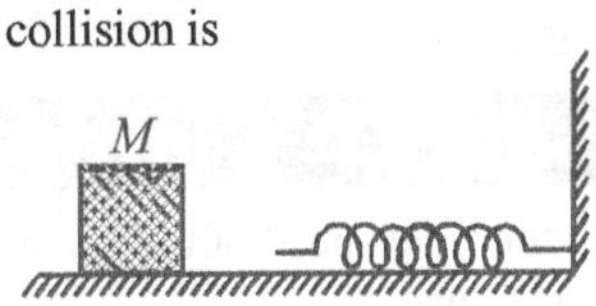

(a) $\frac{kL^2}{2M}$ (b) $\sqrt{Mk}\,L$ (c) $\frac{ML^2}{k}$ (d) zero

52. A mass 'm' moves with a velocity 'v' and collides inelastically with another identical mass. After collision the 1st mass moves with velocity $\frac{v}{\sqrt{3}}$ in a direction perpendicular to the initial direction of motion. Find the speed of the 2nd mass after collision. **[2005]**

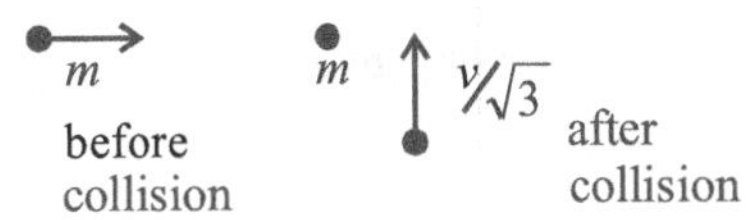

(a) $\sqrt{3}v$ (b) v (c) $\frac{v}{\sqrt{3}}$ (d) $\frac{2}{\sqrt{3}}v$

53. Consider the following two statements : **[2003]**

A. Linear momentum of a system of particles is zero

B. Kinetic energy of a system of particles is zero.

Then

(a) A does not imply B and B does not imply A

(b) A implies B but B does not imply A

(c) A does not imply B but B implies A

(d) A implies B and B implies A

Hints & Solutions

TOPIC-1 : Work

1. (c) Using, $F = ma = m\frac{dV}{dt}$

$$6t = 1.\frac{dV}{dt} \quad [\because \; m = 1 \text{ kg given}]$$

$$\int_0^v dV = \int 6t\, dt$$

$$V = 6\left[\frac{t^2}{2}\right]_0^1 = 3\,\text{ms}^{-1} \quad [\because \; t = 1 \text{ sec given}]$$

From work-energy theorem,

$$W = \Delta KE = \frac{1}{2}m\left(V^2 - u^2\right) = \frac{1}{2}\times 1\times 9 = 4.5\text{ J}$$

2. (c) Acceleration (a) $= \frac{v-4}{t} = \frac{(0-50)}{(10-0)} = -5\text{ m/s}^2$

$u = 50$ m/s

$\therefore v = u + at = 50 - 5t$

Veocity in first two seconds t = 2

$v_{(\text{at } t=2)} = 40$ m/s

From work-energy theorem,

$$\Delta K.E. = W = \frac{1}{2}(40^2 - 50^2)\times 10 = -4500\text{ J}$$

3. (c) Work done in stretching the rubber-band by a distance dx is

$$dW = F\,dx = (ax + bx^2)dx$$

Integrating both sides,

$$W = \int_0^L ax\,dx + \int_0^L bx^2\,dx = \frac{aL^2}{2} + \frac{bL^3}{3}$$

4. (b) Mass of over hanging chain

$$m' = \frac{4}{2}\times(0.6)\text{kg}$$

Let at the surface PE = 0

C.M.of hanging part = 0.3 m below the table

$$U_i = -m'gx = -\frac{4}{2}\times 0.6\times 10\times 0.30$$

$\Delta U = m'gx = 3.6$J = Workdone in putting the entire chain on the table.

5. (b) Workdone in displacing the particle,

$$W = \vec{F}.\vec{x} = (5\hat{i} + 3\hat{j} + 2\hat{k}).(2\hat{i} - \hat{j})$$

$$= 10 - 3 = 7 \text{ joules}$$

6. (b) $k = 5\times 10^3$ N/m

$$W = \frac{1}{2}k\left(x_2^2 - x_1^2\right) = \frac{1}{2}\times 5\times 10^3\left[(0.1)^2 - (0.05)^2\right]$$

$$= \frac{5000}{2}\times 0.15\times 0.05 = 18.75\text{ Nm}$$

7. (b) Small amount of work done in extending the spring by dx is

$$dW = k\,x\,dx$$

$$\therefore W = k\int_{0.05}^{0.15} x\,dx$$

$$= \frac{800}{2}\left[(0.15)^2 - (0.05)^2\right]$$

$$= 400\,[(0.15 + 0.05)(0.15 - 0.05)]$$

$$= 400\times 0.2\times 0.1 = 8\text{ J}$$

TOPIC-2 : Energy

8. (a) Let V_f is the final speed of the body.

From questions,

$$\frac{1}{2}mV_f^2 = \frac{1}{8}mV_0^2 \Rightarrow V_f = \frac{V_0}{2} = 5\,m/s$$

$$F = m\left(\frac{dV}{dt}\right) = -kV^2 \quad \therefore \; (10^{-2})\frac{dV}{dt} = -kV^2$$

$$\int_{10}^{5}\frac{dV}{V^2} = -100K\int_0^{10} dt$$

$$\frac{1}{5} - \frac{1}{10} = 100K(10) \text{ or, } K = 10^{-4}\,kgm^{-1}$$

9. (a) (K.E.)' = 50% of K.E. after hit i.e.,

$$\frac{1}{2}mv'^2 = \frac{50}{100}\times\frac{1}{2}mv^2 \Rightarrow v' = \frac{v}{\sqrt{2}}$$

Coefficient of restitution $= \frac{1}{\sqrt{2}}$

Now, total distance travelled by object is

$$H = h\left(\frac{1+e^2}{1-e^2}\right) = h\left(\frac{1+\frac{1}{2}}{1-\frac{1}{2}}\right) = 3h$$

10. (a) Loss in P.E. = Work done against friction from p $\rightarrow$ Q + work done against friction from Q $\rightarrow$ R

mgh = μ(mg cos θ) PQ + μmg (QR)

h = μ cos θ $\times$ PQ + μ(QR)

$$2=\mu\times\frac{\sqrt{3}}{2}\times\frac{2}{\sin 30^\circ}+\mu x$$

$$2=2\sqrt{3}\,\mu+\mu x \quad \text{---(i)} \quad [\sin 30^\circ=\frac{2}{PQ}]$$

Also work done $P\to Q$ = work done $Q\to R$

$\therefore\ 2\sqrt{3}\,\mu=\mu x$

$\therefore\ x\approx 3.5\text{m}$

From (i) $2=2\sqrt{3}\,\mu+2\sqrt{3}\,\mu=4\sqrt{3}\,\mu$

$$\mu=\frac{2}{4\sqrt{3}}=\frac{1}{2\times 1.732}=0.29$$

11. (b) $n=\frac{W}{\text{input}}=\frac{mgh\times 1000}{\text{input}}=\frac{10\times 9.8\times 1\times 1000}{\text{input}}$

$$\text{Input}=\frac{98000}{0.2}=49\times 10^4\text{J}$$

$$\text{Fat used}=\frac{49\times 10^4}{3.8\times 10^7}=12.89\times 10^{-3}\text{kg.}$$

12. (b) As we know, $dU = F.dr$

$$U=\int_0^r \alpha r^2 dr=\frac{\alpha r^3}{3} \quad \text{...(i)}$$

As, $\frac{mv^2}{r}=\alpha r^2$

$m^2v^2=m\alpha r^3$

or, $2m(KE)=\frac{1}{2}\alpha r^3$ ...(ii)

Total energy = Potential energy + kinetic energy

Now, from eqn (i) and (ii)

Total energy = K.E. + P.E.

$$=\frac{\alpha r^3}{3}+\frac{\alpha r^3}{2}=\frac{5}{6}\alpha r^3$$

13. (b) Applying momentum conservation

$m_1u_1+m_2u_2=m_1v_1+m_2v_2$

$0.1u+m(0)=0.1(0)+m(3)$

$0.1u=3m$

$$\frac{1}{2}0.1u^2=\frac{1}{2}m(3)^2$$

Solving we get, $u = 3$

$$\frac{1}{2}kx^2=\frac{1}{2}K\left(\frac{x}{2}\right)^2+\frac{1}{2}(0.1)3^2$$

$$\Rightarrow\ \frac{3}{4}kx^2=0.9$$

$$\Rightarrow\ \frac{3}{2}\times\frac{1}{2}kx^2=0.9$$

$\therefore\ \frac{1}{2}Kx^2=0.6$ J (total initial energy of the spring)

14. (a) Let u be the initial velocity of the bullet of mass m. After passing through a plank of width x, its velocity decreases to v.

$$\therefore\quad u-v=\frac{4}{n}\ \text{or, } v=u-\frac{4}{n}=\frac{u(n-1)}{n}$$

If F be the retarding force applied by each plank, then using work – energy theorem,

$$Fx=\frac{1}{2}mu^2-\frac{1}{2}mv^2=\frac{1}{2}mu^2-\frac{1}{2}mu^2\frac{(n-1)^2}{n^2}$$

$$=\frac{1}{2}mu^2\left[\frac{1-(n-1)^2}{n^2}\right]$$

$$Fx=\frac{1}{2}mu^2\left(\frac{2n-1}{n^2}\right)$$

Let P be the number of planks required to stop the bullet.

Total distance travelled by the bullet before coming to rest = Px

Using work-energy theorem again,

$$F(Px)=\frac{1}{2}mu^2-0$$

$$\text{or, } P(Fx)=P\left[\frac{1}{2}mu^2\frac{(2n-1)}{n^2}\right]=\frac{1}{2}mu^2$$

$$\therefore\ P=\frac{n^2}{2n-1}$$

15. (d)

16. (a) Given : $k_A=300\,\text{N/m},\ k_B=400\,\text{N/m}$

Let when the combination of springs is compressed by force F. Spring A is compressed by x. Therefore compression in spring B

$x_B=(8.75-x)$ cm

$F=300\times x=400(8.75-x)$

Solving we get, x = 5 cm

$x_B=8.75-5=3.75$cm

$$\frac{E_A}{E_B}=\frac{\frac{1}{2}k_A(x_A)^2}{\frac{1}{2}k_B(x_B)^2}=\frac{300\times(5)^2}{400\times(3.75)^2}=\frac{4}{3}$$

17. (d)

18. (a) According to work-energy theorem,

Change in kinetic energy = work done

$$=\vec{F}.\Delta\vec{r}=(7\hat{i}+4\hat{j}+3\hat{k}).(2\hat{i}+3\hat{j}+4\hat{k})$$

$=14+12+12=38$ J

19. (c) K.E. $\propto t$ or K. E. $= ct$

$$\Rightarrow \frac{1}{2}mv^2 = ct$$

$$\Rightarrow \frac{p^2}{2m} = ct \ (\because p = mv)$$

$$\Rightarrow p = \sqrt{2ctm}$$

$$\Rightarrow F = \sqrt{2\,cm} \times \frac{1}{2\sqrt{t}}$$

$$\Rightarrow F \propto \frac{1}{\sqrt{t}}$$

20. (c) At equilibrium : $\frac{dU(x)}{dx} = 0$

$$\Rightarrow \frac{-12a}{x^{11}} = \frac{-6b}{x^5} \Rightarrow x = \left(\frac{2a}{b}\right)^{\frac{1}{6}}$$

$$\therefore U_{\text{at equilibrium}} = \frac{a}{\left(\frac{2a}{b}\right)^2} - \frac{b}{\left(\frac{2a}{b}\right)} = -\frac{b^2}{4a} \text{ and } U_{(x=\infty)} = 0$$

$$\therefore D = 0 - \left(-\frac{b^2}{4a}\right) = \frac{b^2}{4a}$$

21. (d) The average speed of the athelete

$$v = \frac{100}{10} = 10\,\text{m/s}$$

$$\therefore \text{K.E.} = \frac{1}{2}mv^2$$

If mass is 40 kg then,

$$\text{K.E.} = \frac{1}{2} \times 40 \times (10)^2 = 2000\,\text{J}$$

If mass is 100 kg then,

$$\text{K.E.} = \frac{1}{2} \times 100 \times (10)^2 = 5000\,\text{J}$$

22. (b) Let the block compress the spring by x before stopping. kinetic energy of the block = (P.E of compressed spring) + work done against friction.

$$\frac{1}{2} \times 2 \times (4)^2 = \frac{1}{2} \times 10{,}000 \times x^2 + 15 \times x$$

$$10{,}000\,x^2 + 30x - 32 = 0$$

$$\Rightarrow 5000x^2 + 15x - 16 = 0$$

$$\therefore x = \frac{-15 \pm \sqrt{(15)^2 - 4 \times (5000)(-16)}}{2 \times 5000}$$

$$= 0.055\text{m} = 5.5\text{cm}.$$

23. (d) Let u be the velocity with which the particle is thrown and m be the mass of the particle. Then

$$K = \frac{1}{2}mu^2. \quad \text{...(1)}$$

At the highest point the velocity is u cos 60° (only the horizontal component remains, the vertical component being zero at the top-most point). Therefore kinetic energy at the highest point.

$$K' = \frac{1}{2}m(u\cos 60°)^2 = \frac{1}{2}mu^2\cos^2 60° = \frac{K}{4} \quad \text{[From 1]}$$

24. (b) $\text{K.E} = \frac{1}{2}mv^2 = \frac{1}{2} \times 0.1 \times 25 = 1.25\text{ J}$

$$W = -mgh = -\left(\frac{1}{2}mv^2\right) = -1.25\text{ J}$$

$$\left[\because mgh = \frac{1}{2}mv^2 \text{ by energy conservation}\right]$$

25. (a) Velocity is maximum when K.E. is maximum For minimum. P.E.,

$$\frac{dV}{dx} = 0 \Rightarrow x^3 - x = 0 \Rightarrow x = \pm 1$$

$$\Rightarrow \text{Min. P.E.} = \frac{1}{4} - \frac{1}{2} = -\frac{1}{4}\text{ J}$$

$$\text{K.E.}_{(\text{max.})} + \text{P.E.}_{(\text{min.})} = 2 \text{ (Given)}$$

$$\therefore \text{K.E.}_{(\text{max.})} = 2 + \frac{1}{4} = \frac{9}{4}$$

$$\text{K.E.}_{\text{max.}} = \frac{1}{2}mv^2_{\text{max.}}$$

$$\Rightarrow \frac{1}{2} \times 1 \times v^2_{\text{max.}} = \frac{9}{4} \Rightarrow v_{\text{max.}} = \frac{3}{\sqrt{2}}$$

26. (d) Work done by tension + Work done by force (applied) + Work done by gravitational force = change in kinetic energy

Work done by tension is zero

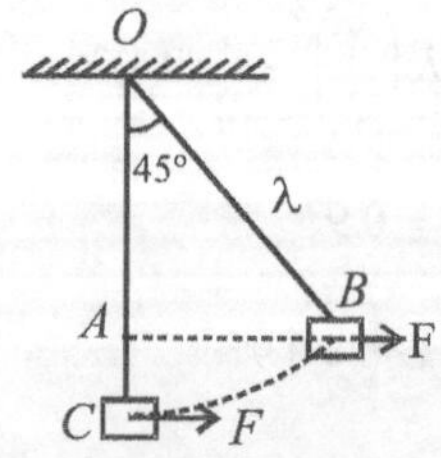

$$\Rightarrow 0 + F \times AB - Mg \times AC = 0$$

$$\Rightarrow F = Mg\left(\frac{AC}{AB}\right) = Mg\left[\frac{1-\frac{1}{\sqrt{2}}}{\frac{1}{\sqrt{2}}}\right]$$

$[\because AB = \ell \sin 45° = \frac{\ell}{\sqrt{2}}$ and

$AC = OC - OA = \ell - \ell \cos 45° = \ell\left(1-\frac{1}{\sqrt{2}}\right)$

where ℓ = length of the string.]

$\Rightarrow F = Mg(\sqrt{2}-1)$

27. (b)

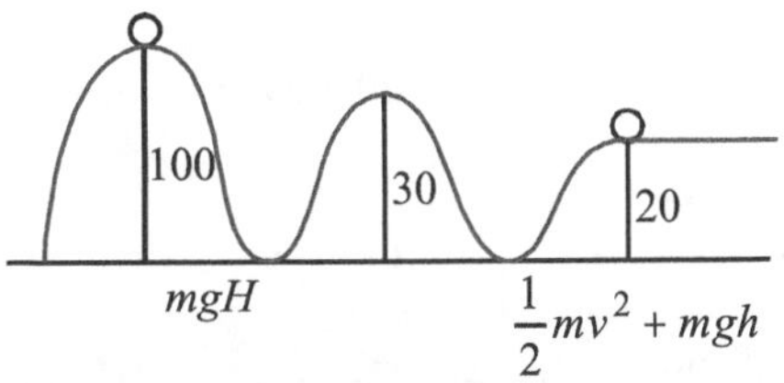

Using conservation of energy,
Loss in potential energy = gain in kinetic energy

$$m(10 \times 100) = m\left(\frac{1}{2}v^2 + 10 \times 20\right)$$

or $\frac{1}{2}v^2 = 800$ or $v = \sqrt{1600} = 40$ m/s

28. (c) Given : retardation $\propto$ displacement
i.e., $a = -x$

But $a = v\frac{dv}{dx}$

$$\therefore \frac{vdv}{dx} = -x \Rightarrow \int_{v_1}^{v_2} v\,dv = -\int_0^x xdx$$

$$\left(v_2^2 - v_1^2\right) = -\frac{x^2}{2}$$

$$\Rightarrow \frac{1}{2}m\left(v_2^2 - v_1^2\right) = \frac{1}{2}m\left(\frac{-x^2}{2}\right)$$

$\therefore$ Loss in kinetic energy, $\therefore \Delta K \propto x^2$

29. (a) Work done by such force is always zero since force is acting in a direction perpendicular to velocity.
$\therefore$ from work-energy theorem = $\Delta K = 0$
K remains constant.

30. (d) The elastic potential energy

$$= \frac{1}{2} \times \text{Force} \times \text{extension}$$

$$= \frac{1}{2} \times 200 \times 0.001 = 0.1 \text{ J}$$

31. (c) Let u be the speed with which the ball of mass m is projected. Then the kinetic energy (E) at the point of projection is

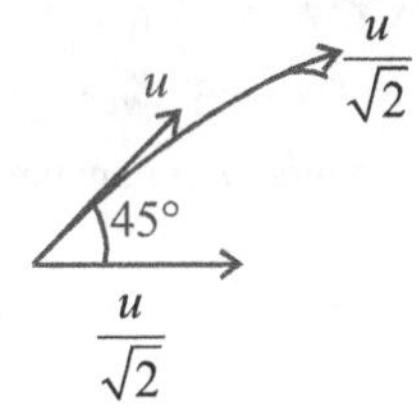

$$E = \frac{1}{2}mu^2 \qquad \text{...(i)}$$

When the ball is at the highest point of its flight, the speed of the ball is $\frac{u}{\sqrt{2}}$ (Remember that the horizontal component of velocity does not change during a projectile motion).
$\therefore$ The kinetic energy at the highest point

$$= \frac{1}{2}m\left(\frac{u}{\sqrt{2}}\right)^2 = \frac{1}{2}\frac{mu^2}{2} = \frac{E}{2} \qquad \text{[From (i)]}$$

TOPIC-3 : Power

32. (b) Centripetel acceleration $a_c = n^2Rt^2$

$$a_c = \frac{v^2}{R} = n^2Rt^2$$

$$v^2 = n^2R^2t^2$$

$$v = nRt$$

$$a_c = \frac{dv}{dt} = nR$$

Power = $ma_t v = m\,nR\,nRt = Mn^2R^2t$.

33. (c) While moving downhill power

$$P = \left(w\sin\theta + \frac{w}{20}\right)10$$

$$P = \left(\frac{w}{10} + \frac{w}{20}\right)10 = \frac{3w}{2}$$

$$\frac{P}{2} = \frac{3w}{4} = \left(\frac{w}{10} - \frac{w}{20}\right)V$$

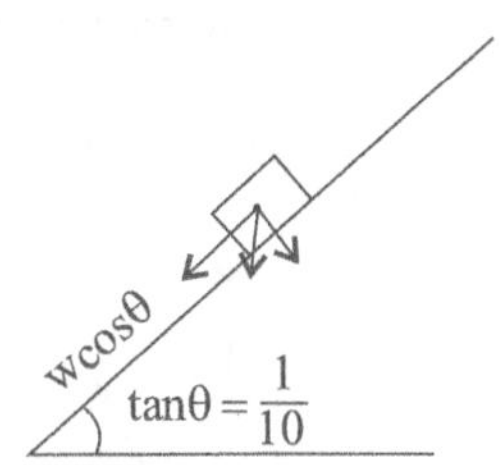

$$\frac{3}{4} = \frac{v}{20} \Rightarrow v = 15 \text{ m/s}$$

$\therefore$ Speed of car while moving downhill v = 15 m/s.

34. (d)

35. (b)

36. (b) Let acceleration of body be a

$$\therefore v_1 = 0 + at_1 \Rightarrow a = \frac{v_1}{t_1}$$

$$\therefore v = at \Rightarrow v = \frac{v_1 t}{t_1}$$

$P_{inst} = \vec{F}.\vec{v} = (m\vec{a}).\vec{v}$

$= \left(\frac{mv_1}{t_1}\right)\left(\frac{v_1 t}{t_1}\right) = m\left(\frac{v_1}{t_1}\right)^2 t$

37. (b) We know that $F \times v = \text{Power}$

$\therefore F \times v = c$ where c = constant

$\therefore m\frac{dv}{dt} \times v = c \quad \left(\because F = ma = \frac{mdv}{dt}\right)$

$\therefore m\int_0^v vdv = c\int_0^t dt \quad \therefore \frac{1}{2}mv^2 = ct$

$\therefore v = \sqrt{\frac{2c}{m}} \times t^{1/2}$

$\therefore \frac{dx}{dt} = \sqrt{\frac{2c}{m}} \times t^{1/2}$ where $v = \frac{dx}{dt}$

$\therefore \int_0^x dx = \sqrt{\frac{2c}{m}} \times \int_0^t t^{1/2}dt$

$x = \sqrt{\frac{2c}{m}} \times \frac{2t^{3/2}}{3} \Rightarrow x \propto t^{3/2}$

TOPIC-4 : Collisions

38. (a) For particle C,
According to law of conservation of linear momentum, verticle component,

$2mv'\sin\theta = mv\sin 60° + mv\sin 45°$

$2mv'\sin\theta = \frac{mv}{\sqrt{2}} + \frac{mv\sqrt{3}}{2}$ ...... (i)

Horizontal component,

$2mv'\cos\theta = mv\sin 60° - mv\cos 45°$

$2mv'\cos\theta = \frac{mv}{2} + \frac{mv}{\sqrt{2}}$ ...... (ii)

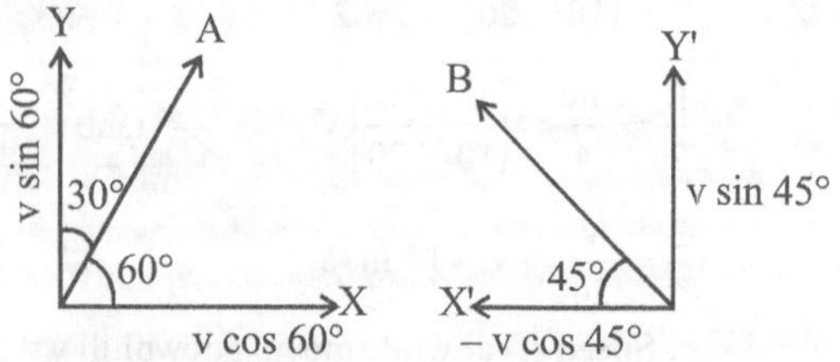

For particle A **For particle B**

Dividing eq^n (i) by eq^n (ii),

$\tan\theta = \frac{\frac{1}{\sqrt{2}} + \frac{\sqrt{3}}{2}}{\frac{1}{2} - \frac{1}{\sqrt{2}}} = \frac{\sqrt{2}+\sqrt{3}}{1-\sqrt{2}}$

39. (a) For inelastic collision $v' = \frac{m_1}{(m_1 + m_2)}v$

$= \frac{1}{(1+1)}v = \frac{v}{2}$

$n \rightarrow v(H)$ Before

$(n)(H) \rightarrow \frac{v}{2}$ After

Loss in K.E. $= \frac{1}{2}mv^2 - \frac{1}{2}(2m)\left(\frac{v}{2}\right)^2 = \frac{1}{4}mv^2$

K.E. lost is used to jump from 1st orbit to 2nd orbit
ΔK.E. = 10.2ev
Minimum K.E. of neutron for inelastic collision

$\frac{1}{2}mv^2 = 2 \times 10.2 = 20.4$ eV

40. (a)

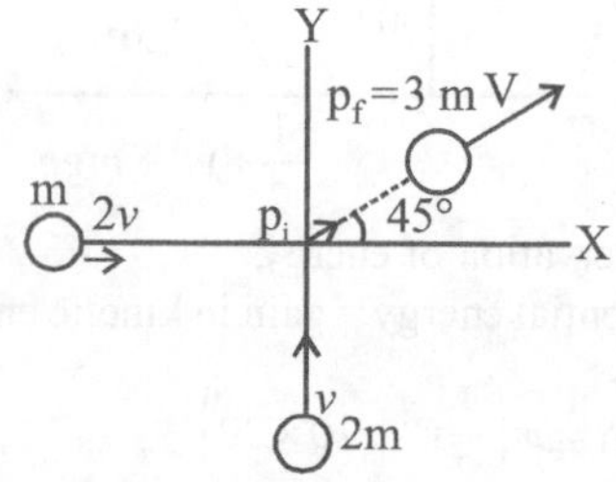

Initial momentum of the system

$p_i = \sqrt{[m(2V)^2 \times m(2V)^2]}$

$= \sqrt{2}m \times 2V$

Final momentum of the system = 3mV
By the law of conservation of momentum

$2\sqrt{2}mv = 3mV$

$\Rightarrow \frac{2\sqrt{2}v}{3} = V_{combined}$

Loss in energy

$\Delta E = \frac{1}{2}m_1V_1^2 + \frac{1}{2}m_2V_2^2 - \frac{1}{2}(m_1 + m_2)V_{combined}^2$

$\Delta E = 3mv^2 - \frac{4}{3}mv^2 = \frac{5}{3}mv^2 = 55.55\%$

Percentage loss in energy during the collision $\simeq$ 56%

41. (b) Given, $m_1 = 4g, u_1 = 300$ m/s

$m_2 = 0.8$ kg $= 800$ g, $u_2 = 0$ m/s

From law of conservation of momentum,

$m_1u_1 + m_2u_2 = m_1v_1 + m_2v_2$

Let the velocity of combined system = v m/s
then,

$4 \times 300 + 800 \times 0 = (800 + 4) \times v$

$v = \frac{1200}{804} = 1.49$ m/s

Now, $\mu = 0.3$ (given)

$a = \mu g$

$a = 0.3 \times 10$ (take $g = 10$ m/s^2)

$= 3$ m/s^2

then, from $v^2 = u^2 + 2as$

$$(1.49)^2 = 0 + 2 \times 3 \times s$$

$$s = \frac{(1.49)^2}{6}$$

$$s = \frac{2.22}{6}$$

$$= 0.379\,m$$

42. (d) From the law of conservation of momentum we know that,

$m_1u_1 + m_2u_2 + ... = m_1v_1 + m_2v_2 + ...$

Given $m_1 = m$, $m_2 = 2m$ and $m_3 = 3m$

and $u_1 = 3u$, $u_2 = 2u$ and $u_3 = u$

Let the velocity when they stick $= \vec{v}$

Then, according to question,

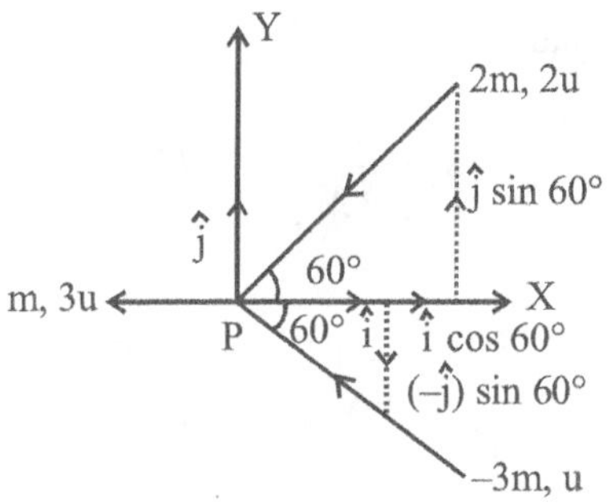

$$m \times 3u\left(\hat{i}\right) + 2m \times 2u\left(-\hat{i}\cos 60° - \hat{j}\sin 60°\right)$$

$$+3\,m \times u\left(-\hat{i}\cos 60° + \hat{j}\sin 60°\right) = (m + 2m + 3m)\,\vec{v}$$

$$\Rightarrow\ 3mu\hat{i} - 4mu\frac{\hat{i}}{2} - 4mu\left(\frac{\sqrt{3}}{2}\hat{j}\right) - 3mu\frac{\hat{i}}{2}$$

$$+3mu\left(\frac{\sqrt{3}}{2}\hat{j}\right) = 6m\,\vec{v}$$

$$\Rightarrow\ mu\hat{i} - \frac{3}{2}mu\hat{i} - \frac{\sqrt{3}}{2}mu\hat{j} = 6m\,\vec{v}$$

$$\Rightarrow\ -\frac{1}{2}mu\hat{i} - \frac{\sqrt{3}}{2}mu\hat{j} = 6m\,\vec{v}$$

$$\Rightarrow\ \vec{v} = \frac{u}{12}\left(-\hat{i} - \sqrt{3}\hat{j}\right)$$

43. (d) Maximum energy loss $= \dfrac{P^2}{2m} - \dfrac{P^2}{2(m+M)}$

$$\left[\because K.E. = \frac{P^2}{2m} = \frac{1}{2}mv^2\right]$$

$$= \frac{P^2}{2m}\left[\frac{M}{(m+M)}\right] = \frac{1}{2}mv^2\left\{\frac{M}{m+M}\right\}$$

Statement II is a case of perfectly inelastic collision.

By comparing the equation given in statement I with above equation, we get

$$f = \left(\frac{M}{m+M}\right) \text{ instead of } \left(\frac{m}{M+m}\right)$$

Hence statement I is wrong and statement II is correct.

44. (c)

45. (c) Fractional decrease in kinetic energy of mass m

$$= 1 - \left(\frac{m_2 - m_1}{m_2 + m_1}\right)^2 = 1 - \left(\frac{2-1}{2+1}\right)^2$$

$$= 1 - \left(\frac{1}{3}\right)^2 = 1 - \frac{1}{9} = \frac{8}{9}$$

Percentage loss in energy

$$= \frac{8}{9} \times 100 \simeq 90\%$$

46. (d)

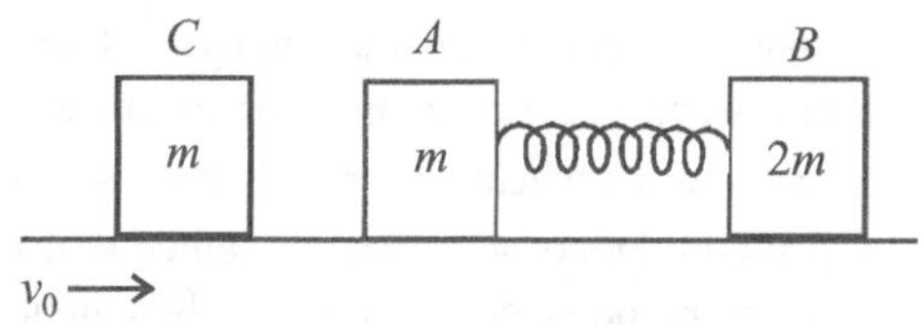

Initial momentum of the system block (C) $= mv_0$. After striking with A, the block C comes to rest and now both block A and B moves with velocity v when compression in spring is x_0.

By the law of conservation of linear momentum

$$mv_0 = (m + 2m)\,v \Rightarrow v = \frac{v_0}{3}$$

By the law of conservation of energy

K.E. of block C = K.E. of system + P.E. of system

$$\frac{1}{2}mv_0^2 = \frac{1}{2}(3m)\left(\frac{v_0}{3}\right)^2 + \frac{1}{2}kx_0^2$$

$$\Rightarrow\ \frac{1}{2}mv_0^2 = \frac{1}{6}mv_0^2 + \frac{1}{2}kx_0^2$$

$$\Rightarrow\ \frac{1}{2}kx_0^2 = \frac{1}{2}mv_0^2 - \frac{1}{6}mv_0^2 = \frac{mv_0^2}{3}$$

$$\therefore\ \ k = \frac{2}{3}m\left(\frac{v_0}{x_0}\right)^2$$

47. (c)

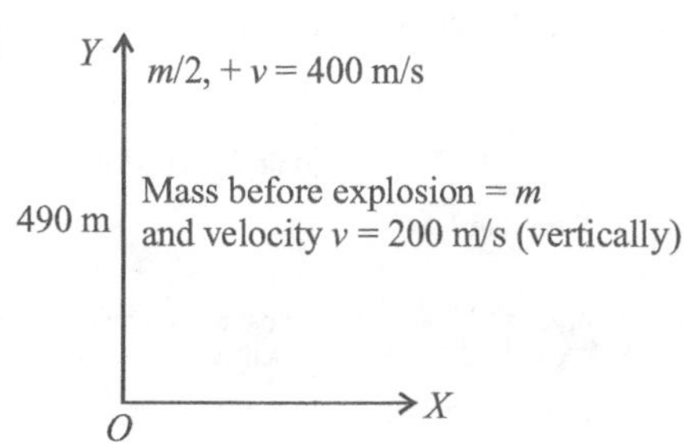

Momentum before explosion
= Momentum after explosion

$$m \times 200\hat{j} = \frac{m}{2} \times 400\hat{j} + \frac{m}{2} v$$

$$= \frac{m}{2}\left(400\hat{j} + v\right)$$

$$\Rightarrow \quad 400\hat{j} - 400\hat{j} = v$$

$\therefore \quad v = 0$

i.e., the velocity of the other part of the mass, $v = 0$

Let time taken to reach the earth by this part be t

Applying formula, $h = ut + \frac{1}{2}gt^2$

$$490 = 0 + \frac{1}{2} \times 9.8 \times t^2$$

$$\Rightarrow \quad t^2 = \frac{980}{9.8} = 100$$

$$\therefore \quad t = \sqrt{100} = 10 \sec$$

48. (a) In completely inelastic collision, all energy is not lost (so, statement -1 is true) and the principle of conservation of momentum holds good for all kinds of collisions (so, statement -2 is true). Statement -2 explains statement -1 correctly because applying the principle of conservation of momentum, we can get the common velocity and hence the kinetic energy of the combined body.

49. (c) Initial kinetic energy of the system

$$\text{K.E}_i = \frac{1}{2}mu^2 + \frac{1}{2}M(0)^2$$

$$= \frac{1}{2} \times 0.5 \times 2 \times 2 + 0 = 1\text{J}$$

For collision, applying conservation of linear momentum

$$m \times u = (m + M) \times v$$

$$\therefore \; 0.5 \times 2 = (0.5 + 1) \times v \Rightarrow v = \frac{2}{3}\text{m/s}$$

Final kinetic energy of the system is

$$\text{K.E}_f = \frac{1}{2}(m + M)v^2$$

$$= \frac{1}{2}(0.5 + 1) \times \frac{2}{3} \times \frac{2}{3} = \frac{1}{3}\text{J}$$

$\therefore$ Energy loss during collision

$$= \left(1 - \frac{1}{3}\right)\text{J} = 0.67\text{J}$$

50. (b) Let the velocity and mass of 4 kg piece be v_1 and m_1 and that of 12 kg piece be v_2 and m_2.

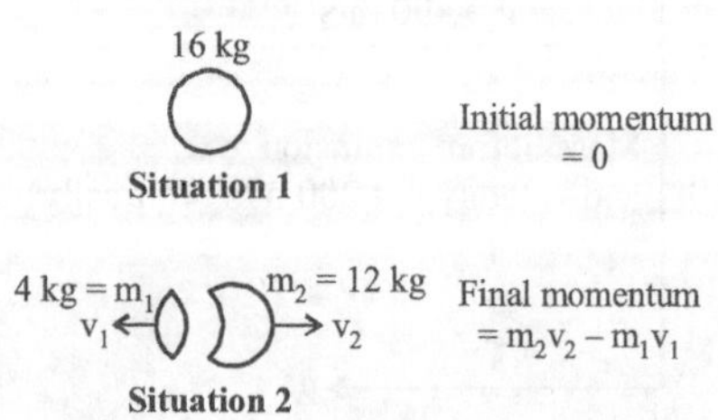

Applying conservation of linear momentum

$$m_2 v_2 = m_1 v_1$$

$$\Rightarrow v_1 = \frac{12 \times 4}{4} = 12\ ms^{-1}$$

$$\therefore K.E._1 = \frac{1}{2}m_1 v_1^2 = \frac{1}{2} \times 4 \times 144 = 288\ J$$

51. (b) $\frac{1}{2}Mv^2 = \frac{1}{2}kL^2$

$$\Rightarrow v = \sqrt{\frac{k}{M}}.L$$

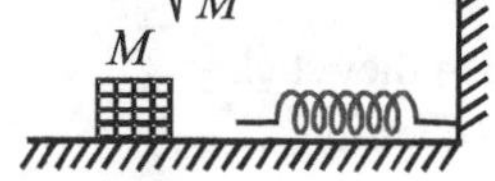

Momentum $= M \times v$

$$= M \times \sqrt{\frac{k}{M}}.L = \sqrt{kM}.L$$

52. (d)

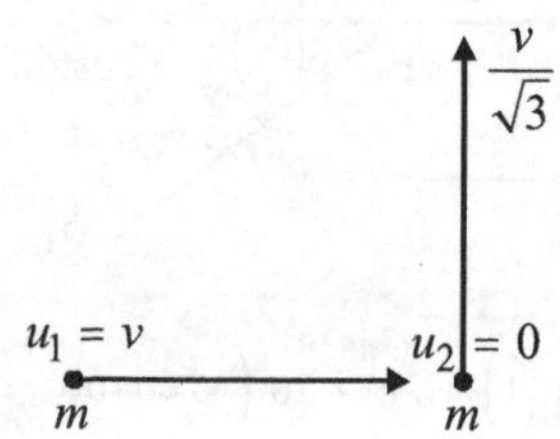

In x-direction : $mv + 0 = m(0) + m(v_2)_x$

In y-direction : $0 + 0 = m\left(\frac{v}{\sqrt{3}}\right) + m(v_2)_y$ is

$$\Rightarrow (v_2)_y = \frac{v}{\sqrt{3}} \text{ and } (v_2)_x = v$$

$$\therefore \; v_2 = \sqrt{\left(\frac{v}{\sqrt{3}}\right)^2 + v^2}$$

$$\Rightarrow v_2 = \sqrt{\frac{v^2}{3} + v^2} = v\sqrt{\frac{4}{3}} = \frac{2v}{\sqrt{3}}$$

53. (c) Kinetic energy of a system of particle is zero only when the speed of each particles is zero. And if speed of each particle is zero, the linear momentum of the system of particle has to be zero.

Also the linear momentum of the system may be zero even when the particles are moving. This is because linear momentum is a vector quantity. In this case the kinetic energy of the system of particles will not be zero.

$\therefore$ A does not imply B but B implies A.

Chapter 6

System of Particles and Rotational Motion

TOPIC-1 : Centre of Mass, Centre of Gravity & Principle of Moments

1. In a physical balance working on the principle of moments, when 5 mg weight is placed on the left pan, the beam becomes horizontal. Both the empty pans of the balance are of equal mass. Which of the following statements is correct? **[Online April 8, 2017]**
   (a) Left arm is longer than the right arm
   (b) Both the arms are of same length
   (c) Left arm is shorter than the right arm
   (d) Every object that is weighed using this balance appears lighter than its actual weight.

2. In the figure shown ABC is a uniform wire. If centre of mass of wire lies vertically below point A, then $\frac{BC}{AB}$ is close to : **[Online April 10, 2016]**

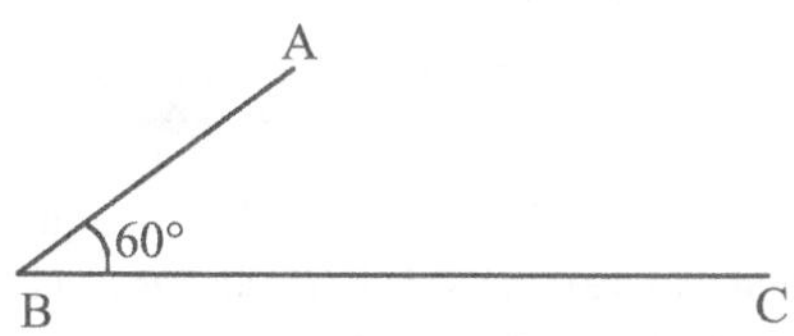

   (a) 1.85 (b) 1.5
   (c) 1.37 (d) 3

3. Distance of the centre of mass of a solid uniform cone from its vertex is z_0. If the radius of its base is R and its height is h then z_0 is equal to : **[2015]**
   (a) $\frac{5h}{8}$ (b) $\frac{3h^2}{8R}$ (c) $\frac{h^2}{4R}$ (d) $\frac{3h}{4}$

4. A uniform thin rod AB of length L has linear mass density $\mu(x) = a + \frac{bx}{L}$, where x is measured from A. If the CM of the rod lies at a distance of $\left(\frac{7}{12}\right)L$ from A, then a and b are related as : **[Online April 11, 2015]**
   (a) $a = 2b$ (b) $2a = b$
   (c) $a = b$ (d) $3a = 2b$

5. A thin bar of length L has a mass per unit length λ, that increases linearly with distance from one end. If its total mass is M and its mass per unit length at the lighter end is λ_0, then the distance of the centre of mass from the lighter end is: **[Online April 11, 2014]**
   (a) $\frac{L}{2}-\frac{\lambda_0 L^2}{4M}$ (b) $\frac{L}{3}+\frac{\lambda_0 L^2}{8M}$
   (c) $\frac{L}{3}+\frac{\lambda_0 L^2}{4M}$ (d) $\frac{2L}{3}-\frac{\lambda_0 L^2}{6M}$

6. A boy of mass 20 kg is standing on a 80 kg free to move long cart. There is negligible friction between cart and ground. Initially, the boy is standing 25 m from a wall. If he walks 10 m on the cart towards the wall, then the final distance of the boy from the wall will be **[Online April 23, 2013]**
   (a) 15m (b) 12.5m (c) 15.5m (d) 17m

7. A thin rod of length 'L' is lying along the x-axis with its ends at $x = 0$ and $x = L$. Its linear density (mass/length) varies with x as $k\left(\frac{x}{L}\right)^n$, where n can be zero or any positive number. If the position x_{CM} of the centre of mass of the rod is plotted against 'n', which of the following graphs best approximates the dependence of x_{CM} on n? **[2008]**

(a)
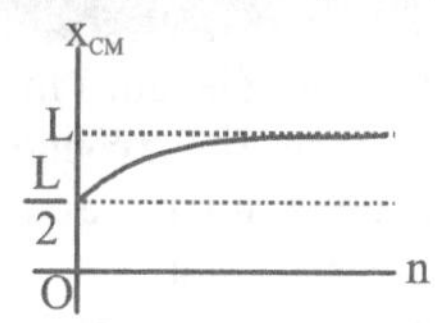

(b)
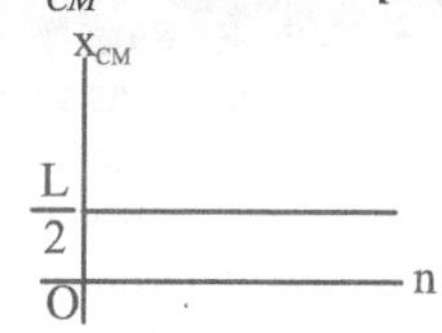

(c)
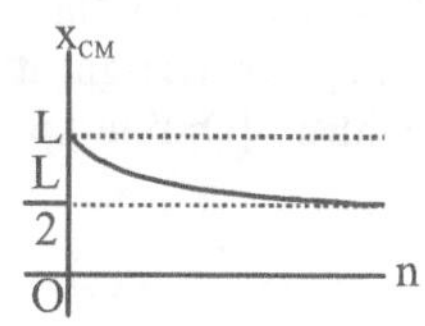

(d)
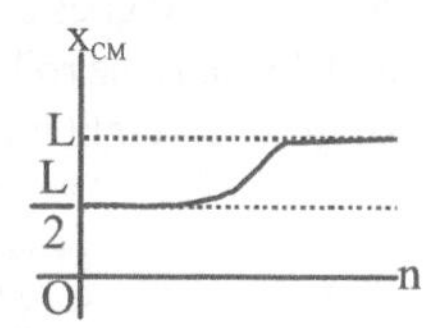

8. A circular disc of radius R is removed from a bigger circular disc of radius $2R$ such that the circumferences of the discs coincide. The centre of mass of the new disc is α / R form the centre of the bigger disc. The value of α is **[2007]**
   (a) 1/4 (b) 1/3 (c) 1/2 (d) 1/6

9. Consider a two particle system with particles having masses m_1 and m_2. If the first particle is pushed towards the centre of mass through a distance d, by what distance should the second particle is moved, so as to keep the centre of mass at the same position? **[2006]**
   (a) $\frac{m_2}{m_1}d$ (b) $\frac{m_1}{m_1+m_2}d$
   (c) $\frac{m_1}{m_2}d$ (d) d

10. A body A of mass M while falling vertically downwards under gravity breaks into two parts; a body B of mass $\frac{1}{3}M$ and a body C of mass $\frac{2}{3}M$. The centre of mass of bodies B and C taken together shifts compared to that of body A towards **[2005]**
(a) does not shift
(b) depends on height of breaking
(c) body B
(d) body C

11. A 'T' shaped object with dimensions shown in the figure, is lying on a smooth floor. A force '$\vec{F}$' is applied at the point P parallel to AB, such that the object has only the translational motion without rotation. Find the location of P with respect to C. **[2005]**

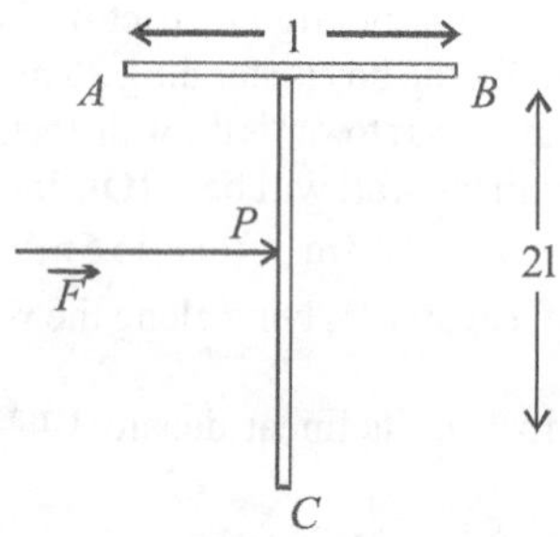

(a) $\frac{3}{2}\ell$ (b) $\frac{2}{3}\ell$ (c) ℓ (d) $\frac{4}{3}\ell$

TOPIC-2 : Angular Displacement, Velocity and Acceleration

12. The machine as shown has 2 rods of length 1 m connected by a pivot at the top. The end of one rod is connected to the floor by a stationary pivot and the end of the other rod has a roller that rolls along the floor in a slot.
As the roller goes back and forth, a 2 kg weight moves up and down. If the roller is moving towards right at a constant speed, the weight moves up with a : **[Online April 9, 2017]**

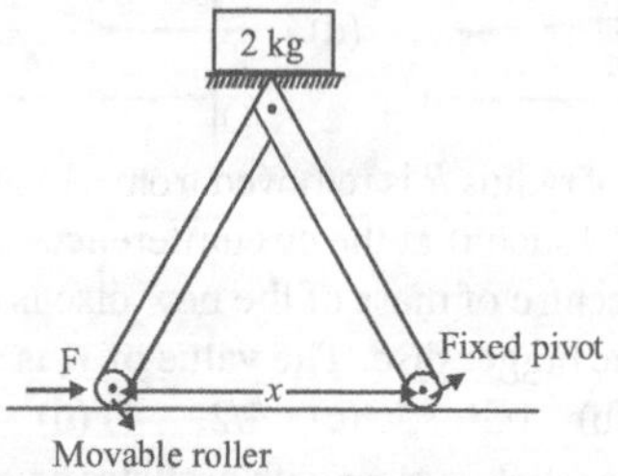

(a) constant speed
(b) decreasing speed
(c) increasing speed
(d) speed which is $\frac{3}{4}$th of that of the roller when the weight is 0.4 m above the ground

13. A slender uniform rod of mass M and length ℓ is pivoted at one end so that it can rotate in a vertical plane (see figure). There is negligible friction at the pivot. The free end is held vertically above the pivot and then released. The angular acceleration of the rod when it makes an angle θ with the vertical is **[2017]**

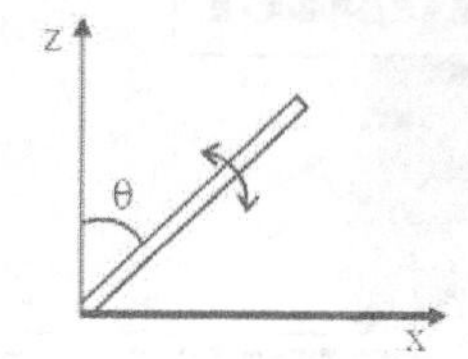

(a) $\frac{3g}{2\ell}\cos\theta$ (b) $\frac{2g}{3\ell}\cos\theta$
(c) $\frac{3g}{2\ell}\sin\theta$ (d) $\frac{2g}{2\ell}\sin\theta$

14. Concrete mixture is made by mixing cement, stone and sand in a rotating cylindrical drum. If the drum rotates too fast, the ingredients remain stuck to the wall of the drum and proper mixing of ingredients does not take place. The maximum rotational speed of the drum in revolutions per minute (rpm) to ensure proper mixing is close to :
(Take the radius of the drum to be 1.25 m and its axle to be horizontal): **[Online April 10, 2016]**
(a) 27.0 (b) 0.4 (c) 1.3 (d) 8.0

15. A cubical block of side 30 cm is moving with velocity 2 ms^{-1} on a smooth horizontal surface. The surface has a bump at a point O as shown in figure. The angular velocity (in rad/s) of the block immediately after it hits the bump, is : **[Online April 9, 2016]**

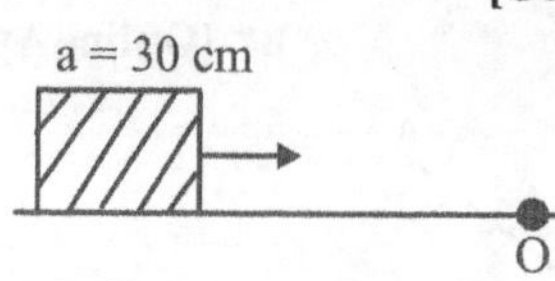

(a) 13.3 (b) 5.0 (c) 9.4 (d) 6.7

16. Two point masses of mass $m_1 = fM$ and $m_2 = (1-f)M$ $(f < 1)$ are in outer space (far from gravitational influence of other objects) at a distance R from each other. They move in circular orbits about their centre of mass with angular velocities ω_1 for m_1 and ω_2 for m_2. In that case **[Online May 19, 2012]**
(a) $(1-f)\,\omega_1 = f\omega$
(b) $\omega_1 = \omega_2$ and independent of f
(c) $f\omega_1 = (1-f)\omega_2$
(d) $\omega_1 = \omega_2$ and depend on f

TOPIC-3 : Torque, Couple and Angular Momentum

17. A particle of mass m is moving along the side of a square of side 'a', with a uniform speed v in the x-y plane as shown in the figure : **[2016]**

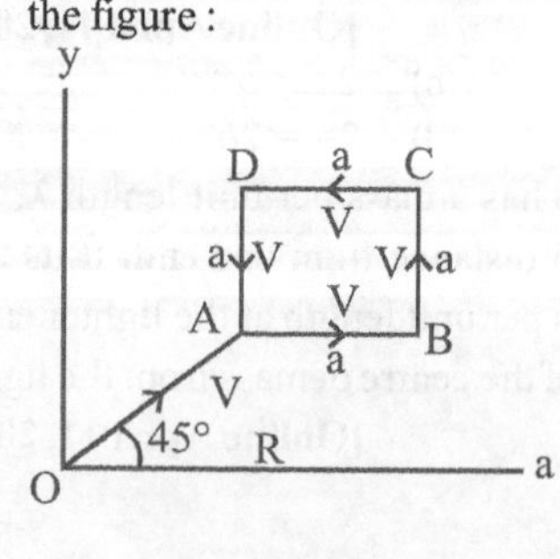

Which of the following statements is false for the angular momentum $\vec{L}$ about the origin?

(a) $\vec{L} = mv\left[\frac{R}{\sqrt{2}} + a\right]\hat{k}$ when the particle is moving from B to C.

(b) $\vec{L} = \frac{mv}{\sqrt{2}}R\hat{k}$ when the particle is moving from D to A.

(c) $\vec{L} = -\frac{mv}{\sqrt{2}}R\hat{k}$ when the particle is moving from A to B.

(d) $\vec{L} = mv\left[\frac{R}{\sqrt{2}} - a\right]\hat{k}$ when the particle is moving from C to D.

18. A particle of mass 2 kg is on a smooth horizontal table and moves in a circular path of radius 0.6 m. The height of the table from the ground is 0.8 m. If the angular speed of the particle is 12 rad s^{-1}, the magnitude of its angular momentum about a point on the ground right under the centre of the circle is : **[Online April 11, 2015]**

(a) 14.4 kg m^2s^{-1} (b) 8.64 kg m^2s^{-1}
(c) 20.16 kg m^2s^{-1} (d) 11.52 kg m^2s^{-1}

19. A bob of mass m attached to an inextensible string of length l is suspended from a vertical support. The bob rotates in a horizontal circle with an angular speed ω rad/s about the vertical. About the point of suspension: **[2014]**

(a) angular momentum is conserved.
(b) angular momentum changes in magnitude but not in direction.
(c) angular momentum changes in direction but not in magnitude.
(d) angular momentum changes both in direction and magnitude.

20. A ball of mass 160 g is thrown up at an angle of 60° to the horizontal at a speed of 10 ms^{-1}. The angular momentum of the ball at the highest point of the trajectory with respect to the point from which the ball is thrown is nearly ($g = 10\ ms^{-2}$) **[Online April 19, 2014]**

(a) 1.73 kg m^2/s (b) 3.0 kg m^2/s
(c) 3.46 kg m^2/s (d) 6.0 kg m^2/s

21. A particle is moving in a circular path of radius a, with a constant velocity v as shown in the figure. The centre of circle is marked by 'C'. The angular momentum from the origin O can be written as: **[Online April 12, 2014]**

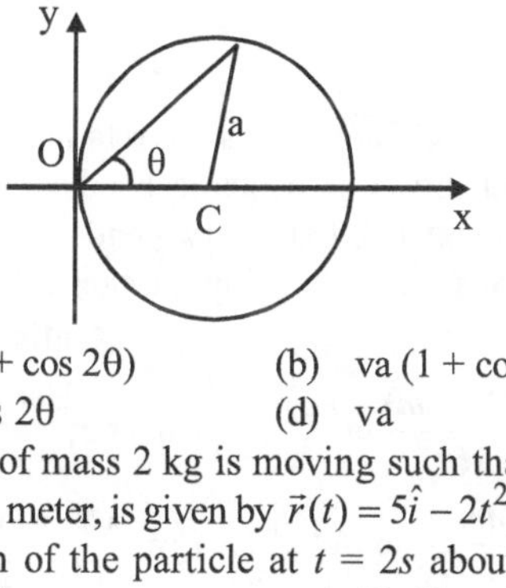

(a) va (1 + cos 2θ) (b) va (1 + cos θ)
(c) va cos 2θ (d) va

22. A particle of mass 2 kg is moving such that at time t, its position, in meter, is given by $\vec{r}(t) = 5\hat{i} - 2t^2\hat{j}$. The angular momentum of the particle at $t = 2s$ about the origin in kg m^{-2} s^{-1} is : **[Online April 23, 2013]**

(a) $-80\hat{k}$ (b) $(10\hat{i} - 16\hat{j})$
(c) $-40\hat{k}$ (d) $40\hat{k}$

23. A bullet of mass 10 g and speed 500 m/s is fired into a door and gets embedded exactly at the centre of the door. The door is 1.0 m wide and weighs 12 kg. It is hinged at one end and rotates about a vertical axis practically without friction. The angular speed of the door just after the bullet embeds into it will be: **[Online April 9, 2013]**

(a) 6.25 rad/sec (b) 0.625 rad/sec
(c) 3.35 rad/sec (d) 0.335 rad/sec

24. A stone of mass m, tied to the end of a string, is whirled around in a circle on a horizontal frictionless table. The length of the string is reduced gradually keeping the angular momentum of the stone about the centre of the circle constant. Then, the tension in the string is given by $T = Ar^n$, where A is a constant, r is the instantaneous radius of the circle. The value of n is equal to **[Online May 26, 2012]**

(a) −1 (b) −2 (c) −4 (d) −3

25. A thin horizontal circular disc is rotating about a vertical axis passing through its centre. An insect is at rest at a point near the rim of the disc. The insect now moves along a diameter of the disc to reach its other end. During the journey of the insect, the angular speed of the disc. **[2011]**

(a) continuously decreases
(b) continuously increases
(c) first increases and then decreases
(d) remains unchanged

26. A small particle of mass m is projected at an angle θ with the x-axis with an initial velocity v_0 in the x-y plane as shown in the figure. At a time $t < \frac{v_0 \sin\theta}{g}$, the angular momentum of the particle is **[2010]**

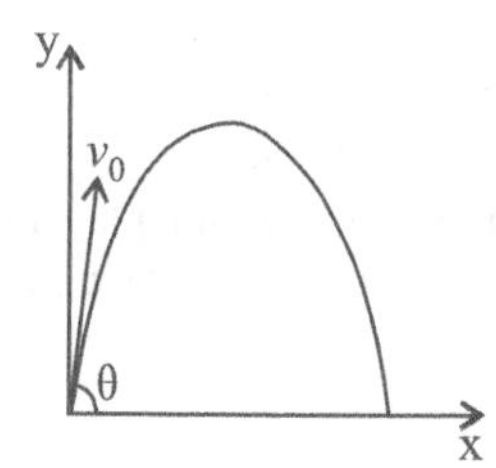

(a) $-mg\, v_0 t^2 \cos\theta\, \hat{j}$ (b) $mg\, v_0 t \cos\theta \hat{k}$

(c) $-\frac{1}{2}mg v_0 t^2 \cos\theta\, \hat{k}$ (d) $\frac{1}{2}mg v_0 t^2 \cos\theta\, \hat{i}$

where $\hat{i}, \hat{j}$ and $\hat{k}$ are unit vectors along x, y and z-axis respectively.

27. Angular momentum of the particle rotating with a central force is constant due to **[2007]**

(a) constant torque
(b) constant force
(c) constant linear momentum
(d) zero torque

28. A thin circular ring of mass m and radius R is rotating about its axis with a constant angular velocity ω. Two objects each of mass M are attached gently to the opposite ends of a diameter of the ring. The ring now rotates with an angular velocity ω' = **[2006]**

(a) $\frac{\omega(m+2M)}{m}$ (b) $\frac{\omega(m-2M)}{(m+2M)}$

(c) $\frac{\omega m}{(m+M)}$ (d) $\frac{\omega m}{(m+2M)}$

29. A force of $-F\hat{k}$ acts on O, the origin of the coordinate system. The torque about the point (1, –1) is **[2006]**

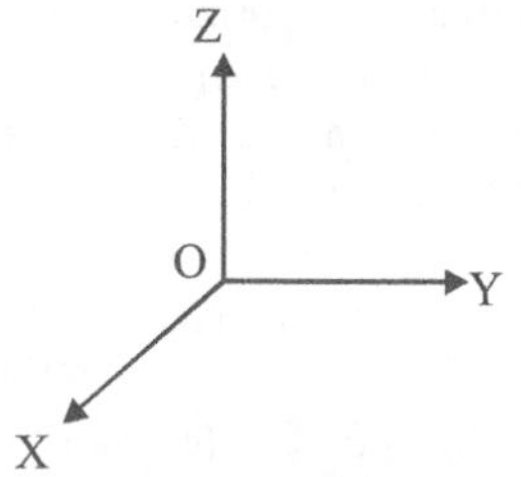

(a) $F(\hat{i}-\hat{j})$ (b) $-F(\hat{i}+\hat{j})$

(c) $F(\hat{i}+\hat{j})$ (d) $-F(\hat{i}-\hat{j})$

30. A solid sphere is rotating in free space. If the radius of the sphere is increased keeping mass same, which one of the following will not be affected ? **[2004]**

(a) Angular velocity
(b) Angular momentum
(c) Moment of inertia
(d) Rotational kinetic energy

31. Let $\vec{F}$ be the force acting on a particle having position vector $\vec{r}$, and $\vec{T}$ be the torque of this force about the origin. Then **[2003]**

(a) $\vec{r}.\vec{T}=0$ and $\vec{F}.\vec{T}\neq 0$
(b) $\vec{r}.\vec{T}\neq 0$ and $\vec{F}.\vec{T}=0$
(c) $\vec{r}.\vec{T}\neq 0$ and $\vec{F}.\vec{T}\neq 0$
(d) $\vec{r}.\vec{T}=0$ and $\vec{F}.\vec{T}=0$

32. A particle of mass m moves along line PC with velocity v as shown. What is the angular momentum of the particle about P? **[2002]**

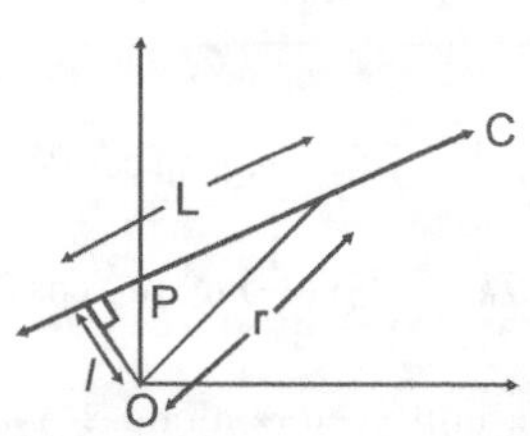

(a) mvL (b) mvl (c) mvr (d) zero.

TOPIC-4 : Moment of Inertia and Rotational K.E.

33. The moment of inertia of a uniform cylinder of length ℓ and radius R about its perpendicular bisector is I. What is the ratio ℓ/R such that the moment of inertia is minimum ? **[2017]**

(a) 1 (b) $\frac{3}{\sqrt{2}}$ (c) $\sqrt{\frac{3}{2}}$ (d) $\frac{\sqrt{3}}{2}$

34. Moment of inertia of an equilateral triangular lamina ABC, about the axis passing through its centre O and perpendicular to its plane is I_o as shown in the figure. A cavity DEF is cut out from the lamina, where D, E, F are the mid points of the sides. Moment of inertia of the remaining part of lamina about the same axis is : **[Online April 8, 2017]**

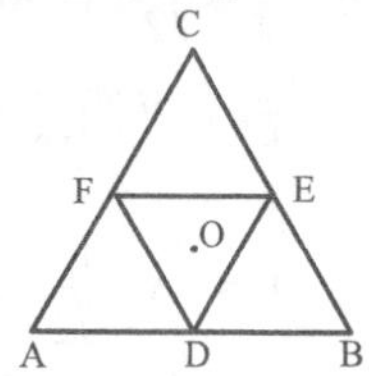

(a) $\frac{7}{8}I_o$ (b) $\frac{15}{16}I_o$

(c) $\frac{3I_o}{4}$ (d) $\frac{31I_o}{32}$

35. A circular hole of radius $\frac{R}{4}$ is made in a thin uniform disc having mass M and radius R, as shown in figure. The moment of inertia of the remaining portion of the disc about an axis passing through the point O and perpendicular to the plane of the disc is : **[Online April 9, 2017]**

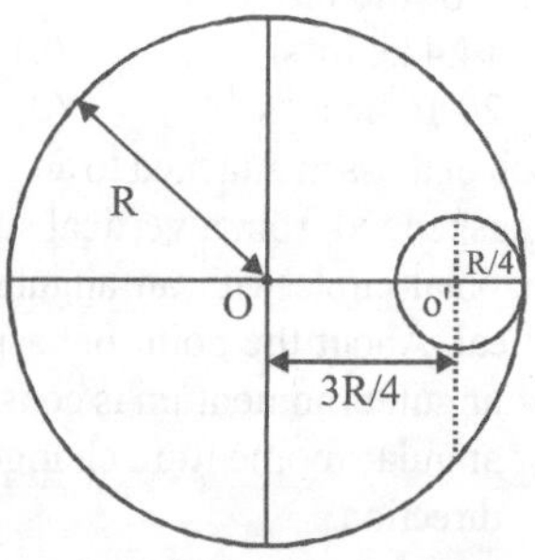

(a) $\frac{219MR^2}{256}$

(b) $\frac{237MR^2}{512}$

(c) $\frac{19MR^2}{512}$

(d) $\frac{197MR^2}{256}$

36. From a solid sphere of mass M and radius R a cube of maximum possible volume is cut. Moment of inertia of cube about an axis passing through its center and perpendicular to one of its faces is : **[2015]**

(a) $\frac{4MR^2}{9\sqrt{3}\pi}$ (b) $\frac{4MR^2}{3\sqrt{3}\pi}$

(c) $\frac{MR^2}{32\sqrt{2}\pi}$ (d) $\frac{MR^2}{16\sqrt{2}\pi}$

37. Consider a thin uniform square sheet made of a rigid material. If its side is 'a' mass m and moment of inertia I about one of its diagonals, then : **[Online April 10, 2015]**

(a) $I>\frac{ma^2}{12}$ (b) $\frac{ma^2}{24}<I<\frac{ma^2}{12}$

(c) $I=\frac{ma^2}{24}$ (d) $I=\frac{ma^2}{12}$

38. A ring of mass M and radius R is rotating about its axis with angular velocity ω. Two identical bodies each of mass m are now gently attached at the two ends of a diameter of the ring. Because of this, the kinetic energy loss will be : **[Online April 25, 2013]**

(a) $\frac{m(M+2m)}{M}\omega^2R^2$ (b) $\frac{Mm}{(M+m)}\omega^2R^2$

(c) $\frac{Mm}{(M+2m)}\omega^2R^2$ (d) $\frac{(M+m)M}{(M+2m)}\omega^2R^2$

39. This question has Statement 1 and Statement 2. Of the four choices given after the Statements, choose the one that best describes the two Statements.
Statement 1: When moment of inertia I of a body rotating about an axis with angular speed ω increases, its angular momentum L is unchanged but the kinetic energy K increases if there is no torque applied on it.
Statement 2: $L = I\omega$, kinetic energy of rotation $= \frac{1}{2}I\omega^2$ **[Online May 12, 2012]**
(a) Statement 1 is true, Statement 2 is true, Statement 2 is not the correct explanation of Statement 1.
(b) Statement 1 is false, Statement 2 is true.
(c) Statement 1 is true, Statement 2 is true, Statement 2 is correct explanation of the Statement 1.
(d) Statement 1 is true, Statement 2 is false.

40. A solid sphere having mass m and radius r rolls down an inclined plane. Then its kinetic energy is **[Online May 7, 2012]**
(a) $\frac{5}{7}$ rotational and $\frac{2}{7}$ translational
(b) $\frac{2}{7}$ rotational and $\frac{5}{7}$ translational
(c) $\frac{2}{5}$ rotational and $\frac{3}{5}$ translational
(d) $\frac{1}{2}$ rotational and $\frac{1}{2}$ translational

41. A circular hole of diameter R is cut from a disc of mass M and radius R; the circumference of the cut passes through the centre of the disc. The moment of inertia of the remaining portion of the disc about an axis perpendicular to the disc and passing through its centre is **[Online May 7, 2012]**
(a) $\left(\frac{15}{32}\right)MR^2$ (b) $\left(\frac{1}{8}\right)MR^2$
(c) $\left(\frac{3}{8}\right)MR^2$ (d) $\left(\frac{13}{32}\right)MR^2$

42. A mass m hangs with the help of a string wrapped around a pulley on a frictionless bearing. The pulley has mass m and radius R. Assuming pulley to be a perfect uniform circular disc, the acceleration of the mass m, if the string does not slip on the pulley, is: **[2011]**
(a) g (b) $\frac{2}{3}g$ (c) $\frac{g}{3}$ (d) $\frac{3}{2}g$

43. A pulley of radius 2 m is rotated about its axis by a force $F = (20t - 5t^2)$ newton (where t is measured in seconds) applied tangentially. If the moment of inertia of the pulley about its axis of rotation is 10 kg-m^2 the number of rotations made by the pulley before its direction of motion is reversed, is: **[2011]**
(a) more than 3 but less than 6
(b) more than 6 but less than 9
(c) more than 9
(d) less than 3

44. A thin uniform rod of length l and mass m is swinging freely about a horizontal axis passing through its end. Its maximum angular speed is ω. Its centre of mass rises to a maximum height of **[2009]**
(a) $\frac{1}{6}\frac{l\omega}{g}$ (b) $\frac{1}{2}\frac{l^2\omega^2}{g}$
(c) $\frac{1}{6}\frac{l^2\omega^2}{g}$ (d) $\frac{1}{3}\frac{l^2\omega^2}{g}$

45. Consider a uniform square plate of side 'a' and mass 'M'. The moment of inertia of this plate about an axis perpendicular to its plane and passing through one of its corners is **[2008]**
(a) $\frac{5}{6}Ma^2$ (b) $\frac{1}{12}Ma^2$ (c) $\frac{7}{12}Ma^2$ (d) $\frac{2}{3}Ma^2$

46. For the given uniform square lamina $ABCD$, whose centre is O, **[2007]**

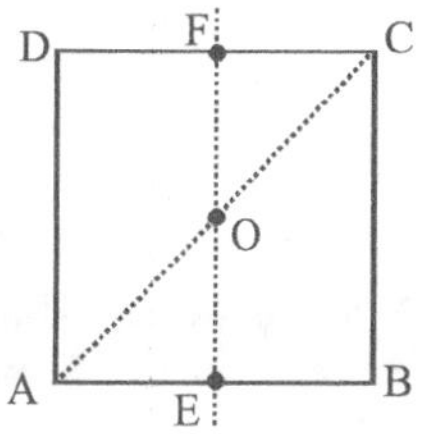

(a) $I_{AC} = \sqrt{2}\, I_{EF}$ (b) $\sqrt{2}I_{AC} = I_{EF}$
(c) $I_{AD} = 3I_{EF}$ (d) $I_{AC} = I_{EF}$

47. Four point masses, each of value m, are placed at the corners of a square $ABCD$ of side ℓ. The moment of inertia of this system about an axis passing through A and parallel to BD is **[2006]**
(a) $2m\ell^2$ (b) $\sqrt{3}m\ell^2$ (c) $3m\ell^2$ (d) $m\ell^2$

48. The moment of inertia of a uniform semicircular disc of mass M and radius r about a line perpendicular to the plane of the disc through the centre is **[2005]**
(a) $\frac{2}{5}Mr^2$ (b) $\frac{1}{4}Mr$
(c) $\frac{1}{2}Mr^2$ (d) Mr^2

49. One solid sphere A and another hollow sphere B are of same mass and same outer radii. Their moment of inertia about their diameters are respectively I_A and I_B Such that **[2004]**
(a) $I_A < I_B$ (b) $I_A > I_B$
(c) $I_A = I_B$ (d) $\frac{I_A}{I_B} = \frac{d_A}{d_B}$
where d_A and d_B are their densities.

50. A circular disc X of radius R is made from an iron plate of thickness t, and another disc Y of radius $4R$ is made from an

iron plate of thickness $\frac{t}{4}$. Then the relation between the moment of inertia I_X and I_Y is **[2003]**

(a) $I_Y = 32 I_X$ (b) $I_Y = 16 I_X$
(c) $I_Y = I_X$ (d) $I_Y = 64 I_X$

51. A particle performing uniform circular motion has angular frequency is doubled & its kinetic energy halved, then the new angular momentum is **[2003]**

(a) $\frac{L}{4}$ (b) $2L$ (c) $4L$ (d) $\frac{L}{2}$

52. Moment of inertia of a circular wire of mass M and radius R about its diameter is **[2002]**

(a) $MR^2/2$ (b) MR^2 (c) $2MR^2$ (d) $MR^2/4$

53. Initial angular velocity of a circular disc of mass M is ω_1. Then two small spheres of mass m are attached gently to diametrically opposite points on the edge of the disc. What is the final angular velocity of the disc? **[2002]**

(a) $\left(\frac{M+m}{M}\right)\omega_1$ (b) $\left(\frac{M+m}{m}\right)\omega_1$
(c) $\left(\frac{M}{M+4m}\right)\omega_1$ (d) $\left(\frac{M}{M+2m}\right)\omega_1$

TOPIC-5 : Rolling Motion

54. A roller is made by joining together two cones at their vertices O. It is kept on two rails AB and CD, which are placed asymmetrically (see figure), with its axis perpendicular to CD and its centre O at the centre of line joining AB and Cd (see figure). It is given a light push so that it starts rolling with its centre O moving parallel to CD in the direction shown. As it moves, the roller will tend to : **[2016]**

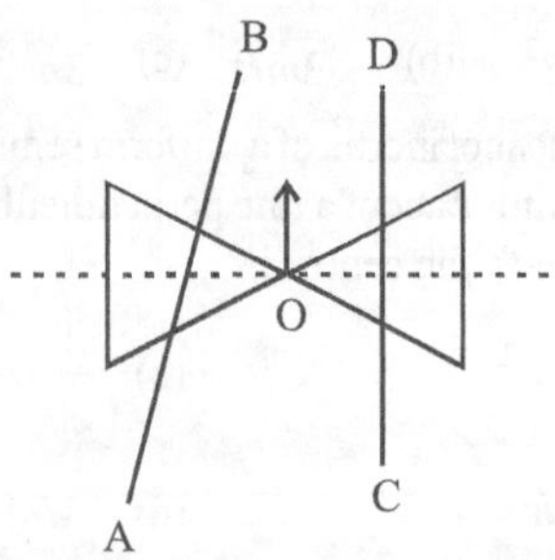

(a) go straight.
(b) turn left and right alternately.
(c) turn left.
(d) turn right.

55. A uniform solid cylindrical roller of mass 'm' is being pulled on a horizontal surface with force F parallel to the surface and applied at its centre. If the acceleration of the cylinder is 'a' and it is rolling without slipping then the value of 'F' is : **[Online April 10, 2015]**

(a) ma (b) $\frac{5}{3}$ma
(c) $\frac{3}{2}$ma (d) 2ma

56. A cylinder of mass M_c and sphere of mass M_s are placed at points A and B of two inclines, respectively (See Figure). If they roll on the incline without slipping such that their accelerations are the same, then the ratio $\frac{\sin\theta_c}{\sin\theta_s}$ is: **[Online April 9, 2014]**

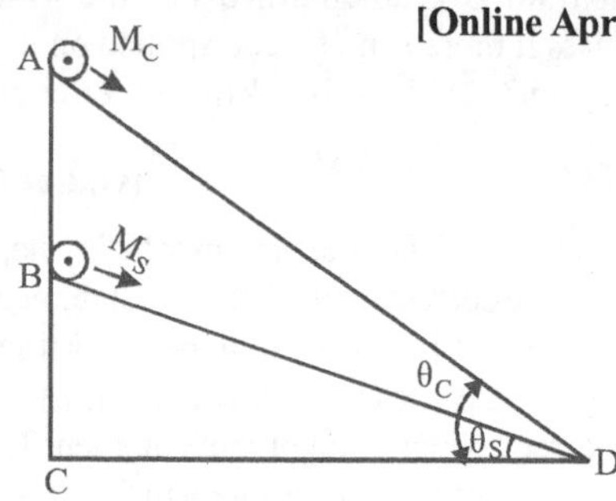

(a) $\sqrt{\frac{8}{7}}$ (b) $\sqrt{\frac{15}{14}}$
(c) $\frac{8}{7}$ (d) $\frac{15}{14}$

57. A loop of radius r and mass m rotating with an angular velocity ω_0 is placed on a rough horizontal surface. The initial velocity of the centre of the hoop is zero. What will be the velocity of the centre of the hoop when it ceases to slip ? **[2013]**

(a) $\frac{r\omega_0}{4}$ (b) $\frac{r\omega_0}{3}$ (c) $\frac{r\omega_0}{2}$ (d) $r\omega_0$

58. A tennis ball (treated as hollow spherical shell) starting from O rolls down a hill. At point A the ball becomes air borne leaving at an angle of 30° with the horizontal. The ball strikes the ground at B. What is the value of the distance AB ?
(Moment of inertia of a spherical shell of mass m and radius R about its diameter $= \frac{2}{3}mR^2$) **[Online April 22, 2013]**

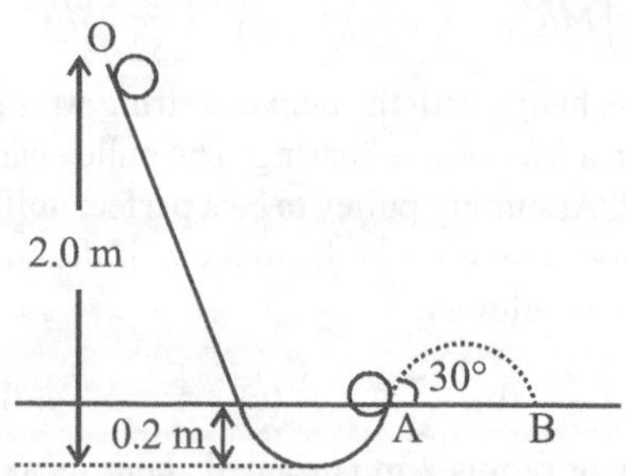

(a) 1.87m (b) 2.08m (c) 1.57m (d) 1.77m

59. A thick-walled hollow sphere has outside radius R_0. It rolls down an incline without slipping and its speed at the bottom is v_0. Now the incline is waxed, so that it is practically frictionless and the sphere is observed to slide down (without any rolling). Its speed at the bottom is observed to be $5v_0/4$. The radius of gyration of the hollow sphere about an axis through its centre is **[Online May 26, 2012]**

(a) $3R_0/2$ (b) $3R_0/4$
(c) $9R_0/16$ (d) $3R_0$

60. A solid sphere is rolling on a surface as shown in figure, with a translational velocity v ms^{-1}. If it is to climb the inclined surface continuing to roll without slipping, then minimum velocity for this to happen is **[Online May 12, 2012]**

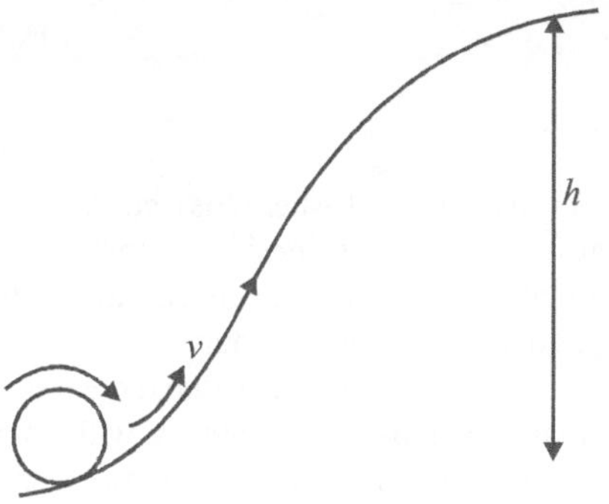

(a) $\sqrt{2gh}$ (b) $\sqrt{\frac{7}{5}gh}$

(c) $\sqrt{\frac{7}{2}gh}$ (d) $\sqrt{\frac{10}{7}gh}$

61. A round uniform body of radius R, mass M and moment of inertia I rolls down (without slipping) an inclined plane making an angle θ with the horizontal. Then its acceleration is **[2007]**

(a) $\dfrac{g\sin\theta}{1-MR^2/I}$ (b) $\dfrac{g\sin\theta}{1+I/MR^2}$

(c) $\dfrac{g\sin\theta}{1+MR^2/I}$ (d) $\dfrac{g\sin\theta}{1-I/MR^2}$

Hints & Solutions

TOPIC-1 : Centre of Mass, Centre of Gravity & Principle of Moments

1. **(c)** According to principle of moments when a system is stable or balance, the anti-clockwise moment is equal to clockwise moment.
i.e., load × load arm = effort × effort arm
When 5 mg weight is placed, load arm shifts to left side, hence left arm becomes shorter than right arm.

2. **(c)** Centre of mass $x_{cm} = \frac{x}{2}\frac{(\rho x)\left(\frac{x}{2}\right)\frac{1}{2} + \rho y^{y/2}}{\rho(x+y)}$

$\Rightarrow \frac{1}{2} + \frac{y}{x} = \frac{y^2}{x^2}$

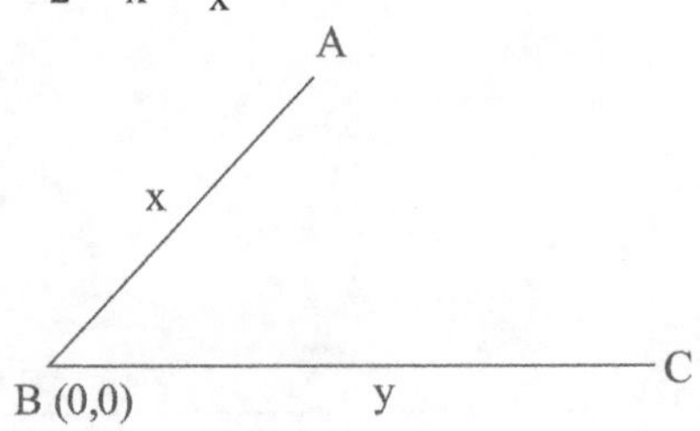

$\therefore \frac{Bc}{AB}\frac{y}{x} = \frac{1+\sqrt{3}}{2} = 1.37$

3. **(d)** $y_{cm} = \frac{\int y dm}{\int dm}$

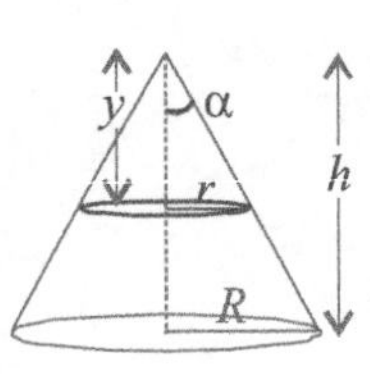

$= \frac{\int_0^h \pi r^2 dy \rho \times y}{\frac{1}{3}\pi R^2 h\rho} = \frac{3h}{4}$

4. **(b)** Centre of mass of the rod is given by:

$x_{cm} = \frac{\int_0^L (ax + \frac{bx^2}{L})dx}{\int_0^L (a + \frac{bx}{L})dx}$

$= \frac{\frac{aL^2}{2} + \frac{bL^2}{3}}{aL + \frac{bL}{2}} = \frac{L\left(\frac{a}{2} + \frac{b}{3}\right)}{a + \frac{b}{2}}$

Now $\frac{7L}{12} = \frac{\frac{a}{2} + \frac{b}{3}}{a + \frac{b}{2}}$

On solving we get, $b = 2a$

5. **(c)**
6. **(d)**
7. **(a)** • When $n = 0, x = k$ where k is a constant. This means that the linear mass density is constant. In this case the centre of mass will be at the midelle of the rod ie at $L/2$. Therefore (c) is ruled out
• n is positive and as its value increases, the rate of increase of linear mass density with increase in x increases. This shows that the centre of mass will shift towards that end of the rod where $n = L$ as the value of n increases. Therefore graph (b) is ruled out.
• The linear mass density $\lambda = k\left(\frac{x}{L}\right)^n$

Here $\frac{x}{L} \le 1$

With increase in the value of n, the centre of mass shift towards the end $x = L$ such that first the shifting is at a higher rate with increase in the value of n and then the rate decreases with the value of n.
These characteristics are represented by graph (a).

$x_{CM} = \frac{\int_0^L x dm}{\int_0^L dm} = \frac{\int_0^L x(\lambda dx)}{\int_0^L \lambda\, dx} = \frac{\int_0^L k\left(\frac{x}{L}\right)^n xdx}{\int_0^L k\left(\frac{x}{L}\right)^n dx}$

$= \frac{k\left[\frac{x^{n+2}}{(n+2)L^n}\right]_0^L}{\left[\frac{kx^{n+1}}{(n+1)L^n}\right]_0^L} = \frac{L(n+1)}{n+2}$

For $n = 0, x_{CM} = \frac{L}{2}; n = 1,$

$x_{CM} = \frac{2L}{3}; n = 2,\ x_{CM} = \frac{3L}{4};....$

8. **(b)** Let the mass per unit area be σ.
Then the mass of the complete disc
$= \sigma[\pi(2R)^2] = 4\pi\sigma R^2$

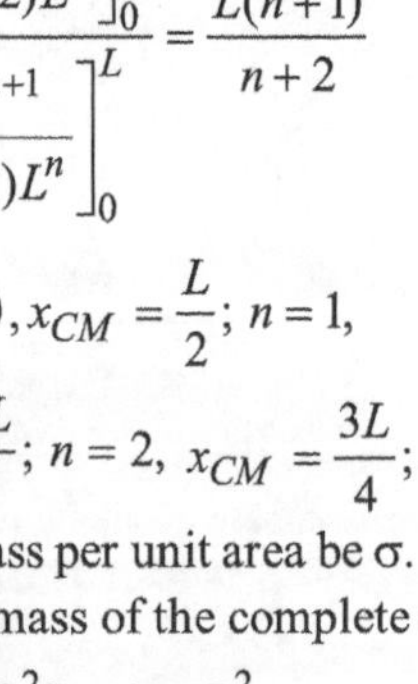

The mass of the removed disc $= \sigma(\pi R^2) = \pi\sigma R^2$

Let us consider the above situation to be a complete disc of radius $2R$ on which a disc of radius R of negative mass is superimposed. Let O be the origin. Then the above figure can be redrawn keeping in mind the concept of centre of mass as :

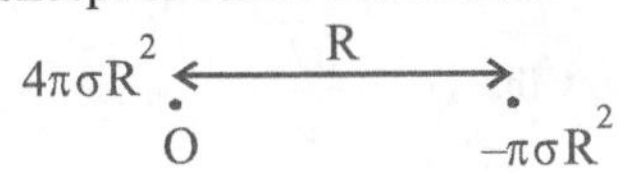

$$x_{c.m} = \frac{\left(4\pi\sigma R^2\right)\times 0 + \left(-\pi\sigma R^2\right)R}{4\pi\sigma R^2 - \pi\sigma R^2}$$

$$\therefore\ x_{c.m} = \frac{-\pi\sigma R^2 \times R}{3\pi\sigma R^2}$$

$$\therefore\ x_{c.m} = -\frac{R}{3} \Rightarrow \alpha = \frac{1}{3}$$

9. (c) Initially,

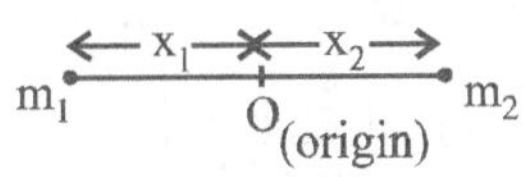

$$0 = \frac{m_1(-x_1) + m_2 x_2}{m_1 + m_2} \Rightarrow m_1 x_1 = m_2 x_2 \ ...(1)$$

Finally,
The centre of mass is at the origin

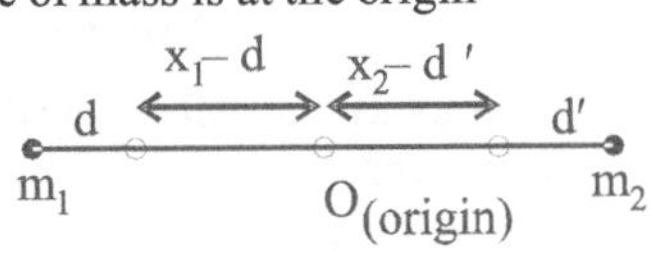

$$\therefore 0 = \frac{m_1(d - x_1) + m_2(x_2 - d')}{m_1 + m_2}$$

$$\Rightarrow 0 = m_1 d - m_1 x_1 + m_2 x_2 - m_2 d'$$

$$\Rightarrow d' = \frac{m_1}{m_2} d$$

[From (1).]

10. (a) Does not shift as no external force acts. The centre of mass of the system continues its original path. It is only the internal forces which comes into play while breaking.

11. (d)

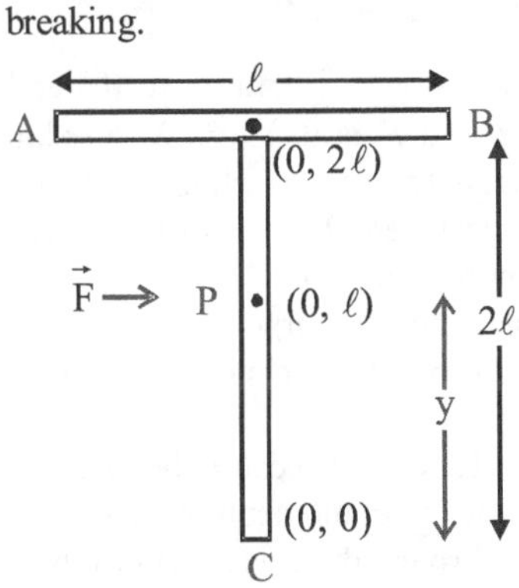

To have linear motion, the force $\vec{F}$ has to be applied at centre of mass.
i.e. the point 'P' has to be at the centre of mass

$$y = \frac{m_1 y_1 + m_2 y_2}{m_1 + m_2} = \frac{m \times 2\ell + 2m \times \ell}{3m} = \frac{4\ell}{3}$$

TOPIC-2 : Angular Displacement, Velocity and Acceleration

12. (b) decreasing speed

13. (c) Torque at angle θ

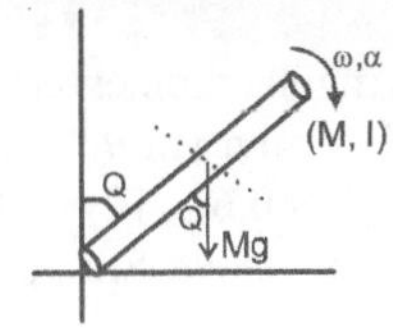

$$\tau = Mg\sin\theta.\frac{l}{2}$$

Also $\tau = I\alpha$

$$\therefore\quad I\alpha = Mg\sin\theta\frac{l}{2}$$

$$\frac{Ml^2}{3}.\alpha = Mg\sin\theta\frac{l}{2} \quad \left[\because I_{rod} = \frac{Ml^2}{3}\right]$$

$$\Rightarrow\quad \frac{l\alpha}{3} = g\frac{\sin\theta}{2} \quad \therefore\quad \alpha = \frac{3g\sin\theta}{2l}$$

14. (a) For just complete rotation

$v = \sqrt{Rg}$ at top point

The rotational speed of the drum

$$\Rightarrow \omega = \frac{v}{R} = \sqrt{\frac{g}{R}} = \sqrt{\frac{10}{1.25}}$$

The maximum rotational speed of the drum in revolutions per minute

$$\omega(\text{rpm}) = \frac{60}{2\pi}\sqrt{\frac{10}{1.25}} = 27.$$

15. (b) Angular momentum, $mvr = I\omega$

Moment of Inertia (I) of cubical block is given by

$$I = m\left(\frac{R^2}{6} + \left(\frac{R}{\sqrt{2}}\right)^2\right)$$

$$\therefore\ \omega = \frac{m.2\frac{R}{2}}{m\left[\frac{R^2}{6} + \left(\frac{R}{\sqrt{2}}\right)^2\right]}$$

$$\Rightarrow \omega = \frac{12}{8R} = \frac{3}{2\times 0.3} = \frac{10}{2} = 5\ \text{rad/s}.$$

16. (b) Angular velocity is the angular displacement per unit time i.e., $\omega = \frac{\Delta\theta}{\Delta t}$

Here $\omega_1 = \omega_2$ and independent of f.

TOPIC-3 : Torque, Couple and Angular Momentum

17. (a) We know that $|L| = mvr_{\perp}$

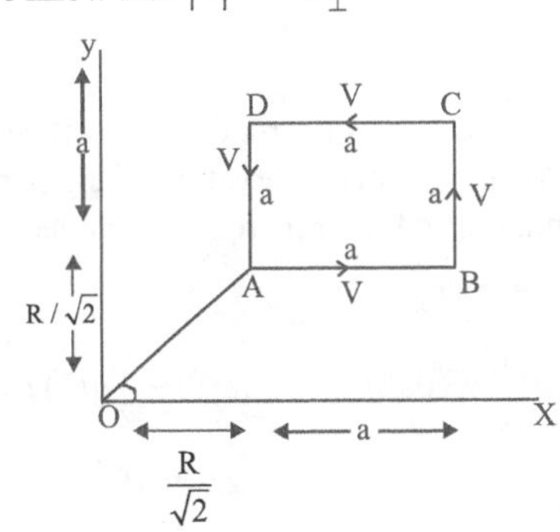

In none of the cases, the perpendicular distance $r_\perp$ is $\left(\frac{R}{\sqrt{2}} - a\right)$

18. **(a)** Angular momentum,
$L_0 = mvr \sin 90°$
$= 2 \times 0.6 \times 12 \times 1 \times 1$
[As $V = r\omega$, Sin 90° = 1]
So, $L_0 = 14.4$ kgm^2/s

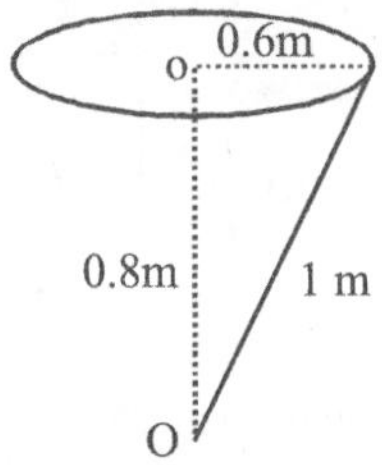

19. **(c)** Torque working on the bob of mass m is, $\tau = mg \times \ell \sin \theta$. (Direction parallel to plane of rotation of particle)

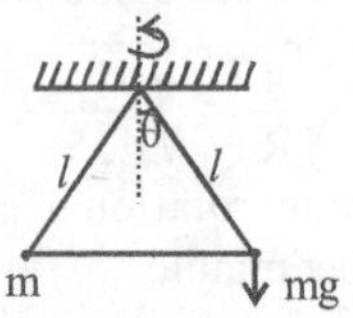

As τ is perpendicular to $\vec{L}$, direction of L changes but magnitude remains same.

20. **(c)** Given : m = 0.160 kg
$\theta = 60°$
v = 10 m/s

Angular momentum $L = \vec{r} \times m\vec{v}$
$= H\,mv \cos\theta$

$$= \frac{v^2 \sin^2\theta}{2g} \cos\theta \qquad \left[H = \frac{v^2 \sin^2\theta}{2g}\right]$$

$$= \frac{10^2 \times \sin^2 60° \times \cos 60°}{2 \times 10}$$

$= 3.46$ kg m^2/s

21. **(a)**

22. **(a)** Angular momentum $L = m(v \times r)$

$$= 2\,\text{kg}\left(\frac{dr}{dt} \times r\right) = 2\,\text{kg}(4t\,j \times 5i - 2t^2\hat{j})$$

$$= 2\,\text{kg}\,(-20\,t\,\hat{k}) = 2\,\text{kg} \times -20 \times 2\,\text{m}^{-2}\,\text{s}^{-1}\,\hat{k}$$

$= -80\,\hat{k}$

23. **(b)**

24. **(d)**

25. **(c)** As insect moves along a diameter, the effective mass and hence the M.I. first decreases then increases so from principle of conservation of angular momentum, angular speed, first increases then decreases.

26. **(c)** $\vec{L} = m(\vec{r} \times \vec{v})$

$$\vec{L} = m\left[v_0 \cos\theta t\,\hat{i} + (v_0 \sin\theta t - \frac{1}{2}gt^2)\hat{j}\right] \times \left[v_0 \cos\theta\,\hat{i} + (v_0 \sin\theta - gt)\hat{j}\right]$$

$$= mv_0 \cos\theta t\left[-\frac{1}{2}gt\right]\hat{k}$$

$$= -\frac{1}{2}mgv_0 t^2 \cos\theta\,\hat{k}$$

27. **(d)** We know that $\vec{\tau_c} = \frac{d\vec{L_c}}{dt}$

where $\vec{\tau_c}$ torque about the center of mass of the body

and $\vec{L_c}$ = Angular momentum about the center of mass of the body. Central forces act along the center of mass. Therefore torque about center of mass is zero.

When $\vec{\tau_c} = 0$ then $\vec{L_c}$ = constt.

28. **(d)** Applying conservation of angular momentum $I'\omega' = I\omega$

$$(mR^2 + 2MR^2)\omega' = mR^2\omega$$

$$\Rightarrow \omega' = \omega\left[\frac{m}{m + 2M}\right]$$

29. **(c)** Torque $\vec{\tau} = \vec{r} \times \vec{F} = (\hat{i} - \hat{j}) \times (-F\hat{k})$

$$= F[-\hat{i} \times \hat{k} + \hat{j} \times \hat{k}] = F(\hat{j} + \hat{i}) = F(\hat{i} + \hat{j})$$

$\left[\text{Since } \hat{k} \times \hat{i} = \hat{j} \text{ and } \hat{j} \times \hat{k} = \hat{i}\right]$

30. **(b)** Angular momentum will remain the same since external torque is zero.

31. **(d)** We know that $\vec{\tau} = \vec{r} \times \vec{F}$

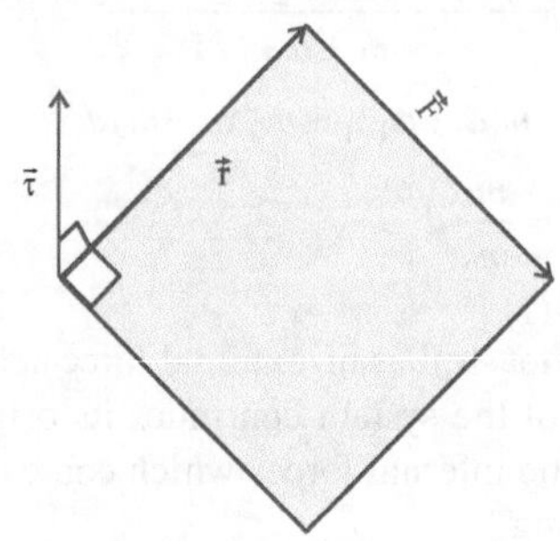

The angle between $\vec{\tau}$ and $\vec{r}$ is 90° and the angle between $\vec{\tau}$ and $\vec{F}$ is also 90°. We also know that the dot product of two vectors which have an angle of 90° between them is zero. Therefore (d) is the correct option.

32. **(d)** Angular momentum (L)
= (linear momentum) × (perpendicular distance of the line of action of momentum from the axis of rotation)

$= mv \times r$ [Here $r = 0$ because the line of
$= mv \times 0$ action of momentum passes
$= 0$ through the axis of rotation]

TOPIC-4 : Moment of Inertia and Rotational K.E.

33. **(c)** As we know, moment of inertia of a solid cylinder about an axis which is perpendicular bisector

$$I = \frac{mR^2}{4} + \frac{ml^2}{12}$$

$$I = \frac{m}{4}\left[R^2 + \frac{l^2}{3}\right]$$

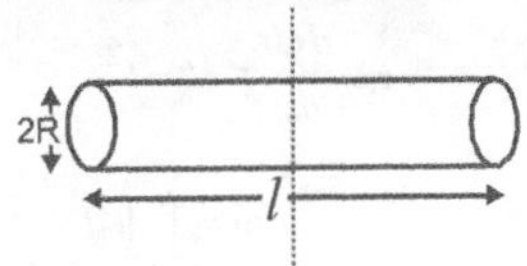

Let V = Volume of cylinder = $\pi R^2 l$

$$= \frac{m}{4}\left[\frac{V}{\pi l} + \frac{l^2}{3}\right] \Rightarrow \frac{dI}{dl} = \frac{m}{4}\left[\frac{-V}{\pi l^2} + \frac{2l}{3}\right] = 0$$

$$\frac{V}{\pi l^2} = \frac{2l}{3} \quad \Rightarrow V = \frac{2\pi l^3}{3}$$

$$\pi R^2 l = \frac{2\pi l^3}{3} \Rightarrow \frac{l^2}{R^2} = \frac{3}{2} \text{ or, } \frac{l}{R} = \sqrt{\frac{3}{2}}$$

34. (b) According to theorem of perpendicular axes, moment of inertia of triangle (ABC)

$I_0 = kml^2$ ..... (i)

BC = 1

Moment of inertia of a cavity DEF

$$I_{DEF} = K\frac{m}{4}\left(\frac{l}{2}\right)^2$$

$$= \frac{k}{16}ml^2$$

From equation (i),

$$I_{DEF} = \frac{I_0}{16}$$

Moment of inertia of remaining part

$$I_{remain} = I_0 - \frac{I_0}{16} = \frac{15I_0}{16}$$

35. (b) Moment of Inertia of complete disc about 'O' point

$$I_{total} = \frac{MR^2}{2}$$

Radius of removed disc = R/4

∴ Mass of removed disc = M/16 [As $M \propto R^2$]

M.I of removed disc about its own axis (O')

$$= \frac{1}{2}\frac{M}{16}\left(\frac{R}{4}\right)^2 = \frac{MR^2}{512}$$

M.I of removed disc about O

$$I_{removed\ disc} = I_{cm} + mx^2$$

$$= \frac{MR^2}{512} + \frac{M}{16}\left(\frac{3R}{4}\right)^2 = \frac{19\,MR^2}{512}$$

M.I of remaining disc

$$I_{remaining} = \frac{MR^2}{2} - \frac{19}{512}MR^2 = \frac{237}{512}MR^2$$

36. (a) Here $a = \frac{2}{\sqrt{3}}R$

$$\text{Now, } \frac{M}{M'} = \frac{\frac{4}{3}\pi R^3}{a^3}$$

$$= \frac{\frac{4}{3}\pi R^3}{\left(\frac{2}{\sqrt{3}}R\right)^3} = \frac{\sqrt{3}}{2}\pi.$$

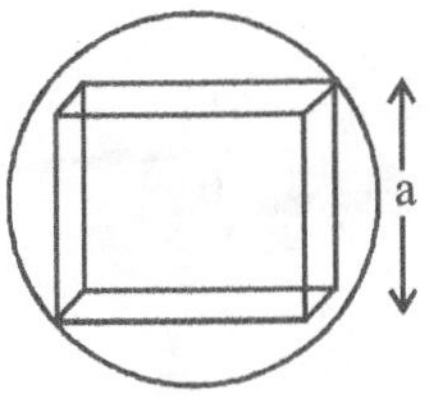

$$M' = \frac{2M}{\sqrt{3}\pi}$$

Moment of inertia of the cube about the given axis,

$$I = \frac{M'a^2}{6}$$

$$= \frac{\frac{2M}{\sqrt{3}\pi} \times \left(\frac{2}{\sqrt{3}}R\right)^2}{6} = \frac{4MR^2}{9\sqrt{3}\pi}$$

37. (d) For a thin uniform square sheet

$$I_1 = I_2 = I_3 = \frac{ma^2}{12}$$

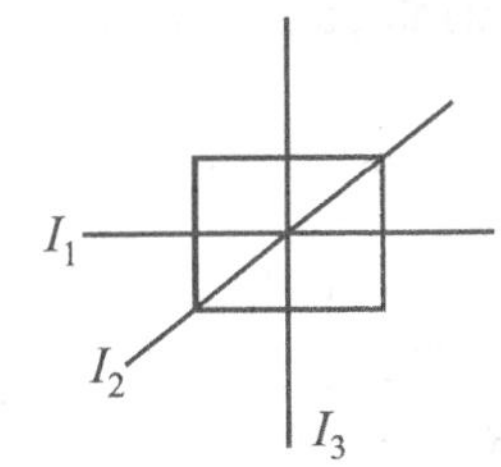

38. (c) Kinetic energy $_{(rotational)}$ $K_R = \frac{1}{2}I\omega^2$

Kinetic energy $_{(translational)}$ $K_T = \frac{1}{2}Mv^2$

(v = Rω)

M.I.$_{(initial)}$ $I_{ring} = MR^2$; $\omega_{initial} = \omega$

M.I.$_{(new)}$ $I'_{(system)} = MR^2 + 2mR^2$

$$\omega'_{(system)} = \frac{M\omega}{M + 2m}$$

Solving we get loss in K.E.

$$= \frac{Mm}{(M + 2m)}\omega^2 R^2$$

39. (b) As $L = I\omega$ so L increases with increase in ω.

Kinetic energy$_{(rotational)}$ depends on an angular velocity 'ω' and moment of inertia of the body I.

i.e., $K.E._{(rotational)} = \frac{1}{2}I\omega^2$

40. (b) $K.E_{rotational} = \frac{1}{2}I\omega^2$

$$= \frac{1}{2}\frac{2}{5}\omega r^2 d^2 \left(\because I_{Solid\ sphere} = \frac{2}{5}mr^2\right)$$

$$K.E_{translational} = \frac{1}{2}mv^2$$

$$\therefore \frac{K.E_{rotational}}{K.E_{translational}} = \frac{2}{5}$$

Hence option (b) is correct

41. (d) M.I. of complete disc about its centre O.

$$I_{Total} = \frac{1}{2}MR^2 \quad ...(i)$$

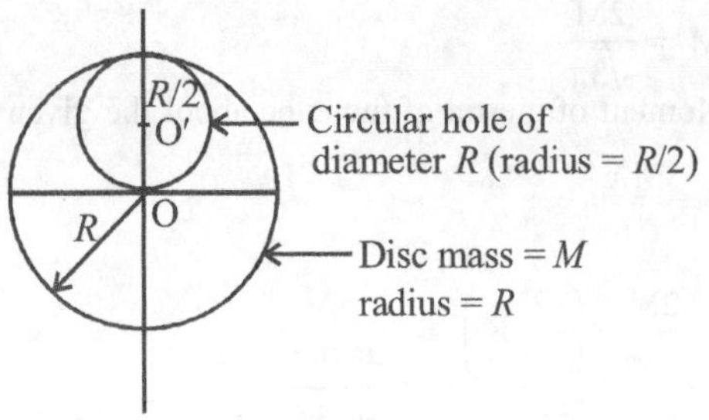

Mass of circular hole (removed)

$= \frac{M}{4}$ $\left(\text{As } M = \pi R^2 t \therefore M \propto R^2\right)$

M.I. of removed hole about its own axis

$$= \frac{1}{2}\left(\frac{M}{4}\right)\left(\frac{R}{2}\right)^2 = \frac{1}{32}MR^2$$

M.I. of removed hole about O'

$$I_{\text{removed hole}} = I_{\text{cm}} + mx^2$$

$$= \frac{MR^2}{32} + \frac{M}{4}\left(\frac{R}{2}\right)^2$$

$$= \frac{MR^2}{32} + \frac{MR^2}{16} = \frac{3MR^2}{32}$$

M.I. of complete disc can also be written as

$$I_{\text{Total}} = I_{\text{removed hole}} + I_{\text{remaining disc}}$$

$$I_{\text{Total}} = \frac{3MR^2}{32} + I_{\text{remaining disc}} \quad \text{...(ii)}$$

From eq. (i) and (ii),

$$\frac{1}{2}MR^2 = \frac{3MR^2}{32} + I_{\text{remaining disc}}$$

$$\Rightarrow I_{\text{remaining disc}}$$

$$= \frac{MR^2}{2} - \frac{3MR^2}{32} = \left(\frac{13}{32}\right)MR^2$$

42. (b) For translational motion,

$mg - T = ma$ .....(1)

For rotational motion,

$T.R = I\alpha = I\frac{\alpha}{R}$ ....(2)

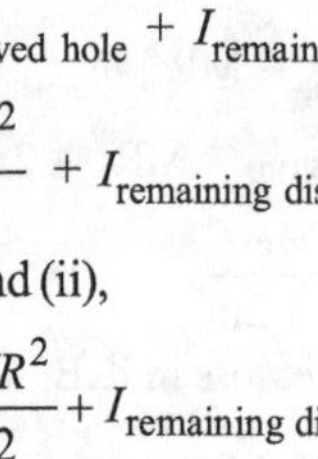

Solving (1) & (2),

$$a = \frac{mg}{\left(m + \frac{I}{R^2}\right)} = \frac{mg}{m + \frac{mR^2}{2R^2}} = \frac{2mg}{3m} = \frac{2g}{3}$$

43. (a) $F = 20t - 5t^2$

$$\therefore \alpha = \frac{FR}{I} = 4t - t^2$$

$$\Rightarrow \frac{d\omega}{dt} = 4t - t^2$$

$$\Rightarrow \int_0^{\omega} d\omega = \int_0^{t} \left(4t - t^2\right)dt$$

$$\Rightarrow \omega = 2t^2 - \frac{t^3}{3} \quad (\text{as } \omega = 0 \text{ at } t = 0, 6\text{s})$$

$$\int_0^{\theta} d\theta = \int_0^{6} \left(2t^2 - \frac{t^3}{3}\right)dt$$

$$\Rightarrow \theta = 36 \text{ rad}$$

$$\Rightarrow n = \frac{36}{2\pi} < 6$$

44. (c)

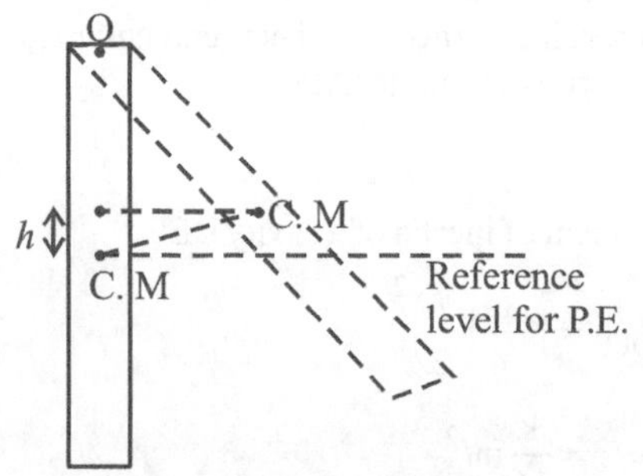

The moment of inertia of the rod about O is $\frac{1}{3}m\ell^2$.

The maximum angular speed of the rod is when the rod is instantaneously vertical. The energy of the rod in this condition is $\frac{1}{2}I\omega^2$ where I is the moment of inertia of the rod about O. When the rod is in its extreme portion, its angular velocity is zero momentarily. In this case, the energy of the rod is mgh where h is the maximum height to which the centre of mass (C.M) rises

$$\therefore mgh = \frac{1}{2}I\omega^2 = \frac{1}{2}\left(\frac{1}{3}ml^2\right)\omega^2$$

$$\Rightarrow h = \frac{\ell^2\omega^2}{6g}$$

45. (d) $I_{nn'} = \frac{1}{12}M(a^2 + a^2) = \frac{Ma^2}{6}$

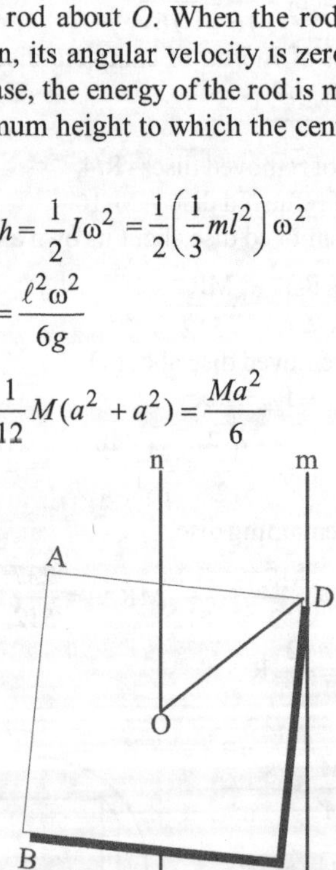

Also, $DO = \frac{DB}{2} = \frac{\sqrt{2}a}{2} = \frac{a}{\sqrt{2}}$

According to parallel axis theorem

$$I_{mm'} = I_{nn'} + M\left(\frac{a}{\sqrt{2}}\right)^2 = \frac{Ma^2}{6} + \frac{Ma^2}{2}$$

$$= \frac{Ma^2 + 3Ma^2}{6} = \frac{2}{3}Ma^2$$

46. (d) By the theorem of perpendicular axes,

$I_z = I_x + I_y$ or, $I_z = 2I_y$

($\because I_x = I_y$ by symmetry of the figure)

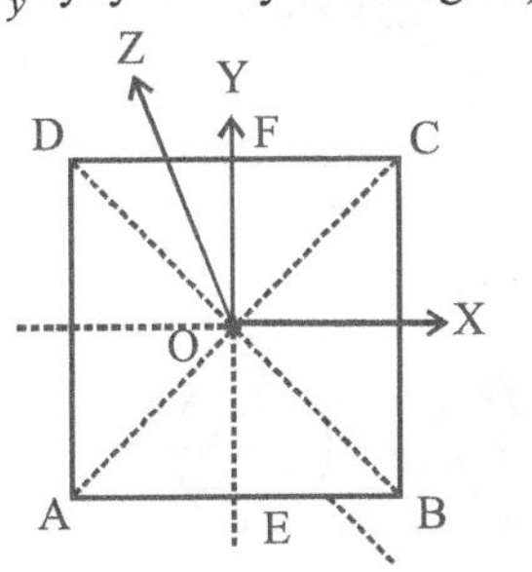

$\therefore\ I_{EF} = \frac{I_z}{2}$ ...(i)

Again, by the same theorem $I_z = I_{AC} + I_{BD} = 2I_{AC}$

($\therefore I_{AC} = I_{BD}$ by symmetry of the figure)

$\therefore\ I_{AC} = \frac{I_z}{2}$ ...(ii)

From (i) and (ii), we get

$I_{EF} = I_{AC}$.

47. (c)

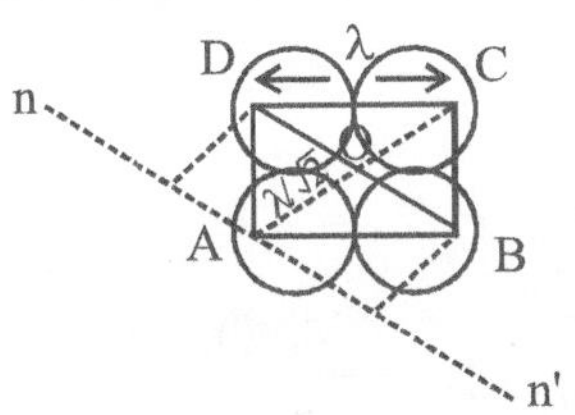

$I_{nn'}$ = M.I due to the point mass at B +
M.I due to the point mass at D +
M.I due to the point mass at C.

$$I_{nn'} = 2 \times m\left(\frac{\ell}{\sqrt{2}}\right)^2 + m(\sqrt{2}\ell)^2$$

$$= m\ell^2 + 2m\ell^2 = 3m\ell^2$$

48. (c) The disc may be assumed as combination of two semi circular parts.
Let I be the moment of inertia of the uniform semicircular disc

$$\Rightarrow 2I = \frac{2Mr^2}{2} \Rightarrow I = \frac{Mr^2}{2}$$

49. (a) The moment of inertia of solid sphere A about its diameter $I_A = \frac{2}{5}MR^2$.

The moment of inertia of a hollow sphere B about its diameter $I_B = \frac{2}{3}MR^2$.

$\therefore I_A < I_B$

50. (d) We know that density $(d) = \frac{mass(M)}{volume(V)}$

$\therefore\ M = d \times V = d \times (\pi R^2 \times t)$.

The moment of inertia of a disc is given by $I = \frac{1}{2}MR^2$

$$\therefore\ I = \frac{1}{2}(d \times \pi R^2 \times t)R^2 = \frac{\pi d}{2} t \times R^4$$

$$\therefore\ \frac{I_X}{I_Y} = \frac{t_X R_X^4}{t_Y R_Y^4} = \frac{t \times R^4}{\frac{t}{4} \times (4R)^4} = \frac{1}{64}$$

51. (a) $K.E. \frac{1}{2}I\omega^2$, but $L = I\omega \Rightarrow I = \frac{L}{\omega}$

$$\therefore\ K.E. = \frac{1}{2}\frac{L}{\omega} \times \omega^2 = \frac{1}{2}L\omega$$

$$\therefore\ \frac{K.E}{K.E'} = \frac{L \times \omega}{L' \times \omega'} \Rightarrow \frac{K.E}{\frac{K.E}{2}} = \frac{L \times \omega}{L' \times 2\omega}$$

$$\therefore\ L' = \frac{L}{4}$$

52. (a) M. I of a circular wire about an axis nn' passing through the centre of the circle and perpendicular to the plane of the circle = MR^2

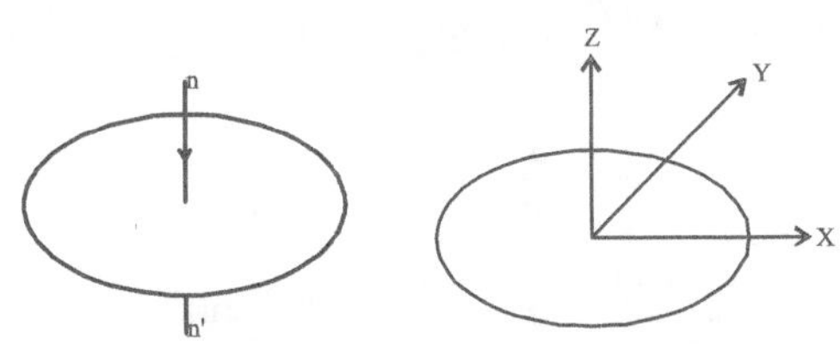

As shown in the figure, X-axis and Y-axis lie in the plane of the ring. Then by perpendicular axis theorem

$I_X + I_Y = I_Z$

$\Rightarrow 2I_X = MR^2$ [$\because I_X = I_Y$ (by symmetry) and $I_Z = MR^2$]

$\therefore I_X = \frac{1}{2}MR^2$

53. (c) When two small spheres of mass m are attached gently, the external torque, about the axis of rotation, is zero and therefore the angular momentum about the axis of rotation is constant.

$$\therefore\ I_1\omega_1 = I_2\omega_2 \Rightarrow \omega_2 = \frac{I_1}{I_2}\omega_1$$

Here $I_1 = \frac{1}{2}MR^2$

and $I_2 = \frac{1}{2}MR^2 + 2mR^2$

$$\therefore\ \omega_2 = \frac{\frac{1}{2}MR^2}{\frac{1}{2}MR^2 + 2mR^2} \times \omega_1 = \frac{M}{M+4m}\omega_1$$

TOPIC-5 : Rolling Motion

54. **(c)** As shown in the diagram, the normal reaction of AB on roller will shift towards O.
This will lead to tending of the system of cones to turn left.

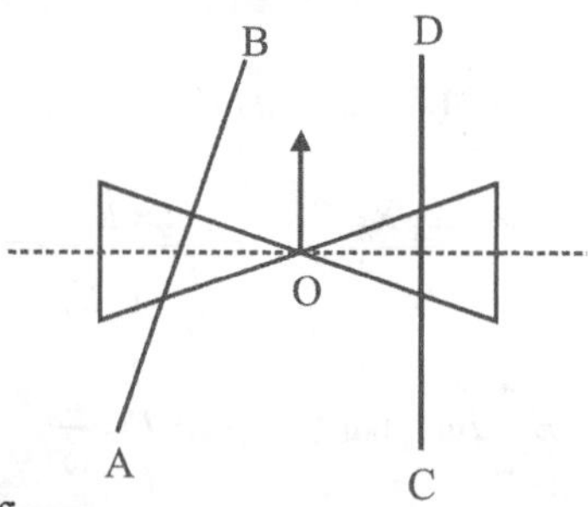

55. **(c)** From figure,
$ma = F - f$ ....(i)

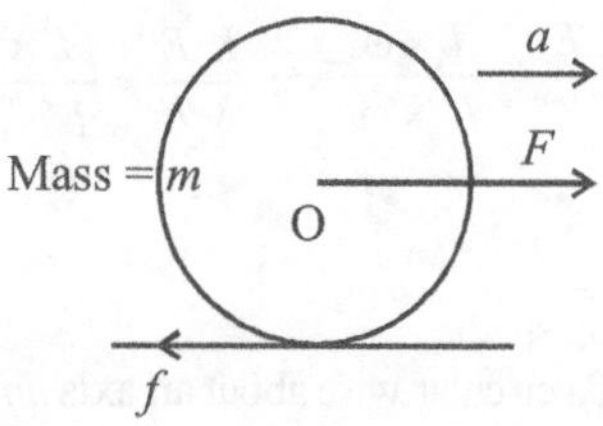

And, torque $\tau = I\alpha$

$$\frac{mR^2}{2}\alpha = fR$$

$$\frac{mR^2}{2}\frac{a}{R} = fR \quad \left[\because \alpha = \frac{a}{R}\right]$$

$$\frac{ma}{2} = f \qquad \text{...(ii)}$$

Put this value in equation (i),

$$ma = F - \frac{ma}{2} \text{ or } F = \frac{3ma}{2}$$

56. **(d)** As we know,

$$\text{Acceleration, } a = \frac{mg\sin\theta}{m + \frac{I}{r^2}}$$

$$\text{For cylinder, } a_c = \frac{M_c g \sin\theta_c}{M_c + \frac{1}{2}\frac{M_c R^2}{R^2}}$$

$$= \frac{M_c g\sin\theta_c}{M_c + \frac{M_c R^2}{2R^2}}$$

$$\text{or, } a_c = \frac{2}{3} g\sin\theta_c$$

For sphere,

$$a_s = \frac{M_s g\sin\theta_s}{M_s + \frac{I_s}{r^2}}$$

$$= \frac{M_s g\sin\theta_s}{M_s + \frac{2}{5}\frac{MR^2}{R^2}}$$

$$\text{or, } a_s = \frac{5}{7} g\sin\theta_s$$

given, $a_c = a_s$

$$\text{i.e., } \frac{2}{3} g\sin\theta_c = \frac{5}{7} g\sin\theta_s$$

$$\therefore\ \frac{\sin\theta_c}{\sin\theta_s} = \frac{\frac{5}{7}g}{\frac{2}{3}g} = \frac{15}{14}$$

57. **(c)**

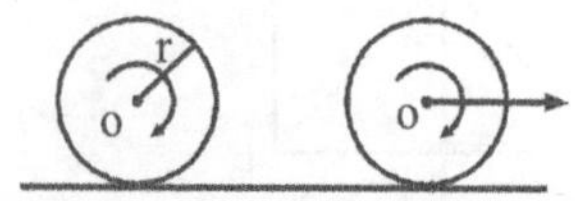

From conservation of angular momentum about any fix point on the surface,

$$mr^2\omega_0 = 2mr^2\omega$$

$$\Rightarrow \omega = \omega_0/2 \Rightarrow v = \frac{\omega_0 r}{2} \quad [\because v = r\omega]$$

58. **(b)** Velocity of the tennis ball on the surface of the earth or ground

$$v = \sqrt{\frac{2gh}{1+\frac{k^2}{R^2}}}$$ (where k = radius of gyration of spherical shell $= \sqrt{\frac{2}{3}}R$)

$$\text{Horizontal range AB} = \frac{v^2\sin 2\theta}{g}$$

$$= \frac{\left(\sqrt{\frac{2gh}{1+k^2/R^2}}\right)^2 \sin(2\times 30°)}{g} = 2.08\,\text{m}$$

59. **(b)** When body rolls dawn on inclined plane with velocity V_0 at bottom then body has both rotational and translational kinetic energy.
Therefore, by law of conservation of energy,

$$P.E. = K.E._{trans} + K.E._{rotational}$$

$$= \frac{1}{2}mV_0^2 + \frac{1}{2}I\omega^2$$

$$= \frac{1}{2}mV_0^2 + \frac{1}{2}mk^2\frac{V_0^2}{R_0^2} \qquad \text{...(i)}$$

$$\left[\because I = mk^2, \omega = \frac{V}{R_0}\right]$$

When body is sliding down then body has only translatory motion.

$\therefore P.E. = K.E_{trans}$

$$= \frac{1}{2}m\left(\frac{5}{4}v_0\right)^2 \quad ...(ii)$$

Dividing (i) by (ii) we get

$$\frac{P.E.}{P.E.} = \frac{\frac{1}{2}mv_0^2\left[1+\frac{K^2}{R_0^2}\right]}{\frac{1}{2}\times\frac{25}{16}\times mV_0^2}$$

$$= \frac{25}{16} = 1+\frac{K^2}{R_0^2} \Rightarrow \frac{K^2}{R_0^2} = \frac{9}{16}$$

or, $K = \frac{3}{4}R_0$.

60. **(d)** Minimum velocity for a body rolling without slipping

$$v = \sqrt{\frac{2gh}{1+\frac{K^2}{R^2}}}$$

For solid sphere, $\frac{K^2}{R^2} = \frac{2}{5}$

$$\therefore \quad v = \sqrt{\frac{2gh}{1+\frac{K^2}{R^2}}} = \sqrt{\frac{10}{7}gh}$$

61. **(b)** This is a standard formula and should be memorized.

$$a = \frac{g\sin\theta}{1+\frac{I}{MR^2}}$$

Chapter 7

Gravitation

TOPIC-1 : Kepler's Laws of Planetary Motion

1. Figure shows elliptical path abcd of a planet around the sun S such that the area of triangle csa is $\frac{1}{4}$ the area of the ellipse. (See figure) With db as the semimajor axis, and ca as the semiminor axis. If t_1 is the time taken for planet to go over path abc and t_2 for path taken over cda then: **[Online April 9, 2016]**

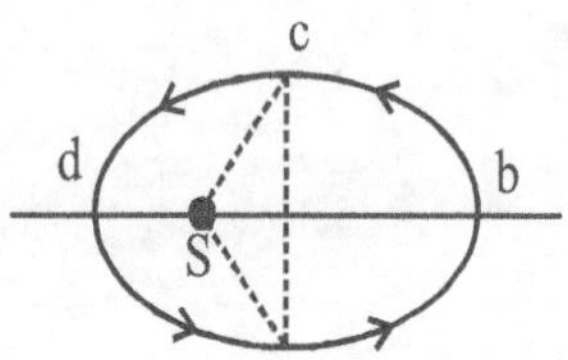

(a) $t_1 = 4t_2$ (b) $t_1 = 2t_2$
(c) $t_1 = 3t_2$ (d) $t_1 = t_2$

2. India's Mangalyan was sent to the Mars by launching it into a transfer orbit EOM around the sun. It leaves the earth at E and meets Mars at M. If the semi-major axis of Earth's orbit is $a_e = 1.5 \times 10^{11}$ m, that of Mars orbit $a_m = 2.28 \times 10^{11}$ m, taken Kepler's laws give the estimate of time for Mangalyan to reach Mars from Earth to be close to: **[Online April 9, 2014]**

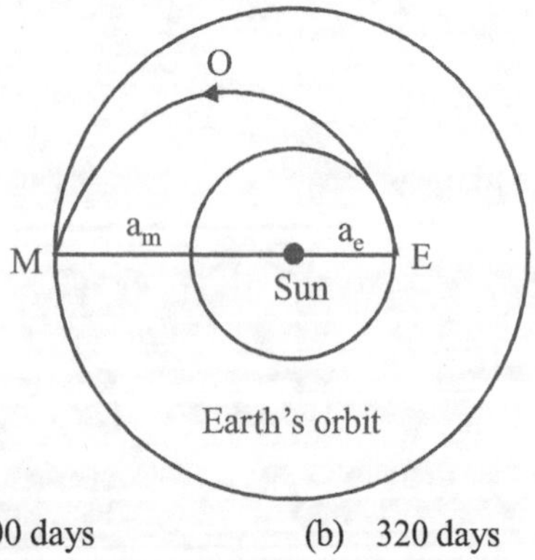

(a) 500 days (b) 320 days
(c) 260 days (d) 220 days

3. The time period of a satellite of earth is 5 hours. If the separation between the earth and the satellite is increased to 4 times the previous value, the new time period will become **[2003]**
(a) 10 hours (b) 80 hours
(c) 40 hours (d) 20 hours

TOPIC-2 : Newton's Universal Law of Gravitation

4. Four particles, each of mass M and equidistant from each other, move along a circle of radius R under the action of their mutual gravitational attraction. The speed of each particle is: **[2014]**
(a) $\sqrt{\frac{GM}{R}}$ (b) $\sqrt{2\sqrt{2}\frac{GM}{R}}$
(c) $\sqrt{\frac{GM}{R}\left(1+2\sqrt{2}\right)}$ (d) $\frac{1}{2}\sqrt{\frac{GM}{R}\left(1+2\sqrt{2}\right)}$

5. From a sphere of mass M and radius R, a smaller sphere of radius $\frac{R}{2}$ is carved out such that the cavity made in the original sphere is between its centre and the periphery (See figure). For the configuration in the figure where the distance between the centre of the original sphere and the removed sphere is 3R, the gravitational force between the two sphere is: **[Online April 11, 2014]**

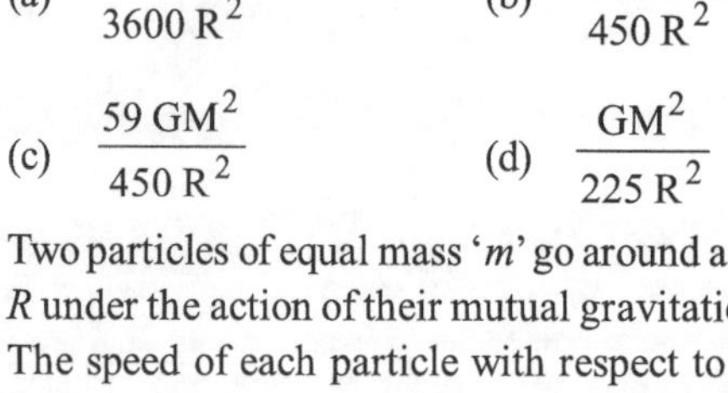

(a) $\frac{41\,GM^2}{3600\,R^2}$ (b) $\frac{41\,GM^2}{450\,R^2}$
(c) $\frac{59\,GM^2}{450\,R^2}$ (d) $\frac{GM^2}{225\,R^2}$

6. Two particles of equal mass 'm' go around a circle of radius R under the action of their mutual gravitational attraction. The speed of each particle with respect to their centre of mass is **[2011 RS]**
(a) $\sqrt{\frac{Gm}{4R}}$ (b) $\sqrt{\frac{Gm}{3R}}$ (c) $\sqrt{\frac{Gm}{2R}}$ (d) $\sqrt{\frac{Gm}{R}}$

7. Two spherical bodies of mass M and $5M$ & radii R & $2R$ respectively are released in free space with initial separation between their centres equal to $12\,R$. If they attract each other due to gravitational force only, then the distance covered by the smaller body just before collision is **[2003]**
(a) $2.5\,R$ (b) $4.5\,R$ (c) $7.5\,R$ (d) $1.5\,R$

TOPIC-3 : Acceleration due to Gravity

8. The variation of acceleration due to gravity g with distance d from centre of the earth is best represented by (R = Earth's radius): **[2017, Online May 7, 2012]**

(a) 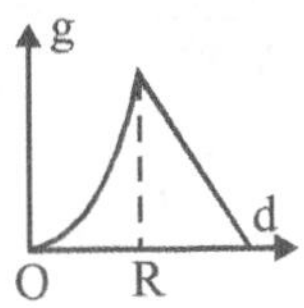

(b) 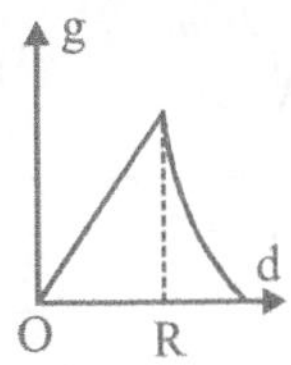

(c) 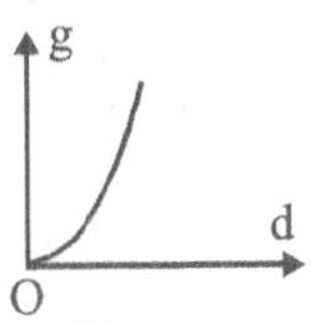

(d) 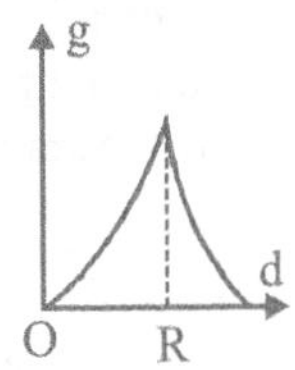

9. The mass density of a spherical body is given by $\rho(r) = \frac{k}{r}$ for $r \le R$ and $\rho(r) = 0$ for $r > R$,
where r is the distance from the centre.
The correct graph that describes qualitatively the acceleration, a, of a test particle as a function of r is : **[Online April 9, 2017]**

(a) 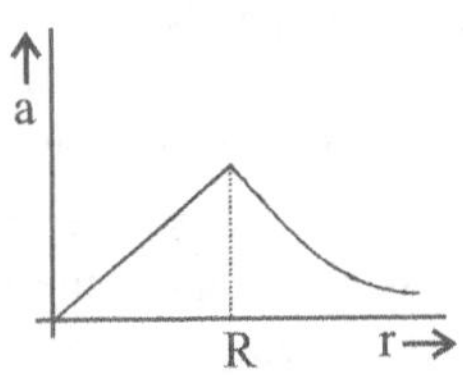

(b) 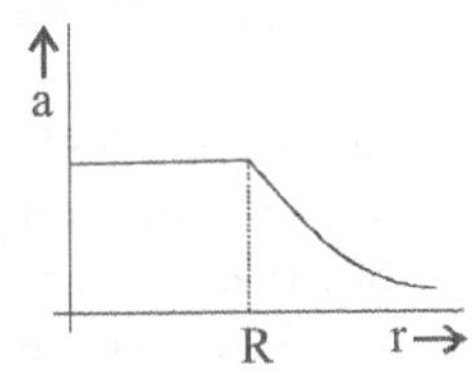

(c) 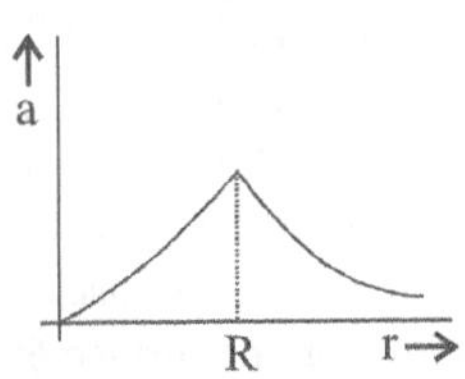

(d) 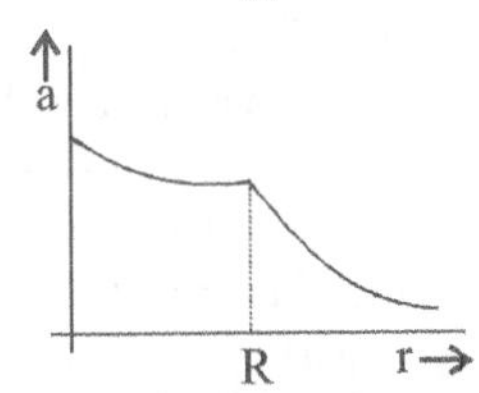

10. If the Earth has no rotational motion, the weight of a person on the equator is W. Determine the speed with which the earth would have to rotate about its axis so that the person at the equator will weight $\frac{3}{4}$W. Radius of the Earth is 6400 km and g = 10 m/s^2. **[Online April 8, 2017]**
(a) 1.1×10^{-3} rad/s (b) 0.83×10^{-3} rad/s
(c) 0.63×10^{-3} rad/s (d) 0.28×10^{-3} rad/s

11. The change in the value of acceleration of earth towards sun, when the moon comes from the position of solar eclipse to the position on the other side of earth in line with sun is: (mass of the moon = 7.36×10^{22} kg, radius of the moon's orbit = 3.8×10^8 m). **[Online April 22, 2013]**
(a) 6.73×10^{-5} m/s^2 (b) 6.73×10^{-3} m/s^2
(c) 6.73×10^{-2} m/s^2 (d) 6.73×10^{-4} m/s^2

12. Assuming the earth to be a sphere of uniform density, the acceleration due to gravity inside the earth at a distance of r from the centre is proportional to **[Online May 12, 2012]**
(a) r (b) r^{-1} (c) r^2 (d) r^{-2}

13. The height at which the acceleration due to gravity becomes $\frac{g}{9}$ (where g = the acceleration due to gravity on the surface of the earth) in terms of R, the radius of the earth, is **[2009]**
(a) $\frac{R}{\sqrt{2}}$ (b) $R/2$ (c) $\sqrt{2}R$ (d) 2R

14. The change in the value of 'g' at a height 'h' above the surface of the earth is the same as at a depth 'd' below the surface of earth. When both 'd' and 'h' are much smaller than the radius of earth, then which one of the following is correct? **[2005]**
(a) $d = \frac{3h}{2}$ (b) $d = \frac{h}{2}$
(c) $d = h$ (d) $d = 2h$

15. Average density of the earth **[2005]**
(a) is a complex function of g
(b) does not depend on g
(c) is inversely proportional to g
(d) is directly proportional to g

TOPIC-4 : Gravitational Field and Potential Energy

16. From a solid sphere of mass M and radius R, a spherical portion of radius R/2 is removed, as shown in the figure. Taking gravitational potential V = 0 at r = ∞, the potential at the centre of the cavity thus formed is :
(*G = gravitational constant*) **[2015]**

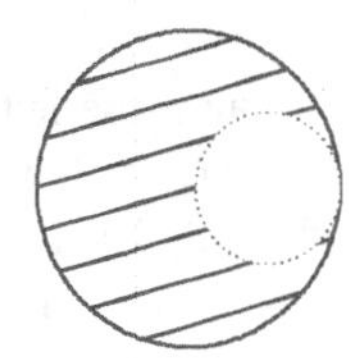

(a) $\frac{-2GM}{3R}$ (b) $\frac{-2GM}{R}$ (c) $\frac{-GM}{2R}$ (d) $\frac{-GM}{R}$

17. Which of the following most closely depicts the correct variation of the gravitational potential V(r) due to a large planet of radius R and uniform mass density ? (figures are not drawn to scale) **[Online April 11, 2015]**

(a) 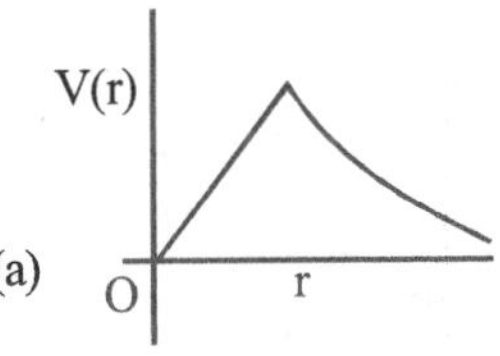

(b) 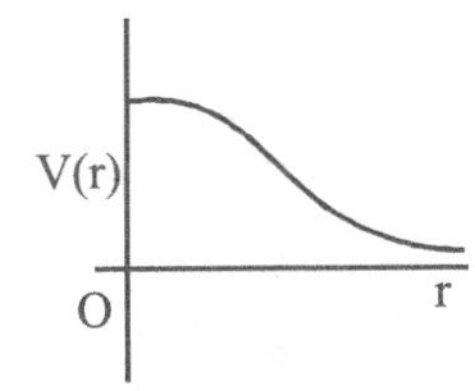

(c) 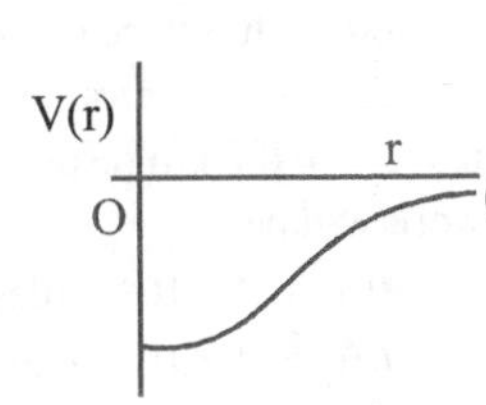

(d) 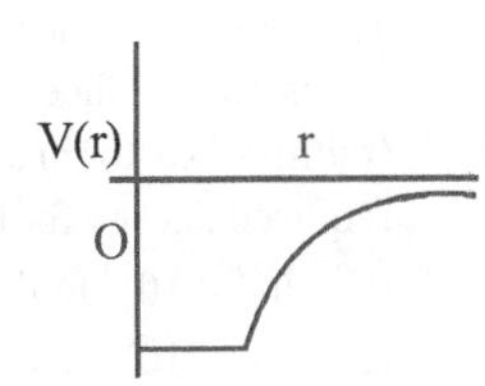

18. The gravitational field in a region is given by $\vec{g} = 5\text{N/kg}\hat{i} + 12\text{N/kg}\hat{j}$. The change in the gravitational potential energy of a particle of mass 1 kg when it is taken from the origin to a point (7 m, – 3 m) is: **[Online April 19, 2014]**

(a) 71 J (b) $13\sqrt{58}$J (c) -71 J (d) 1 J

19. 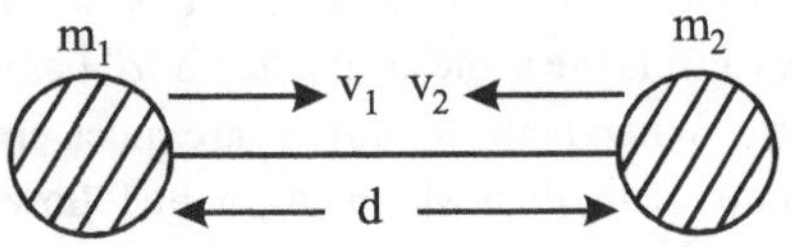

Two hypothetical planets of masses m_1 and m_2 are at rest when they are infinite distance apart. Because of the gravitational force they move towards each other along the line joining their centres. What is their speed when their separation is 'd'? **[Online April 12, 2014]**

(Speed of m_1 is v_1 and that of m_2 is v_2)

(a) $v_1 = v_2$

(b) $v_1 = m_2\sqrt{\frac{2G}{d(m_1+m_2)}}$ $v_2 = m_1\sqrt{\frac{2G}{d(m_1+m_2)}}$

(c) $v_1 = m_1\sqrt{\frac{2G}{d(m_1+m_2)}}$ $v_2 = m_2\sqrt{\frac{2G}{d(m_1+m_2)}}$

(d) $v_1 = m_2\sqrt{\frac{2G}{m_1}}$ $v_2 = m_2\sqrt{\frac{2G}{m_2}}$

20. The gravitational field, due to the 'left over part' of a uniform sphere (from which a part as shown, has been 'removed out'), at a very far off point, P, located as shown, would be (nearly): **[Online April 9, 2013]**

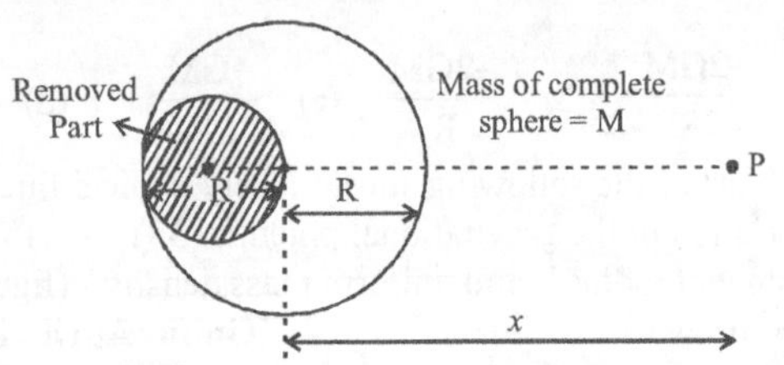

(a) $\frac{5}{6}\frac{GM}{x^2}$ (b) $\frac{8}{9}\frac{GM}{x^2}$

(c) $\frac{7}{8}\frac{GM}{x^2}$ (d) $\frac{6}{7}\frac{GM}{x^2}$

21. The mass of a spaceship is 1000 kg. It is to be launched from the earth's surface out into free space. The value of g and R (radius of earth) are 10 m/s^2 and 6400 km respectively. The required energy for this work will be **[2012]**

(a) 6.4×10^{11} Joules (b) 6.4×10^{8} Joules

(c) 6.4×10^{9} Joules (d) 6.4×10^{10} Joules

22. A point particle is held on the axis of a ring of mass m and radius r at a distance r from its centre C. When released, it reaches C under the gravitational attraction of the ring. Its speed at C will be **[Online May 26, 2012]**

(a) $\sqrt{\frac{2Gm}{r}\left(\sqrt{2}-1\right)}$ (b) $\sqrt{\frac{Gm}{r}}$

(c) $\sqrt{\frac{2Gm}{r}\left(1-\frac{1}{\sqrt{2}}\right)}$ (d) $\sqrt{\frac{2Gm}{r}}$

23. Two bodies of masses m and 4 m are placed at a distance r. The gravitational potential at a point on the line joining them where the gravitational field is zero is: **[2011]**

(a) $-\frac{4Gm}{r}$ (b) $-\frac{6Gm}{r}$ (c) $-\frac{9Gm}{r}$ (d) zero

24. This question contains Statement-1 and Statement-2. Of the four choices given after the statements, choose the one that best describes the two statements. **[2008]**

Statement-1 : For a mass M kept at the centre of a cube of side 'a', the flux of gravitational field passing through its sides 4 π GM. and

Statement-2: If the direction of a field due to a point source is radial and its dependence on the distance 'r' from the source is given as $\frac{1}{r^2}$, its flux through a closed surface depends only on the strength of the source enclosed by the surface and not on the size or shape of the surface.

(a) Statement -1 is false, Statement-2 is true
(b) Statement -1 is true, Statement-2 is true; Statement -2 is a correct explanation for Statement-1
(c) Statement -1 is true, Statement-2 is true; Statement -2 is not a correct explanation for Statement-1
(d) Statement -1 is true, Statement-2 is false

25. A particle of mass 10 g is kept on the surface of a uniform sphere of mass 100 kg and radius 10 cm. Find the work to be done against the gravitational force between them to take the particle far away from the sphere

(you may take $G = 6.67 \times 10^{-11}$ Nm^2/kg^2) **[2005]**

(a) 3.33×10^{-10} J (b) 13.34×10^{-10} J

(c) 6.67×10^{-10} J (d) 6.67×10^{-9} J

26. If 'g' is the acceleration due to gravity on the earth's surface, the gain in the potential energy of an object of mass 'm' raised from the surface of the earth to a height equal to the radius 'R' of the earth is **[2004]**

(a) $\frac{1}{4}mgR$ (b) $\frac{1}{2}mgR$

(c) 2 mgR (d) mgR

27. Energy required to move a body of mass m from an orbit of radius 2R to 3R is **[2002]**

(a) $GMm/12R^2$ (b) $GMm/3R^2$

(c) $GMm/8R$ (d) $GMm/6R$.

TOPIC-5 : Motion of Satellites, Escape Speed and Orbital Velocity

28. A satellite is revolving in a circular orbit at a height 'h' from the earth's surface (radius of earth R; h << R). The minimum increase in its orbital velocity required, so that the satellite could escape from the earth's gravitational field, is close to : (Neglect the effect of atmosphere.) **[2016]**

(a) $\sqrt{gR/2}$ (b) $\sqrt{gR}\left(\sqrt{2}-1\right)$

(c) $\sqrt{2gR}$ (d) $\sqrt{gR}$

29. An astronaut of mass m is working on a satellite orbiting the earth at a distance h from the earth's surface. The radius of the earth is R, while its mass is M. The gravitational pull F_G on the astronaut is : **[Online April 10, 2016]**

(a) Zero since astronaut feels weightless

(b) $\frac{GMm}{(R+h)^2} < F_G < \frac{GMm}{R^2}$

(c) $F_G = \frac{GMm}{(R+h)^2}$

(d) $0 < F_G < \frac{GMm}{R^2}$

30. A very long (length L) cylindrical galaxy is made of uniformly distributed mass and has radius R(R << L). A star outside the galaxy is orbiting the galaxy in a plane perpendicular to the galaxy and passing through its centre. If the time period of star is T and its distance from the galaxy's axis is *r*, then : **[Online April 10, 2015]**

(a) $T \propto r$ (b) $T \propto \sqrt{r}$

(c) $T \propto r^2$ (d) $T^2 \propto r^3$

31. What is the minimum energy required to launch a satellite of mass m from the surface of a planet of mass M and radius R in a circular orbit at an altitude of 2R? **[2013]**

(a) $\frac{5GmM}{6R}$ (b) $\frac{2GmM}{3R}$ (c) $\frac{GmM}{2R}$ (d) $\frac{GmM}{2R}$

32. A planet in a distant solar system is 10 times more massive than the earth and its radius is 10 times smaller. Given that the escape velocity from the earth is 11 km s^{-1}, the escape velocity from the surface of the planet would be **[2008]**

(a) 1.1 km s^{-1} (b) 11 km s^{-1}

(c) 110 km s^{-1} (d) 0.11 km s^{-1}

33. Suppose the gravitational force varies inversely as the nth power of distance. Then the time period of a planet in circular orbit of radius '*R*' around the sun will be proportional to

(a) R^n (b) $R^{\left(\frac{n-1}{2}\right)}$ **[2004]**

(c) $R^{\left(\frac{n+1}{2}\right)}$ (d) $R^{\left(\frac{n-2}{2}\right)}$

34. The time period of an earth satellite in circular orbit is independent of **[2004]**

(a) both the mass and radius of the orbit

(b) radius of its orbit

(c) the mass of the satellite

(d) neither the mass of the satellite nor the radius of its orbit.

35. A satellite of mass *m* revolves around the earth of radius *R* at a height *x* from its surface. If *g* is the acceleration due to gravity on the surface of the earth, the orbital speed of the satellite is **[2004]**

(a) $\frac{gR^2}{R+x}$ (b) $\frac{gR}{R-x}$

(c) gx (d) $\left(\frac{gR^2}{R+x}\right)^{1/2}$

36. The escape velocity for a body projected vertically upwards from the surface of earth is 11 km/s. If the body is projected at an angle of 45° with the vertical, the escape velocity will be

(a) $11\sqrt{2}$ km/s (b) 22 km/s **[2003]**

(c) 11 km/s (d) $\frac{11}{\sqrt{2}}$ km/s

37. The kinetic energy needed to project a body of mass *m* from the earth surface (radius *R*) to infinity is **[2002]**

(a) *mgR*/2 (b) 2*mgR* (c) *mgR* (d) *mgR*/4.

38. If suddenly the gravitational force of attraction between Earth and a satellite revolving around it becomes zero, then the satellite will **[2002]**

(a) continue to move in its orbit with same velocity

(b) move tangentially to the original orbit in the same velocity

(c) become stationary in its orbit

(d) move towards the earth

39. The escape velocity of a body depends upon mass as **[2002]**

(a) m^0 (b) m^1 (c) m^2 (d) m^3

Hints & Solutions

TOPIC-1 : Kepler's Laws of Planetary Motion

1. **(c)** Let area of ellipse abcd = x

Area of SabcS $= \frac{x}{2} + \frac{x}{4}$ (i.e., ar of abca + SacS)

(Area of half ellipse + Area of triangle)

$$= \frac{3x}{4}$$

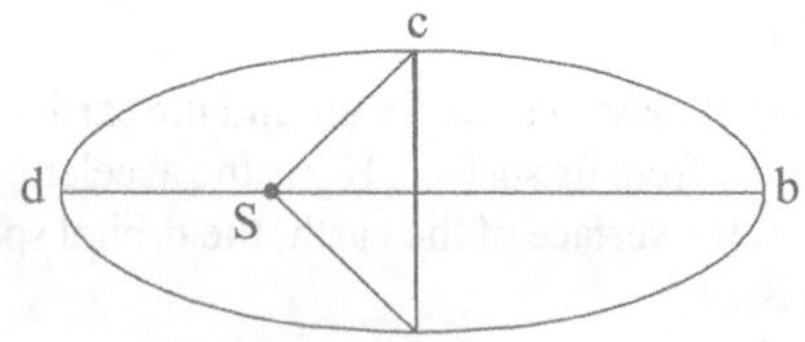

Area of SadcS $= x - \frac{3x}{4} = \frac{x}{4}$

$$\frac{\text{Area of SabcS}}{\text{Area of SadcS}} = \frac{3x/4}{x/4} = \frac{t_1}{t_2}$$

$\frac{t_1}{t_2} = 3$ or, $t_1 = 3t_2$

2. **(b)**

3. **(c)** According to Kepler's law of planetary motion $T^2 \propto R^3$

$$\therefore \; T_2 = T_1\left(\frac{R_2}{R_1}\right)^{3/2} = 5 \times \left[\frac{4R}{R}\right]^{3/2} = 5 \times 2^3 = 40 \text{ hour}$$

TOPIC-2 : Newton's Universal Law of Gravitation

4. **(d)** $2F\cos 45° + F' = \frac{Mv^2}{R}$ (From figure)

Where $F = \frac{GM^2}{(\sqrt{2}R)^2}$ and $F' = \frac{GM^2}{4R^2}$

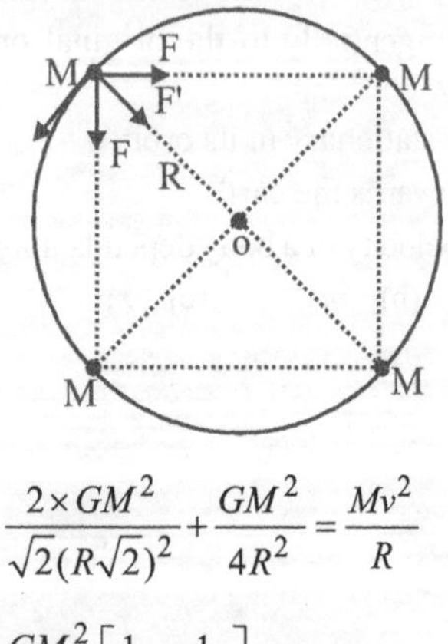

$$\Rightarrow \frac{2 \times GM^2}{\sqrt{2}(R\sqrt{2})^2} + \frac{GM^2}{4R^2} = \frac{Mv^2}{R}$$

$$\Rightarrow \frac{GM^2}{R}\left[\frac{1}{4} + \frac{1}{\sqrt{2}}\right] = Mv^2$$

$$\therefore \; v = \sqrt{\frac{GM}{R}\left(\frac{\sqrt{2}+4}{4\sqrt{2}}\right)} = \frac{1}{2}\sqrt{\frac{GM}{R}(1+2\sqrt{2})}$$

5. **(a)** Volume of removed sphere

$$V_{remo} = \frac{4}{3}\pi\left(\frac{R}{2}\right)^3 = \frac{4}{3}\pi R^3\left(\frac{1}{8}\right)$$

Volume of the sphere (remaining)

$$V_{remain} = \frac{4}{3}\pi R^3 - \frac{4}{3}\pi R^3\left(\frac{1}{8}\right)$$

$$= \frac{4}{3}\pi R^3\left(\frac{7}{8}\right)$$

Therefore mass of sphere carved and remaining sphere are at respectively $\frac{1}{8}$M and $\frac{7}{8}$M.

Therefore, gravitational force between these two sphere,

$$F = \frac{GMm}{r^2}$$

$$= \frac{G\frac{7M}{8} \times \frac{1}{8}M}{(3R)^2} = \frac{7}{64 \times 9}\frac{GM^2}{R^2}$$

$$\simeq \frac{41}{3600}\frac{GM^2}{R^2}$$

6. **(a)** Here, centripetal force will be given by the gravitational force between the two particles.

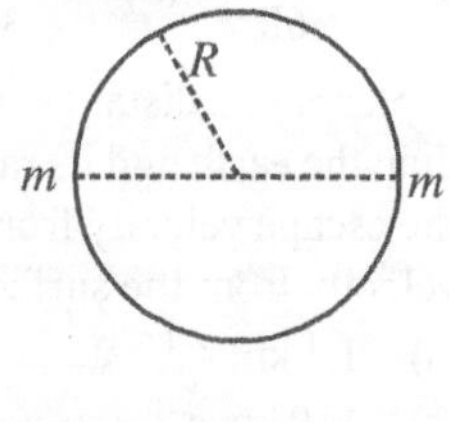

$$\frac{Gm^2}{(2R)^2} = m\omega^2 R$$

$$\Rightarrow \frac{Gm}{4R^3} = \omega^2$$

$$\Rightarrow \omega = \sqrt{\frac{Gm}{4R^3}}$$

If the velocity of the two particles with respect to the centre of gravity is v then

$v = \omega R$

$$v = \sqrt{\frac{Gm}{4R^3}} \times R = \sqrt{\frac{Gm}{4R}}$$

7. (c) The gravitational force acting on both the masses is the same. We know that
Force = mass × acceleration.

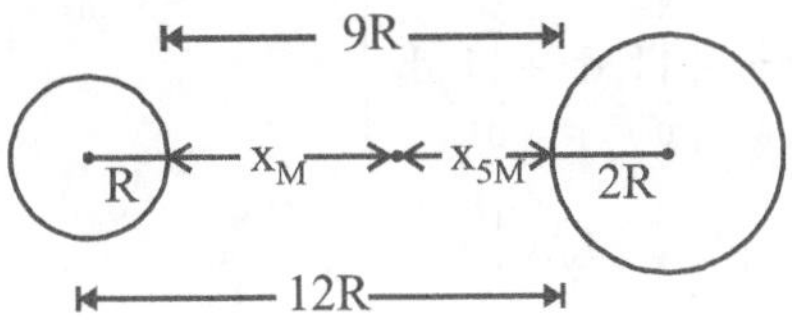

For same force, acceleration $\propto \frac{1}{\text{mass}}$

$\therefore \frac{a_{5M}}{a_M} = \frac{M}{5M} = \frac{1}{5}$ .....(i)

Let t be the time taken for the two masses to collide and x_{5M}, x_M be the distance travelled by the mass 5*M* and *M* respectively.

For mass 5*M*

$u = 0,\ S = x_{5M},\ t = t,\ a = a_{5M}$

$S = ut + \frac{1}{2}at^2$

$\therefore x_{5M} = \frac{1}{2}a_{5M}t^2$ ....(ii)

For mass *M*

$u = 0, s = x_M, t = t,\ a = a_M$

$\therefore s = ut + \frac{1}{2}at^2$

$\Rightarrow x_M = \frac{1}{2}a_M t^2$ ...(iii)

Dividing (ii) by (iii)

$$\frac{x_{5M}}{x_M} = \frac{\frac{1}{2}a_{5M}t^2}{\frac{1}{2}a_M t^2} = \frac{a_{5M}}{a_M} = \frac{1}{5} \quad \text{[From (i)]}$$

$\therefore 5x_{5M} = x_M$ ....(iv)

From the figure it is clear that

$x_{5M} + x_M = 9R$ ....(v)

Where *O* is the point where the two spheres collide.

From (iv) and (v)

$\frac{x_M}{5} + x_M = 9R$

$\therefore 6x_M = 45R \qquad \therefore x_M = \frac{45}{6}R = 7.5R$

TOPIC-3 : Acceleration due to Gravity

8. (b) Variation of acceleration due to gravity, *g* with distance '*d*' from centre of the earth

If $d < R, g = \frac{Gm}{R^2}.d \qquad$ *i.e.*, $g \propto d$ (straight line)

If $d = R, g_s = \frac{Gm}{R^2}$

If $d > R, g = \frac{Gm}{d^2} \qquad$ *i.e.*, $g \propto \frac{1}{d^2}$

9. (b) Given that, mass density $\left(\frac{\text{mass}}{\text{volume}}\right)$ of a spherical body $\rho(r) = \frac{k}{r}$

$\frac{M}{V} = \frac{k}{r}$ for inside $r \le R$

$M = \frac{kv}{r}$ ..... (i)

Inside the surface of sphere Intensity

$I = \frac{GMr}{R^3} \qquad \because I = \frac{F}{m}$

$g_{inside} = \frac{GMr}{R^3} \qquad$ or $\quad I = \frac{mg}{m} = g$

$= \frac{G}{R^3}.\frac{kv}{r}.r = \text{constant} \qquad$ From eq. (i),

Similarly, $g_{out} = \frac{GM}{r^2}$

Hence, option (2) is correct graph.

10. (c) We know, $g' = g - \omega^2 R\cos^2\theta$

$\frac{3g}{4} = g - \omega^2 R$

Given, $g' = \frac{3}{4}g$

$\omega^2 R = \frac{g}{4}$

$\omega = \sqrt{\frac{g}{4R}} = \sqrt{\frac{10}{4 \times 6400 \times 10^3}}$

$= \frac{1}{2 \times 8 \times 100} = 0.6 \times 10^{-3}$ rad/s

11. (a)

12. (a) Acceleration due to gravity at depth d from the surface of the earth or at a distance r from the centre '*O*' of the earth $g' = \frac{4}{3}\pi\rho Gr$

Hence $g' \propto r$

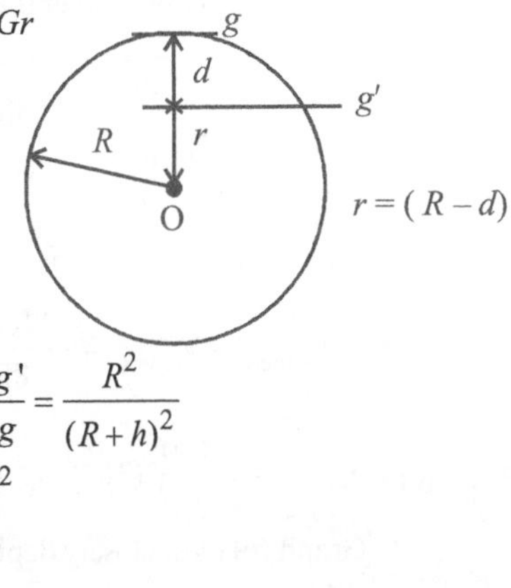

13. (d) We know that $\frac{g'}{g} = \frac{R^2}{(R+h)^2}$

$\therefore \frac{g/9}{g} = \left[\frac{R}{R+h}\right]^2$

$\therefore \frac{R}{R+h} = \frac{1}{3}$

$\therefore h = 2R$

14. **(d)** Variation of g with altitude is, $g_h = g\left[1-\frac{2h}{R}\right]$;

variation of g with depth is, $g_d = g\left[1-\frac{d}{R}\right]$

Equating g_h and g_d, we get $d = 2h$

15. **(d)** $g = \frac{GM}{R^2} = \frac{G\rho \times V}{R^2} \Rightarrow g = \frac{G\times\rho\times\frac{4}{3}\pi R^3}{R^2}$

$g = \frac{4}{3}\rho\pi G.R$ where $\rho \rightarrow$ average density

$\rho = \left(\frac{3g}{4\pi GR}\right)$

$\Rightarrow \rho$ is directly proportional to g.

TOPIC-4 : Gravitational Field and Potential Energy

16. **(d)** Due to complete solid sphere, potential at point P

$$V_{sphere} = \frac{-GM}{2R^3}\left[3R^2 - \left(\frac{R}{2}\right)^2\right]$$

$$= \frac{-GM}{2R^3}\left(\frac{11R^2}{4}\right) = -11\frac{GM}{8R}$$

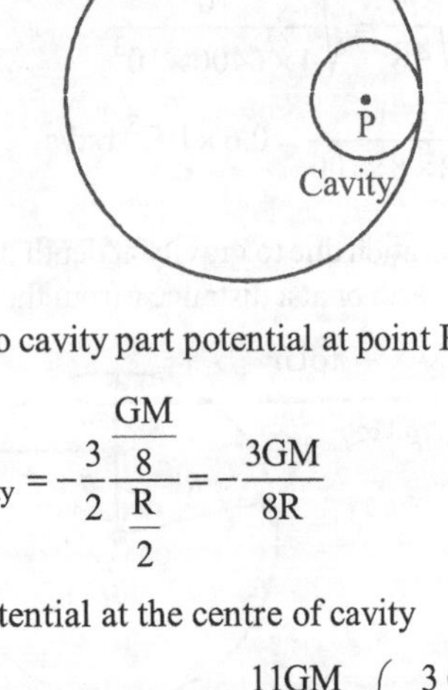

Due to cavity part potential at point P

$$V_{cavity} = -\frac{3}{2}\frac{\frac{GM}{8}}{\frac{R}{2}} = -\frac{3GM}{8R}$$

So potential at the centre of cavity

$$= V_{sphere} - V_{cavity} = -\frac{11GM}{8R} - \left(-\frac{3}{8}\frac{GM}{R}\right) = \frac{-GM}{R}$$

17. **(c)** As, $V = -\frac{GM}{2R^3}(3R^2 - r^2)$

Graph (c) most closely depicts the correct variation of $v(r)$.

18. **(d)** Gravitational field, $I = (5\hat{i} + 12\hat{j})$ N/kg

$$I = -\frac{dv}{dr}$$

$$v = -\left[\int_0^x I_x dx + \int_0^y I_y dy\right]$$

$$= -\left[I_x.x + I_y.y\right]$$

$$= -\left[5(7-0) + 12(-3-0)\right]$$

$$= -\left[35 + (-36)\right] = 1\ \text{J/kg}$$

i.e., change in gravitational potential 1 J/kg.
Hence change in gravitational potential energy 1 J

19. **(b)** We choose reference point, infinity, where total energy of the system is zero.
So, initial energy of the system = 0

Final energy $= \frac{1}{2}m_1v_1^2 + \frac{1}{2}m_2v_2^2 - \frac{Gm_1m_2}{d}$

From conservation of energy,
Initial energy = Final energy

$$\therefore 0 = \frac{1}{2}m_1{v_1}^2 + \frac{1}{2}m_2{v_2}^2 - \frac{Gm_1m_2}{d}$$

or $\frac{1}{2}m_1v_1^2 + \frac{1}{2}m_1v_2^2 = \frac{Gm_1m_2}{d}$ ...(1)

By conservation of linear momentum

$$m_1v_1 + m_2v_2 = 0 \text{ or } \frac{v_1}{v_2} = -\frac{m_2}{m_1} \Rightarrow v_2 = -\frac{m_1}{m_2}v_1$$

Putting value of v_2 in equation (1), we get

$$m_1v_1^2 + m_2\left(-\frac{m_1v_1}{m_2}\right)^2 = \frac{2Gm_1m_2}{d}$$

$$\frac{m_1m_2v_1^2 + m_1^2v_1^2}{m_2} = \frac{2Gm_1m_2}{d}$$

$$v_1 = \sqrt{\frac{2Gm_2^2}{d(m_1+m_2)}} = m_2\sqrt{\frac{2G}{d(m_1+m_2)}}$$

Similarly $v_2 = -m_1\sqrt{\frac{2G}{d(m_1+m_2)}}$

20. **(c)** Let mass of smaller sphere (which has to be removed) is m

$\Rightarrow$ Radius $= \frac{R}{2}$ (from figure)

$$\frac{M}{\frac{4}{3}\pi R^3} = \frac{m}{\frac{4}{3}\pi\left(\frac{R}{2}\right)^3}$$

$$\Rightarrow m = \frac{M}{8}$$

Mass of the left over part of the sphere

$$M' = M - \frac{M}{8} = \frac{7}{8}M$$

Therefore gravitational field due to the left over part of the sphere

$$= \frac{GM'}{x^2} = \frac{7}{8}\frac{GM}{x^2}$$

21. **(d)** The work done to launch the spaceship

$$W = -\int_R^{\infty} \vec{F}.\vec{dr} = -\int_R^{\infty} \frac{GMm}{r^2} dr$$

$$W = +\frac{GMm}{R} \quad \ldots (i)$$

The force of attraction of the earth on the spaceship, when it was on the earth's surface

$$F = \frac{GMm}{R^2}$$

$$\Rightarrow mg = \frac{GMm}{R^2} \Rightarrow g = \frac{GM}{R^2} \quad \ldots (ii)$$

The required energy for this work is given by

$$= U - W = mgR$$

$$= 1000 \times 10 \times 6400 \times 10^3$$

$$= 6.4 \times 10^{10} \text{ Joule}$$

22. **(c)** Let 'M' be the mass of the particle

Now, $E_{initial} = E_{final}$

i.e. $\frac{GMm}{\sqrt{2}r} + 0 = \frac{GMm}{r} + \frac{1}{2}MV^2$

or, $\frac{1}{2}MV^2 = \frac{GMm}{r}\left[1 - \frac{1}{\sqrt{2}}\right]$

$$\Rightarrow \frac{1}{2}V^2 = \frac{Gm}{r}\left[1 - \frac{1}{\sqrt{2}}\right]$$

or, $V = \sqrt{\frac{2Gm}{r}\left(1 - \frac{1}{\sqrt{2}}\right)}$

23. **(c)** Let the gravitational field at P, distant x from mass m, be zero.

$$\therefore \frac{Gm}{x^2} = \frac{4Gm}{(r-x)^2}$$

$$\Rightarrow \frac{1}{x} = \frac{2}{r-x}$$

$$\therefore r - x = 2x$$

$$x = \frac{r}{3}$$

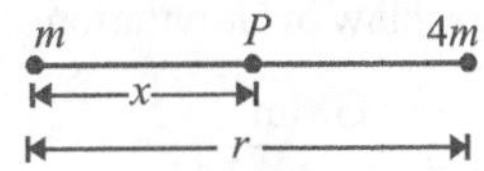

Gravitational potential at P,

$$V = -\frac{Gm}{\frac{r}{3}} - \frac{4Gm}{\frac{2r}{3}} = -\frac{9Gm}{r}$$

24. **(b)** Gravitational flux through a closed surface is given by

$$\int \vec{E_g} \cdot \vec{dS} = -4\pi GM$$

where, M = mass enclosed in the closed surface

This relationship is valid when $|\vec{E}_g| \propto \frac{1}{r^2}$.

25. **(c)** Workdone,

$$W = \Delta U = U_f - U_i = 0 - \left[\frac{-GMm}{R}\right]$$

$$W = \frac{6.67 \times 10^{-11} \times 100}{0.1} \times \frac{10}{1000} = 6.67 \times 10^{-10} \text{ J}$$

26. **(b)** At earth surface, $P.E.$ of system is $-\frac{GmM}{R}$

At a distance R from the earth's surface, $P.E$ .of system is $-\frac{GmM}{2R}$

$$\therefore \Delta U = \frac{-GmM}{2R} + \frac{GmM}{R}; \quad \Delta U = \frac{GmM}{2R}$$

$$\text{Now } \frac{GM}{R^2} = g; \therefore \frac{GM}{R} = gR$$

$$\therefore \Delta U = \frac{1}{2}mgR$$

27. **(d)** Energy required = (Potential energy of the Earth -mass system when mass is at distance $3R$) – (Potential energy of the Earth -mass system when mass is at distance $2R$)

$$= \frac{-GMm}{3R} - \left(\frac{-GMm}{2R}\right) = \frac{-GMm}{3R} + \frac{GMm}{2R}$$

$$= \frac{-2GMm + 3GMm}{6R} = \frac{GMm}{6R}$$

TOPIC-5 : Motion of Satellites, Escape Speed and Orbital Velocity

28. **(b)** For h << R, the orbital velocity is $\sqrt{gR}$

Escape velocity = $\sqrt{2gR}$

$\therefore$ The minimum increase in its orbital velocity

$$= \sqrt{2gR} - \sqrt{gR} = \sqrt{gR}\ (\sqrt{2} - 1)$$

29. **(c)** According to universal law of Gravitation,

Gravitational force $F = \dfrac{GMm}{(R+h)^2}$

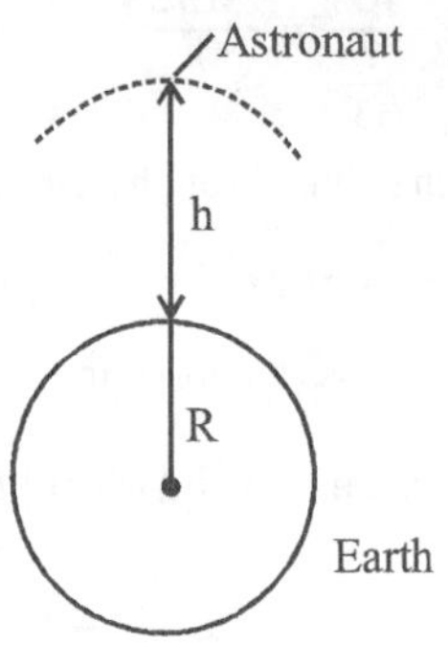

30. **(a)** $F = \dfrac{2GM}{Lr}m$ or, $\dfrac{mv^2}{r} = \dfrac{2GM}{Lr}m$

$mr\left(\dfrac{2\pi}{T}\right)^2 = \dfrac{2GMm}{Lr}\left[\because v = r\omega \text{ and } \omega = \dfrac{2\pi}{T}\right]$

$\Rightarrow T \propto r$

31. **(a)** As we know,

Gravitational potential energy $= \dfrac{-GMm}{r}$

and orbital velocity, $v_0 = \sqrt{GM/R+h}$

$E_f = \dfrac{1}{2}mv_0^2 - \dfrac{GMm}{3R} = \dfrac{1}{2}m\dfrac{GM}{3R} - \dfrac{GMm}{3R}$

$= \dfrac{GMm}{3R}\left(\dfrac{1}{2}-1\right) = \dfrac{-GMm}{6R}$

$E_i = \dfrac{-GMm}{R} + K$

$E_i = E_f$

Therefore minimum required energy, $K = \dfrac{5GMm}{6R}$

32. **(c)** $\dfrac{(v_e)_p}{(v_e)_e} = \dfrac{\sqrt{\dfrac{2GM_p}{R_p}}}{\sqrt{\dfrac{2GM_e}{R_e}}} = \sqrt{\dfrac{M_p}{M_e} \times \dfrac{R_e}{R_p}}$

$= \sqrt{\dfrac{10M_e}{M_e} \times \dfrac{R_e}{R_e/10}} = 10$

$\therefore (v_e)_p = 10 \times (v_e)_e = 10 \times 11 = 110\ km/s$

33. **(c)** $F = KR^{-n} = MR\omega^2 \Rightarrow \omega^2 = KR^{-(n+1)}$

or $\omega = KR^{\frac{-(n+1)}{2}}$

$\dfrac{2\pi}{T} \propto R^{\frac{-(n+1)}{2}}$ $\quad\therefore T \propto R^{\frac{+(n+1)}{2}}$

34. **(c)** We have, $\dfrac{mv^2}{R+x} = \dfrac{GmM}{(R+x)^2}$

x = height of satellite from earth surface
m = mass of satellite

$\Rightarrow v^2 = \dfrac{GM}{(R+x)}$ or $v = \sqrt{\dfrac{GM}{R+x}}$

$T = \dfrac{2\pi(R+x)}{v} = \dfrac{2\pi(R+x)}{\sqrt{\dfrac{GM}{R+x}}}$

which is independent of mass of satellite

35. **(d)** Gravitational force provides the necessary centripetal force.

$\therefore \dfrac{mv^2}{(R+x)} = \dfrac{GmM}{(R+x)^2}$ also $g = \dfrac{GM}{R^2}$

$\therefore \dfrac{mv^2}{(R+x)} = m\left(\dfrac{GM}{R^2}\right)\dfrac{R^2}{(R+x)^2}\dfrac{n!}{r!(n-r)!}$

$\therefore \dfrac{mv^2}{(R+x)} = mg\dfrac{R^2}{(R+x)^2}$

$\therefore v^2 = \dfrac{gR^2}{R+x} \Rightarrow v = \left(\dfrac{gR^2}{R+x}\right)^{1/2}$

36. **(c)** $v_e = \sqrt{2gR}$

The escape velocity is independent of the angle at which the body is projected.

37. **(c)** $K.E = \dfrac{1}{2}mv_e^2$ where v_e = escape velocity = $\sqrt{2gR}$

$\therefore K.E = \dfrac{1}{2}m \times 2gR = mgR$

38. **(c)** Due to inertia of motion it will move tangentially to the original orbit in the same velocity.

39. **(a)** Escape velocity, $v_e = \sqrt{2gR} = \sqrt{\dfrac{2GM}{R}} \Rightarrow v_e \propto m^0$

Where M, R are the mass and radius of the planet respectively. In this expression the mass of the body (m) is not present showing that the escape velocity is independent of the mass.

Chapter 8

Mechanical Properties of Solids

TOPIC-1 : Hooke's Law & Young's Modulus

1. A thin 1 m long rod has a radius of 5 mm. A force of 50 πkN is applied at one end to determine its Young's modulus. Assume that the force is exactly known. If the least count in the measurement of all lengths is 0.01 mm, which of the following statements is false ? **[Online April 10, 2016]**
   (a) The maximum value of Y that can be determined is $2 \times 10^{14} N/m^2$.
   (b) $\frac{\Delta Y}{Y}$ gets minimum contribution from the uncertainty in the length
   (c) $\frac{\Delta Y}{Y}$ gets its maximum contribution from the uncertainty in strain
   (d) The figure of merit is the largest for the length of the rod.

2. A uniformly tapering conical wire is made from a material of Young's modulus Y and has a normal, unextended length L. The radii, at the upper and lower ends of this conical wire, have values R and 3R, respectively. The upper end of the wire is fixed to a rigid support and a mass M is suspended from its lower end. The equilibrium extended length, of this wire, would equal : **[Online April 9, 2016]**
   (a) $L\left(1+\frac{2}{9}\frac{Mg}{\pi YR^2}\right)$ (b) $L\left(1+\frac{1}{9}\frac{Mg}{\pi YR^2}\right)$
   (c) $L\left(1+\frac{1}{3}\frac{Mg}{\pi YR^2}\right)$ (d) $L\left(1+\frac{2}{3}\frac{Mg}{\pi YR^2}\right)$

3. The pressure that has to be applied to the ends of a steel wire of length 10 cm to keep its length constant when its temperature is raised by 100°C is:
   (For steel Young's modulus is $2\times10^{11} Nm^{-2}$ and coefficient of thermal expansion is $1.1\times10^{-5} K^{-1}$) **[2014]**
   (a) 2.2×10^8 Pa (b) 2.2×10^9 Pa
   (c) 2.2×10^7 Pa (d) 2.2×10^6 Pa

4. Two blocks of masses m and M are connected by means of a metal wire of cross-sectional area A passing over a frictionless fixed pulley as shown in the figure. The system is then released. If M = 2 m, then the stress produced in the wire is : **[Online April 25, 2013]**

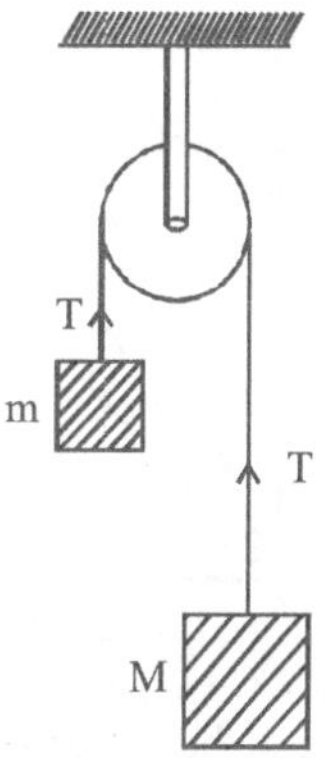

   (a) $\frac{2mg}{3A}$ (b) $\frac{4mg}{3A}$ (c) $\frac{mg}{A}$ (d) $\frac{3mg}{4A}$

5. A copper wire of length 1.0 m and a steel wire of length 0.5 m having equal cross-sectional areas are joined end to end. The composite wire is stretched by a certain load which stretches the copper wire by 1 mm. If the Young's modulii of copper and steel are respectively $1.0 \times 10^{11} Nm^{-2}$ and $2.0 \times 10^{11} Nm^{-2}$, the total extension of the composite wire is : **[Online April 23, 2013]**
   (a) 1.75 mm (b) 2.0 mm (c) 1.50 mm (d) 1.25 mm

6. A uniform wire (Young's modulus $2 \times 10^{11} Nm^{-2}$) is subjected to longitudinal tensile stress of $5 \times 10^7 Nm^{-2}$. If the overall volume change in the wire is 0.02%, the fractional decrease in the radius of the wire is close to : **[Online April 22, 2013]**
   (a) 1.0×10^{-4} (b) 1.5×10^{-4}
   (c) 0.25×10^{-4} (d) 5×10^{-4}

7. If the ratio of lengths, radii and Young's moduli of steel and brass wires in the figure are *a*, *b* and *c* respectively, then the corresponding ratio of increase in their lengths is : **[Online April 9, 2013]**

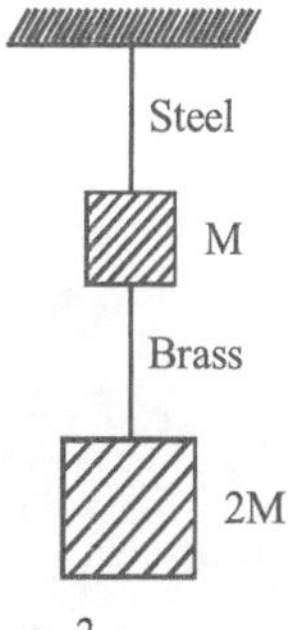

   (a) $\frac{3c}{2ab^2}$ (b) $\frac{2a^2c}{b}$ (c) $\frac{3a}{2b^2c}$ (d) $\frac{2ac}{b^2}$

8. A steel wire can sustain 100 kg weight without breaking. If the wire is cut into two equal parts, each part can sustain a weight of **[Online May 19, 2012]**
(a) 50 kg (b) 400 kg (c) 100 kg (d) 200 kg

9. A structural steel rod has a radius of 10 mm and length of 1.0 m. A 100 kN force stretches it along its length. Young's modulus of structural steel is $2 \times 10^{11}\ Nm^{-2}$. The percentage strain is about **[Online May 7, 2012]**
(a) 0.16% (b) 0.32% (c) 0.08% (d) 0.24%

10. The load versus elongation graphs for four wires of same length and made of the same material are shown in the figure. The thinnest wire is represented by the line **[Online May 7, 2012]**

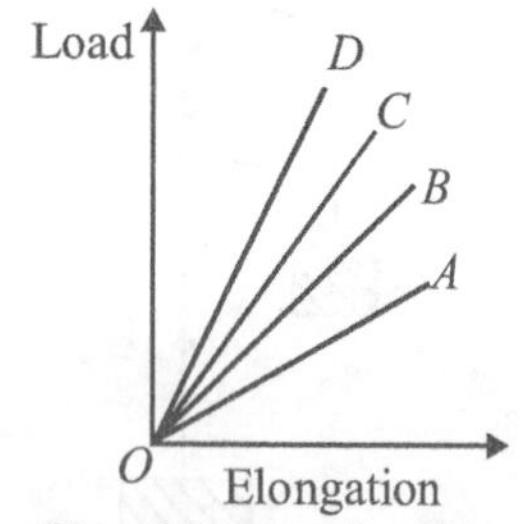

(a) OA (b) OC (c) OD (d) OB

11. Two wires are made of the same material and have the same volume. However wire 1 has cross-sectional area A and wire 2 has cross-sectional area $3A$. If the length of wire 1 increases by Δx on applying force F, how much force is needed to stretch wire 2 by the same amount? **[2009]**
(a) $4F$ (b) $6F$ (c) $9F$ (d) F

12. A wire elongates by l mm when a load W is hanged from it. If the wire goes over a pulley and two weights W each are hung at the two ends, the elongation of the wire will be (in mm) **[2006]**
(a) l (b) $2l$ (c) zero (d) $l/2$

TOPIC-2 : Bulk and Rigidity Modulus and Work Done in Stretching a Wire

13. A bottle has an opening of radius a and length b. A cork of length b and radius $(a + \Delta a)$ where $(\Delta a << a)$ is compressed to fit into the opening completely (see figure). If the bulk modulus of cork is B and frictional coefficient between the bottle and cork is μ then the force needed to push the cork into the bottle is : **[Online April 10, 2016]**

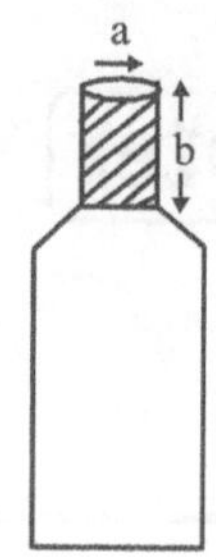

(a) $(\pi\mu B\, b)\, a$ (b) $(2\pi\mu Bb)\, \Delta a$
(c) $(\pi\mu B\, b)\, \Delta a$ (d) $(4\, \pi\mu B\, b)\, \Delta a$

14. Steel ruptures when a shear of $3.5 \times 10^8\ N\ m^{-2}$ is applied. The force needed to punch a 1 cm diameter hole in a steel sheet 0.3 cm thick is nearly: **[Online April 12, 2014]**
(a) 1.4×10^4 N (b) 2.7×10^4 N
(c) 3.3×10^4 N (d) 1.1×10^4 N

15. The bulk moduli of ethanol, mercury and water are given as 0.9, 25 and 2.2 respectively in units of $10^9\ Nm^{-2}$. For a given value of pressure, the fractional compression in volume is $\frac{\Delta V}{V}$. Which of the following statements about $\frac{\Delta V}{V}$ for these three liquids is correct ? **[Online April 11, 2014]**
(a) Ethanol > Water > Mercury
(b) Water > Ethanol > Mercury
(c) Mercury > Ethanol > Water
(d) Ethanol > Mercury > Water

16. In materials like aluminium and copper, the correct order of magnitude of various elastic moduli is: **[Online April 9, 2014]**
(a) Young's modulus < shear modulus < bulk modulus.
(b) Bulk modulus < shear modulus < Young's modulus
(c) Shear modulus < Young's modulus < bulk modulus.
(d) Bulk modulus < Young's modulus < shear modulus.

17. If 'S' is stress and 'Y' is young's modulus of material of a wire, the energy stored in the wire per unit volume is **[2005]**
(a) $\frac{S^2}{2Y}$ (b) $2S^2Y$ (c) $\frac{S}{2Y}$ (d) $\frac{2Y}{S^2}$

18. A wire fixed at the upper end stretches by length ℓ by applying a force F. The work done in stretching is **[2004]**
(a) $2F\ell$ (b) $F\ell$ (c) $\frac{F}{2\ell}$ (d) $\frac{F\ell}{2}$

Hints & Solutions

TOPIC-1 : Hooke's Law & Young's Modulus

1. **(a)** Young's modulus $Y = \frac{F}{A} / \frac{\Delta\ell}{\ell}$

$$Y = \frac{F\ell}{\pi r^2 \Delta\ell}$$

Given, radius r = 5mm, force F = 50πk N,

$$\frac{\ell}{\Delta\ell} = 0.01 \text{ mm}$$

$$\therefore\ Y = \frac{F}{\pi r^2}\frac{\ell}{\Delta\ell} = 2 \times 10^{14}\,\text{N/m}^2.$$

2. **(c)** Consider a small element dx of radius r,

$$r = \frac{2R}{L}x + R$$

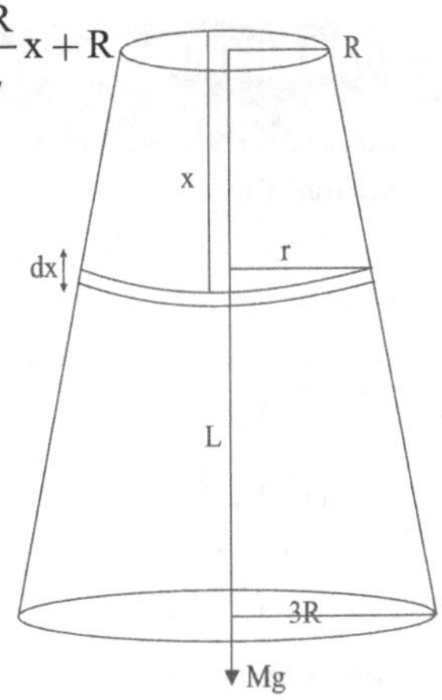

At equilibrium change in length of the wire

$$\int_0^1 dL = \int \frac{Mg\,dx}{\pi\left[\frac{2R}{L}x + R\right]^2 y}$$

Taking limit from 0 to L

$$\Delta L = \frac{Mg}{\pi y}\left[-\frac{1}{\left[\frac{2Rx}{L} + R\right]_0^L} \times \frac{L}{2R}\right] = \frac{MgL}{3\pi R^2 y}$$

The equilibrium extended length of wire = L + ΔL

$$= L + \frac{MgL}{3\pi R^2 Y} = L\left(1 + \frac{1}{3}\frac{Mg}{\pi Y R^2}\right)$$

3. **(a)** Young's modulus $Y = \frac{\text{stress}}{\text{strain}}$

stress = Y × strain

Stress in steel wire = Applied pressure

Pressure = stress = Y × strain

$$\text{Strain} = \frac{\Delta L}{L} = \alpha\Delta T \text{ (As length is constant)}$$

$$= 2 \times 10^{11} \times 1.1 \times 10^{-5} \times 100 = 2.2 \times 10^8\,\text{Pa}$$

4. **(b)** Tension in the wire, $T = \left(\frac{2mM}{m+M}\right)g$

$$\text{Stress} = \frac{\text{Force / Tension}}{\text{Area}} = \frac{2mM}{A(m+M)}g$$

$$= \frac{2(m \times 2m)g}{A(m+2m)} \quad (M = 2\text{ m given})$$

$$= \frac{4m^2}{3mA}g = \frac{4mg}{3A}$$

5. **(d)** $Y_c \times (\Delta L_c / L_c) = Y_s \times (\Delta L_s / L_s)$

$$\Rightarrow 1\times10^{11} \times \left(\frac{1\times10^{-3}}{1}\right) = 2\times10^{11} \times \left(\frac{\Delta L_s}{0.5}\right)$$

$$\therefore\ \Delta L_s = \frac{0.5\times10^{-3}}{2} = 0.25\text{ mm}$$

Therefore, total extension of the composite wire

$= \Delta L_c + \Delta L_s$

$= 1\text{ mm} + 0.25\text{ m} = 1.25\text{ m}$

6. **(c)** Given, $y = 2\times10^{11}\,\text{Nm}^{-2}$

$$\text{Stress}\left(\frac{F}{A}\right) = 5\times10^7\,\text{Nm}^{-2}$$

$$\Delta V = 0.02\% = 2 \times 10^{-4}\,\text{m}^3$$

$$\frac{\Delta r}{r} = ?$$

$$\gamma = \frac{\text{stress}}{\text{strain}} \Rightarrow \text{strain}\left(\frac{\Delta\ell}{\ell_0}\right) = \frac{\gamma}{\text{stress}} \quad \ldots \text{(i)}$$

$$\Delta V = 2\pi r\ell_0\Delta r - \pi r^2\Delta\ell \quad \ldots \text{(ii)}$$

From eqns (i) and (ii) putting the value of $\Delta\ell$, ℓ_0 and ΔV and solving we get

$$\frac{\Delta r}{r} = 0.25\times10^{-4}$$

7. **(c)** According to questions,

$$\frac{\ell_s}{\ell_b} = a,\ \frac{r_s}{r_b} = b,\ \frac{y_s}{y_b} = c,\ \frac{\Delta\ell s}{\Delta\ell_b} = ?$$

$$\text{As, } y = \frac{F\ell}{A\Delta\ell} \Rightarrow \Delta\ell = \frac{F\ell}{Ay}$$

$$\Delta\ell_s = \frac{3mg\ell_s}{\pi r_s^2 . y_s} \quad [\because F_s = (M+2M)g]$$

$$\Delta\ell_b = \frac{2Mg\ell_b}{\pi r_b^2 . y_b} \quad [\because F_b = 2Mg]$$

$$\therefore \frac{\Delta\ell_s}{\Delta\ell_b} = \frac{\frac{3Mg\ell_s}{\pi r_s^2 . y_s}}{\frac{2Mg.\ell_b}{\pi r_b^2 . y_b}} = \frac{3a}{2b^2C}$$

8. (c) Breaking force α area of cross section of wire
Load hold by wire is independent of length of the wire.

9. (a) Given: $F = 100\text{ kN} = 10^5\text{ N}$
$Y = 2\times10^{11}\text{ Nm}^{-2}$
$\ell_0 = 1.0\text{ m}$
radius $r = 10\text{ mm} = 10^{-2}\text{ m}$

From formula, $Y = \frac{\text{Stress}}{\text{Strain}}$

$$\Rightarrow \text{Strain} = \frac{\text{Stress}}{Y} = \frac{F}{AY}$$

$$= \frac{10^5}{\pi r^2 Y} = \frac{10^5}{3.14\times10^{-4}\times2\times10^{11}}$$

$$= \frac{1}{628}$$

Therefore % strain $= \frac{1}{628}\times100 = 0.16\%$

10. (a) From the graph, it is clear that for the same value of load, elongation is maximum for wire *OA*. Hence *OA* is the thinnest wire among the four wires.

11. (c)

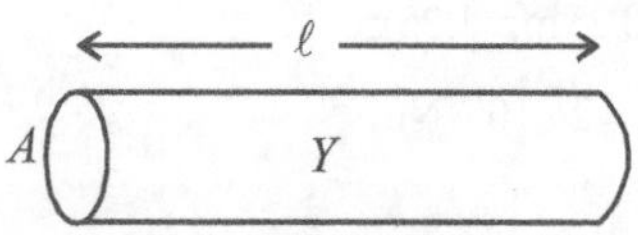

Wire (1)

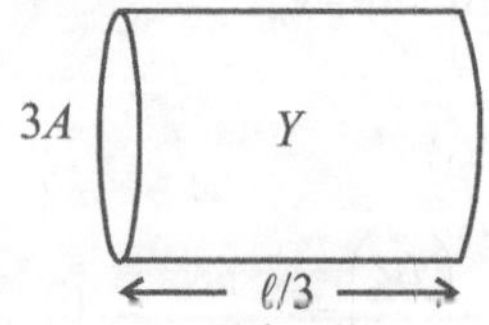

Wire (2)

As shown in the figure, the wires will have the same Young's modulus (same material) and the length of the wire of area of cross-section 3*A* will be $\ell/3$ (same volume as wire 1).

For wire 1,

$$Y = \frac{F/A}{\Delta x/\ell} \quad ...(i)$$

For wire 2,

$$Y = \frac{F'/3A}{\Delta x/(\ell/3)} \quad ...(ii)$$

From (i) and (ii), $\frac{F}{A}\times\frac{\ell}{\Delta x} = \frac{F'}{3A}\times\frac{\ell}{3\Delta x} \Rightarrow F' = 9F$

12. (a) Case (i)

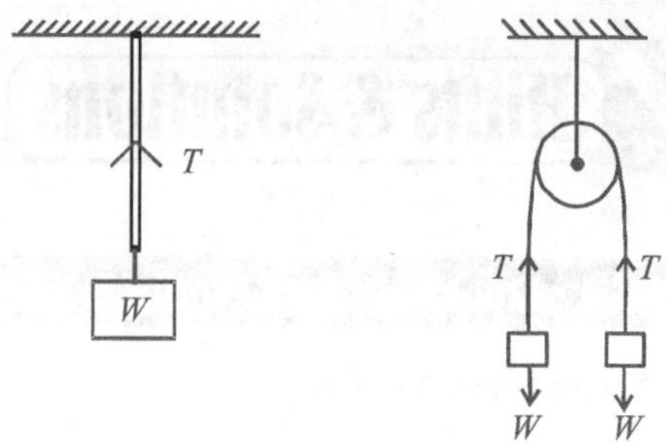

At equilibrium, $T = W$

$$Y = \frac{W/A}{\ell/L} \quad .....(1)$$

Case (ii) At equilibrium $T = W$

$$\therefore Y = \frac{W/A}{\frac{\ell/2}{L/2}} \Rightarrow Y = \frac{W/A}{\ell/L}$$

⇒ Elongation is the same.

TOPIC-2 : Bulk and Rigidity Modulus and Work Done in stretching a wire

13. (d) $\text{Stress} = \frac{\text{Normal force}}{\text{Area}} = \frac{N}{A} = \frac{N}{(2\pi a)b}$

Stress = B×strain

$$\frac{N}{(2\pi a)b} = B\frac{2\pi a\Delta a\times b}{\pi a^2 b}$$

$$\Rightarrow N = B\frac{(2\pi a)^2\Delta ab^2}{\pi a^2 b}$$

Force needed to push the cork.

$$f = \mu N = \mu 4\pi b\Delta aB = (4\pi\mu Bb)\Delta a$$

14. (c)

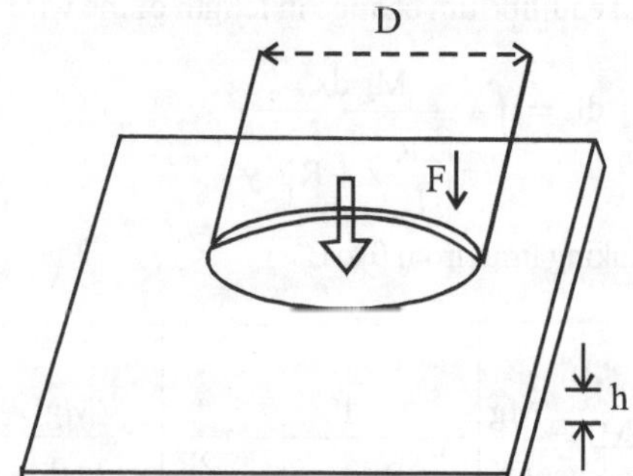

Shearing strain is created along the side surface of the punched disk. Note that the forces exerted on the disk are exerted along the circumference of the disk, and the total force exerted on its center only.

Let us assume that the shearing stress along the side surface of the disk is uniform, then

$$F = \int_{\text{surface}} dF_{max} = \int_{\text{surface}} \sigma_{max}\, dA = \sigma_{max}\int_{\text{surface}} dA$$

$= \int \sigma_{max}.A = \sigma_{max}.2\pi\left(\frac{D}{2}\right)h$

$= 3.5\times10^8\times\left(\frac{1}{2}\times10^{-2}\right)\times0.3\times10^{-2}\times2\pi$

$= 3.297\times10^4 \simeq 3.3\times10^4\,N$

15. (a) Compressibility $= \frac{1}{\text{Bulk modulus}}$

As bulk modulus is least for ethanol (0.9) and maximum for mercury (25) among ehtanol, mercury and water.

Hence compression in volume $\frac{\Delta V}{V}$

Ethanol > Water > Mercury

16. (c) Poisson's ratio, $\sigma = \frac{\text{lateral strain }(\beta)}{\text{longitudinal strain }(\alpha)}$

For material like copper, $\sigma = 0.33$

And, $Y = 3k(1-2\sigma)$

Also, $\frac{9}{Y} = \frac{1}{k} + \frac{3}{\eta}$

$Y = 2\eta(1+\sigma)$

Hence, $\eta < Y < k$

17. (a) Energy stored per unit volume,

$E = \frac{1}{2}\times \text{stress}\times\text{strain}$

We know that,

$Y = \frac{\text{stress}}{\text{strain}}$ or $\text{strain} = \frac{\text{stress}}{Y}$

$E = \frac{1}{2}\times\text{stress}\times\frac{\text{stress}}{Y} = \frac{1}{2}.\frac{S^2}{Y}$

18. (d) Work done by constant force in displacing the object by a distance ℓ.

= change in potential energy

$= \frac{1}{2}\times \text{stress}\times\text{strain}\times\text{volume}$

$= \frac{1}{2}\times\frac{F}{A}\times\frac{\ell}{L}\times A\times L = \frac{F\ell}{2}$

Chapter 9

Mechanical Properties of Fluids

TOPIC-1 : Pressure, Density, Pascal's Law and Archimedes' Principle

1. There is a circular tube in a vertical plane. Two liquids which do not mix and of densities d_1 and d_2 are filled in the tube. Each liquid subtends 90° angle at centre. Radius joining their interface makes an angle α with vertical. Ratio $\frac{d_1}{d_2}$ is: **[2014]**

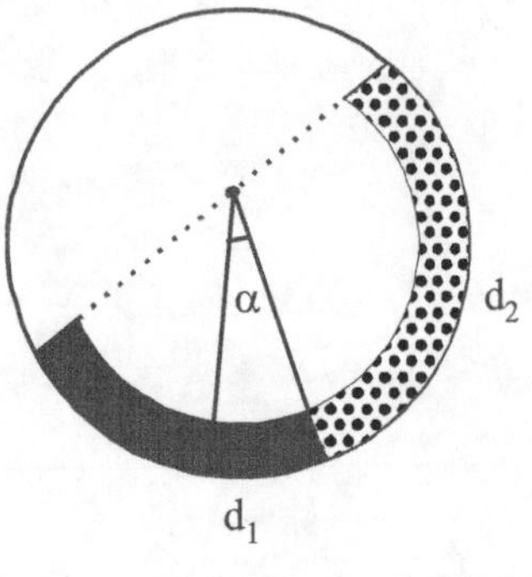

(a) $\frac{1+\sin\alpha}{1-\sin\alpha}$ (b) $\frac{1+\cos\alpha}{1-\cos\alpha}$

(c) $\frac{1+\tan\alpha}{1-\tan\alpha}$ (d) $\frac{1+\sin\alpha}{1-\cos\alpha}$

2. A uniform cylinder of length L and mass M having cross-sectional area A is suspended, with its length vertical, from a fixed point by a massless spring such that it is half submerged in a liquid of density σ at equilibrium position. The extension x_0 of the spring when it is in equilibrium is:

(a) $\frac{Mg}{k}$ (b) $\frac{Mg}{k}\left(1-\frac{LA\sigma}{M}\right)$ **[2013]**

(c) $\frac{Mg}{k}\left(1-\frac{LA\sigma}{2M}\right)$ (d) $\frac{Mg}{k}\left(1+\frac{LA\sigma}{M}\right)$

3. A ball is made of a material of density ρ where $\rho_{oil} < \rho < \rho_{water}$ with ρ_{oil} and ρ_{water} represe-nting the densities of oil and water, respectively. The oil and water are immiscible. If the above ball is in equilibrium in a mixture of this oil and water, which of the following pictures represents its equilibrium position ? **[2010]**

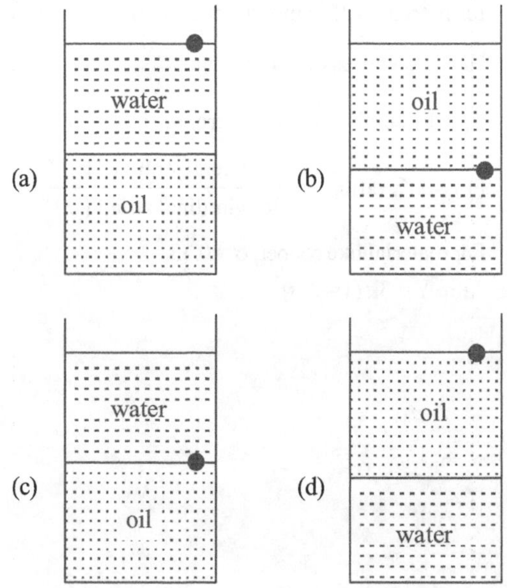

4. Two identical charged spheres are suspended by strings of equal lengths. The strings make an angle of 30° with each other. When suspended in a liquid of density $0.8 g\ cm^{-3}$, the angle remains the same. If density of the material of the sphere is $1.6\ g\ cm^{-3}$, the dielectric constant of the liquid is **[2010]**

(a) 4 (b) 3 (c) 2 (d) 1

5. A jar is filled with two non-mixing liquids 1 and 2 having densities ρ_1 and, ρ_2 respectively. A solid ball, made of a material of density ρ_3, is dropped in the jar. It comes to equilibrium in the position shown in the figure. Which of the following is true for ρ_1, ρ_2 and ρ_3? **[2008]**

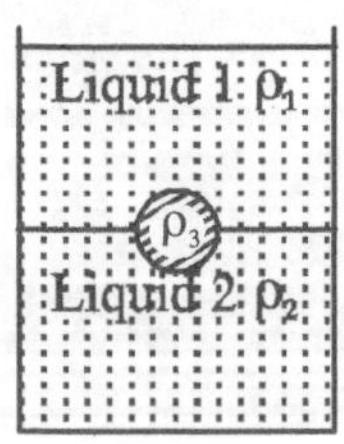

(a) $\rho_3 < \rho_1 < \rho_2$ (b) $\rho_1 > \rho_3 > \rho_2$

(c) $\rho_1 < \rho_2 < \rho_3$ (d) $\rho_1 < \rho_3 < \rho_2$

TOPIC-2 : Fluid Flow, Reynold's Number and Bernoulli's Principle

6. Two tubes of radii r_1 and r_2, and lengths l_1 and l_2, respectively, are connected in series and a liquid flows through each of them in streamline conditions. P_1 and P_2 are pressure differences across the two tubes. If P_2 is $4P_1$ and l_2 is $\frac{l_1}{4}$, then the radius r_2 will be equal to : **[Online April 9, 2017]**

(a) r_1 (b) $2r_1$ (c) $4r_1$ (d) $\frac{r_1}{2}$

7. Consider a water jar of radius R that has water filled up to height H and is kept on a stand of height h (see figure). Through a hole of radius r (r << R) at its bottom, the water leaks out and the stream of water coming down towards the ground has a shape like a funnel as shown in the figure. If the radius of the cross–section of water stream when it hits the ground is x. Then : **[Online April 9, 2016]**

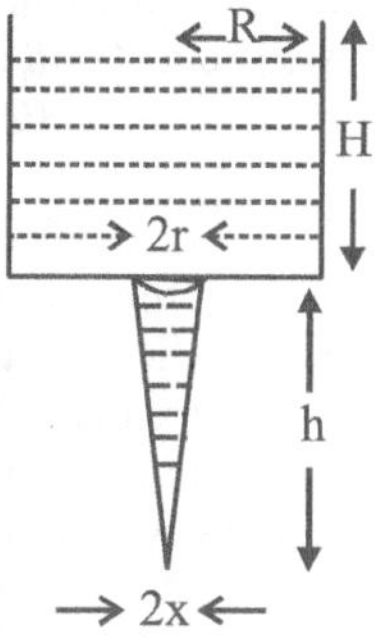

(a) $x = r\left(\frac{H}{H+h}\right)^{\frac{1}{4}}$ (b) $x = r\left(\frac{H}{H+h}\right)$

(c) $x = r\left(\frac{H}{H+h}\right)^{2}$ (d) $x = r\left(\frac{H}{H+h}\right)^{\frac{1}{2}}$

8. If it takes 5 minutes to fill a 15 litre bucket from a water tap of diameter $\frac{2}{\sqrt{\pi}}$ cm then the Reynolds number for the flow is (density of water = 10^3 kg/m^3) and viscosity of water = 10^{-3} Pa.s) close to : **[Online April 10, 2015]**

(a) 1100 (b) 11,000
(c) 550 (d) 5500

9. An open glass tube is immersed in mercury in such a way that a length of 8 cm extends above the mercury level. The open end of the tube is then closed and sealed and the tube is raised vertically up by additional 46 cm. What will be length of the air column above mercury in the tube now? (Atmospheric pressure = 76 cm of Hg) **[2014]**

(a) 16 cm (b) 22 cm
(c) 38 cm (d) 6 cm

10. In the diagram shown, the difference in the two tubes of the manometer is 5 cm, the cross section of the tube at A and B is 6 mm^2 and 10 mm^2 respectively. The rate at which water flows through the tube is ($g = 10$ ms^{-2}) **[Online April 19, 2014]**

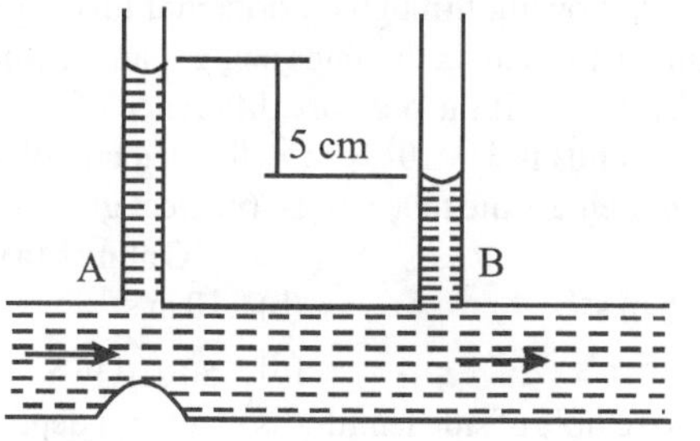

(a) 7.5 cc/s (b) 8.0 cc/s
(c) 10.0 cc/s (d) 12.5 cc/s

11. A cylindrical vessel of cross-section A contains water to a height h. There is a hole in the bottom of radius 'a'. The time in which it will be emptied is: **[Online April 12, 2014]**

(a) $\frac{2A}{\pi a^2}\sqrt{\frac{h}{g}}$ (b) $\frac{\sqrt{2}A}{\pi a^2}\sqrt{\frac{h}{g}}$

(c) $\frac{2\sqrt{2}A}{\pi a^2}\sqrt{\frac{h}{g}}$ (d) $\frac{A}{\sqrt{2}\pi a^2}\sqrt{\frac{h}{g}}$

12. Water is flowing at a speed of 1.5 ms^{-1} through horizontal tube of cross-sectional area 10^{-2} m^2 and you are trying to stop the flow by your palm. Assuming that the water stops immediately after hitting the palm, the minimum force that you must exert should be (density of water = 10^3 kgm^{-3}) **[Online April 9, 2014]**

(a) 15N (b) 22.5N (c) 33.7N (d) 45N

13. Air of density 1.2 kg m^{-3} is blowing across the horizontal wings of an aeroplane in such a way that its speeds above and below the wings are 150 ms^{-1} and 100 ms^{-1}, respectively. The pressure difference between the upper and lower sides of the wings, is : **[Online April 22, 2013]**

(a) 60 Nm^{-2} (b) 180 Nm^{-2}
(c) 7500 Nm^{-2} (d) 12500 Nm^{-2}

14. In a cylindrical water tank, there are two small holes *A* and *B* on the wall at a depth of h_1, from the surface of water and at a height of h_2 from the bottom of water tank. Surface of water is at height of h_2 from the bottom of water tank. Surface of water is at heigh *H* from the bottom of water tank. Water coming out from both holes strikes the ground at the same point *S*. Find the ratio of h_1 and h_2 **[Online May 26, 2012]**

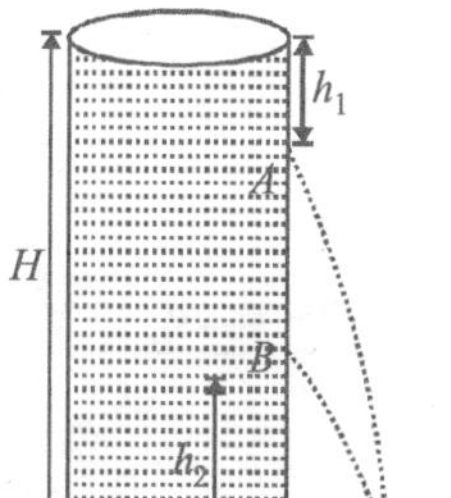

(a) Depends on *H* (b) 1 : 1
(c) 2 : 2 (d) 1 : 2

15. Water is flowing through a horizontal tube having cross-sectional areas of its two ends being A and A' such that the ratio A/A' is 5. If the pressure difference of water between the two ends is 3×10^5 N m^{-2}, the velocity of water with which it enters the tube will be (neglect gravity effects) **[Online May 12, 2012]**

(a) 5 m s^{-1} (b) 10 m s^{-1}
(c) 25 m s^{-1} (d) $50\sqrt{10}$ m s^{-1}

16. A square hole of side length ℓ is made at a depth of h and a circular hole of radius r is made at a depth of 4h from the surface of water in a water tank kept on a horizontal surface. If $\ell << h, r << h$ and the rate of water flow from the holes is the same, then r is equal to **[May 7, 2012]**

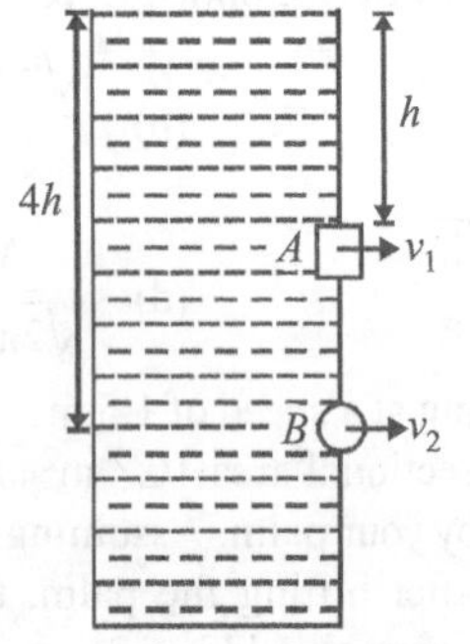

(a) $\frac{\ell}{\sqrt{2\pi}}$ (b) $\frac{\ell}{\sqrt{3\pi}}$ (c) $\frac{\ell}{3\pi}$ (d) $\frac{\ell}{2\pi}$

17. Water is flowing continuously from a tap having an internal diameter 8×10^{-3} m. The water velocity as it leaves the tap is 0.4 ms^{-1}. The diameter of the water stream at a distance 2×10^{-1} m below the tap is close to: **[2011]**

(a) 7.5×10^{-3} m (b) 9.6×10^{-3} m
(c) 3.6×10^{-3} m (d) 5.0×10^{-3} m

18. A cylinder of height 20 m is completely filled with water. The velocity of efflux of water (in ms^{-1}) through a small hole on the side wall of the cylinder near its bottom is **[2002]**

(a) 10 (b) 20 (c) 25.5 (d) 5

TOPIC-3 : Viscosity and Terminal Velocity

19. Which of the following option correctly describes the variation of the speed v and acceleration 'a' of a point mass falling vertically in a viscous medium that applies a force F = –kv, where 'k' is a constant, on the body? (Graphs are schematic and not drawn to scale) **[Online April 9, 2016]**

(a)
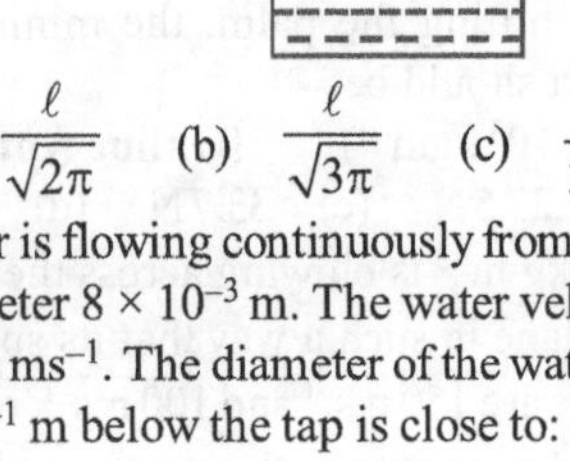

(b)
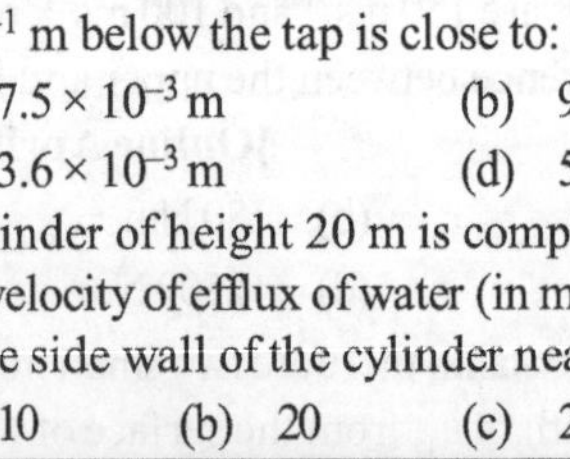

(c)
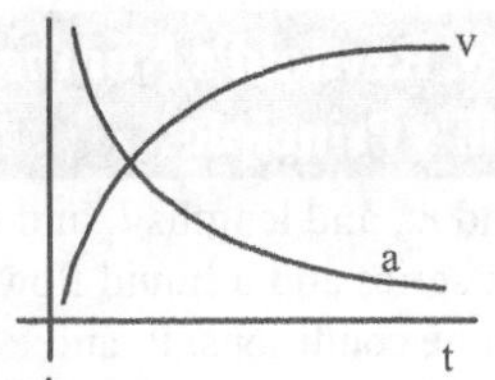

(d)
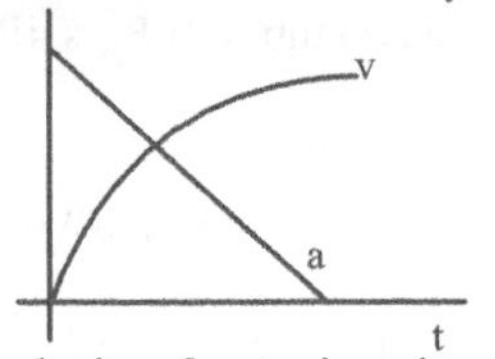

20. The velocity of water in a river is 18 km/hr near the surface. If the river is 5 m deep, find the shearing stress between the horizontal layers of water. The co-efficient of viscosity of water = 10^{-2} poise. **[Online April 19, 2014]**

(a) 10^{-1} N/m^2 (b) 10^{-2} N/m^2
(c) 10^{-3} N/m^2 (d) 10^{-4} N/m^2

21. The average mass of rain drops is 3.0×10^{-5} kg and their avarage terminal velocity is 9 m/s. Calculate the energy transferred by rain to each square metre of the surface at a place which receives 100 cm of rain in a year. **[Online April 11, 2014]**

(a) 3.5×10^5 J (b) 4.05×10^4 J
(c) 3.0×10^5 J (d) 9.0×10^4 J

22. A tank with a small hole at the bottom has been filled with water and kerosene (specific gravity 0.8). The height of water is 3m and that of kerosene 2m. When the hole is opened the velocity of fluid coming out from it is nearly: (take g = 10 ms^{-2} and density of water = 10^3 kg m^{-3}) **[Online April 11, 2014]**

(a) 10.7 ms^{-1} (b) 9.6 ms^{-1}
(c) 8.5 ms^{-1} (d) 7.6 ms^{-1}

23. In an experiment, a small steel ball falls through a liquid at a constant speed of 10 cm/s. If the steel ball is pulled upward with a force equal to twice its effective weight, how fast will it move upward ? **[Online April 25, 2013]**

(a) 5 cm/s (b) Zero (c) 10 cm/s (d) 20 cm/s

24. The terminal velocity of a small sphere of radius a in a viscous liquid is proportional to **[Online May 26, 2012]**

(a) a^2 (b) a^3 (c) a (d) a^{-1}

25. If a ball of steel (density $\rho = 7.8$ g cm^{-3}) attains a terminal velocity of 10 cm s^{-1} when falling in water (Coefficient of viscosity $\eta_{water} = 8.5 \times 10^{-4}$ Pa.s), then, its terminal velocity in glycerine ($\rho = 1.2$ g cm^{-3}, $\eta = 13.2$ Pa.s) would be, nearly **[2011 RS]**

(a) 6.25×10^{-4} cm s^{-1} (b) 6.45×10^{-4} cm s^{-1}
(c) 1.5×10^{-5} cm s^{-1} (d) 1.6×10^{-5} cm s^{-1}

26. A spherical solid ball of volume V is made of a material of density ρ_1. It is falling through a liquid of density ρ_1 $(\rho_2 < \rho_1)$. Assume that the liquid applies a viscous force on the ball that is proportional to the square of its speed v, i.e., $F_{viscous} = -kv^2$ $(k > 0)$. The terminal speed of the ball is **[2008]**

(a) $\sqrt{\frac{Vg(\rho_1 - \rho_2)}{k}}$ (b) $\frac{Vg\rho_1}{k}$

(c) $\sqrt{\frac{Vg\rho_1}{k}}$ (d) $\frac{Vg(\rho_1 - \rho_2)}{k}$

27. If the terminal speed of a sphere of gold (density = 19.5 kg/m^3) is 0.2 m/s in a viscous liquid (density = 1.5 kg/m^3), find the terminal speed of a sphere of silver (density = 10.5 kg/m^3) of the same size in the same liquid **[2006]**

(a) 0.4 m/s (b) 0.133 m/s
(c) 0.1 m/s (d) 0.2 m/s

28. Spherical balls of radius 'R' are falling in a viscous fluid of viscosity 'η' with a velocity 'v'. The retarding viscous force acting on the spherical ball is **[2004]**

(a) inversely proportional to both radius 'R' and velocity 'v'
(b) directly proportional to both radius 'R' and velocity 'v'
(c) directly proportional to 'R' but inversely proportional to 'v'
(d) inversely proportional to 'R' but directly proportional to velocity 'v'

TOPIC-4 : Surface Tension, Surface Energy and Capillarity

29. If two glass plates have water between them and are separated by very small distance (see figure), it is very difficult to pull them apart. It is because the water in between forms cylindrical surface on the side that gives rise to lower pressure in the water in comparison to atmosphere. If the radius of the cylindrical surface is R and surface tension of water is T then the pressure in water between the plates is lower by : **[Online April 10, 2015]**

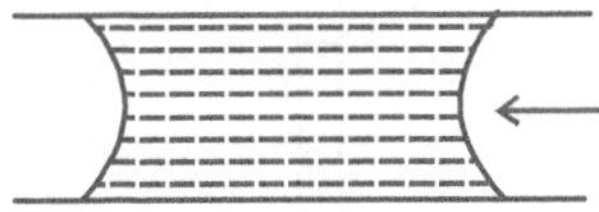

(a) $\frac{2T}{R}$ (b) $\frac{4T}{R}$
(c) $\frac{T}{4R}$ (d) $\frac{T}{R}$

30. On heating water, bubbles being formed at the bottom of the vessel detach and rise. Take the bubbles to be spheres of radius R and making a circular contact of radius r with the bottom of the vessel. If r ≪ R and the surface tension of water is T, value of r just before bubbles detach is: (density of water is ρ_w) **[2014]**

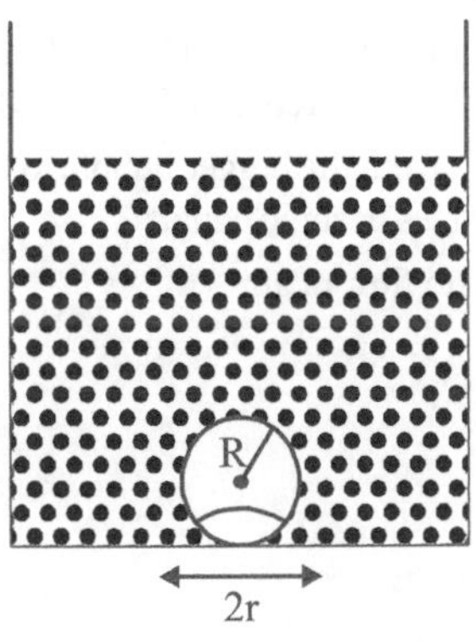

(a) $R^2\sqrt{\frac{2\rho_w g}{3T}}$ (b) $R^2\sqrt{\frac{\rho_w g}{6T}}$
(c) $R^2\sqrt{\frac{\rho_w g}{T}}$ (d) $R^2\sqrt{\frac{3\rho_w g}{T}}$

31. A large number of liquid drops each of radius r coalesce to from a single drop of radius R. The energy released in the process is converted into kinetic energy of the big drop so formed. The speed of the big drop is (given, surface tension of liquid T, density ρ) **[Online April 19, 2014, 2012]**

(a) $\sqrt{\frac{T}{\rho}\left(\frac{1}{r}-\frac{1}{R}\right)}$ (b) $\sqrt{\frac{2T}{\rho}\left(\frac{1}{r}-\frac{1}{R}\right)}$
(c) $\sqrt{\frac{4T}{\rho}\left(\frac{1}{r}-\frac{1}{R}\right)}$ (d) $\sqrt{\frac{6T}{\rho}\left(\frac{1}{r}-\frac{1}{R}\right)}$

32. Two soap bubbles coalesce to form a single bubble. If V is the subsequent change in volume of contained air and S change in total surface area, T is the surface tension and P atmospheric pressure, then which of the following relation is correct? **[Online April 12, 2014]**

(a) $4PV+3ST=0$ (b) $3PV+4ST=0$
(c) $2PV+3ST=0$ (d) $3PV+2ST=0$

33. An air bubble of radius 0.1 cm is in a liquid having surface tension 0.06 N/m and density 10^3 kg/m^3. The pressure inside the bubble is 1100 Nm^{-2} greater than the atmospheric pressure. At what depth is the bubble below the surface of the liquid? ($g = 9.8$ ms^{-2}) **[Online April 11, 2014]**

(a) 0.1m (b) 0.15m (c) 0.20m (d) 0.25m

34. A capillary tube is immersed vertically in water and the height of the water column is x. When this arrangement is taken into a mine of depth d, the height of the water column is y. If R is the radius of earth, the ratio $\frac{x}{y}$ is: **[Online April 9, 2014]**

(a) $\left(1-\frac{d}{R}\right)$ (b) $\left(1-\frac{2d}{R}\right)$
(c) $\left(\frac{R-d}{R+d}\right)$ (d) $\left(\frac{R+d}{R-d}\right)$

35. Wax is coated on the inner wall of a capillary tube and the tube is then dipped in water. Then, compared to the unwaxed capillary, the angle of contact θ and the height h upto which water rises change. These changes are : **[Online April 23, 2013]**

(a) θ increases and h also increases
(b) θ decreases and h also decreases
(c) θ increases and h decreases
(d) θ decreases and h increases

36. A thin tube sealed at both ends is 100 cm long. It lies horizontally, the middle 20 cm containing mercury and two equal ends containing air at standard atmospheric pressure. If the tube is now turned to a vertical position, by what amount will the mercury be displaced? **[Online April 23, 2013]**

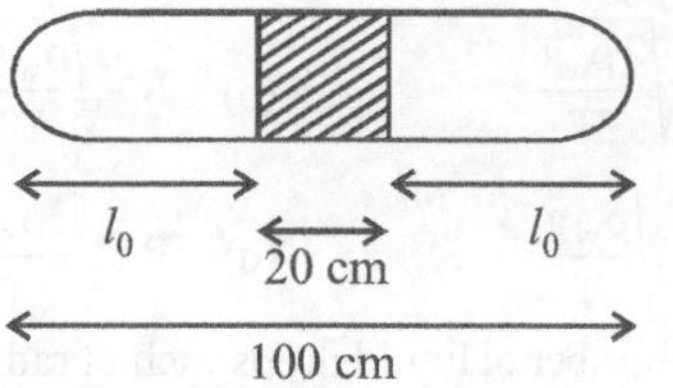

(Given : cross-section of the tube can be assumed to be uniform)

(a) 2.95 cm (b) 5.18 cm
(c) 8.65 cm (d) 0.0 cm

37. This question has Statement-1 and Statement-2. Of the four choices given after the Statements, choose the one that best describes the two Statetnents.

Statement-1: A capillary is dipped in a liquid and liquid rises to a height h in it. As the temperature of the liquid is raised, the height h increases (if the density of the liquid and the angle of contact remain the same).

Statement-2: Surface tension of a liquid decreases with the rise in its temperature. **[Online April 9, 2013]**

(a) Statement-1 is true, Statement-2 is true; Statement-2 is **not** the correct explanation for Statement-1.
(b) Statement-1 is false, Statement-2 is true.
(c) Statement-1 is true, Statement-2 is false.
(d) Statement-1 is true, Statement-2 is true; Statement-2 is the correct explanation for Statement-1.

38. A thin liquid film formed between a U-shaped wire and a light slider supports a weight of 1.5×10^{-2} N (see figure). The length of the slider is 30 cm and its weight is negligible. The surface tension of the liquid film is **[2012]**

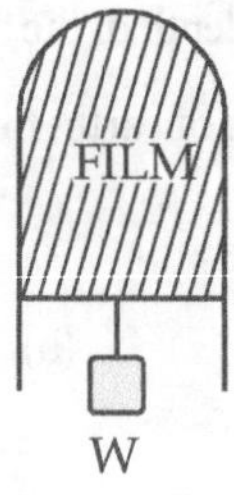

(a) $0.0125\ Nm^{-1}$ (b) $0.1\ Nm^{-1}$
(c) $0.05\ Nm^{-1}$ (d) $0.025\ Nm^{-1}$

39. Work done in increasing the size of a soap bubble from a radius of 3 cm to 5 cm is nearly (Surface tension of soap solution = $0.03\ Nm^{-1}$) **[2011]**

(a) $0.2\ \pi$mJ (b) 2πmJ
(c) 0.4πmJ (d) 4πmJ

40. Two mercury drops (each of radius 'r') merge to form bigger drop. The surface energy of the bigger drop, if T is the surface tension, is : **[2011 RS]**

(a) $4\pi r^2 T$ (b) $2\pi r^2 T$
(c) $2^{8/3}\pi r^2 T$ (d) $2^{5/3}\pi r^2 T$

41. A capillary tube (A) is dipped in water. Another identical tube (B) is dipped in a soap-water solution. Which of the following shows the relative nature of the liquid columns in the two tubes? **[2008]**

(a)
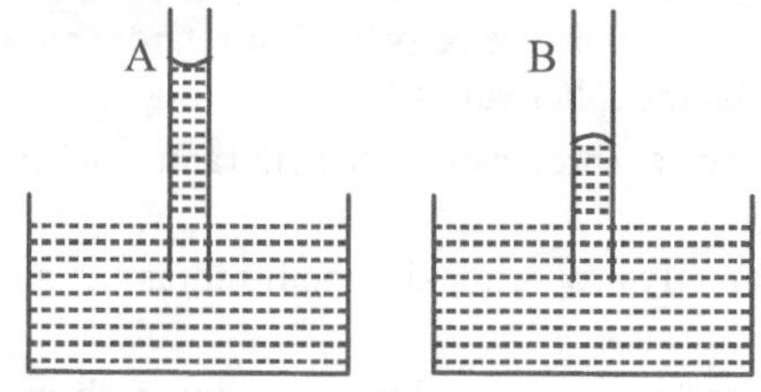

(b)
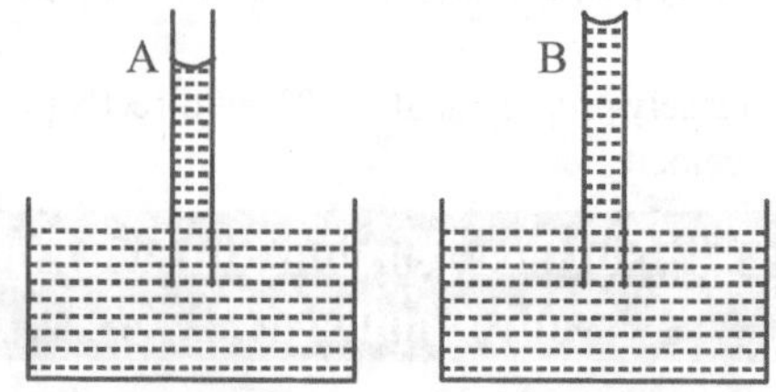

(c)
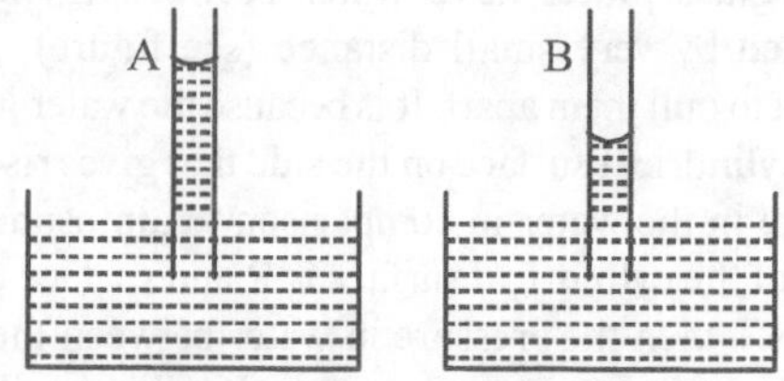

(d)
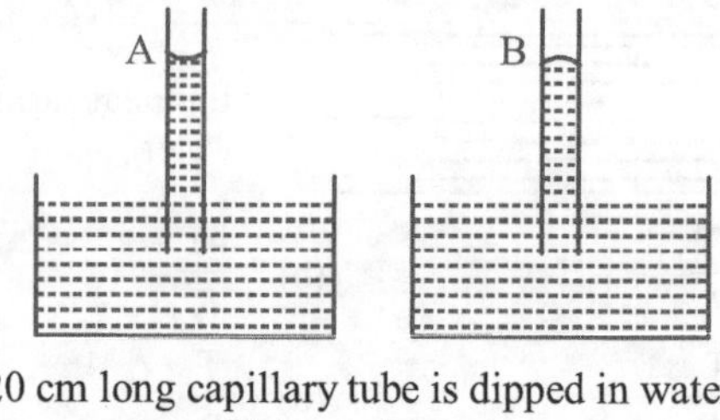

42. A 20 cm long capillary tube is dipped in water. The water rises up to 8 cm. If the entire arrangement is put in a freely falling elevator the length of water column in the capillary tube will be **[2005]**

(a) 10 cm (b) 8 cm (c) 20 cm (d) 4 cm

43. If two soap bubbles of different radii are connected by a tube **[2004]**

(a) air flows from the smaller bubble to the bigger
(b) air flows from bigger bubble to the smaller bubble till the sizes are interchanged
(c) air flows from the bigger bubble to the smaller bubble till the sizes become equal
(d) there is no flow of air.

Hints & Solutions

TOPIC-1 : Pressure, Density, Pascal's Law and Archimedes' Principle

1. **(c)** Pressure at interface A must be same from both the sides to be in equilibrium.

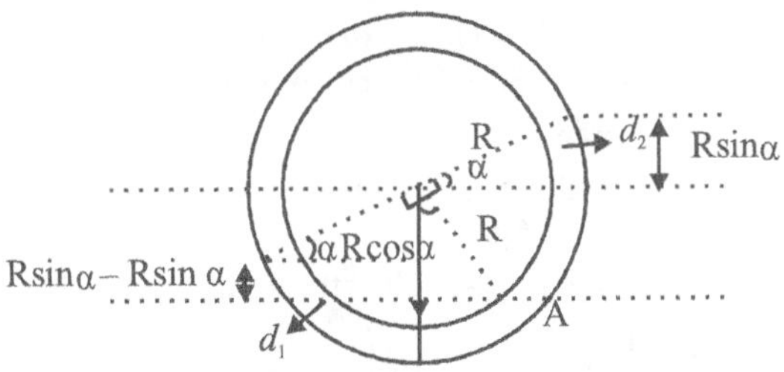

$\therefore \quad (R\cos\alpha + R\sin\alpha)d_2 g = (R\cos\alpha - R\sin\alpha)d_1 g$

$$\Rightarrow \frac{d_1}{d_2} = \frac{\cos\alpha + \sin\alpha}{\cos\alpha - \sin\alpha} = \frac{1+\tan\alpha}{1-\tan\alpha}$$

2. **(c)** From figure, $kx_0 + F_B = Mg$

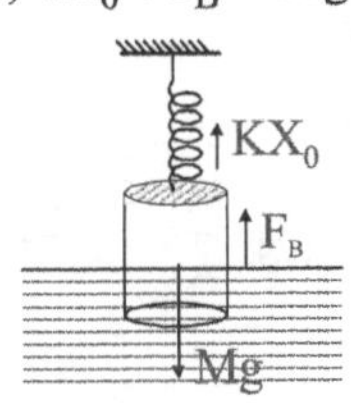

$$kx_0 + \sigma\frac{L}{2}Ag = Mg$$

[$\because$ mass = density × volume]

$$\Rightarrow kx_0 = Mg - \sigma\frac{L}{2}Ag$$

$$\Rightarrow x_0 = \frac{Mg - \frac{\sigma LAg}{2}}{k} = \frac{Mg}{k}\left(1-\frac{LA\sigma}{2M}\right)$$

Hence, extension of the spring when it is in equilibrium is, $x_0 = \frac{Mg}{k}\left(1-\frac{LA\sigma}{2M}\right)$

3. **(b)** Oil will float on water so, (2) or (4) is the correct option. But density of ball is more than that of oil,, hence it will sink in oil.

4. **(c)**

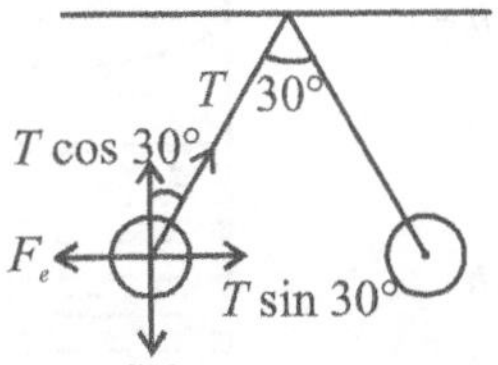

$F_e = T\sin 30°$

$mg = T\cos 30°$

$\Rightarrow \tan 30° = \frac{F_e}{mg}$ ...(1)

In liquid ,

$F_e' = T'\sin 30°$ ...(A)

$mg = F_B + T'\cos 30°$

But F_B = Buoyant force

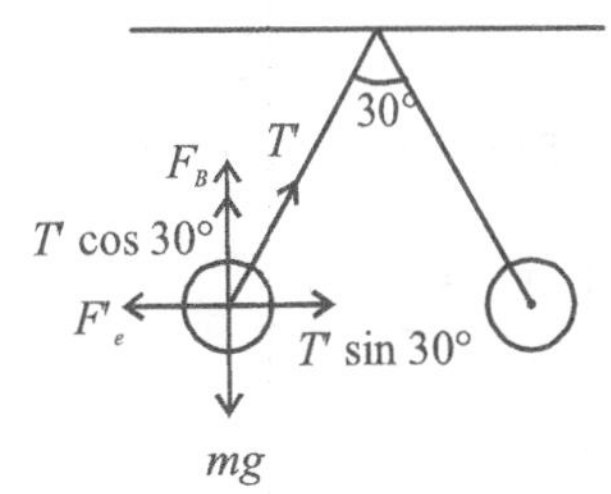

$= V(d-\rho)g = V(1.6-0.8)g = 0.8\,Vg$

$= 0.8\frac{m}{d}g = \frac{0.8mg}{1.6} = \frac{mg}{2}$

$\therefore mg = \frac{mg}{2} + T'\cos 30°$

$\Rightarrow \frac{mg}{2} = T'\cos 30°$ ...(B)

From (A) and (B), $\tan 30° = \frac{2F_e'}{mg}$

From (1) and (2)

$\frac{F_e}{mg} = \frac{2F_e'}{mg}$ (2)

$\Rightarrow F_e = 2F_e'$

If K be the dielectric constant, then

$F_e' = \frac{F_e}{K}$

$\therefore F_e = \frac{2F_e}{K} \Rightarrow K = 2$

5. **(d)** From the figure it is clear that liquid 1 floats on liquid 2. The lighter liquid floats over heavier liquid. Therefore we can conclude that $\rho_1 < \rho_2$

Also $\rho_3 < \rho_2$ otherwise the ball would have sink to the bottom of the jar.

Also $\rho_3 > \rho_1$ otherwise the ball would have floated in liquid 1. From the above discussion we conclude that

$$\rho_1 < \rho_3 < \rho_2.$$

TOPIC-2 : Fluid Flow, Reynold's Number and Bernoulli's Principle

6. **(d)** The volume of liquid flowing through both the tubes i.e., rate of flow of liquid is same.

Therefore, $V = V_1 = V_2$

i.e., $\dfrac{\pi P_1 r_1^4}{8\eta l_1} = \dfrac{\pi P_2 r_2^4}{8\eta l_2}$

or $\dfrac{P_1 r_1^4}{l_1} = \dfrac{P_2 r_2^4}{l_2}$

$\because$ $P_2 = 4P_1$ and $l_2 = l_1/4$

$$\frac{P_1 r_1^4}{l_1} = \frac{4P_1 r_2^4}{l_1/4} \Rightarrow r_2^4 = \frac{r_1^4}{16}$$

$$r_2 = r_1/2$$

7. **(a)** According to Bernoulli's Principle,

$$\frac{1}{2}\rho v_1^2 + \rho g h = \frac{1}{2}\rho v_2^2$$

$$v_1^2 + 2gh = v_2^2$$

$$2gH + 2gh = v_2^2 \qquad \text{...(i)}$$

$$a_1 v_1 = a_2 v_2$$

$$\pi r^2 \sqrt{2gh} = \pi x^2 v_2$$

$$\frac{r^2}{x^2}\sqrt{2gh} = v_2$$

Substituting the value of v_2 in equation (i)

$$2gH + 2gh = \frac{r^4}{x^4} 2gh \text{ or, } x = r\left[\frac{H}{H+h}\right]^{\frac{1}{4}}$$

8. **(d)** Given: Diameter of water tap $= \dfrac{2}{\sqrt{\pi}}$ cm

$\therefore$ Radius, $r = \dfrac{1}{\sqrt{\pi}} \times 10^{-2}$ m

$$\frac{dm}{dt} = \rho A V$$

$$\frac{15}{5 \times 60} = 10^3 \times \pi \left(\frac{1}{\sqrt{\pi}}\right)^2 \times 10^{-4} V$$

$$\Rightarrow V = 0.05 \text{ m/s}$$

Reynold's number, $R_e = \dfrac{\rho V r}{n}$

$$= \frac{10^3 \times 0.5 \times \frac{2}{\sqrt{\pi}} 10^{-2}}{10^{-3}} \cong 5500$$

9. **(a)**

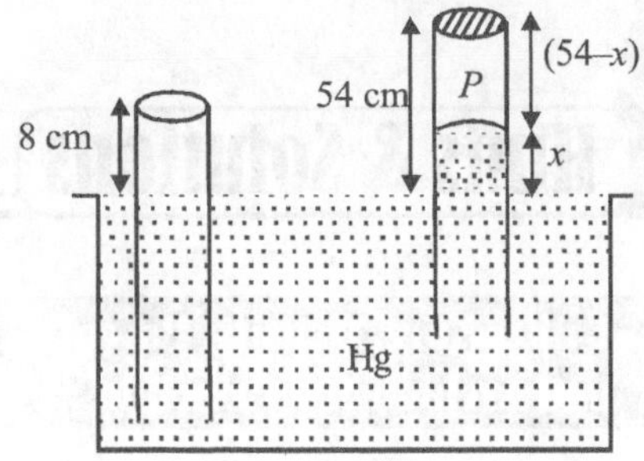

Length of the air column above mercury in the tube is,

$P + x = P_0$

$\Rightarrow P = (76 - x)$

$\Rightarrow 8 \times A \times 76 = (76 - x) \times A \times (54 - x)$

$\therefore x = 38$

Thus, length of air column $= 54 - 38 = 16$ cm.

10. **(a)** According to Bernoulli's theorem,

$$P_1 + \frac{1}{2}\rho v_1^2 = P_2 + \frac{1}{2}\rho v_2^2$$

$$\therefore v_2^2 - v_1^2 = 2gh \qquad \text{...(1)}$$

According to the equation of continuty

$$A_1 v_1 = A_2 v_2 \qquad \text{...(2)}$$

$$\frac{A_1}{A_2} = \frac{6 \text{ mm}^2}{10 \text{ mm}^2}$$

From equation (2), $\dfrac{A_1}{A_2} = \dfrac{v_2}{v_1} = \dfrac{6}{10}$

or, $v_2 = \dfrac{6}{10} v_1$

Putting this value of v_2 in equation (1)

$$\left(\frac{6}{10} v_1\right)^2 - (v_1)^2 = 2 \times 10^3 \times 5$$

$$\left[\begin{array}{l}\because g = 10 \text{m/s}^2 = 10^3 \text{cm/s}^2 \\ \text{and } h = 5 \text{ cm}\end{array}\right]$$

Solving we get $v_1 = \dfrac{10}{8}$

Therefore the rate at which water flows through the tube $= A_1 v_1 = A_2 v_2 = \dfrac{6 \times 10}{8} = 7.5 \text{cc/s}$

11. **(b)** Let the rate of falling water level be $-\dfrac{dh}{dt}$

Initially at $t = 0; h = h$

$t = t; h = 0$

Then, $A\left(-\dfrac{dh}{dt}\right) = \pi a^2 . v$

$$dt = -\frac{A}{\pi a^2 \sqrt{2gh}} dh$$

[$\because$ velocity of efflux of liquid $v = \sqrt{2gh}$]

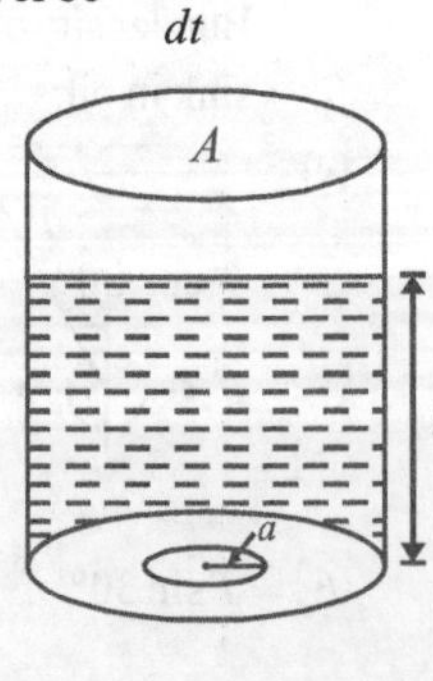

Integrating both sides

$$\int_0^t dt = -\frac{A}{\sqrt{2g}\pi a^2}\int_h^0 h^{-1/2}dh$$

$$[t]_0^t = -\frac{A}{\sqrt{2g}\pi a^2}\cdot\left[\frac{h^{1/2}}{1/2}\right]_h^0$$

$$t = \frac{\sqrt{2}A}{\pi a^2}\sqrt{\frac{h}{g}}$$

12. (a) For 1 m length of horizontal tube

Mass of water M = density × volume

$= 10^3 \times$ area × length

$= 10^3 \times 10^{-2} \times 1 = 10$ kg

Therefore minimum force = $\frac{\Delta p}{\Delta t}$ (rate of change of momentum)

$= 10 \times 1.5 = 15\,N$

13. (c) Pressure difference

$$P_2 - P_1 = \frac{1}{2}\rho\left(v_2^2 - v_1^2\right)$$

$$= \frac{1}{2}\times 1.2\left((150)^2 - (100)^2\right)$$

$$= \frac{1}{2}\times 1.2(22500 - 10000)$$

$= 7500$ Nm^{-2}

14. (a) Range is same for both holes

$\therefore\ 2\sqrt{(H-h_1)h_1} = 2\sqrt{(H-h_2)h_2}$

Squaring both sides,

$4(H - h_1)h_1 = 4(H - h_2)h_2$

$Hh_1 - h_1^2 = Hh_2 - h_2^2$

On solving we get,

$H = h_1 + h_2$

Hence, the ratio of $\frac{h_1}{h_2}$ depends on H.

15. (a) According to Bernoulli's theorem

$$P_1 + \frac{1}{2}\rho v_1^2 = P_2 + \frac{1}{2}\rho v_2^2 \quad \text{...(i)}$$

From question,

$$P_1 - P_2 = 3\times 10^5,\ \frac{A_1}{A_2} = 5$$

According to equation of continuity

$A_1 v_1 = A_2 v_2$

or, $\frac{A_1}{A_2} = \frac{v_2}{v_1} = 5$

$\Rightarrow\ v_2 = 5v_1$

From equation (i)

$$P_1 - P_2 = \frac{1}{2}\rho\left(v_2^2 - v_1^2\right)$$

or $3\times 10^5 = \frac{1}{2}\times 1000\left(5v_1^2 - v_1^2\right)$

$\Rightarrow\ 600 = 6v_1 \times 4v_1$

$\Rightarrow\ v_1^2 = 25$

$\therefore\ v_1 = 5$ m/s

16. (a) As $A_1v_1 = A_2v_2$ (Principle of continuity)

or, $\ell^2\sqrt{2gh} = \pi r^2\sqrt{2g\times 4h}$

(Efflux velocity = $\sqrt{2gh}$)

$\therefore\ r^2 = \frac{\ell^2}{2\pi}$ or $r = \sqrt{\frac{\ell^2}{2\pi}} = \frac{\ell}{\sqrt{2\pi}}$

17. (c) From Bernoulli's theorem,

$$P_0 + \frac{1}{2}\rho v_1^2 \rho gh = P_0 + \frac{1}{2}\rho v_2^2 + 0$$

$$v_2 = \sqrt{v_1^2 + 2gh} = \sqrt{0.16 + 2\times 10\times 0.2}$$

$= 2.03$ m/s

From equation of continuity

$A_2v_2 = A_1v_1$

$$\pi\frac{D_2^2}{4}\times v_2 = \pi\frac{D_1^2}{4}v_1$$

$$\Rightarrow D_1 D_2\sqrt{\frac{v_1}{v_2}} = 3.55\times 10^{-3}\text{ m}$$

18. (b) The velocity of efflux is given

$v = \sqrt{2gh}$

Where h is the height of the free surface of liquid from the hole

$\therefore\ v = \sqrt{2\times 10\times 20} = 20$ m/s

TOPIC-3 : Viscosity and Terminal velocity

19. (c) When a point mass is falling vertically in a viscous medium, the medium or viscous fluid exerts drag force on the body to oppose its motion and at one stage body falling with constant terminal velocity.

20. (b) $\eta = 10^{-2}$ poise

$v = 18$ km/h $= \frac{18000}{3600} = 5$ m/s

$l = 5$ m

Strain rate $= \frac{v}{l}$

Coefficient of viscosity, $\eta = \frac{\text{shearing stress}}{\text{strain rate}}$

$\therefore$ Shearing stress = η × strain rate

$$= 10^{-2}\times\frac{5}{5} = 10^{-2}\text{ Nm}^{-2}$$

21. (b) Total volume of rain drops, received 100 cm in a year by area 1 m^2

$= 1m^2 \times \frac{100}{100} m = 1\ m^3$

As we know, density of water,

$d = 10^3\ kg/m^3$

Therefore, mass of this volume of water

$M = d \times v = 10^3 \times 1 = 10^3\ kg$

Average terminal velocity of rain drop

$v = 9$ m/s (given)

Therefore, energy transferred by rain,

$$E = \frac{1}{2} mv^2$$

$$= \frac{1}{2} \times 10^3 \times (9)^2$$

$$= \frac{1}{2} \times 10^3 \times 81 = 4.05 \times 10^4\ J$$

22. (b) According to Toricelli's theorem,

Velocity of efflex,

$$V_{eff} = \sqrt{2gh} = \sqrt{2 \times 9.8 \times 5} \cong 9.8\ ms^{-1}$$

23. (c)

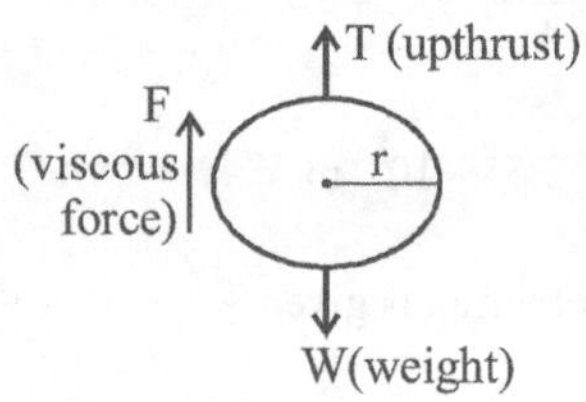

Weight of the body

$W = mg = \frac{4}{3}\pi r^3 \rho g$

$T = \frac{4}{3}\pi r^3 \sigma g$

and $F = 6\pi\eta vr$

When the body attains terminal velocity net force acting on the body is zero. i.e.,

$W - T - F = 0$

And terminal velocity $v = \frac{2}{9}\frac{r^2(\rho - \sigma)g}{\eta}$

As in case of upward motion upward force is twice its effective weight, therefore, it will move with same speed 10 cm/s

24. (a) Terminal velocity in a viscous medium is given by:

$$V_T = \frac{2a^2(\rho - \sigma)g}{9\eta}$$

$\therefore V_T \propto a^2$

25. (a) $V\rho g = 6\pi\eta rv + V\rho_\ell g$

$\Rightarrow Vg(\rho - \rho_\ell) = 6\pi\eta rv$

Also $Vg(\rho - \rho_i') = 6\pi\eta' rv'$

$$\therefore\ v'\eta' = \frac{(\rho - \rho_\ell')}{(\rho - \rho_\ell)} \times v\eta$$

$$\Rightarrow v' = \frac{(\rho - \rho_\ell')}{(\rho - \rho_\ell)} \times \frac{v\eta}{\eta'}$$

$$= \frac{(7.8 - 1.2)}{(7.8 - 1)} \times \frac{10 \times 8.5 \times 10^{-4}}{13.2}$$

$\therefore\ v' = 6.25 \times 10^{-4}$ cm/s

26. (a) The condition for terminal speed (v_t) is

Weight = Buoyant force + Viscous force

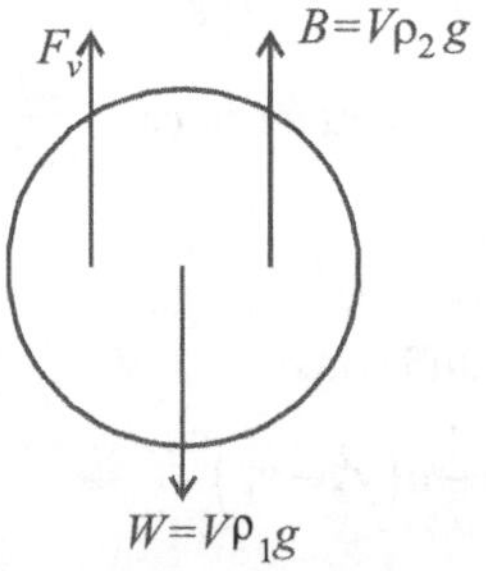

$\therefore V\rho_1 g = V\rho_2 g + kv_t^2 \qquad \therefore v_t = \sqrt{\frac{Vg(\rho_1 - \rho_2)}{k}}$

27. (c) Terminal velocity, $v_T = \frac{2r^2(d_1 - d_2)g}{9\eta}$

$$\frac{v_{T_2}}{0.2} = \frac{(10.5 - 1.5)}{(19.5 - 1.5)} \Rightarrow v_{T_2} = 0.2 \times \frac{9}{18}$$

$\therefore v_{T_2} = 0.1$ m/s

28. (b) From Stoke's law,

viscous force $F = \pi\eta rv$

hence F is directly proportional to radius & velocity.

TOPIC-4 : Surface Tension, Surface Energy and Capillarity

29. (d) Here excess pressure, $P_{excess} = \frac{T}{r_1} + \frac{T}{r_2}$

$$P_{excess} = \frac{T}{R} \qquad \because \begin{pmatrix} r_1 = R \\ r_2 = O \end{pmatrix}$$

30. (a) When the bubble gets detached,

Buoyant force = force due to surface tension

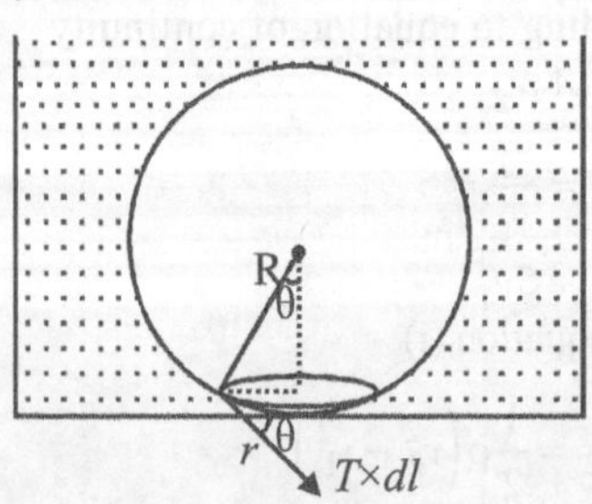

Force due to excess pressure = upthrust

Access pressure in air bubble = $\frac{2T}{R}$

$$\frac{2T}{R}(\pi r^2) = \frac{4\pi R^3}{3}\rho_w g$$

$$\Rightarrow \ r^2 = \frac{2R^4 \rho_w g}{3T} \Rightarrow r = R^2\sqrt{\frac{2\rho_w g}{3T}}$$

31. (d) When drops combine to form a single drop of radius R.

Then energy released, $E = 4\pi TR^3\left[\frac{1}{r}-\frac{1}{R}\right]$

If this energy is converted into kinetic energy then

$$\frac{1}{2}mv^2 = 4\pi R^3 T\left[\frac{1}{r}-\frac{1}{R}\right]$$

$$\frac{1}{2}\times\left[\frac{4}{3}\pi R^3\rho\right]v^2 = 4\pi R^3 T\left[\frac{1}{r}-\frac{1}{R}\right]$$

$$v^2 = \frac{6T}{\rho}\left[\frac{1}{r}-\frac{1}{R}\right]$$

$$v = \sqrt{\frac{6T}{\rho}\left[\frac{1}{r}-\frac{1}{R}\right]}$$

32. (b)

33. (a) **Given:** Radius of air bubble,

$r = 0.1$ cm $= 10^{-3}$ m

Surface tension of liquid,

$S = 0.06$ N/m $= 6\times10^{-2}$ N/m

Density of liquid, $\rho = 10^3$ kg/m^3

Excess pressure inside the bubble,

$\rho_{exe} = 1100$ Nm^{-2}

Depth of bubble below the liquid surface,

$h = ?$

As we know,

$$\rho_{Excess} = h\rho g + \frac{2s}{r}$$

$$\Rightarrow \ 1100 = h\times10^3\times9.8 + \frac{2\times6\times10^{-2}}{10^{-3}}$$

$$\Rightarrow \ 1100 = 9800\,h + 120$$

$$\Rightarrow \ 9800h = 1100 - 120$$

$$\Rightarrow \ h = \frac{980}{9800} = 0.1\text{ m}$$

34. (a) Acceleration due to gravity changes with the depth,

$$g' = g\left(1-\frac{d}{R}\right)$$

Pressure, $P = \rho gh$

Hence ratio, $\frac{x}{y}$ is $\left(1-\frac{d}{R}\right)$

35. (c) Angle of contact θ

$$\cos\theta = \frac{T_{SA}-T_{SL}}{T_{LA}}$$

when water is on a waxy or oily surface

$T_{SA} < T_{SL}$ cos θ is negative i.e.,

$90° < \theta < 180°$

i.e., angle of contact θ increases

And for $\theta > 90°$ liquid level in capillary tube fall. i.e., h decreases

36. (b)

37. (b) Surface tension of a liquid decreases with the rise in temperture. At the boiling point of liquid, surface tension is zero.

Capillary rise $h = \frac{2T\cos\theta}{rdg}$

As surface tension T decreases with rise in temperature hence capillary rise also decreases.

38. (d) The surface tension of the liquid film is given as

$T = \frac{F}{2l}$, where F is the force, and l = length of the slider.

$F = 2lT$

At equilibrium, $F = W$

$2Tl = mg$

$$T = \frac{mg}{2l} = \frac{1.5\times10^{-2}}{2\times30\times10^{-2}} = \frac{1.5}{60}$$

$= 0.025$ Nm^{-1}

39. (c) $W = 2T\Delta V$

$W = 2T4\pi[(5^2)-(3)^2]\times10^{-4}$

$= 2\times0.03\times4\pi[25-9]\times10^{-4}$ J

$= 0.4\pi\times10^{-3}$ J

$= 0.4\pi$ mJ

40. (c) Sum of volumes of 2 smaller drops = Volume of the bigger drop

$$2.\frac{4}{3}\pi r^3 = \frac{4}{3}\pi R^3 \Rightarrow R = 2^{1/3}\, r$$

Surface energy $= T.4\pi R^2$

$$= T4\pi 2^{2/3} r^2 = T.2^{8/3}\pi r^2.$$

41. (c) In case of water, the meniscus shape is concave upwards. Also according to ascent formula

$$h = \frac{2T\cos\theta}{r\rho g}$$

The surface tension (T) of soap solution is less than water. Therefore rise of soap solution in the capillary tube is less as compared to water. As in the case of water, the meniscus shape of soap solution is also concave upwards.

42. (c) Water fills the tube entirely in gravityless condition i.e., 20 cm.

43. (a) Let pressure outside be P_0.

$\therefore P_1$ (in smaller bubble) $= P_0 + \frac{2T}{r}$

P_2 (in bigger bubble) $= P_0 + \frac{2T}{R}$ $\quad (R > r)$

$\therefore P_1 > P_2$

hence air moves from smaller bubble to bigger bubble.

Chapter 10

Thermal Properties of Matter

TOPIC-1 : Thermometer & Thermal Expansion

1. An external pressure P is applied on a cube at 0°C so that it is equally compressed from all sides. K is the bulk modulus of the material of the cube and α is its coefficient of linear expansion. Suppose we want to bring the cube to its original size by heating. The temperature should be raised by : **[2017]**

(a) $\frac{3\alpha}{PK}$ (b) $3PK\alpha$

(c) $\frac{P}{3\alpha K}$ (d) $\frac{P}{\alpha K}$

2. A steel rail of length 5 m and area of cross-section 40 cm^2 is prevented from expanding along its length while the temperature rises by 10°C. If coefficient of linear expansion and Young's modulus of steel are $1.2 \times 10^{-5} K^{-1}$ and $2 \times 10^{11} Nm^{-2}$ respectively, the force developed in the rail is approximately: **[Online April 9, 2017]**

(a) 2×10^7 N (b) 1×10^5 N

(c) 2×10^9 N (d) 3×10^{-5} N

3. A compressive force, F is applied at the two ends of a long thin steel rod. It is heated, simultaneously, such that its temperature increases by ΔT. The net change in its length is zero. Let l be the length of the rod, A its area of cross–section, Y its Young's modulus, and α its coefficient of linear expansion. Then, F is equal to : **[Online April 8, 2017]**

(a) $l^2 Y\alpha\Delta T$ (b) $lAY\alpha\Delta T$

(c) $AY\alpha\Delta T$ (d) $\frac{AY}{\alpha\Delta T}$

4. The ratio of the coefficient of volume expansion of a glass container to that of a viscous liquid kept inside the container is 1 : 4. What fraction of the inner volume of the container should the liquid occupy so that the volume of the remaining vacant space will be same at all temperatures ? **[Online April 23, 2013]**

(a) 2 : 5 (b) 1 : 4 (c) 1 : 64 (d) 1 : 8

5. On a linear temperature scale Y, water freezes at – 160° Y and boils at – 50° Y. On this Y scale, a temperature of 340 K would be read as : (water freezes at 273 K and boils at 373 K) **[Online April 9, 2013]**

(a) – 73.7° Y (b) – 233.7° Y

(c) – 86.3° Y (d) – 106.3° Y

6. A wooden wheel of radius R is made of two semicircular part (see figure). The two parts are held together by a ring made of a metal strip of cross sectional area S and length L. L is slightly less than $2\pi R$. To fit the ring on the wheel, it is heated so that its temperature rises by ΔT and it just steps over the wheel. As it cools down to surrounding temperature, it presses the semicircular parts together. If the coefficient of linear expansion of the metal is α, and its Young's modulus is Y, the force that one part of the wheel applies on the other part is : **[2012]**

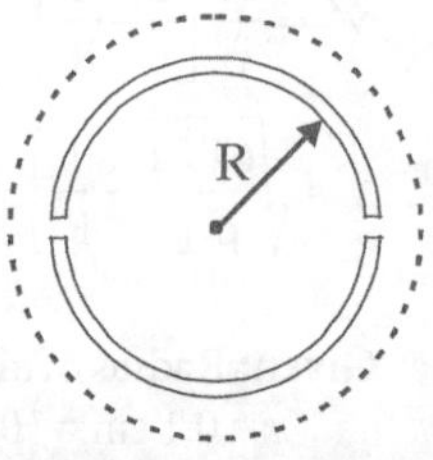

(a) $2\pi SY\alpha\Delta T$

(b) $SY\alpha\Delta T$

(c) $\pi SY\alpha\Delta T$

(d) $2SY\alpha\Delta T$

TOPIC-2 : Calorimetry and Heat Transfer

7. A copper ball of mass 100 gm is at a temperature T. It is dropped in a copper calorimeter of mass 100 gm, filled with 170 gm of water at room temperature. Subsequently, the temperature of the system is found to be 75°C. T is given by (Given : room temperature = 30° C, specific heat of copper = 0.1 cal/gm°C **[2017]**

(a) 1250°C (b) 825°C (c) 800°C (d) 885° C

8. In an experiment a sphere of aluminium of mass 0.20 kg is heated upto 150°C. Immediately, it is put into water of volume 150 cc at 27°C kept in a calorimeter of water equivalent to 0.025 kg. Final temperature of the system is 40°C. The specific heat of aluminium is : **[Online April 8, 2017]**

(take 4.2 Joule=1 calorie)

(a) 378 J/kg – °C (b) 315 J/kg – °C

(c) 476 J/kg – °C (d) 434 J/kg – °C

9. An experiment takes 10 minutes to raise the temperature of water in a container from 0°C to 100°C and another 55 minutes to convert it totally into steam by a heater supplying heat at a uniform rate. Neglecting the specific heat of the container and taking specific heat of water to be 1 cal / g °C, the heat of vapourization according to this experiment will come out to be : **[Online April 11, 2015]**

(a) 560 cal/ g (b) 550 cal/ g

(c) 540 cal/ g (d) 530 cal/ g

10. Three rods of Copper, Brass and Steel are welded together to form a Y shaped structure. Area of cross - section of each rod = 4 cm^2. End of copper rod is maintained at 100ºC where as ends of brass and steel are kept at 0ºC. Lengths of the copper, brass and steel rods are 46, 13 and 12 cms respectively. The rods are thermally insulated from surroundings excepts at ends. Thermal conductivities of copper, brass and steel are 0.92, 0.26 and 0.12 CGS units respectively. Rate of heat flow through copper rod is: **[2014]**

(a) 1.2 cal/s (b) 2.4 cal/s
(c) 4.8 cal/s (d) 6.0 cal/s

11. A black coloured solid sphere of radius R and mass M is inside a cavity with vacuum inside. The walls of the cavity are maintained at temperature T_0. The initial temperature of the sphere is $3T_0$. If the specific heat of the material of the sphere varies as αT^3 per unit mass with the temperature T of the sphere, where α is a constant, then the time taken for the sphere to cool down to temperature $2T_0$ will be (σ is Stefan Boltzmann constant) **[Online April 19, 2014]**

(a) $\frac{M\alpha}{4\pi R^2\sigma}\ln\left(\frac{3}{2}\right)$ (b) $\frac{M\alpha}{4\pi R^2\sigma}\ln\left(\frac{16}{3}\right)$

(c) $\frac{M\alpha}{16\pi R^2\sigma}\ln\left(\frac{16}{3}\right)$ (d) $\frac{M\alpha}{16\pi R^2\sigma}\ln\left(\frac{3}{2}\right)$

12. Water of volume 2 L in a closed container is heated with a coil of 1 kW. While water is heated, the container loses energy at a rate of 160 J/s. In how much time will the temperature of water rise from 27°C to 77°C? (Specific heat of water is 4.2 kJ/kg and that of the container is negligible). **[Online April 9, 2014]**

(a) 8 min 20 s (b) 6 min 2 s
(c) 7 min (d) 14 min

13. Assume that a drop of liquid evaporates by decrease in its surface energy, so that its temperature remains unchanged. What should be the minimum radius of the drop for this to be possible? The surface tension is T, density of liquid is ρ and L is its latent heat of vaporization. **[2013]**

(a) $\rho L/T$ (b) $\sqrt{T/\rho L}$ (c) $T/\rho L$ (d) $2T/\rho L$

14. A mass of 50g of water in a closed vessel, with surroundings at a constant temperature takes 2 minutes to cool from 30°C to 25°C. A mass of 100g of another liquid in an identical vessel with identical surroundings takes the same time to cool from 30° C to 25° C. The specific heat of the liquid is : (The water equivalent of the vessel is 30g.) **[Online April 25, 2013]**

(a) 2.0 kcal/kg (b) 7 kcal/kg
(c) 3 kcal/kg (d) 0.5 kcal/kg

15. 500 g of water and 100 g of ice at 0°C are in a calorimeter whose water equivalent is 40 g. 10 g of steam at 100°C is added to it. Then water in the calorimeter is : (Latent heat of ice = 80 cal/g, Latent heat of steam = 540 cal/ g) **[Online April 23, 2013]**

(a) 580 g (b) 590 g (c) 600 g (d) 610 g

16. Given that 1 g of water in liquid phase has volume 1 cm^3 and in vapour phase 1671 cm^3 at atmospheric pressure and the latent heat of vaporization of water is 2256 J/g; the change in the internal energy in joules for 1 g of water at 373 K when it changes from liquid phase to vapour phase at the same temperature is : **[Online April 22, 2013]**

(a) 2256 (b) 167 (c) 2089 (d) 1

17. A large cylindrical rod of length L is made by joining two identical rods of copper and steel of length $\left(\frac{L}{2}\right)$ each. The rods are completely insulated from the surroundings. If the free end of copper rod is maintained at 100°C and that of steel at 0°C then the temperature of junction is (Thermal conductivity of copper is 9 times that of steel) **[Online May 19, 2012]**

(a) 90ºC (b) 50ºC (c) 10ºC (d) 67ºC

18. The heat radiated per unit area in 1 hour by a furnace whose temperature is 3000 K is ($\sigma = 5.7 \times 10^{-8}$ W m^{-2} K^{-4}) **[Online May 7, 2012]**

(a) 1.7×10^{10} J (b) 1.1×10^{12} J
(c) 2.8×10^{8} J (d) 4.6×10^{6} J

19. 100g of water is heated from 30°C to 50°C. Ignoring the slight expansion of the water, the change in its internal energy is (specific heat of water is 4184 J/kg/K): **[2011]**

(a) 8.4 kJ (b) 84 kJ (c) 2.1 kJ (d) 4.2 kJ

20. The specific heat capacity of a metal at low temperature (T) is given as

$$C_p(kJK^{-1}kg^{-1}) = 32\left(\frac{T}{400}\right)^3$$

A 100 gram vessel of this metal is to be cooled from 20ºK to 4ºK by a special refrigerator operating at room temperature (27°C). The amount of work required to cool the vessel is **[2011 RS]**

(a) greater than 0.148 kJ
(b) between 0.148 kJ and 0.028 kJ
(c) less than 0.028 kJ
(d) equal to 0.002 kJ

21. A long metallic bar is carrying heat from one of its ends to the other end under steady–state. The variation of temperature θ along the length x of the bar from its hot end is best described by which of the following figures? **[2009]**

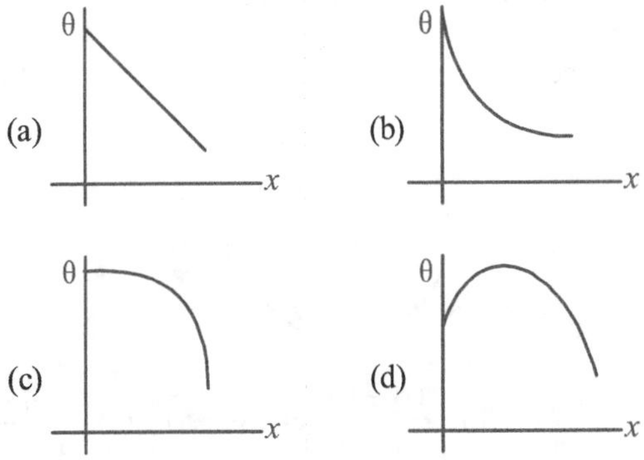

22. One end of a thermally insulated rod is kept at a temperature T_1 and the other at T_2. The rod is composed of two sections of length l_1 and l_2 and thermal conductivities K_1 and K_2 respectively. The temperature at the interface of the two section is **[2007]**

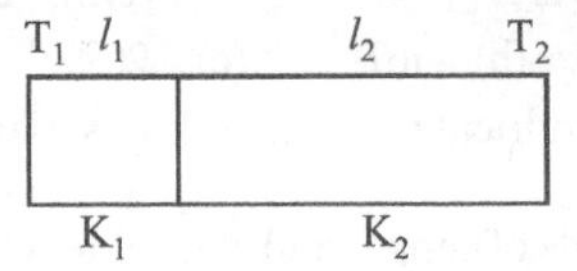

(a) $\frac{(K_1 l_1 T_1 + K_2 l_2 T_2)}{(K_1 l_1 + K_2 l_2)}$ (b) $\frac{(K_2 l_2 T_1 + K_1 l_1 T_2)}{(K_1 l_1 + K_2 l_2)}$

(c) $\frac{(K_2 l_1 T_1 + K_1 l_2 T_2)}{(K_2 l_1 + K_1 l_2)}$ (d) $\frac{(K_1 l_2 T_1 + K_2 l_1 T_2)}{(K_1 l_2 + K_2 l_1)}$

23. Assuming the Sun to be a spherical body of radius R at a temperature of TK, evaluate the total radiant powerd incident of Earth at a distance r from the Sun **[2006]**

(a) $4\pi r_0^2 R^2 \sigma \frac{T^4}{r^2}$ (b) $\pi r_0^2 R^2 \sigma \frac{T^4}{r^2}$

(c) $r_0^2 R^2 \sigma \frac{T^4}{4\pi r^2}$ (d) $R^2 \sigma \frac{T^4}{r^2}$

where r_0 is the radius of the Earth and σ is Stefan's constant.

24. Two rigid boxes containing different ideal gases are placed on a table. Box A contains one mole of nitrogen at temperature T_0, while Box contains one mole of helium at temperature $\left(\frac{7}{3}\right) T_0$. The boxes are then put into thermal contact with each other, and heat flows between them until the gases reach a common final temperature (ignore the heat capacity of boxes). Then, the final temperature of the gases, T_f in terms of T_0 is **[2006]**

(a) $T_f = \frac{3}{7} T_0$ (b) $T_f = \frac{7}{3} T_0$

(c) $T_f = \frac{3}{2} T_0$ (d) $T_f = \frac{5}{2} T_0$

25. The figure shows a system of two concentric spheres of radii r_1 and r_2 are kept at temperatures T_1 and T_2, respectively. The radial rate of flow of heat in a substance between the two concentric spheres is proportional to **[2005]**

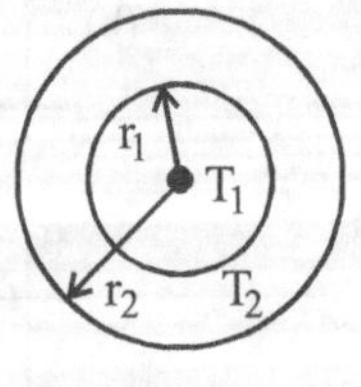

(a) $\ell n\left(\frac{r_2}{r_1}\right)$ (b) $\frac{(r_2 - r_1)}{(r_1 r_2)}$ (c) $(r_2 - r_1)$ (d) $\frac{r_1 r_2}{(r_2 - r_1)}$

26. If the temperature of the sun were to increase from T to $2T$ and its radius from R to $2R$, then the ratio of the radiant energy received on earth to what it was previously will be **[2004]**

(a) 32 (b) 16 (c) 4 (d) 64

27. The temperature of the two outer surfaces of a composite slab, consisting of two materials having coefficients of thermal conductivity K and $2K$ and thickness x and $4x$, respectively, are T_2 and $T_1 (T_2 > T_1)$. The rate of heat transfer through the slab, in a steady state is $\left(\frac{A(T_2 - T_1)K}{x}\right) f$, with f equal to **[2004]**

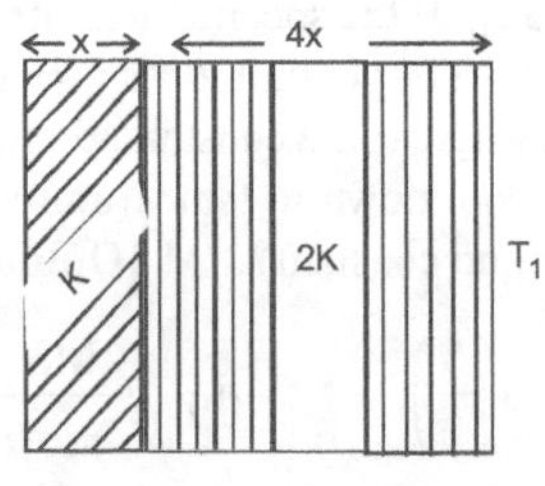

(a) $\frac{2}{3}$ (b) $\frac{1}{2}$ (c) 1 (d) $\frac{1}{3}$

28. The earth radiates in the infra-red region of the spectrum. The spectrum is correctly given by **[2003]**

(a) Rayleigh Jeans law
(b) Planck's law of radiation
(c) Stefan's law of radiation
(d) Wien's law

29. Heat given to a body which raises its temperature by 1°C is

(a) water equivalent **[2002]**
(b) thermal capacity
(c) specific heat
(d) temperature gradient

30. Infrared radiation is detected by **[2002]**

(a) spectrometer (b) pyrometer
(c) nanometer (d) photometer

31. Which of the following is more close to a black body? **[2002]**

(a) black board paint (b) green leaves
(c) black holes (d) red roses

32. If mass-energy equivalence is taken into account, when water is cooled to form ice, the mass of water should **[2002]**

(a) increase
(b) remain unchanged
(c) decrease
(d) first increase then decrease

33. Two spheres of the same material have radii 1 m and 4 m and temperatures 4000 K and 2000 K respectively. The ratio of the energy radiated per second by the first sphere to that by the second is **[2002]**

(a) 1 : 1 (b) 16 : 1 (c) 4 : 1 (d) 1 : 9.

TOPIC-3 : Newton's Law of Cooling

34. Hot water cools from 60°C to 50°C in the first 10 minutes and to 42°C in the next 10 minutes. The temperature of the surroundings is: **[Online April 12, 2014]**
(a) 25°C (b) 10°C (c) 15°C (d) 20°C

35. A hot body, obeying Newton's law of cooling is cooling down from its peak value 80°C to an ambient temperature of 30°C. It takes 5 minutes in cooling down from 80°C to 40°C. How much time will it take to cool down from 62°C to 32°C? (Given In 2 = 0.693, In 5 = 1.609) **[Online April 11, 2014]**
(a) 3.75 minutes (b) 8.6 minutes
(c) 9.6 minutes (d) 6.5 minutes

36. If a piece of metal is heated to temperature θ and then allowed to cool in a room which is at temperature θ_0, the graph between the temperature T of the metal and time t will be closest to **[2013]**

(a)
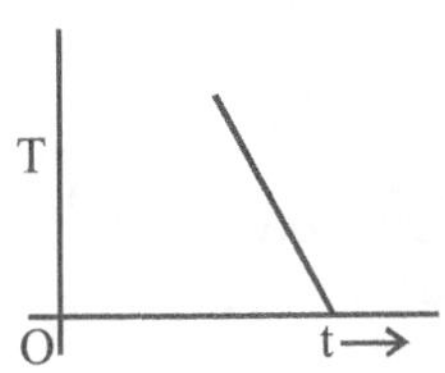

(b)
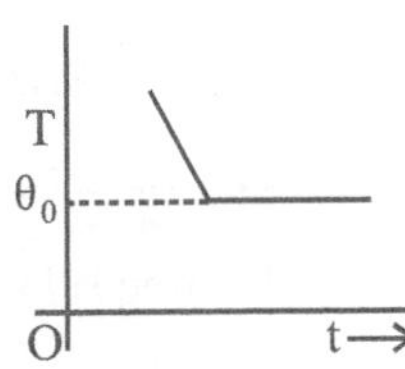

(c)
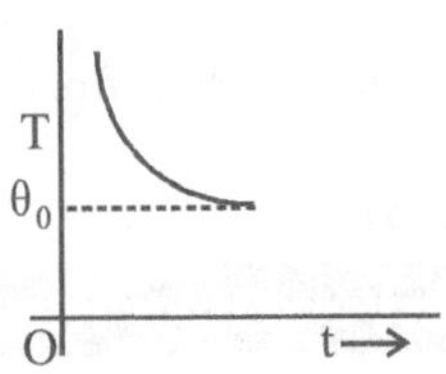

(d)
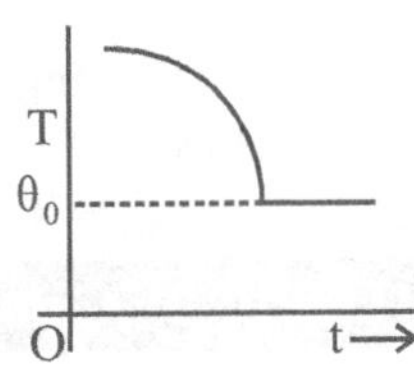

37. A liquid in a beaker has temperature $\theta(t)$ at time t and θ_0 is temperature of surroundings, then according to Newton's law of cooling the correct graph between $\log_e(\theta - \theta_0)$ and t is : **[2012]**

(a)
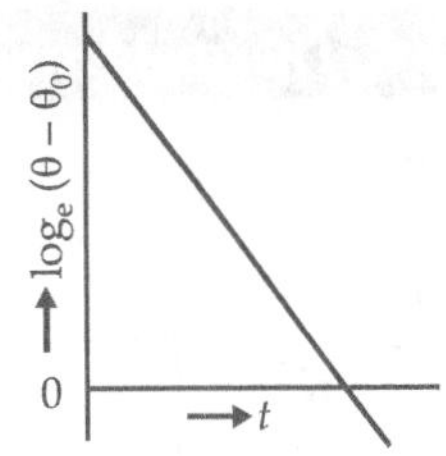

(b)
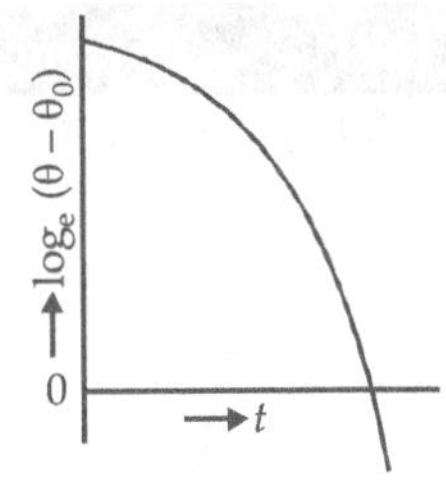

(c)
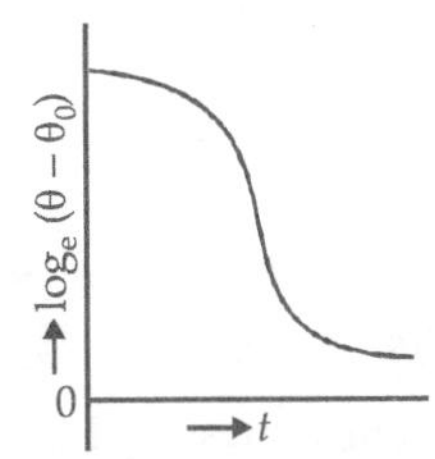

(d)
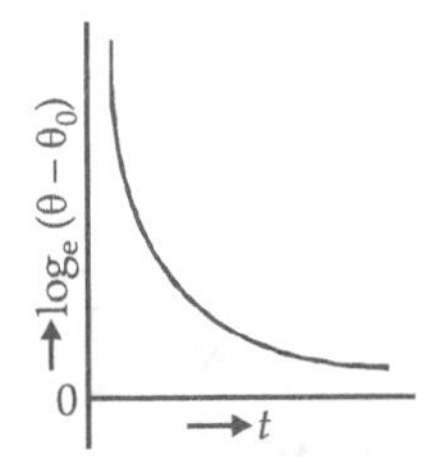

38. According to Newton's law of cooling, the rate of cooling of a body is proportional to $(\Delta\theta)^n$, where $\Delta\theta$ is the difference of the temperature of the body and the surroundings, and n is equal to **[2003]**
(a) two (b) three
(c) four (d) one

Hints & Solutions

TOPIC-1 : Thermometer & Thermal Expansion

1. **(c)** As we know, Bulk modulus

$$K = \frac{\Delta P}{\left(\frac{-\Delta V}{V}\right)} \Rightarrow \frac{\Delta V}{V} = \frac{P}{K}$$

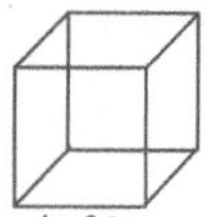

J = 3α

$V = V_0(1 + \gamma \Delta t)$

$$\frac{\Delta V}{V_0} = \gamma \Delta t$$

$$\therefore \frac{P}{K} = \gamma \Delta t \Rightarrow \Delta t = \frac{P}{\gamma K} = \frac{P}{3\alpha K}$$

2. **(b)** Young's modulus $= \frac{\text{Thermal stress}}{\text{Strain}} = \frac{F/A}{\Delta L/L}$

$$Y = \frac{F}{A.\alpha.\Delta\theta} \quad \left(\because \frac{\Delta L}{L} = \alpha \Delta \theta\right)$$

Force developed in the rail $F = YA\alpha\Delta t$

$= 2 \times 10^{11} \times 40 \times 10^{-4} \times 1.2 \times 10^{-5} \times 10$

$= 9.6 \times 10^4 = 1 \times 10^5$ N

3. **(c)** Due to thermal exp., change in length $(\Delta l) = l\,\alpha\,\Delta T$ ... (i)

$$\text{Young's modulus (Y)} = \frac{\text{Normal stress}}{\text{Longitudinal strain}}$$

$$Y = \frac{F/A}{\Delta l/l} \Rightarrow \frac{\Delta l}{l} = \frac{F}{AY}$$

$$\Delta l = \frac{Fl}{AY}$$

From eq^n (i), $\frac{Fl}{AY} = l\,\alpha\,\Delta T$

$F = AY\alpha\Delta T$

4. **(b)** When there is no change in liquid level in vessel then

$\gamma'_{real} = \gamma'_{vessel}$

Change in volume in liquid relative to vessel

$\Delta V_{app} = V\gamma'_{app}\,\Delta\theta = V(\gamma'_{real} - \gamma'_{vessel})$

5. **(c)** $\frac{\text{Reading on any scale} - \text{LFP}}{\text{UFP} - \text{LFP}}$

= constant for all scales

$$\frac{340 - 273}{373 - 273} = \frac{°Y - (-160)}{-50 - (-160)}$$

$$\Rightarrow \frac{67}{100} = \frac{y + 160}{110}$$

$\therefore$ Y = −86.3° Y

6. **(d)** The Young modulus is given as

$$Y = \frac{F/S}{\Delta L/L}$$

Here it is given as

$$Y = \frac{F}{S2\pi\Delta R} \times 2\pi R \quad \{L = 2\pi R\}$$

$$\text{or} \quad Y = \frac{FR}{S.\Delta R} \quad \ldots(i)$$

The coefficient of linear expansion is given as

$$\alpha = \frac{\Delta R}{R\Delta T}$$

$$\Rightarrow \frac{\Delta R}{R} = \alpha.\Delta T \Rightarrow \frac{R}{\Delta R} = \frac{1}{\alpha\Delta T} \quad \ldots(ii)$$

From equation (i) and (ii)

$$Y = \frac{F}{S.\alpha\Delta T} \Rightarrow F = Y.S.\alpha\Delta T$$

$\therefore$ The ring is pressing the wheel from both sides, Thus

$$F_{net} = 2F = 2YS\alpha\Delta T$$

TOPIC-2 : Calorimetry and Heat Transfer

7. **(d)** According to principle of calorimetry,

Heat lost = Heat gain

$100 \times 0.1(-75) = 100 \times 0.1 \times 45 + 170 \times 1 \times 45$

$10 - 750 = 450 + 7650$

$10 = 1200 + 7650 = 8850$

$T = 885°C$

8. **(d)** According to principle of calorimetry,

$Q_{given} = Q_{used}$

$0.2 \times S \times (150 - 40) = 150 \times 1 \times (40 - 27) + 25 \times (40 - 27)$

$0.2 \times S \times 110 = 150 \times 13 + 25 \times 13$

Specific heat of aluminium

$$S = \frac{13 \times 25 \times 7}{0.2 \times 110} = 434 \text{ J/kg-°C}$$

9. **(b)** As $Pt = mC\Delta T$

So, $P \times 10 \times 60 = mC\,100$ ...(i)

and $P \times 55 \times 60 = mL$ ...(ii)

Dividing equation (i) by (ii) we get

$$\frac{10}{55} = \frac{C \times 100}{L}$$

$\therefore L = 550$ cal./g.

10. **(c)** Rate of heat flow is given by,

$$Q = \frac{KA(\theta_1 - \theta_2)}{l}$$

Where, K = coefficient of thermal conductivity
l = length of rod and A = area of cross-section of rod

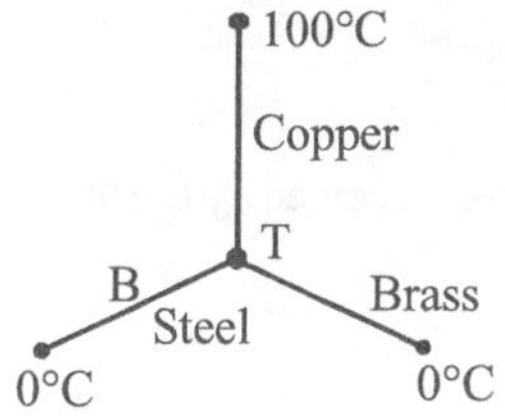

If the junction temperature is T, then

$Q_{Copper} = Q_{Brass} + Q_{Steel}$

$$\frac{0.92 \times 4(100-T)}{46} = \frac{0.26 \times 4 \times (T-0)}{13} + \frac{0.12 \times 4 \times (T-0)}{12}$$

$\Rightarrow$ $200 - 2T = 2T + T$

$\Rightarrow$ $T = 40°C$

$$\therefore \quad Q_{Copper} = \frac{0.92 \times 4 \times 60}{46} = 4.8 \text{ cal/s}$$

11. (c) In the given problem, fall in temperature of sphere,

$dT = (3T_0 - 2T_0) = T_0$

Temperature of surrounding, $T_{surr} = T_0$

Initial temperature of sphere, $T_{initial} = 3T_0$

Specific heat of the material of the sphere varies as,

$c = \alpha T^3$ per unit mass (α = a constant)

Applying formula,

$$\frac{dT}{dt} = \frac{\sigma A}{McJ}\left(T^4 - T_{surr}^4\right)$$

$$\Rightarrow \quad \frac{T_0}{dt} = \frac{\sigma 4\pi R^2}{M\alpha(3T_0)^3 J}\left[(3T_0)^4 - (T_0)^4\right]$$

$$\Rightarrow \quad dt = \frac{M\alpha 27 T_0^4 J}{\sigma 4\pi R^2 \times 80 T_0^4}$$

Solving we get,

Time taken for the sphere to cool down temperature $2T_0$,

$$t = \frac{M\alpha}{16\pi R^2 \sigma} \ln\left(\frac{16}{3}\right)$$

12. (a) From question,

In 1 sec heat gained by water

= 1 KW – 160 J/s

= 1000 J/s – 160 J/s

= 840 J/s

Total heat required to raise the temperature of water (volume 2L) from 27°c to 77°c

$= m_{water} \times$ sp. ht $\times \Delta\theta$

$= 2 \times 10^3 \times 4.2 \times 50$ [$\because$ mass = density $\times$ volume]

And, $840 \times t = 2 \times 10^3 \times 4.2 \times 50$

$$\text{or,} \quad t = \frac{2 \times 10^3 \times 4.2 \times 50}{840}$$

= 500 s = 8 min 20s

13. (d) When radius is decrease by ΔR,

$$4\pi R^2 \Delta R \rho L = 4\pi T[R^2 - (R - \Delta R)^2]$$

$$\Rightarrow \rho R^2 \Delta RL = T[R^2 - R^2 + 2R\Delta R - \Delta R^2]$$

$$\Rightarrow \rho R^2 \Delta RL = T2R\Delta R \qquad [\Delta R \text{ is very small}]$$

$$\Rightarrow R = \frac{2T}{\rho L}$$

14. (d) As the surrounding is identical, vessel is identical time taken to cool both water and liquid (from 30°C to 25°C) is same 2 minutes, therefore

$$\left(\frac{dQ}{dt}\right)_{water} = \left(\frac{dQ}{dt}\right)_{liquid}$$

$$\text{or,} \quad \frac{(m_w C_w + W)\Delta T}{t} = \frac{(m_\ell C_\ell + W)\Delta T}{t}$$

(W = water equivalent of the vessel)

or, $m_w C_w = m_\ell C_\ell$

$$\therefore \text{ Specific heat of liquid}, C_\ell = \frac{m_w C_w}{m_\ell}$$

$$= \frac{50 \times 1}{100} = 0.5 \text{ kcal/kg}$$

15. (b) As 1g of steam at 100°C melts 8g of ice at 0°C.

10 g of steam will melt 8× 10 g of ice at 0°C

Water in calorimeter = 500 + 80 + 10g = 590g

16. (c)

17. (a)

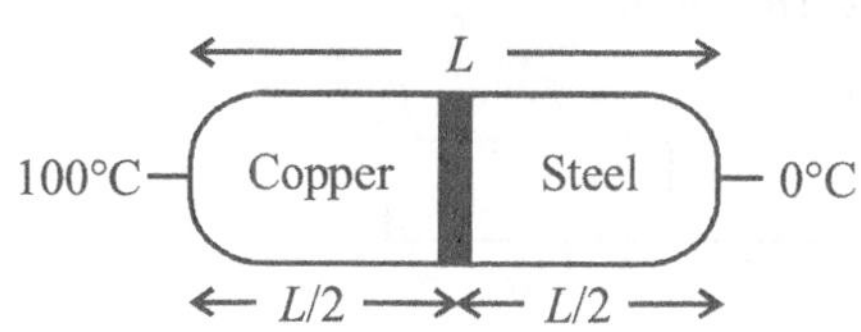

Let conductivity of steel $K_{steel} = k$ then from question

Conductivity of copper $K_{copper} = 9k$

$\theta_{copper} = 100°C$

$\theta_{steel} = 0°C$

$$l_{steel} = l_{copper} = \frac{L}{2}$$

From formula temperature of junction;

$$\theta = \frac{K_{copper}\theta_{copper}\, l_{steel} + K_{steel}\,\theta_{steel}\, l_{copper}}{K_{copper}\, l_{steel} + K_{steel}\, l_{copper}}$$

$$= \frac{9k \times 100 \times \frac{L}{2} + k \times 0 \times \frac{L}{2}}{9k \times \frac{L}{2} + k \times \frac{L}{2}}$$

$$= \frac{\frac{900}{2} kL}{\frac{10kL}{2}} = 90°C$$

18. (a) According to Stefan's law

$E = \sigma T^4$

Heat radiated per unit area in 1 hour (3600s) is

$= 5.7 \times 10^{-8} \times (300)^4 \times 3600 = 1.7 \times 10^{10}$ J

19. (a) $\Delta U = \Delta Q = mc\Delta T$

$= 100 \times 10^{-3} \times 4184\,(50 - 30) \approx 8.4$ kJ

20. (d) Required work = energy released

Here, $Q = \int mc\,dT$

$$= \int_{20}^{4} 0.1 \times 32 \times \left(\frac{T^3}{400^3}\right) dT \approx 0.002 \text{ kJ}.$$

Therefore, required work = 0.002 kJ

21. (a) The heat flow rate is given by

$$\frac{dQ}{dt} = \frac{kA(\theta_1 - \theta)}{x}$$

$$\Rightarrow \theta_1 - \theta = \frac{x}{kA}\frac{dQ}{dt} \Rightarrow \theta = \theta_1 - \frac{x}{kA}\frac{dQ}{dt}$$

where θ_1 is the temperature of hot end and θ is temperature at a distance x from hot end.

The above equation can be graphically represented by option (a).

22. (d) Let T be the temperature of the interface. As the two sections are in series, the rate of flow of heat in them will be equal.

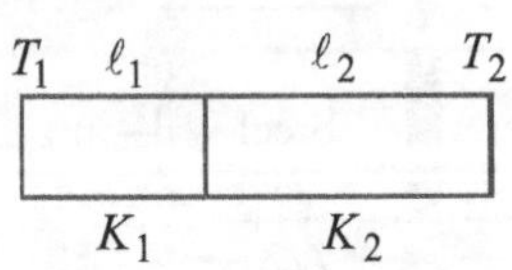

$$\therefore \frac{K_1 A(T_1 - T)}{\ell_1} = \frac{K_2 A(T - T_2)}{\ell_2},$$

where A is the area of cross-section.

or, $K_1 A(T_1 - T)\ell_2 = K_2 A(T - T_2)\ell_1$

or, $K_1 T_1 \ell_2 - K_1 T \ell_2 = K_2 T \ell_1 - K_2 T_2 \ell_1$

or, $(K_2\ell_1 + K_1\ell_2)T = K_1 T_1 \ell_2 + K_2 T_2 \ell_1$

$$\therefore T = \frac{K_1 T_1 \ell_2 + K_2 T_2 \ell_1}{K_2 \ell_1 + K_1 \ell_2} = \frac{K_1 \ell_2 T_1 + K_2 \ell_1 T_2}{K_1 \ell_2 + K_2 \ell_1}.$$

23. (b) Total power radiated by Sun = $\sigma T^4 \times 4\pi R^2$

The intensity of power at earth's surface

$$= \frac{\sigma T^4 \times 4\pi R^2}{4\pi r^2}$$

Total power received by Earth

$$= \frac{\sigma T^4 R^2}{r^2}(\pi r_0^2)$$

24. (c) Heat lost by He = Heat gained by N_2

$n_1 C_{v_1} \Delta T_1 = n_2 C_{v_2} \Delta T_2$

$$\frac{3}{2}R\left[\frac{7}{3}T_0 - T_f\right] = \frac{5}{2}R\left[T_f - T_0\right]$$

$7T_0 - 3T_f = 5T_f - 5T_0$

$$\Rightarrow 12T_0 = 8T_f \Rightarrow T_f = \frac{12}{8}T_0 \Rightarrow T_f = \frac{3}{2}T_0.$$

25. (d)

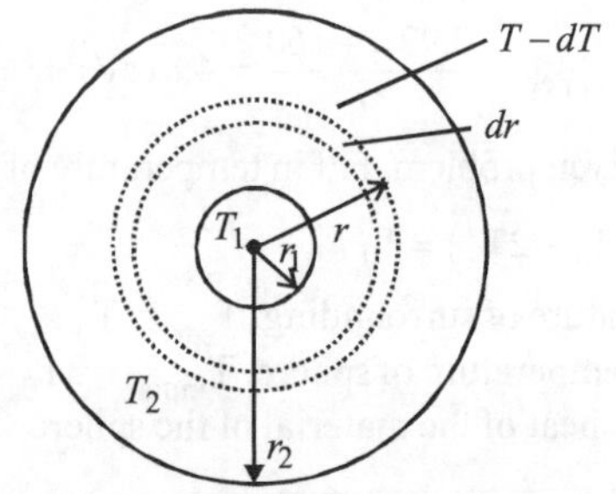

Consider a shell of thickness (dr) and of radiius (r) and let the temperature of inner and outer surfaces of this shell be T and $(T - dT)$ respectively.

$\frac{dQ}{dt}$ = rate of flow of heat through it

$$= \frac{KA[(T - dT) - T]}{dr} = \frac{-KAdT}{dr}$$

$$= -4\pi K r^2 \frac{dT}{dr} \qquad (\because A = 4\pi r^2)$$

To measure the radial rate of heat flow, integration technique is used, since the area of the surface through which heat will flow is not constant.

$$\text{Then, } \left(\frac{dQ}{dt}\right)\int_{r_1}^{r_2} \frac{1}{r^2}dr = -4\pi K \int_{T_1}^{T_2} dT$$

$$\frac{dQ}{dt}\left[\frac{1}{r_1} - \frac{1}{r_2}\right] = -4\pi K\left[T_2 - T_1\right]$$

$$\text{or } \frac{dQ}{dt} = \frac{-4\pi K r_1 r_2 (T_2 - T_1)}{(r_2 - r_1)}$$

$$\therefore \frac{dQ}{dt} \propto \frac{r_1 r_2}{(r_2 - r_1)}$$

26. (d) $E = \sigma A T^4$; $A \propto R^2$ $\therefore E \propto R^2 T^4$

$$\therefore \frac{E_2}{E_1} = \frac{R_2^2 T_2^4}{R_1^2 T_1^4}$$

put $R_2 = 2R, R_1 = R$
$T_2 = 2T, T_1 = T$

$$\Rightarrow \frac{E_2}{E_1} = \frac{(2R)^2 (2T)^4}{R^2 T^4} = 64$$

27. (d) The thermal resistance is given by

$$\frac{x}{KA} + \frac{4x}{2KA} = \frac{x}{KA} + \frac{2x}{KA} = \frac{3x}{KA}$$

$$\therefore \frac{dQ}{dt} = \frac{\Delta T}{\frac{3x}{KA}} = \frac{(T_2 - T_1)KA}{3x}$$

$$= \frac{1}{3}\left\{\frac{A(T_2 - T_1)K}{x}\right\}$$

$$\therefore f = \frac{1}{3}$$

28. (d) Wien's law correctly explains the spectrum

29. (b) Heat required for raising the temperature of the whole body by 1°C is called the thermal capacity of the body.

30. (b) Pyrometer is used to detect infra-red radiation.

31. (a) Black board paint is quite approximately equal to black bodies.

32. (c) When water is cooled to form ice, energy is released from water in the form of heat. As energy is equivalent to mass, therefore, when water is cooled to ice, its mass decreases.

33. (a) The energy radiated per second is given by $E = e\sigma T^4 A$

For same material e is same. σ is stefan's constant

$$\therefore \frac{E_1}{E_2} = \frac{T_1^4 A_1}{T_2^4 A_2} = \frac{T_1^4 4\pi r_1^2}{T_2^4 4\pi r_2^2} = \frac{(4000)^4 \times 1^2}{(2000)^4 \times 4^2} = \frac{1}{1}$$

TOPIC-3 : Newton's Law of Cooling

34. (b) By Newton's law of cooling

$$\frac{\theta_1 - \theta_2}{t} = -K\left[\frac{\theta_1 + \theta_2}{2} - \theta_0\right]$$

where θ_0 is the temperature of surrounding.

Now, hot water cools from 60°C to 50°C in 10 minutes,

$$\frac{60 - 50}{10} = -K\left[\frac{60 + 50}{2} - \theta_0\right] \quad ...(i)$$

Again, it cools from 50°C to 42°C in next 10 minutes.

$$\frac{50 - 42}{10} = -K\left[\frac{50 + 42}{2} - \theta_0\right] \quad ...(ii)$$

Dividing equations (i) by (ii) we get

$$\frac{1}{0.8} = \frac{55 - \theta_0}{46 - \theta_0}$$

$$\frac{10}{8} = \frac{55 - \theta_0}{46 - \theta_0}$$

$$460 - 10\theta_0 = 440 - 8\theta_0$$

$$2\theta_0 = 20$$

$$\theta_0 = 10°C$$

35. (b) From Newton's law of cooling,

$$t = \frac{1}{k}\log_e\left(\frac{\theta_2 - \theta_0}{\theta_1 - \theta_0}\right)$$

From question and above equation,

$$5 = \frac{1}{k}\log_e\frac{(40 - 30)}{(80 - 30)} \quad ...(1)$$

$$\text{And, } t = \frac{1}{k}\log_e\frac{(32 - 30)}{(62 - 30)} \quad ...(2)$$

Dividing equation (2) by (1),

$$\frac{t}{5} = \frac{\frac{1}{k}\log_e\frac{(32 - 30)}{(62 - 30)}}{\frac{1}{k}\log_e\frac{(40 - 30)}{(80 - 30)}}$$

On solving we get, time taken to cool down from 62°C to 32°C, $t = 8.6$ minutes.

36. (c) According to Newton's law of cooling, the temperature goes on decreasing with time non-linearly.

37. (a) Newton's law of cooling

$$\frac{d\theta}{dt} = -k(\theta - \theta_0)$$

$$\Rightarrow \frac{d\theta}{(\theta - \theta_0)} = -k dt$$

Integrating

$\Rightarrow \log(\theta - \theta_0) = -kt + c$

Which represents an equation of straight line.

Thus the option (a) is correct.

38. (d) According to Newton's law of cooling $-\frac{dQ}{dt} \propto (\Delta\theta)$

Chapter 11

Thermodynamics

TOPIC-1 : First Law of Thermodynamics

1. 200g water is heated from 40°C to 60°C. Ignoring the slight expansion of water, the change in its internal energy is close to (Given specific heat of water = 4184 J/kgK): **[Online April 9, 2016]**

(a) 167.4 kJ (b) 8.4 kJ (c) 4.2 kJ (d) 16.7 kJ

2. A gas is compressed from a volume of $2m^3$ to a volume of $1 m^3$ at a constant pressure of $100 N/m^2$. Then it is heated at constant volume by supplying 150 J of energy. As a result, the internal energy of the gas: **[Online April 19, 2014]**

(a) increases by 250 J (b) decreases by 250 J
(c) increases by 50 J (d) decreases by 50 J

3. An insulated container of gas has two chambers separated by an insulating partition. One of the chambers has volume V_1 and contains ideal gas at pressure P_1 and temperature T_1. The other chamber has volume V_2 and contains ideal gas at pressure P_2 and temperature T_2. If the partition is removed without doing any work on the gas, the final equilibrium temperature of the gas in the container will be **[2008]**

(a) $\frac{T_1T_2(P_1V_1+P_2V_2)}{P_1V_1T_2+P_2V_2T_1}$ (b) $\frac{P_1V_1T_1+P_2V_2T_2}{P_1V_1+P_2V_2}$

(c) $\frac{P_1V_1T_2+P_2V_2T_1}{P_1V_1+P_2V_2}$ (d) $\frac{T_1T_2(P_1V_1+P_2V_2)}{P_1V_1T_1+P_2V_2T_2}$

4. When a system is taken from state i to state f along the path iaf, it is found that $Q = 50$ cal and $W = 20$ cal. Along the path ibf $Q = 36$ cal. W along the path ibf is **[2007]**

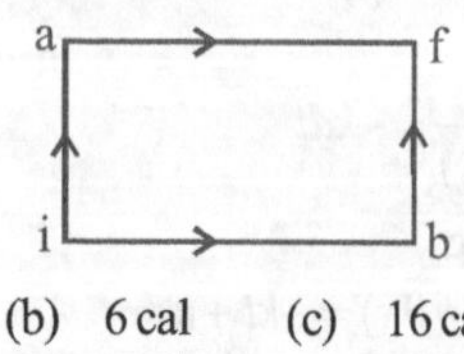

(a) 14 cal (b) 6 cal (c) 16 cal (d) 66 cal

5. A system goes from A to B via two processes I and II as shown in figure. If ΔU_1 and ΔU_2 are the changes in internal energies in the processes I and II respectively, then **[2005]**

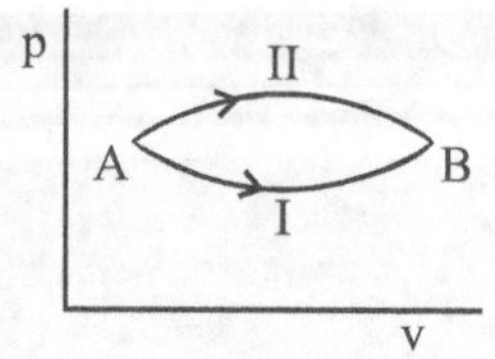

(a) relation between ΔU_1 and ΔU_2 can not be determined

(b) $\Delta U_1 = \Delta U_2$

(c) $\Delta U_2 < \Delta U_1$

(d) $\Delta U_2 > \Delta U_1$

6. Which of the following is incorrect regarding the first law of thermodynamics? **[2005]**

(a) It is a restatement of the principle of conservation of energy
(b) It is not applicable to any cyclic process
(c) It does not introduces the concept of the entropy
(d) It introduces the concept of the internal energy

TOPIC-2 : Specific Heat Capacity and Thermodynamical Processes

7. 'n' moles of an ideal gas undergoes a process A → B as shown in the figure. The maximum temperature of the gas during the process will be : **[2016]**

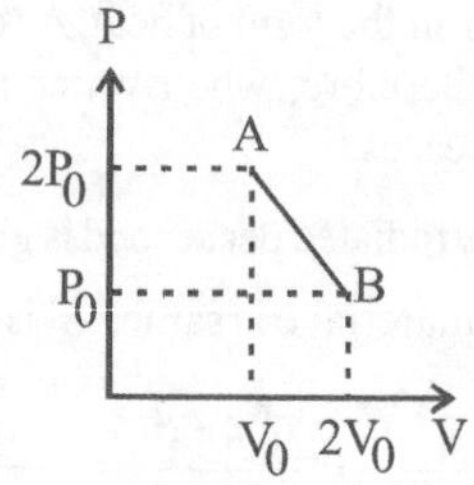

(a) $\frac{9P_0V_0}{2nR}$ (b) $\frac{9P_0V_0}{nR}$ (c) $\frac{9P_0V_0}{4nR}$ (d) $\frac{3P_0V_0}{2nR}$

8. The ratio of work done by an ideal monoatomic gas to the heat supplied to it in an isobaric process is : **[Online April 9, 2016]**

(a) $\frac{2}{5}$ (b) $\frac{3}{2}$ (c) $\frac{3}{5}$ (d) $\frac{2}{3}$

9. Consider an ideal gas confined in an isolated closed chamber. As the gas undergoes an adiabatic expansion, the average time of collision between molecules increases as V^q, where V is the volume of the gas. The value of q is : $\left(\gamma = \frac{C_p}{C_v}\right)$ **[2015]**

(a) $\frac{\gamma+1}{2}$ (b) $\frac{\gamma-1}{2}$ (c) $\frac{3\gamma+5}{6}$ (d) $\frac{3\gamma-5}{6}$

10. Consider a spherical shell of radius R at temperature T. The black body radiation inside it can be considered as an ideal gas of photons with internal energy per unit volume $u = \frac{U}{V} \propto T^4$ and pressure $p = \frac{1}{3}\left(\frac{U}{V}\right)$. If the shell now undergoes an adiabatic expansion the relation between T and R is : **[2015]**

(a) $T \propto \frac{1}{R}$ (b) $T \propto \frac{1}{R^3}$ (c) $T \propto e^{-R}$ (d) $T \propto e^{-3R}$

11. An ideal gas goes through a reversible cycle a→b→c→d has the V - T diagram shown below. Process d→a and b→c are adiabatic.

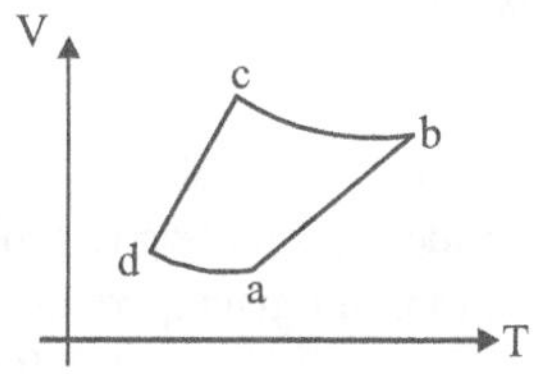

The corresponding P - V diagram for the process is (all figures are schematic and not drawn to scale) : **[Online April 10, 2015]**

(a)
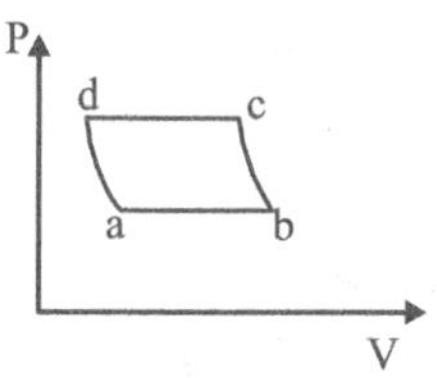

(b)
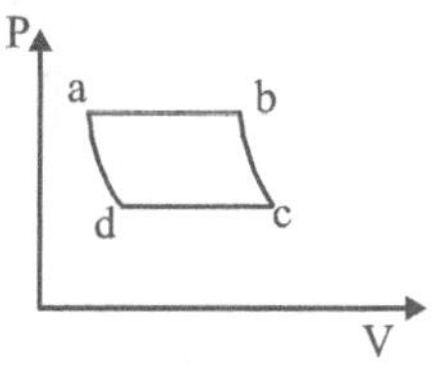

(c)
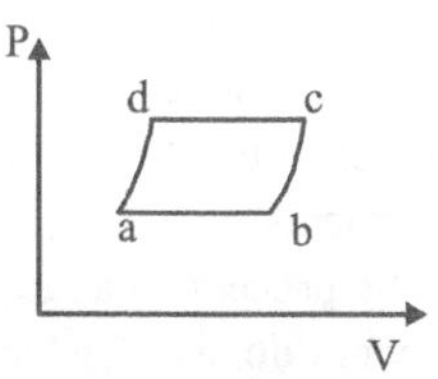

(d)
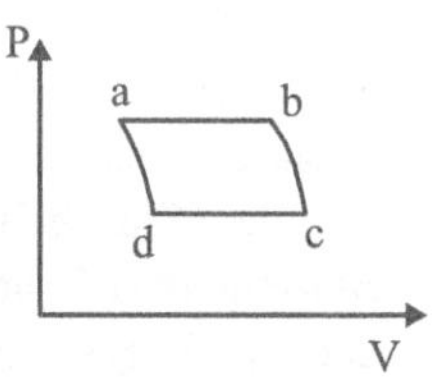

12. One mole of a diatomic ideal gas undergoes a cyclic process ABC as shown in figure. The process BC is adiabatic. The temperatures at A, B and C are 400 K, 800 K and 600 K respectively. Choose the correct statement: **[2014]**

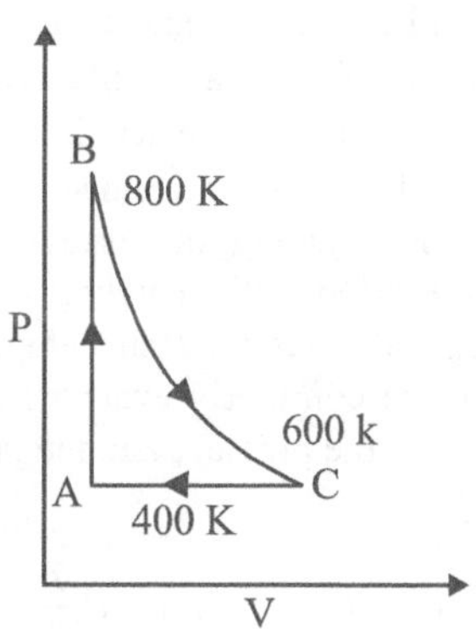

(a) The change in internal energy in whole cyclic process is 250 R.

(b) The change in internal energy in the process CA is 700 R.

(c) The change in internal energy in the process AB is - 350 R.

(d) The change in internal energy in the process BC is – 500 R.

13. An ideal monoatomic gas is confined in a cylinder by a spring loaded piston of cross section 8.0×10^{-3} m^2. Initially the gas is at 300 K and occupies a volume of 2.4×10^{-3} m^3 and the spring is in its relaxed state as shown in figure. The gas is heated by a small heater until the piston moves out slowly by 0.1 m. The force constant of the spring is 8000 N/m and the atmospheric pressure is 1.0×10^5 N/m^2. The cylinder and the piston are thermally insulated. The piston and the spring are massless and there is no friction between the piston and the cylinder. The final temperature of the gas will be:

(Neglect the heat loss through the lead wires of the heater. The heat capacity of the heater coil is also negligible).

[Online April 11, 2014]

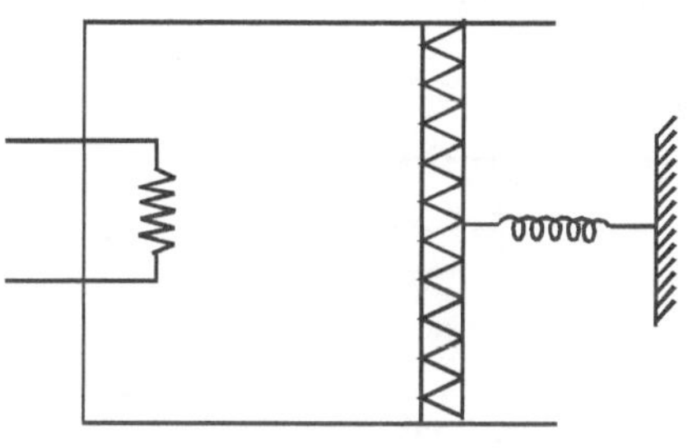

(a) 300 K (b) 800 K

(c) 500 K (d) 1000 K

14. During an adiabatic compression, 830 J of work is done on 2 moles of a diatomic ideal gas to reduce its volume by 50%. The change in its temperature is nearly:

($R = 8.3$ JK^{-1} mol^{-1}) **[Online April 11, 2014]**

(a) 40 K (b) 33 K

(c) 20 K (d) 14 K

15. The equation of state for a gas is given by $PV = nRT + \alpha V$, where n is the number of moles and α is a positive constant. The initial temperature and pressure of one mole of the gas contained in a cylinder are T_o and P_o respectively. The work done by the gas when its temperature doubles isobarically will be: **[Online April 9, 2014]**

(a) $\frac{P_o T_o R}{P_o - \alpha}$ (b) $\frac{P_o T_o R}{P_o + \alpha}$

(c) $P_o T_o R \ln 2$ (d) $P_o T_o R$

16. A certain amount of gas is taken through a cyclic process (A B C D A) that has two isobars, one isochore and one isothermal. The cycle can be represented on a P-V indicator diagram as : **[Online April 22, 2013]**

(a)
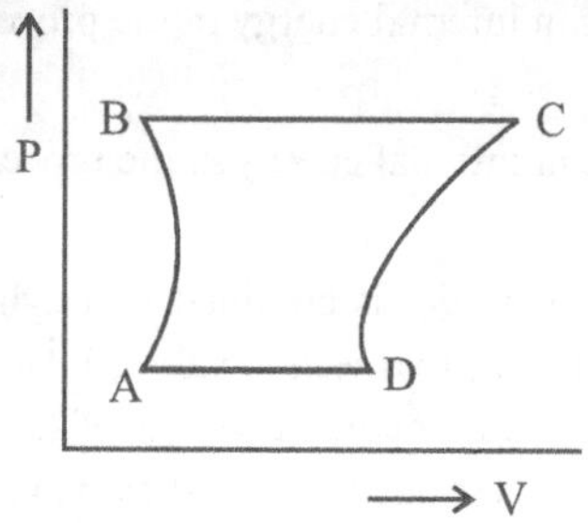

(b)
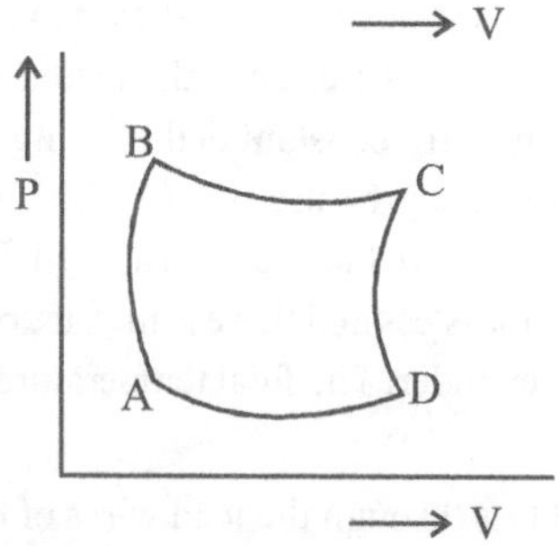

(c)
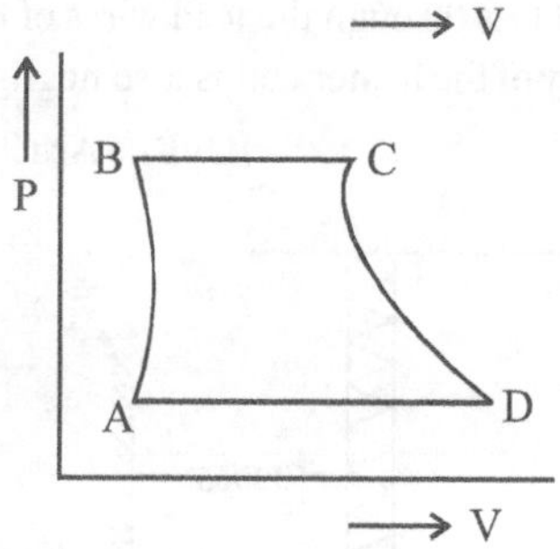

(d)
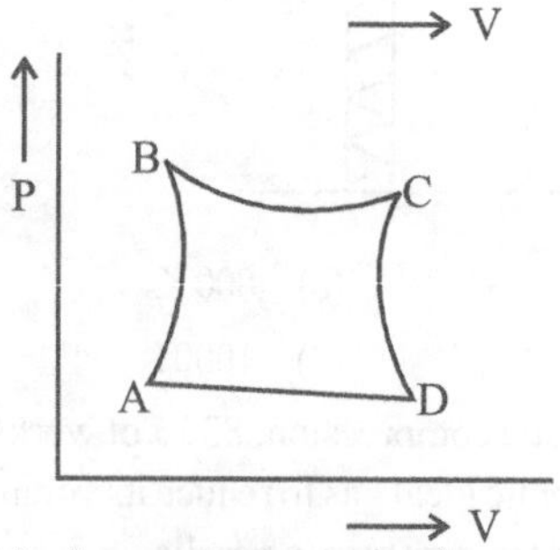

17. An ideal gas at atmospheric pressure is adiabatically compressed so that its density becomes 32 times of its initial value. If the final pressure of gas is 128 atmospheres, the value of 'γ' of the gas is : **[Online April 22, 2013]**
(a) 1.5 (b) 1.4 (c) 1.3 (d) 1.6

18. Helium gas goes through a cycle ABCDA (consisting of two isochoric and isobaric lines) as shown in figure. The efficiency of this cycle is nearly : (Assume the gas to be close to ideal gas) **[2012]**

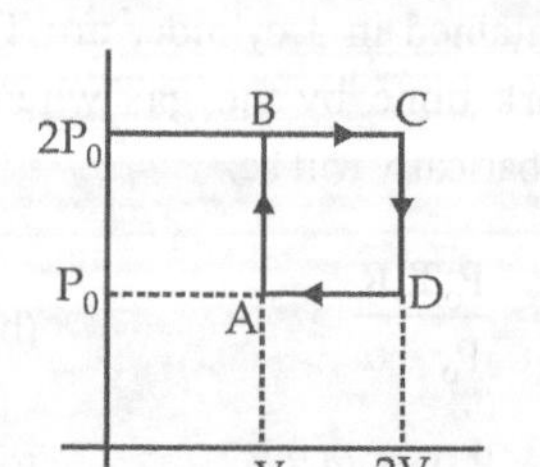

(a) 15.4%
(b) 9.1%
(c) 10.5%
(d) 12.5%

19. An ideal monatomic gas with pressure P, volume V and temperature T is expanded isothermally to a volume $2V$ and a final pressure P_i. If the same gas is expanded adiabatically to a volume $2V$, the final pressure is P_a. The ratio $\frac{P_a}{P_i}$ is **[Online May 26, 2012]**
(a) $2^{-1/3}$ (b) $2^{1/3}$ (c) $2^{2/3}$ (d) $2^{-2/3}$

20. The pressure of an ideal gas varies with volume as $P = \alpha V$, where α is a constant. One mole of the gas is allowed to undergo expansion such that its volume becomes 'm' times its initial volume. The work done by the gas in the process is **[Online May 19, 2012]**

(a) $\frac{\alpha V}{2}\left(m^2-1\right)$ (b) $\frac{\alpha^2 V^2}{2}\left(m^2-1\right)$

(c) $\frac{\alpha}{2}\left(m^2-1\right)$ (d) $\frac{\alpha V^2}{2}\left(m^2-1\right)$

21. n moles of an ideal gas undergo a process $A \to B$ as shown in the figure. Maximum temperature of the gas during the process is **[Online May 12, 2012]**

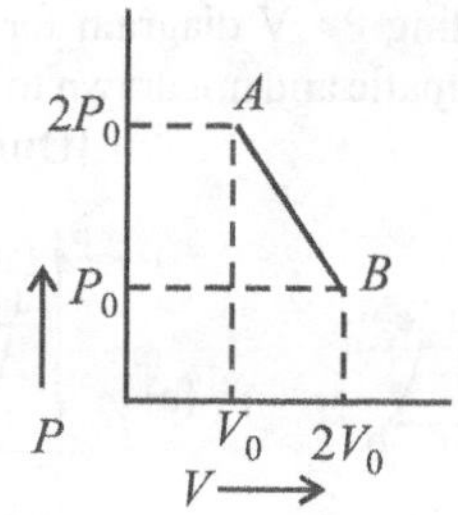

(a) $\frac{9P_0V_0}{nR}$ (b) $\frac{3P_0V_0}{2nR}$ (c) $\frac{9P_0V_0}{2nR}$ (d) $\frac{9P_0V_0}{4nR}$

22. This question has Statement 1 and Statement 2. Of the four choices given after the Statements, choose the one that best describes the two Statements.
Statement 1: In an adiabatic process, change in internal energy of a gas is equal to work done on/by the gas in the process.
Statement 2: The temperature of a gas remains constant in an adiabatic process. **[Online May 7, 2012]**
(a) Statement 1 is true, Statement 2 is true, Statement 2 is a correct explanation of Statement 1.
(b) Statement 1 is true, Statement 2 is false.
(c) Statement 1 is false, Statement 2 is true.
(d) Statement 1 is false, Statement 2 is true, Statement 2 is not a correct explanation of Statement 1.

23. A container with insulating walls is divided into equal parts by a partition fitted with a valve. One part is filled with an ideal gas at a pressure P and temperature T, whereas the other part is completly evacuated. If the valve is suddenly opened, the pressure and temperature of the gas will be : **[2011 RS]**

(a) $\frac{P}{2}, \frac{T}{2}$ (b) P, T (c) $P, \frac{T}{2}$ (d) $\frac{P}{2}, T$

Directions for questions 24 to 26: *Questions are based on the following paragraph.*
Two moles of helium gas are taken over the cycle *ABCDA*, as shown in the *P-T* diagram. **[2009]**

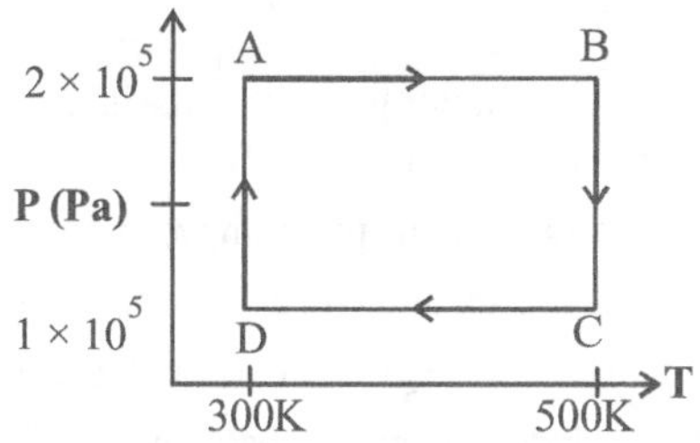

24. Assuming the gas to be ideal the work done on the gas in taking it from *A* to *B* is
(a) 300 R (b) 400 R (c) 500 R (d) 200 R

25. The work done on the gas in taking it from *D* to *A* is
(a) +414 R (b) −690 R (c) +690 R (d) −414 R

26. The net work done on the gas in the cycle *ABCDA* is
(a) 279 R (b) 1076 R (c) 1904 R (d) zero

27. The work of 146 kJ is performed in order to compress one kilo mole of gas adiabatically and in this process the temperature of the gas increases by 7°C. The gas is ($R = 8.3\ J\ mol^{-1}\ K^{-1}$) **[2006]**
(a) diatomic
(b) triatomic
(c) a mixture of monoatomic and diatomic
(d) monoatomic

28. Which of the following parameters does not characterize the thermodynamic state of matter? **[2003]**
(a) Temperature (b) Pressure
(c) Work (d) Volume

TOPIC-3 : Carnot Engine, Refrigerators and Second Law of Thermodynamics

29. An engine operates by taking n moles of an ideal gas through the cycle ABCDA shown in figure. The thermal efficiency of the engine is : (Take $C_v = 1.5\ R$, where R is gas constant) **[Online April 8, 2017]**

(a) 0.24
(b) 0.15
(c) 0.32
(d) 0.08

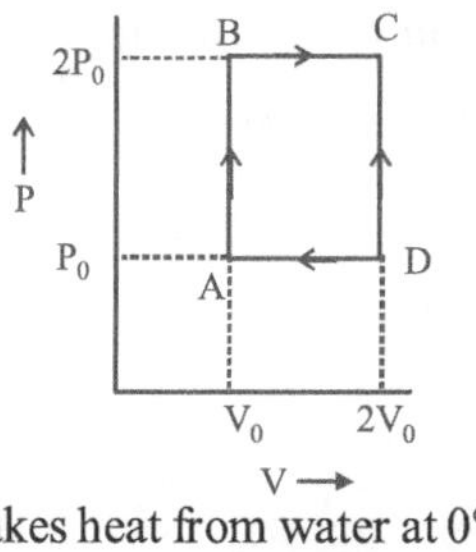

30. A Carnot freezer takes heat from water at 0°C inside it and rejects it to the room at a temperature of 27°C. The latent heat of ice is $336 \times 10^3\ J\ kg^{-1}$. If 5 kg of water at 0°C is converted into ice at 0°C by the freezer, then the energy consumed by the freezer is close to : **[Online April 10, 2016]**
(a) $1.51 \times 10^5\ J$ (b) $1.68 \times 10^6\ J$
(c) $1.71 \times 10^7\ J$ (d) $1.67 \times 10^5\ J$

31. A solid body of constant heat capacity 1 J/°C is being heated by keeping it in contact with reservoirs in two ways : **[2015]**
(i) Sequentially keeping in contact with 2 reservoirs such that each reservoir supplies same amount of heat.
(ii) Sequentially keeping in contact with 8 reservoirs such that each reservoir supplies same amount of heat.

In both the cases body is brought from initial temperature 100°C to final temperature 200°C. Entropy change of the body in the two cases respectively is :
(a) *ln2, 2ln2* (b) *2ln2, 8ln2*
(c) *ln2, 4ln2* (d) *ln2, ln2*

32. A Carnot engine absorbs 1000 J of heat energy from a reservoir at 127°C and rejects 600 J of heat energy during each cycle. The efficiency of engine and temperature of sink will be: **[Online April 12, 2014]**
(a) 20% and −43°C (b) 40% and −33°C
(c) 50% and −20°C (d) 70% and −10°C

33.

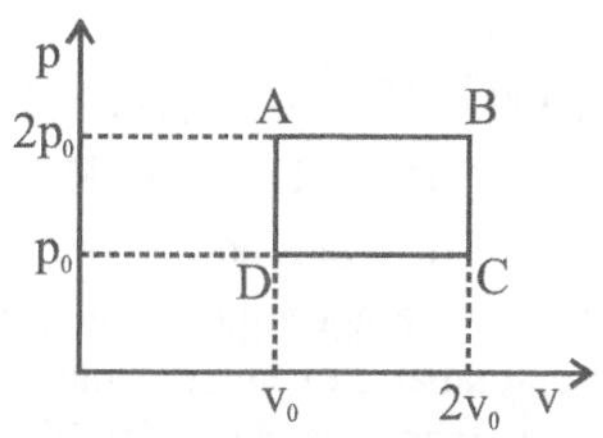

The above p-v diagramrepresents the thermodynamic cycle of an engine, operating with an ideal monatomic gas. The amount of heat, extracted from the source in a single cycle is **[2013]**

(a) $p_0 v_0$ (b) $\left(\frac{13}{2}\right) p_0 v_0$

(c) $\left(\frac{11}{2}\right) p_0 v_0$ (d) $4 p_0 v_0$

34. A Carnot engine, whose efficiency is 40%, takes in heat from a source maintained at a temperature of 500K. It is desired to have an engine of efficiency 60%. Then, the intake temperature for the same exhaust (sink) temperature must be : **[2012]**
(a) efficiency of Carnot engine cannot be made larger than 50%
(b) 1200 K
(c) 750 K
(d) 600 K

35. The door of a working refrigerator is left open in a well insulated room. The temperature of air in the room will **[Online May 26, 2012]**
(a) decrease
(b) increase in winters and decrease in summers
(c) remain the same
(d) increase

36. This question has Statement 1 and Statement 2. Of the four choices given after the Statements, choose the one that best describes the two Statements.
Statement 1: An inventor claims to have constructed an engine that has an efficiency of 30% when operated between the boiling and freezing points of water. This is not possible.
Statement 2: The efficiency of a real engine is always less than the efficiency of a Carnot engine operating between the same two temperatures. **[Online May 19, 2012]**
(a) Statement 1 is true, Statement 2 is true, Statement 2 is not the correct explanation of Statement 1.
(b) Statement 1 is true, Statement 2 is false.
(c) Statement 1 is false, Statement 2 is true.
(d) Statement 1 is true, Statement 2 is true, Statement 2 is the correct explanation of Statement 1.

37. A Carnot engine operating between temperatures T_1 and T_2 has efficiency $\frac{1}{6}$. When T_2 is lowered by 62 K its efficiency increases to $\frac{1}{3}$. Then T_1 and T_2 are, respectively: **[2011]**
(a) 372 K and 310 K (b) 330 K and 268 K
(c) 310 K and 248 K (d) 372 K and 310 K

38. A diatomic ideal gas is used in a Carnot engine as the working substance. If during the adiabatic expansion part of the cycle the volume of the gas increases from V to 32 V, the efficiency of the engine is **[2010]**
(a) 0.5 (b) 0.75 (c) 0.99 (d) 0.25

39. A Carnot engine, having an efficiency of $\eta = 1/10$ as heat engine, is used as a refrigerator. If the work done on the system is 10 J, the amount of energy absorbed from the reservoir at lower temperature is **[2007]**
(a) 100 J (b) 99 J (c) 90 J (d) 1 J

40. The temperature-entropy diagram of a reversible engine cycle is given in the figure. Its efficiency is **[2005]**

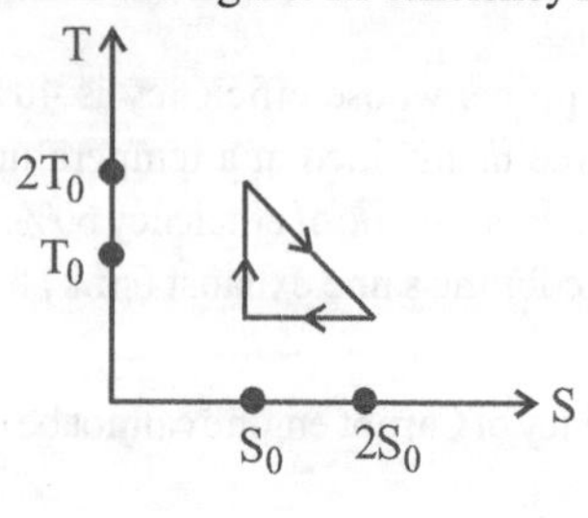

(a) $\frac{1}{4}$ (b) $\frac{1}{2}$
(c) $\frac{2}{3}$ (d) $\frac{1}{3}$

41. Which of the following statements is **correct** for any thermodynamic system ? **[2004]**
(a) The change in entropy can never be zero
(b) Internal energy and entropy are state functions
(c) The internal energy changes in all processes
(d) The work done in an adiabatic process is always zero.

42. "Heat cannot by itself flow from a body at lower temperature to a body at higher temperature" is a statement or consequence of **[2003]**
(a) second law of thermodynamics
(b) conservation of momentum
(c) conservation of mass
(d) first law of thermodynamics

43. A Carnot engine takes 3×10^6 cal of heat from a reservoir at $627^\circ C$, and gives it to a sink at $27^\circ C$. The work done by the engine is **[2003]**
(a) 4.2×10^6 J (b) 8.4×10^6 J
(c) 16.8×10^6 J (d) zero

44. Which statement is incorrect? **[2002]**
(a) All reversible cycles have same efficiency
(b) Reversible cycle has more efficiency than an irreversible one
(c) Carnot cycle is a reversible one
(d) Carnot cycle has the maximum efficiency in all cycles

45. Even Carnot engine cannot give 100% efficiency because we cannot **[2002]**
(a) prevent radiation
(b) find ideal sources
(c) reach absolute zero temperature
(d) eliminate friction

Hints & Solutions

TOPIC-1 : First Law of Thermodynamics

1. (d) Volume of water does not change, no work is done on or by the system (W = 0)
According to first law of thermodynamics
$Q = \Delta U + W$
For Isochoric process $Q = \Delta U$
$\Delta U = \mu c dT = 2 \times 4184 \times 20 = 16.7$ kJ.

2. (a) As we know,
$\Delta Q = \Delta u + \Delta w$ (Ist law of thermodynamics)
$\Rightarrow \Delta Q = \Delta u + P\Delta v$
or $150 = \Delta u + 100(1-2)$
$= \Delta u - 100$
$\therefore \Delta u = 150 + 100 = 250J$
Thus the internal energy of the gas increases by 250 J

3. (a) Here $Q = 0$ and $W = 0$. Therefore from first law of thermodynamics $\Delta U = Q + W = 0$
$\therefore$ Internal energy of the system with partition = Internal energy of the system without partition.
$$n_1 C_v T_1 + n_2 C_v T_2 = (n_1 + n_2) C_v T$$
$$\therefore T = \frac{n_1 T_1 + n_2 T_2}{n_1 + n_2}$$
But $n_1 = \frac{P_1 V_1}{RT_1}$ and $n_2 = \frac{P_2 V_2}{RT_2}$
$$\therefore T = \frac{\frac{P_1 V_1}{RT_1} \times T_1 + \frac{P_2 V_2}{RT_2} \times T_2}{\frac{P_1 V_1}{RT_1} + \frac{P_2 V_2}{RT_2}}$$
$$= \frac{T_1 T_2 (P_1 V_1 + P_2 V_2)}{P_1 V_1 T_2 + P_2 V_2 T_1}$$

4. (b) For path iaf, $Q = 50$ cal, $W = 20$ cal

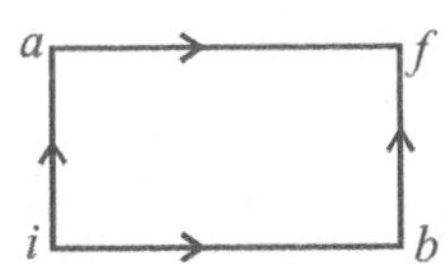

By first law of thermodynamics,
$\Delta U = Q - W = 50 - 20 = 30$ cal.
For path ibf
$Q = 36$ cal
$W = ?$
or, $W = Q - \Delta U$
(Since, the change in internal energy does not depend on the path, therefore $\Delta U = 30$ cal)
$\therefore W = Q - \Delta U = 36 - 30 = 6$ cal.

5. (b) Change in internal energy do not depend upon the path followed by the process. It only depends on initial and final states i.e.,
$$\Delta U_1 = \Delta U_2$$

6. (b) First law is applicable to a cyclic process. Concept of entropy is introduced by the second law.

TOPIC-2 : Specific Heat Capacity and Thermodynamical Processes

7. (c) The equation for the line is

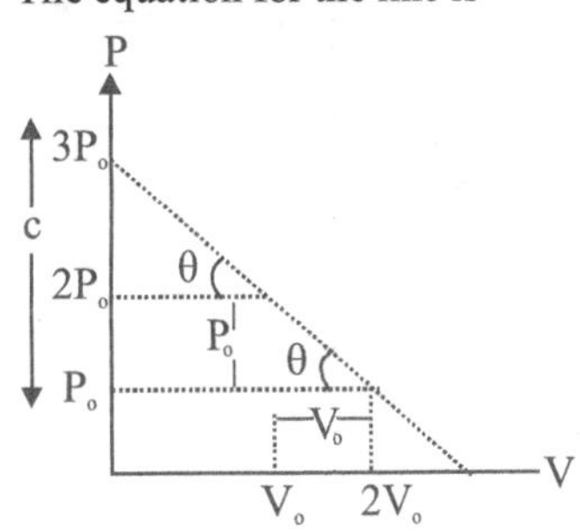

$$P = \frac{-P_0}{V_0} V + 3P$$
$$\left[\text{slope} = \frac{-P_0}{V_0}, \ c = 3P_0\right]$$
$PV_0 + P_0 V = 3P_0 V_0$ ...(i)
But $pv = nRT$
$\therefore p = \frac{nRT}{v}$ ...(ii)
From (i) & (ii) $\frac{nRT}{v} V_0 + P_0 V = 3P_0 V_0$
$\therefore nRT V_0 + P_0 V^2 = 3P_0 V_0$ ...(iii)
For temperature to be maximum $\frac{dT}{dv} = 0$
Differentiating e.q. (iii) by 'v' we get
$$nRV_0 \frac{dT}{dv} + P_0(2v) = 3P_0 V_0$$

$$\therefore nRV_0 \frac{dT}{dv} = 3P_0V_0 - 2P_0V$$

$$\frac{dT}{dv} = \frac{3P_0V_0 - 2P_0V}{nRV_0} = 0$$

$$V = \frac{3V_0}{2} \quad \therefore p = \frac{3P_0}{2}$$ [From (i)]

$$\therefore T_{max} = \frac{9P_0V_0}{4nR}$$ [From (iii)]

8. (a) Efficiency of heat engine is given by

$$\eta = \frac{w}{Q} = 1 - \frac{C_V}{C_P} = \frac{R}{C_p} = \frac{R}{\frac{5R}{2}} = \frac{2}{5}$$

$(\because C_p - C_v = R)$

For monoatomic gas $C_P = \frac{5}{2}R$.

9. (a) $$\tau = \frac{1}{\sqrt{2}\pi d^2 \left(\frac{N}{V}\right)\sqrt{\frac{3RT}{M}}}$$

$$\tau \propto \frac{V}{\sqrt{T}}$$

As, $TV^{\gamma-1} = K$

So, $\tau \propto V^{\gamma + 1/2}$

Therefore, $q = \frac{\gamma+1}{2}$

10. (a) As, $P = \frac{1}{3}\left(\frac{U}{V}\right)$

But $\frac{U}{V} = KT^4$

So, $P = \frac{1}{3}KT^4$

or $\frac{uRT}{V} = \frac{1}{3}KT^4$ [As $PV = uRT$]

$$\frac{4}{3}\pi R^3T^3 = \text{constant}$$

Therefore, $T \propto \frac{1}{R}$

11. (b) In *VT* graph

ab-process : Isobaric, temperature increases.
bc process : Adiabatic, pressure decreases.
cd process : Isobaric, volume decreases.
da process : Adiabatic, pressure increases.
The above processes correctly represented in *P-V* diagram (b).

12. (d) In cyclic process, change in total internal energy is zero.

$$\Delta U_{cyclic} = 0$$

$$\Delta U_{BC} = nC_v\Delta T = 1 \times \frac{5R}{2}\Delta T$$

Where, C_v = molar specific heat at constant volume.

For BC, $\Delta T = -200$ K

$\therefore \Delta U_{BC} = -500R$

13. (c)

14. (c) **Given :** work done, $W = 830$ J

No. of moles of gas, $\mu = 2$

For diatomic gas $\gamma = 1.4$

Work done during an adiabatic change

$$W = \frac{\mu R(T_1 - T_2)}{\gamma - 1}$$

$$\Rightarrow 830 = \frac{2 \times 8.3(\Delta T)}{1.4 - 1} = \frac{2 \times 8.3(\Delta T)}{0.4}$$

$$\Rightarrow \Delta T = \frac{830 \times 0.4}{2 \times 8.3} = 20 \text{ K}$$

15. (a)

16. (c) P-V indicator diagram for isobaric

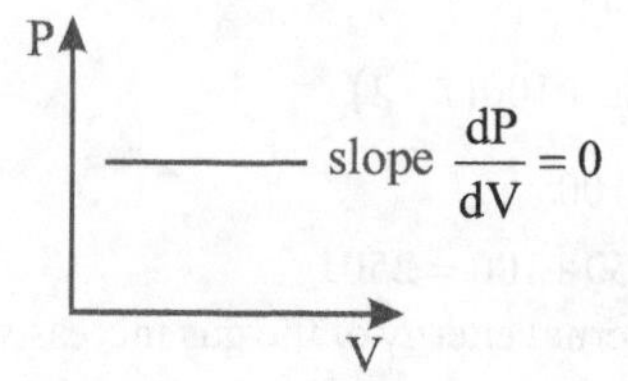

P-V indicator diagram for isochoric process

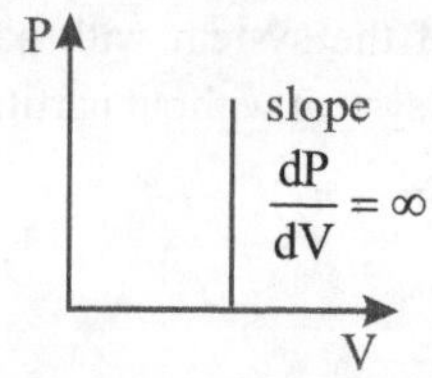

P-V indicator diagram for isothermal process

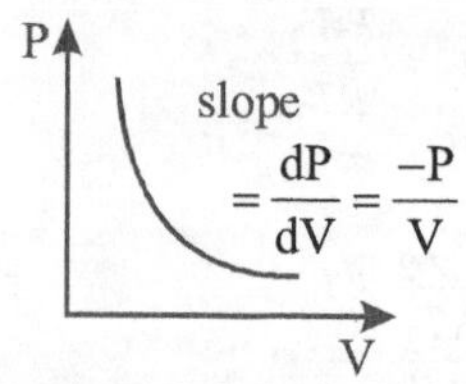

17. (b) Volume of the gas

$V = \frac{m}{d}$ and

using PV^γ = constant

$$\frac{P'}{P} = \frac{V}{V'} = \left(\frac{d'}{d}\right)^\gamma$$

or $128 = (32)^\gamma$

$$\therefore \gamma = \frac{7}{5} = 1.4$$

18. (a) The efficiency $\eta = \frac{\text{output work}}{\text{input work}}$

Input work = Work done in going A to B + workdone in going B to C and the work done in going C to D.

$$W_i = \frac{n}{2}(P_0V_0) + \frac{n}{2}(2P_0V_0) + 2P_0V_0$$

where n = degree of freedom

which is 3 for mono-atomic gases like He

$$= \left(\frac{3}{2} + \frac{3}{2}.2 + 2\right)P_0V_0$$

$$= \left(\frac{3+10}{2}\right)P_0V_0 = \frac{13}{2}P_0V_0$$

and $W_0 = P_0V_0$

$$\eta = \frac{P_0V_0}{\frac{13}{2}P_0V_0} = \frac{2}{13}$$

Efficiency in %

$$\eta = \frac{2}{13} \times 100 = \frac{200}{13} \simeq 15.4\%$$

19. **(d)** For isothermal process :

$PV = P_i\, 2V$

$P = 2P_i$ ...(i)

For adiabatic process

$PV^\gamma = P_a\,(2V)^\gamma$

($\because$ for monatomic gas $\gamma = 5/3$)

or, $2P_iV^{\frac{5}{3}} = P_a(2V)^{\frac{5}{3}}$ [From (i)]

$$\Rightarrow \frac{P_a}{P_i} = \frac{2}{2^{\frac{5}{3}}}$$

$$\Rightarrow \frac{P_a}{P_i} = 2^{\frac{-2}{3}}$$

20. **(d)** Given $P = \alpha V$

Work done, $w = \int_V^{mV} PdV$

$$= \int_V^{mV} \alpha V dV = \frac{\alpha V^2}{2}(m^2 - 1).$$

21. **(b)** Work done during the process $A \to B$

= Area of trapezium (= area bounded by indicator diagram with V-axis)

$$= \frac{1}{2}(2P_0 + P_0)(2V_0 - V_0) = \frac{3}{2}P_0V_0$$

Ideal gas eqn : $PV = nRT$

$$\Rightarrow T = \frac{PV}{nR} = \frac{3P_0V_0}{2nR}$$

22. **(b)** In an adiabatic process, $\delta H = 0$

And according to first law of thermodynamics

$\delta H = \delta U + W$

$\therefore W = -\delta U$

23. **(d)**

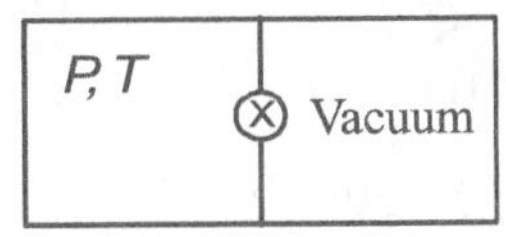

It is the free expansion

$\therefore$ So, T remains constant

$\Rightarrow P_1V_1 = P_2V_2$

$\Rightarrow P\frac{V}{2} = P_2(V)$

$$P_2 = \left(\frac{P}{2}\right)$$

24. **(b)** A to B is an isobaric process. The work done

$W = nR(T_2 - T_1)$

$= 2R(500 - 300) = 400R$

25. **(a)** Work done by the system intheisothermal process

DA is $W = 2.303\,nRT\,\log_{10}\frac{P_D}{P_A}$

$= 2.303 \times 2\ R \times 300$

$\log_{10}\frac{1 \times 10^5}{2 \times 10^5} - 414\text{R}.$

Therefore, work done on the gas is + 414 R.

26. **(a)** The net work in the cycle $ABCDA$ is

$$W = W_{AB} + W_{BC} + W_{CD} + W_{DA}$$

$$= 400R + 2.303nRT\log\frac{P_B}{P_C} + (-400R) - 414R$$

$$= 2.303 \times 2R \times 500\log\frac{2 \times 10^5}{1 \times 10^5} - 414R$$

$= 693.2\,R - 414\,R\quad = 279.2\,R$

27. **(a)** $W = \frac{nR\Delta T}{1-\gamma} \Rightarrow -146000 = \frac{1000 \times 8.3 \times 7}{1-\gamma}$

or $1 - \gamma = -\frac{58.1}{146} \Rightarrow \gamma = 1 + \frac{58.1}{146} = 1.4$

Hence the gas is diatomic.

28. **(c)** Work is a path function. The remaining three parameters are state function.

TOPIC-3 : Carnot Engine, Refrigerators and Second Law of Thermodynamics

29. **(b)** Work-done $(W) = P_0V_0$

According to principle of calorimetry

Heat given $= Q_{AB} = Q_{BC}$

$= nC_v dT_{AB} + nC_p dT_{BC}$

$= \frac{3}{2}(nRT_B - nRT_A) + \frac{5}{2}(nRT_C - nRT_B)$

$= \frac{3}{2}(2P_0V_0 - P_0V_0) + \frac{5}{2}(4P_0V_0 - 2P_0V)$

$= \frac{13}{2}P_0V_0$

Thermal efficiency of engine $(\eta) = \frac{W}{Q_{given}} = \frac{2}{13} = 0.15$

30. **(d)** $\Delta H = mL = 5 \times 336 \times 10^3 = Q_{sink}$

$$\frac{Q_{sink}}{Q_{source}} = \frac{T_{sink}}{T_{source}}$$

$$\therefore Q_{source} = \frac{T_{source}}{T_{sink}} \times Q_{sink}$$

Energy consumed by freezer

$$\therefore W_{output} = Q_{source} - Q_{sink} = Q_{sink}\left(\frac{T_{source}}{T_{sink}} - 1\right)$$

Given: $T_{source} = 27°C + 273 = 300K$,

$T_{sink} = 0°C + 273 = 273\,k$

$$W_{output} = 5 \times 336 \times 10^3\left(\frac{300}{273} - 1\right) = 1.67 \times 10^5\,J$$

31. **(d)** The entropy change of the body in the two cases is same as entropy is a state function.

32. **(b)** Given: $Q_1 = 1000\,J$

$Q_2 = 600\,J$

$T_1 = 127°C = 400\,K$

$T_2 = ?$

$\eta = ?$

Efficiency of carnot engine,

$$\eta = \frac{W}{Q_1} \times 100\%$$

or, $\eta = \frac{Q_2 - Q_1}{Q_1} \times 100\%$

or, $\eta = \frac{1000 - 600}{1000} \times 100\%$

$\eta = 40\%$

Now, for carnot cycle $\frac{Q_2}{Q_1} = \frac{T_2}{T_1}$

$$\frac{600}{1000} = \frac{T_2}{400}$$

$$T_2 = \frac{600 \times 400}{1000}$$

$= 240\,K$

$= 240 - 273$

$\therefore T_2 = -33°C$

33. **(b)** Heat is extracted from the source in path DA and AB is

$$\Delta Q = \frac{3}{2}R\left(\frac{P_0V_0}{R}\right) + \frac{5}{2}R\left(\frac{2P_0V_0}{R}\right)$$

$$\Rightarrow \frac{3}{2}P_0V_0 + \frac{5}{2}2P_0V_0 = \left(\frac{13}{2}\right)P_0V_0$$

34. **(c)** The efficiency of the engine is given as

$$\eta = \left(1 - \frac{T_2}{T_1}\right) \times 100$$

For first case

$T_1 = 500\,K;\ \eta = 40$

$$40 = \left(1 - \frac{T_2}{500}\right) \times 100$$

$$\Rightarrow \frac{40}{100} = 1 - \frac{T_2}{500}$$

$$\Rightarrow \frac{T_2}{500} = \frac{60}{100} \Rightarrow T_2 = 300\,K$$

For second case :

$$\frac{60}{100} = \left(1 - \frac{300}{T_2}\right)$$

$$\frac{300}{T_2} = \frac{40}{100}$$

$$\Rightarrow T_2 = \frac{100 \times 300}{40} \rightarrow T_2 = 750\,K$$

35. **(d)** In a refrigerator, the heat dissipated in the atmosphere is more than that taken from the cooling chamber, therefore the room is heated. If the door of a refrigerator is kept open.

36. **(d)** According to Carnot's theorem - no heat engine working between two given temperatures of source and sink can be more efficient than a perfectly reversible engine i.e. Carnot engine working between the same two temperatures.

Efficiency of Carnot's engine, $n = 1 - \frac{T_2}{T_1}$

where, T_1 = temperature of source

T_2 = temperature of sink

37. **(d)** Efficiency of engine

$\eta_1 = 1 - \frac{T_2}{T_1}$

$\Rightarrow \frac{T_2}{T_1} = \frac{5}{6}$ ....(i)

Again, $\eta_2 = 1 - \frac{T_2 - 62}{T_1} = \frac{1}{3}$ ....(ii)

Solving (i) and (ii), we get,

$T_1 = 372$ K and $T_2 = \frac{5}{6} \times 372 = 310$ K

38. **(b)**

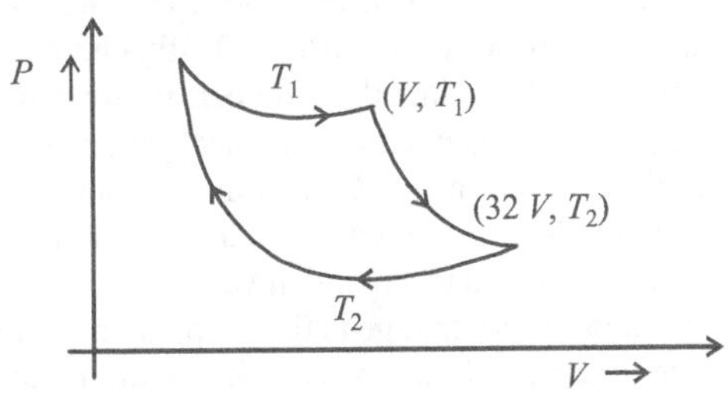

We have, $TV^{\gamma-1}$ = constant

$\Rightarrow T_1 V^{\gamma-1} = T_2 (32V)^{\gamma-1}$

$\Rightarrow T_1 = (32)^{\gamma-1} . T_2$

For diatomic gas, $\gamma = \frac{7}{5}$

$\therefore \gamma - 1 = \frac{2}{5}$

$\therefore T_1 = (32)^{\frac{2}{5}} . T_2 \Rightarrow T_1 = 4T_2$

Now, efficiency $= 1 - \frac{T_2}{T_1}$

$= 1 - \frac{T_2}{4T_2} = 1 - \frac{1}{4} = \frac{3}{4} = 0.75.$

39. **(c)** The efficiency (η) of a Carnot engine and the coefficient of performance (β) of a refrigerator are related as

$\beta = \frac{1-\eta}{\eta}$ Here, $\eta = \frac{1}{10}$

$\therefore \beta = \frac{1 - \frac{1}{10}}{\left(\frac{1}{10}\right)} = 9.$

Also, Coefficient of performance (β) is given by

$\beta = \frac{Q_2}{W}$, where Q_2 is the energy absorbed from the reservoir.

or, $9 = \frac{Q_2}{10}$ $\therefore Q_2 = 90$ J.

40. **(d)** $Q_1 = T_0 S_0 + \frac{1}{2} T_0 S_0$

$= \frac{3}{2} T_0 S_0$

$Q_2 = T_0 (2S_0 - S_0)$
$= T_0 S_0$

and $Q_3 = 0$

$\eta = \frac{W}{Q_1} = \frac{Q_1 - Q_2}{Q_1}$

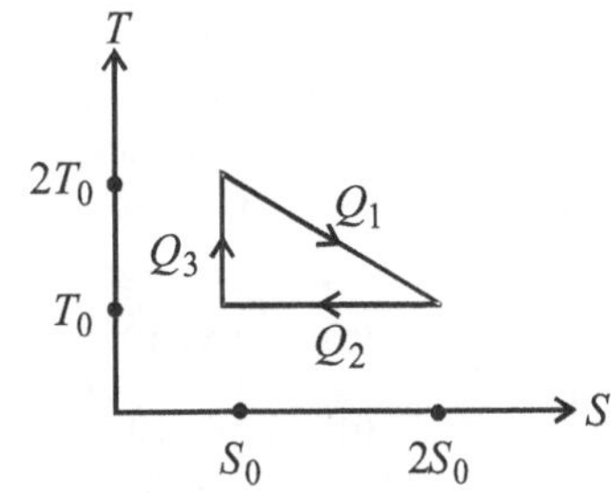

$= 1 - \frac{Q_2}{Q_1} = 1 - \frac{T_0 S_0}{\frac{3}{2} T_0 S_0} = \frac{1}{3}$

41. **(b)** Internal energy and entropy are state function, they do not depend upon path taken.

42. **(a)** This is a statement of second law of thermodynamics

43. **(b)** $\eta = 1 - \frac{T_2}{T_1} = 1 - \frac{(273+27)}{(273+627)} = 1 - \frac{300}{900} = 1 - \frac{1}{3} = \frac{2}{3}$

But $\eta = \frac{W}{Q}$

$\therefore \frac{W}{Q} = \frac{2}{3} \Rightarrow W = \frac{2}{3} \times Q = \frac{2}{3} \times 3 \times 10^6$

$= 2 \times 10^6 \text{cal} = 2 \times 10^6 \times 4.2 \text{ J} = 8.4 \times 10^6 \text{ J}$

44. **(a)** All reversible engines working for the same temperature of source and sink have same efficiencies. If the temperatures are different, the efficiency is different.

45. **(c)** In Carnot's cycle we assume frictionless piston, absolute insulation and ideal source and sink (reservoirs). The efficiency of carnot's cycle is given by $\eta = 1 - \frac{T_2}{T_1}$

For $\eta = 1$ or 100 %, $T_2 = 0$ K.

The temperature of 0 K (absolute zero) can not be obtained .

Chapter 12

Kinetic Theory

TOPIC-1 : Kinetic Theory of an Ideal Gas and Gas Laws

1. The temperature of an open room of volume 30 m^3 increases from 17°C to 27°C due to sunshine. The atmospheric pressure in the room remains 1×10^5 Pa. If n_i and n_f are the number of molecules in the room before and after heating, then $n_f - n_i$ will be : **[2017]**

(a) 2.5×10^{25} (b) -2.5×10^{25}

(c) -1.61×10^{23} (d) 1.38×10^{23}

2. For the P-V diagram given for an ideal gas,

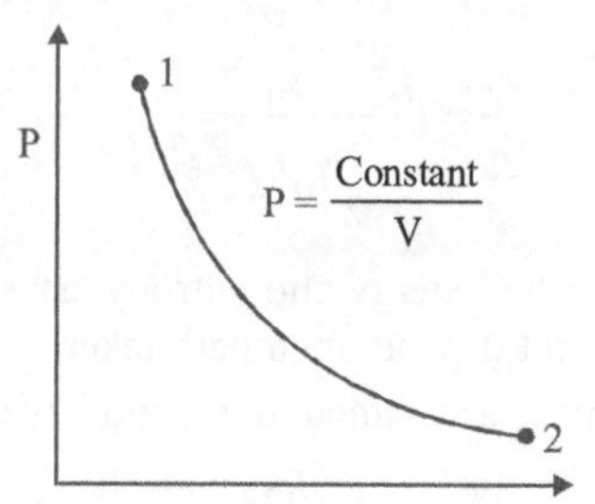

out of the following which one correctly represents the T-P diagram? **[Online April 9, 2017]**

(a) 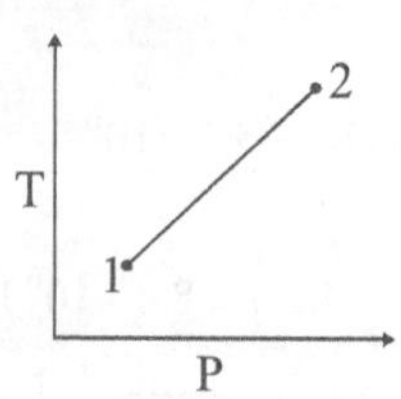

(b) 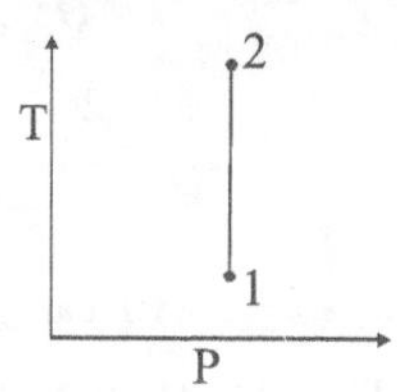

(c) 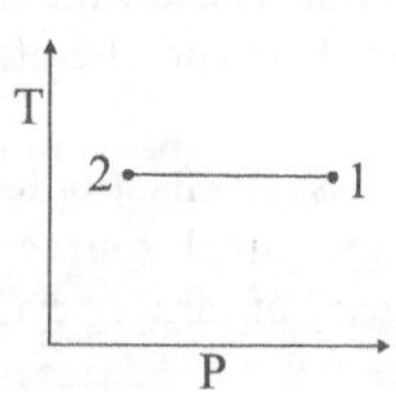

(d) 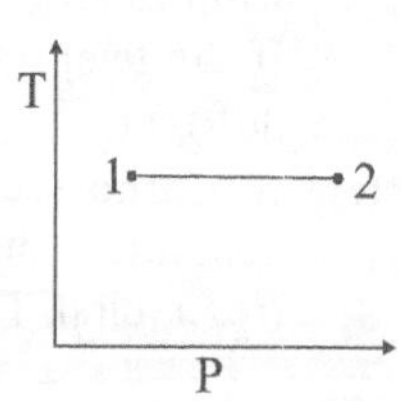

3. 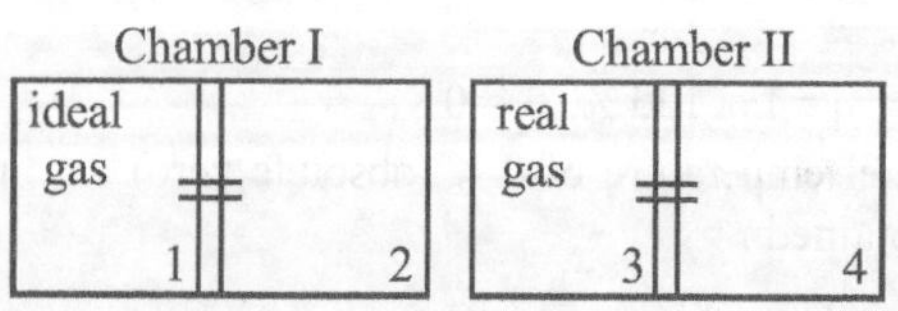

There are two identical chambers, completely thermally insulated from surroundings. Both chambers have a partition wall dividing the chambers in two compartments. Compartment 1 is filled with an ideal gas and Compartment 3 is filled with a real gas. Compartments 2 and 4 are vacuum. A small hole (orifice) is made in the partition walls and the gases are allowed to expand in vacuum.

Statement-1: No change in the temperature of the gas takes place when ideal gas expands in vacuum. However, the temperature of real gas goes down (cooling) when it expands in vacuum.

Statement-2: The internal energy of an ideal gas is only kinetic. The internal energy of a real gas is kinetic as well as potential. **[Online April 9, 2013]**

(a) Statement-1 is false and Statement-2 is true.
(b) Statement-1 and Statement-2 both are true. Statement-2 is the correct explanation of Statement-1.
(c) Statement-1 is true and Statement-2 is false.
(d) Statement-1 and Statement-2 both are true. Statement-2 is **not** correct explanation of Statement-1.

4. Cooking gas containers are kept in a lorry moving with uniform speed. The temperature of the gas molecules inside will **[2002]**

(a) increase
(b) decrease
(c) remain same
(d) decrease for some, while increase for others

TOPIC-2 : Speed of Gas, Pressure and Kinetic Energy

5. N moles of a diatomic gas in a cylinder are at a temperature T. Heat is supplied to the cylinder such that the temperature remains constant but n moles of the diatomic gas get converted into monoatomic gas. What is the change in the total kinetic energy of the gas ? **[Online April 9, 2017]**

(a) $\frac{1}{2}nRT$ (b) 0 (c) $\frac{3}{2}nRT$ (d) $\frac{5}{2}nRT$

6. In an ideal gas at temperature T, the average force that a molecule applies on the walls of a closed container depends on T as T^q. A good estimate for q is: **[Online April 10, 2015]**

(a) $\frac{1}{2}$ (b) 2

(c) 1 (d) $\frac{1}{4}$

7. A gas molecule of mass M at the surface of the Earth has kinetic energy equivalent to 0°C. If it were to go up straight without colliding with any other molecules, how high it would rise? Assume that the height attained is much less than radius of the earth. (k_B is Boltzmann constant). **[Online April 19, 2014]**

(a) 0 (b) $\frac{273k_B}{2Mg}$

(c) $\frac{546k_B}{3Mg}$ (d) $\frac{819k_B}{2Mg}$

8. At room temperature a diatomic gas is found to have an r.m.s. speed of 1930 ms^{-1}. The gas is: **[Online April 12, 2014]**

(a) H_2 (b) Cl_2 (c) O_2 (d) F_2

9. In the isothermal expansion of 10g of gas from volume V to 2V the work done by the gas is 575J. What is the root mean square speed of the molecules of the gas at that temperature? **[Online April 25, 2013]**

(a) 398m/s (b) 520m/s
(c) 499m/s (d) 532m/s

10. A perfect gas at 27°C is heated at constant pressure so as to double its volume. The final temperature of the gas will be, close to **[Online May 7, 2012]**

(a) 327°C (b) 200°C (c) 54°C (d) 300°C

11. A thermally insulated vessel contains an ideal gas of molecular mass M and ratio of specific heats γ. It is moving with speed v and it's suddenly brought to rest. Assuming no heat is lost to the surroundings, its temperature increases by: **[2011]**

(a) $\frac{(\gamma-1)}{2\gamma R}Mv^2K$ (b) $\frac{\gamma M^2 v}{2R}K$

(c) $\frac{(\gamma-1)}{2R}Mv^2K$ (d) $\frac{(\gamma-1)}{2(\gamma+1)R}Mv^2K$

12. Three perfect gases at absolute temperatures T_1, T_2 and T_3 are mixed. The masses of molecules are m_1, m_2 and m_3 and the number of molecules are n_1, n_2 and n_3 respectively. Assuming no loss of energy, the final temperature of the mixture is: **[2011]**

(a) $\frac{n_1T_1+n_2T_2+n_3T_3}{n_1+n_2+n_3}$ (b) $\frac{n_1T_1^2+n_2T_2^2+n_3T_3^2}{n_1T_1+n_2T_2+n_3T_3}$

(c) $\frac{n_1^2T_1^2+n_2^2T_2^2+n_3^2T_3^2}{n_1T_1+n_2T_2+n_3T_3}$ (d) $\frac{(T_1+T_2+T_3)}{3}$

13. One kg of a diatomic gas is at a pressure of $8\times10^4 N/m^2$. The density of the gas is $4 kg/m^3$. What is the energy of the gas due to its thermal motion? **[2009]**

(a) 5×10^4 J (b) 6×10^4 J
(c) 7×10^4 J (d) 3×10^4 J

14. The speed of sound in oxygen (O_2) at a certain temperature is 460 ms^{-1}. The speed of sound in helium (He) at the same temperature will be (assume both gases to be ideal) **[2008]**

(a) 1421 ms^{-1} (b) 500 ms^{-1}
(c) 650 ms^{-1} (d) 330 ms^{-1}

15. At what temperature is the r.m.s velocity of a hydrogen molecule equal to that of an oxygen molecule at 47°C? **[2002]**

(a) 80 K (b) –73 K (c) 3 K (d) 20 K

TOPIC-3 : Degree of Freedom, Specific Heat Capacity, and Mean Free Path

16. C_p and C_v are specific heats at constant pressure and constant volume respectively. It is observed that
$C_p - C_v = a$ for hydrogen gas
$C_p - C_v = b$ for nitrogen gas
The correct relation between a and b is: **[2017]**

(a) a = 14 b (b) a = 28 b
(c) $a = \frac{1}{14}b$ (d) a = b

17. An ideal gas has molecules with 5 degrees of freedom. The ratio of specific heats at constant pressure (C_p) and at constant volume (C_v) is: **[Online April 8, 2017]**

(a) 6 (b) $\frac{7}{2}$ (c) $\frac{5}{2}$ (d) $\frac{7}{5}$

18. An ideal gas undergoes a quasi static, reversible process in which its molar heat capacity C remains constant. If during this process the relation of pressure P and volume V is given by PV^n = constant, then n is given by (Here C_P and C_V are molar specific heat at constant pressure and constant volume, respectively): **[2016]**

(a) $n=\frac{C_P-C}{C-C_V}$ (b) $n=\frac{C-C_V}{C-C_P}$

(c) $n=\frac{C_P}{C_V}$ (d) $n=\frac{C-C_P}{C-C_V}$

19. Using equipartition of energy, the specific heat (in J kg^{-1} K^{-1}) of aluminium at room temperature can be estimated to be (atomic weight of aluminium = 27) **[Online April 11, 2015]**

(a) 410 (b) 25
(c) 1850 (d) 925

20. Modern vacuum pumps can evacuate a vessel down to a pressure of 4.0×10^{-15} atm. at room temperature (300 K). Taking R = 8.0 JK^{-1} $mole^{-1}$, 1 atm = 10^5 Pa and $N_{Avogadro} = 6\times10^{23}$ $mole^{-1}$, the mean distance between molecules of gas in an evacuated vessel will be of the order of: **[Online April 9, 2014]**

(a) 0.2 μm (b) 0.2 mm (c) 0.2 cm (d) 0.2 nm

21. Figure shows the variation in temperature (ΔT) with the amount of heat supplied (Q) in an isobaric process corresponding to a monoatomic (M), diatomic (D) and a polyatomic (P) gas. The initial state of all the gases are the same and the scales for the two axes coincide. Ignoring vibrational degrees of freedom, the lines a, b and c respectively correspond to: **[Online April 9, 2013]**

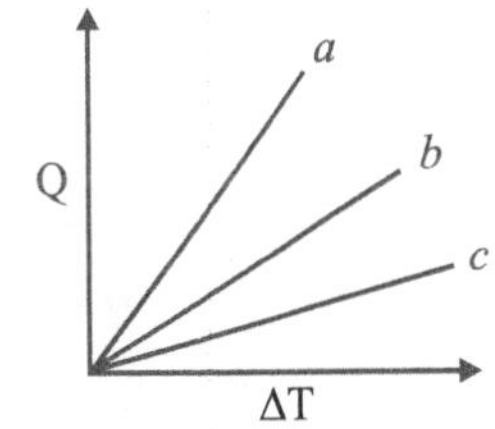

(a) P, M and D (b) M, D and P
(c) P, D and M (d) D, M and P

22. A given ideal gas with $\gamma = \frac{C_p}{C_v} = 1.5$ at a temperature T. If the gas is compressed adiabatically to one-fourth of its initial volume, the final temperature will be **[Online May 12, 2012]**

(a) $2\sqrt{2}T$ (b) $4T$ (c) $2T$ (d) $8T$

23. If C_P and C_V denote the specific heats of nitrogen per unit mass at constant pressure and constant volume respectively, then **[2007]**

(a) $C_P - C_V = 28R$ (b) $C_P - C_V = R/28$

(c) $C_P - C_V = R/14$ (d) $C_P - C_V = R$

24. A gaseous mixture consists of 16 g of helium and 16 g of oxygen. The ratio $\frac{C_p}{C_v}$ of the mixture is **[2005]**

(a) 1.62 (b) 1.59 (c) 1.54 (d) 1.4

25. One mole of ideal monatomic gas $(\gamma = 5/3)$ is mixed with one mole of diatomic gas $(\gamma = 7/5)$. What is γ for the mixture? γ Denotes the ratio of specific heat at constant pressure, to that at constant volume **[2004]**

(a) 35/23 (b) 23/15 (c) 3/2 (d) 4/3

26. During an adiabatic process, the pressure of a gas is found to be proportional to the cube of its absolute temperature. The ratio C_P/C_V for the gas is **[2003]**

(a) $\frac{4}{3}$ (b) 2 (c) $\frac{5}{3}$ (d) $\frac{3}{2}$

Hints & Solutions

TOPIC-1 : Kinetic Theory of an Ideal Gas and Gas Laws

1. (b) Given: Temperature $T_i = 17 + 273 = 290\,K$
Temperature $T_f = 27 + 273 = 300\,K$
Atmospheric pressure, $P_0 = 1 \times 10^5\,Pa$
Volume of room, $V_0 = 30\,m^3$
Difference in number of molecules, $N_f - N_i = ?$
The number of molecules

$$\Rightarrow N = \frac{PV}{RT}(N_0)$$

$$\therefore N_f - N_i = \frac{P_0V_0}{R}\left(\frac{1}{T_f} - \frac{1}{T_i}\right) N_0$$

$$= \frac{1\times10^5\times30}{8.314}\times6.023\times10^{23}\left(\frac{1}{300} - \frac{1}{290}\right)$$

$$= -2.5 \times 10^{25}$$

2. (c) From P-V graph,

$$P \propto \frac{1}{V},\quad T = \text{constant}$$

and Pressure is increasing from 2 to 1 so option (3) represents correct T-P graph.

3. (a) In ideal gases the molecules are considered as point particles and for point particles, there is no internal excitation, no vibration and no rotation. For an ideal gas the internal energy can only be translational kinetic energy and for real gas both kinetic as well as potential energy.

4. (c) Since P and V are not changing, so temperature remain same.

TOPIC-2 : Speed of Gas, Pressure and Kinetic Energy

5. (a) Energy associated with N moles of diatomic gas,

$$U_i = N\frac{5}{2}RT$$

Energy associated with n moles of monoatomic gas

$$= n\frac{3}{2}RT$$

Total energy when n moles of diatomic gas converted into monoatomic $(U_f) = 2n\frac{3}{2}RT + (N-n)\frac{5}{2}RT$

$$= \frac{1}{2}nRT + \frac{5}{2}NRT$$

Now, change in total kinetic energy of the gas

$$\Delta U = Q = \frac{1}{2}nRT$$

6. (c) Pressure, $P = \frac{1}{3}\frac{mN}{V}V_{rms}^2$

or, $P = \frac{(mN)T}{V}$

If the gas mass and temperature are constant then
$P \propto (V_{rms})^2 \propto T$
So, force $\propto (V_{rms})^2 \propto T$
i.e., Value of $q = 1$

7. (d) Kinetic energy of each molecule,

$$K.E. = \frac{3}{2}K_BT$$

In the given problem,
Temperature, T = 0°C = 273 K
Height attained by the gas molecule, h = ?

$$K.E. = \frac{3}{2}K_B(273) = \frac{819K_B}{2}$$

K.E. = P.E.

$$\Rightarrow \frac{819K_B}{2} = Mgh$$

$$\text{or } h = \frac{819K_B}{2Mg}$$

8. (a) $\because \quad C = \sqrt{\frac{3RT}{M}}$

$$(1930)^2 = \frac{3\times8.314\times300}{M}$$

$$M = \frac{3\times8.314\times300}{1930\times1930} \approx 2\times10^{-3}\,kg$$

The gas is H_2.

9. (c) $v_{rms} = \sqrt{\frac{3\rho v}{\text{mass of the gas}}}$

10. (a) Given, $V_1 = V$
$V_2 = 2V$
$T_1 = 27° + 273 = 300\,K$
$T_2 = ?$
From charle's law

$$\frac{V_1}{T_1} = \frac{V_2}{T_2} \quad (\because \text{Pressure is constant})$$

$$\text{or, } \frac{V}{300} = \frac{2V}{T_2}$$

$$\therefore T_2 = 600\,K = 600 - 273 = 327°C$$

11. (c) Here, work done is zero.
So, loss in kinetic energy = change in internal energy of gas

$$\frac{1}{2}mv^2 = nC_v\Delta T = n\frac{R}{\gamma-1}\Delta T$$

$$\frac{1}{2}mv^2 = \frac{m}{M}\frac{R}{\gamma-1}\Delta T$$

$$\therefore \Delta T = \frac{Mv^2(\gamma-1)}{2R}K$$

12. (a) Number of moles of first gas $= \frac{n_1}{N_A}$

Number of moles of second gas $= \frac{n_2}{N_A}$

Number of moles of third gas $= \frac{n_3}{N_A}$

If there is no loss of energy then
$P_1V_1 + P_2V_2 + P_3V_3 = PV$

$$\frac{n_1}{N_A}RT_1 + \frac{n_2}{N_A}RT_2 + \frac{n_3}{N_A}RT_3 = \frac{n_1+n_2+n_3}{N_A}RT_{mix}$$

$$T_{mix} = \frac{n_1T_1 + n_2T_2 + n_3T_3}{n_1+n_2+n_3}$$

13. (a) $K.E = \frac{5}{2}nRT = \frac{5}{2}\frac{m}{M}RT = \frac{5}{2}\frac{m}{M}\times\frac{PM}{d}$ $[\because PM = dRT]$

$$= \frac{5}{2}\frac{mP}{d} = \frac{5}{2}\times\frac{1\times8\times10^4}{4} = 5\times10^4\,J$$

14. (a) The speed of sound in a gas is given by $v = \sqrt{\frac{\gamma RT}{M}}$

$$\therefore \frac{v_{O_2}}{v_{He}} = \sqrt{\frac{\gamma_{O_2}}{M_{O_2}}\times\frac{M_{He}}{\gamma_{He}}}$$

$$= \sqrt{\frac{1.4}{32}\times\frac{4}{1.67}} = 0.3237$$

$$\therefore v_{He} = \frac{v_{O_2}}{0.3237} = \frac{460}{0.3237} = 1421\ \text{m/s}$$

15. (d) $v_{rms} = \sqrt{\frac{8RT}{\pi M}}$

For v_{rms} to be equal $\frac{T_{H_2}}{M_{H_2}} = \frac{T_{O_2}}{M_{O_2}}$

Here $M_{H_2} = 2;\ M_{O_2} = 32;$

$T_{O_2} = 47 + 273 = 320\,K$

$$\therefore \frac{T_{H_2}}{2} = \frac{320}{32} \Rightarrow T_{H_2} = 20\,K$$

TOPIC-3 : Degree of Freedom, Specific Heat Capacity, and Mean Free Path

16. (a) As we know, $C_p - C_v = R$ where C_p and C_v are molar specific heat capacities

or, $C_p - C_v = \frac{R}{M}$

For hydrogen ($M = 2$) $C_p - C_v = a = \frac{R}{2}$

For nitrogen ($M = 28$) $C_p - C_v = b = \frac{R}{28}$

$$\therefore \frac{a}{b} = 14 \text{ or, } a = 14b$$

17. (d) The ratio of specific heats at constant pressure (C_p) and constant volume (C_v)

$$\frac{C_p}{C_v} = \gamma = \left(1+\frac{2}{f}\right)$$

where f is degree of freedom

$$\frac{C_p}{C_v} = \left(1+\frac{2}{5}\right) = \frac{7}{5}$$

18. (d) For a polytropic process

$$C = C_v + \frac{R}{1-n} \quad \therefore C - C_v = \frac{R}{1-n}$$

$$\therefore 1-n = \frac{R}{C-C_v} \quad \therefore 1-\frac{R}{C-C_v} = n$$

$$\therefore n = \frac{C-C_v-R}{C-C_v} = \frac{C-C_v-C_p+C_v}{C-C_v}$$

$$= \frac{C-C_p}{C-C_v} \quad (\because C_p - C_{v=R})$$

19. (d) Using equipartition of energy, we have

$$\frac{6}{2}KT = mCT$$

$$C = \frac{3\times1.38\times10^{-23}\times6.02\times10^{23}}{27\times10^{-3}}$$

$\therefore C = 925$ J/kgK

20. (b)

21. (b) On giving same amount of heat at constant pressure, there is no change in temperature for mono, dia and polyatomic.

$$(\Delta Q)_P = \mu C_p\Delta T\left(\mu = \frac{\text{No. of molecules}}{\text{Avogedro's no.}}\right)$$

or $\Delta T \propto \frac{1}{\text{no. of molecules}}$

22. (c) $TV^{\gamma-1} = \text{constant}$

$$T_1V_1^{\gamma-1} = T_2V_2^{\gamma-1}$$

$$\Rightarrow T(V)^{1/2} = T_2\left(\frac{V}{4}\right)^{1/2}$$

$$\left[\because \gamma = 1.5, T_1 = T, V_1 = V \text{ and } V_2 = \frac{V}{4}\right]$$

$$\therefore T_2 = \left(\frac{4V}{V}\right)^{1/2}T = 2T$$

23. (b) According to Mayer's relationship

$C_P - C_V = R$, as per the question $(C_P - C_V)M = R$

$\Rightarrow C_P - C_V = R/28$

Here M = 28 = mass of 1 unit of N_2

24. (a) For mixture of gas, $C_v = \dfrac{n_1 C_{v_1} + n_2 C_{v_2}}{n_1 + n_2}$

$$= \frac{4 \times \frac{3}{2}R + \frac{1}{2} \times \frac{5}{2}R}{\left(4 + \frac{1}{2}\right)} = \frac{6R + \frac{5}{4}R}{\frac{9}{2}} = \frac{29R \times 23}{9 \times 4} = \frac{29R}{18}$$

and $C_p = \dfrac{n_1 C_{p_1} + n_2 C_{p_2}}{(n_1 + n_2)} = \dfrac{4 \times \frac{5R}{2} + \frac{1}{2} \times \frac{7R}{2}}{\left(4 + \frac{1}{2}\right)}$

$$= \frac{10R + \frac{7}{4}R}{\frac{9}{2}} = \frac{47R}{18}$$

$$\therefore \frac{C_p}{C_v} = \frac{47R}{18} \times \frac{18}{29R} = 1.62$$

25. (c) $\gamma_1 = \frac{5}{3}\ \gamma_2 = \frac{7}{5}$

$n_1 = 1, n_2 = 1$

$$\frac{n_1 + n_2}{\gamma - 1} = \frac{n_1}{\gamma_1 - 1} + \frac{n_2}{\gamma_2 - 1}$$

$$\Rightarrow \frac{1+1}{\gamma - 1} = \frac{1}{\frac{5}{3} - 1} + \frac{1}{\frac{7}{5} - 1} = \frac{3}{2} + \frac{5}{2} = 4$$

$$\therefore \frac{2}{\gamma - 1} = 4 \Rightarrow \gamma = \frac{3}{2}$$

26. (d) $P \propto T^3 \Rightarrow PT^{-3} = \text{constant}$ ....(i)

But for an adiabatic process, the pressure temperature relationship is given by

$P^{1-\gamma}\ T^{\gamma} = \text{constant}$

$\Rightarrow PT^{\frac{\gamma}{1-\gamma}} = \text{constt.}$ ....(ii)

From (i) and (ii) $\dfrac{\gamma}{1-\gamma} = -3 \Rightarrow \gamma = -3 + 3\gamma \Rightarrow \gamma = \dfrac{3}{2}$

Chapter 13

Oscillations

TOPIC-1 : Displacement, Phase, Velocity and Acceleration in S.H.M.

1. The ratio of maximum acceleration to maximum velocity in a simple harmonic motion is $10\ s^{-1}$. At, t = 0 the displacement is 5 m. What is the maximum acceleration ? The initial phase is $\frac{\pi}{4}$ **[Online April 8, 2017]**

(a) $500\ m/s^2$ (b) $500\sqrt{2}\ m/s^2$

(c) $750\ m/s^2$ (d) $750\sqrt{2}\ m/s^2$

2. A particle performs simple harmonic mition with amplitude A. Its speed is trebled at the instant that it is at a distance $\frac{2A}{3}$ from equilibrium position. The new amplitude of the motion is : **[2016]**

(a) $A\sqrt{3}$ (b) $\frac{7A}{3}$ (c) $\frac{A}{3}\sqrt{41}$ (d) 3A

3. Two particles are performing simple harmonic motion in a straight line about the same equilibrium point. The amplitude and time period for both particles are same and equal to A and T, respectively. At time t=0 one particle has displacement A while the other one has displacement $\frac{-A}{2}$ and they are moving towards each other. If they cross each other at time t, then t is: **[Online April 9, 2016]**

(a) $\frac{5T}{6}$ (b) $\frac{T}{3}$ (c) $\frac{T}{4}$ (d) $\frac{T}{6}$

4. A simple harmonic oscillator of angular frequency 2 rad s^{-1} is acted upon by an external force F = sin *t* N. If the oscillator is at rest in its equilibrium position at *t* = 0, its position at later times is proportional to : **[Online April 10, 2015]**

(a) $\sin t + \frac{1}{2}\cos 2t$ (b) $\cos t - \frac{1}{2}\sin 2t$

(c) $\sin t - \frac{1}{2}\sin 2t$ (d) $\sin t + \frac{1}{2}\sin 2t$

5. *x* and *y* displacements of a particle are given as $x(t) = a \sin \omega t$ and $y(t) = a \sin 2\omega t$. Its trajectory will look like : **[Online April 10, 2015]**

(a) 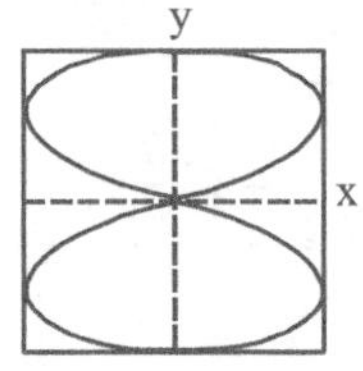

(b) 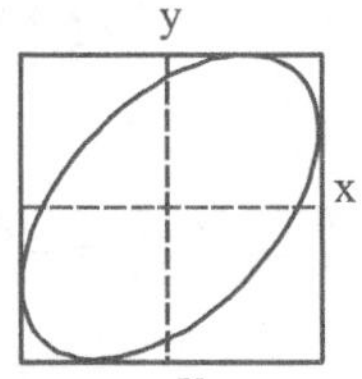

(c) 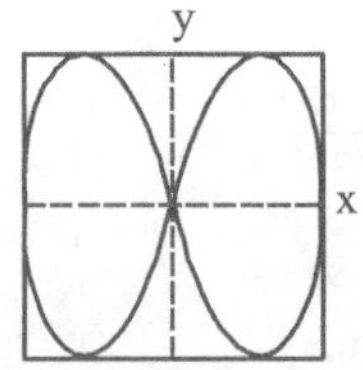

(d) 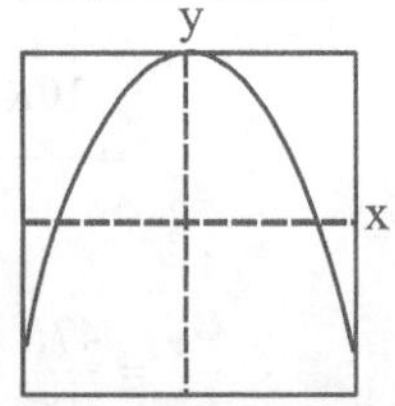

6. A body is in simple harmonic motion with time period half second (T = 0.5 s) and amplitude one cm (A = 1 cm). Find the average velocity in the interval in which it moves form equilibrium position to half of its amplitude. **[Online April 19, 2014]**

(a) 4 cm/s (b) 6 cm/s (c) 12 cm/s (d) 16 cm/s

7. Which of the following expressions corresponds to simple harmonic motion along a straight line, where x is the displacement and a, b, c are positive constants? **[Online April 12, 2014]**

(a) $a + bx - cx^2$ (b) bx^2

(c) $a - bx + cx^2$ (d) $-bx$

8. A particle which is simultaneously subjected to two perpendicular simple harmonic motions represented by; $x = a_1 \cos \omega t$ and $y = a_2 \cos 2\omega t$ traces a curve given by: **[Online April 9, 2014]**

(a) 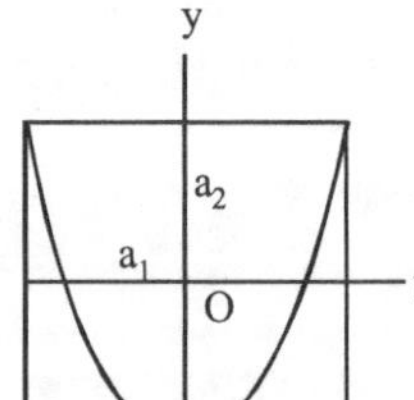

(b) 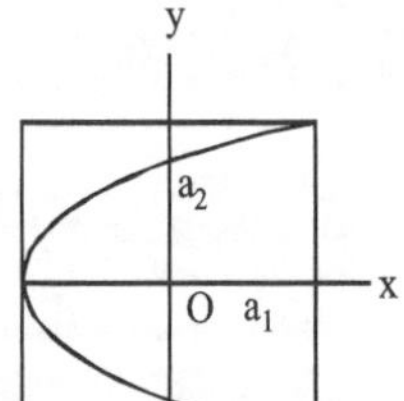

(c) 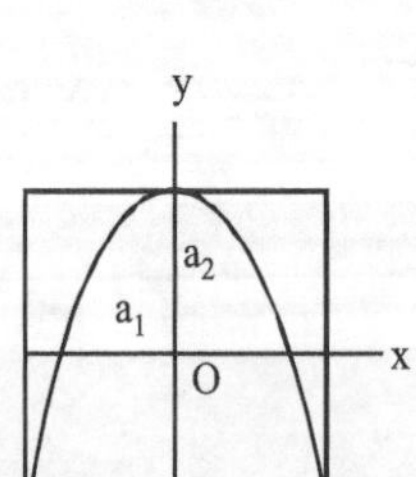

(d) 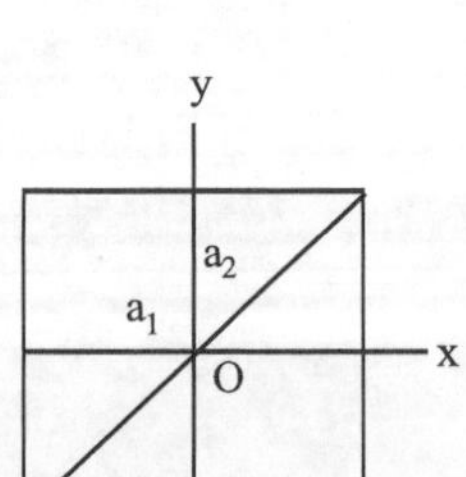

9. The displacement $y(t) = A \sin(\omega t + \phi)$ of a pendulum for $\phi = \frac{2\pi}{3}$ is correctly represented by **[Online May 19, 2012]**

(a) 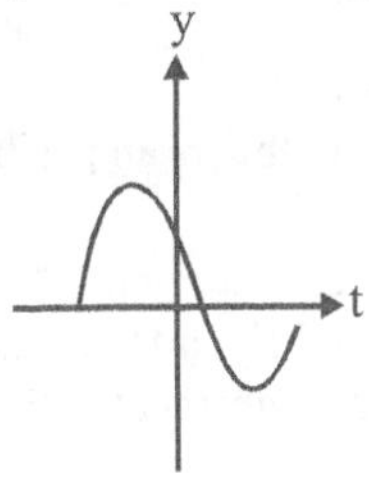

(b) 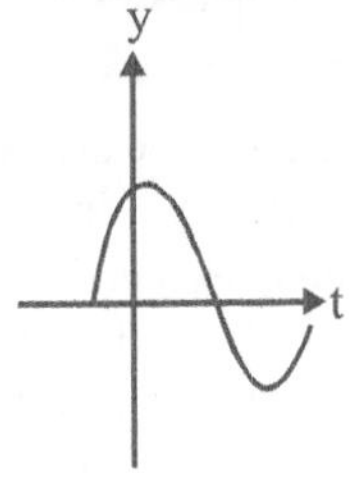

(c) 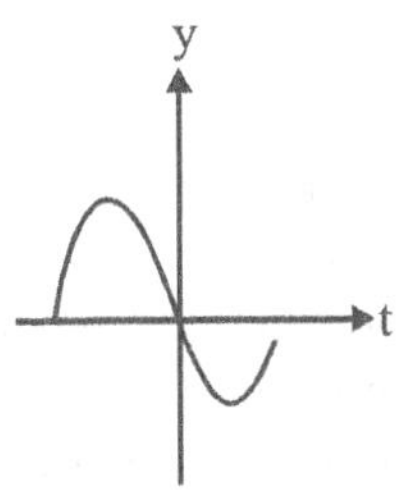

(d) 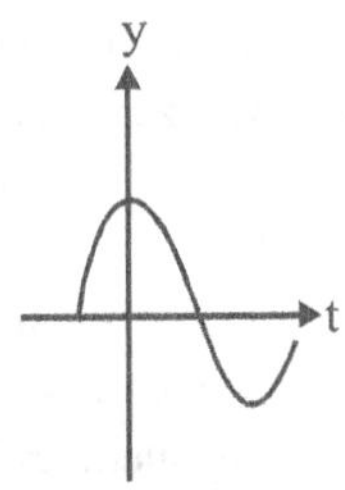

10. Two particles are executing simple harmonic motion of the same amplitude A and frequency ω along the x-axis. Their mean position is separated by distance $X_0 (X_0 > A)$. If the maximum separation between them is $(X_0 + A)$, the phase difference between their motion is: **[2011]**

(a) $\frac{\pi}{3}$ (b) $\frac{\pi}{4}$ (c) $\frac{\pi}{6}$ (d) $\frac{\pi}{2}$

11. A mass M, attached to a horizontal spring, executes S.H.M. with amplitude A_1. When the mass M passes through its mean position then a smaller mass m is placed over it and both of them move together with amplitude A_2. The ratio of $\left(\frac{A_1}{A_2}\right)$ is: **[2011]**

(a) $\frac{M+m}{M}$ (b) $\left(\frac{M}{M+m}\right)^{\frac{1}{2}}$

(c) $\left(\frac{M+m}{M}\right)^{\frac{1}{2}}$ (d) $\frac{M}{M+m}$

12. A point mass oscillates along the x-axis according to the law $x = x_0 \cos(\omega t - \pi/4)$. If the acceleration of the particle is written as $a = A\cos(\omega t + \delta)$, then **[2007]**

(a) $A = x_0\omega^2,\ \delta = 3\pi/4$

(b) $A = x_0,\ \delta = -\pi/4$

(c) $A = x_0\omega^2,\ \delta = \pi/4$

(d) $A = x_0\omega^2,\ \delta = -\pi/4$

13. A coin is placed on a horizontal platform which undergoes vertical simple harmonic motion of angular frequency ω. The amplitude of oscillation is gradually increased. The coin will leave contact with the platform for the first time

(a) at the mean position of the platform **[2006]**

(b) for an amplitude of $\frac{g}{\omega^2}$

(c) for an amplitude of $\frac{g^2}{\omega^2}$

(d) at the highest position of the platform

14. The maximum velocity of a particle, executing simple harmonic motion with an amplitude 7 mm, is 4.4 m/s. The period of oscillation is **[2006]**

(a) 0.01 s (b) 10 s (c) 0.1 s (d) 100 s

15. The function $\sin^2(\omega t)$ represents **[2005]**

(a) a periodic, but not simple harmonic motion with a period $\frac{\pi}{\omega}$

(b) a periodic, but not simple harmonic motion with a period $\frac{2\pi}{\omega}$

(c) a simple harmonic motion with a period $\frac{\pi}{\omega}$

(d) a simple harmonic motion with a period $\frac{2\pi}{\omega}$

16. Two simple harmonic motions are represented by the equations $y_1 = 0.1 \sin\left(100\pi t + \frac{\pi}{3}\right)$ and $y_2 = 0.1 \cos \pi t$. The phase difference of the velocity of particle 1 with respect to the velocity of particle 2 is **[2005]**

(a) $\frac{\pi}{3}$ (b) $\frac{-\pi}{6}$ (c) $\frac{\pi}{6}$ (d) $\frac{-\pi}{3}$

17. Two particles A and B of equal masses are suspended from two massless springs of spring constants k_1 and k_2, respectively. If the maximum velocities, during oscillation, are equal, the ratio of amplitude of A and B is **[2003]**

(a) $\sqrt{\frac{k_1}{k_2}}$ (b) $\frac{k_2}{k_1}$ (c) $\sqrt{\frac{k_2}{k_1}}$ (d) $\frac{k_1}{k_2}$

18. The displacement of a particle varies according to the relation $x = 4(\cos \pi t + \sin \pi t)$. The amplitude of the particle is **[2003]**

(a) -4 (b) 4 (c) $4\sqrt{2}$ (d) 8

TOPIC-2 : Energy in Simple Harmonic Motion

19. A particle is executing simple harmonic motion with a time period T. At time t = 0, it is at its position of equilibrium. The kinetic energy-time graph of the particle will look like: **[2017]**

(a) 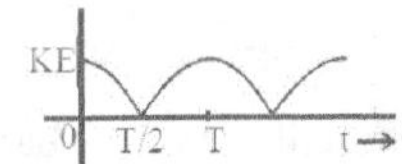

(b) 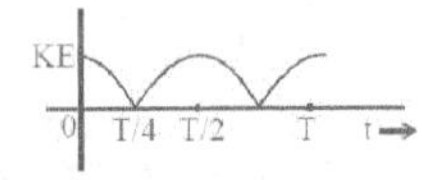

(c) 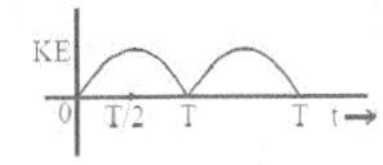

(d) 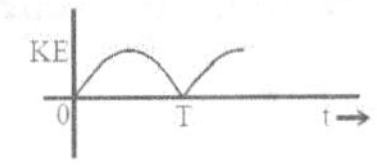

20. A block of mass 0.1 kg is connected to an elastic spring of spring constant 640 Nm^{-1} and oscillates in a medium of constant 10^{-2} kg s^{-1}. The system dissipates its energy gradually. The time taken for its mechanical energy of vibration to drop to half of its initial value, is closest to : **[Online April 9, 2017]**

(a) 2 s (b) 3.5 s (c) 5 s (d) 7 s

21. For a simple pendulum, a graph is plotted between its kinetic energy (KE) and potential energy (PE) against its displacement d. Which one of the following represents these correctly? (*graphs are schematic and not drawn to scale*) **[2015]**

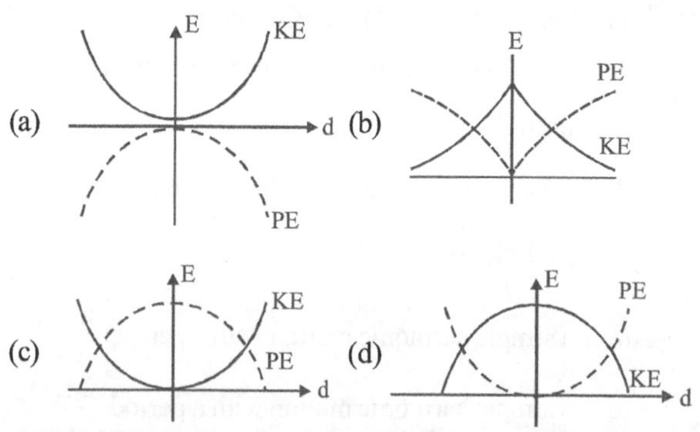

22. A pendulum with time period of 1s is losing energy. At certain time its energy is 45 J. If after completing 15 oscillations, its energy has become 15 J, its damping constant (in s^{-1}) is : **[Online April 11, 2015]**

(a) $\frac{1}{2}$ (b) $\frac{1}{30}\ln 3$ (c) 2 (d) $\frac{1}{15}\ln 3$

23. This question has Statement 1 and Statement 2. Of the four choices given after the Statements, choose the one that best describes the two Statements.

If two springs S_1 and S_2 of force constants k_1 and k_2 respectively, are stretched by the same force, it is found that more work is done on spring S_1 than on spring S_2.

Statement 1 : If stretched by the same amount work done on S_1

Statement 2 : $k_1 < k_2$ **[2012]**

(a) Statement 1 is false, Statement 2 is true.
(b) Statement 1 is true, Statement 2 is false.
(c) Statement 1 is true, Statement 2 is true, Statement 2 is the correct explanation for Statement 1
(d) Statement 1 is true, Statement 2 is true, Statement 2 is not the correct explanation for Statement 1

24. A particle of mass m executes simple harmonic motion with amplitude a and frequency ν. The average kinetic energy during its motion from the position of equilibrium to the end is **[2007]**

(a) $2\pi^2 ma^2\nu^2$ (b) $\pi^2 ma^2\nu^2$

(c) $\frac{1}{4}ma^2\nu^2$ (d) $4\pi^2 ma^2\nu^2$

25. Starting from the origin a body oscillates simple harmonically with a period of 2 s. After what time will its kinetic energy be 75% of the total energy? **[2006]**

(a) $\frac{1}{6}$s (b) $\frac{1}{4}$s (c) $\frac{1}{3}$s (d) $\frac{1}{12}$s

26. The total energy of a particle, executing simple harmonic motion is **[2004]**

(a) independent of x (b) $\propto x^2$

(c) $\propto x$ (d) $\propto x^{1/2}$

where x is the displacement from the mean position, hence total energy is independent of x.

27. A body executes simple harmonic motion. The potential energy (P.E), the kinetic energy (K.E) and total energy (T.E) are measured as a function of displacement x. Which of the following statements is true ? **[2003]**

(a) K.E. is maximum when $x=0$
(b) T.E is zero when $x=0$
(c) K.E is maximum when x is maximum
(d) P.E is maximum when $x=0$

28. In a simple harmonic oscillator, at the mean position **[2002]**

(a) kinetic energy is minimum, potential energy is maximum
(b) both kinetic and potential energies are maximum
(c) kinetic energy is maximum, potential energy is minimum
(d) both kinetic and potential energies are minimum

TOPIC-3 : Time Period, Frequency, Simple Pendulum and Spring Pendulum

29. In an experiment to determine the period of a simple pendulum of length 1 m, it is attached to different spherical bobs of radii r_1 and r_2. The two spherical bobs have uniform mass distribution. If the relative difference in the periods, is found to be 5×10^{-4} s, the difference in radii, $|r_1 - r_2|$ is best given by: **[Online April 9, 2017]**

(a) 1 cm (b) 0.1 cm (c) 0.5 cm (d) 0.01 cm

30. A 1 kg block attached to a spring vibrates with a frequency of 1 Hz on a frictionless horizontal table. Two springs identical to the original spring are attached in parallel to an 8 kg block placed on the same table. So, the frequency of vibration of the 8 kg block is : **[Online April 8, 2017]**

(a) $\frac{1}{4}$Hz (b) $\frac{1}{2\sqrt{2}}$Hz (c) $\frac{1}{2}$Hz (d) 2 Hz

31. A pendulum clock loses 12 s a day if the temperature is 40°C and gains 4 s a day if the temperature is 20° C. The temperature at which the clock will show correct time, and the co-efficient of linear expansion (α) of the metal of the pendulum shaft are respectively : **[2016]**

(a) 30°C; $\alpha = 1.85 \times 10^{-3}$/°C
(b) 55°C; $\alpha = 1.85 \times 10^{-2}$/°C
(c) 25°C; $\alpha = 1.85 \times 10^{-5}$/°C
(d) 60°C; $\alpha = 1.85 \times 10^{-4}$/°C

32. In an engine the piston undergoes vertical simple harmonic motion with amplitude 7 cm. A washer rests on top of the piston and moves with it. The motor speed is slowly increased. The frequency of the piston at which the washer no longer stays in contact with the piston, is close to : **[Online April 10, 2016]**

(a) 0.7 Hz (b) 1.9 Hz (c) 1.2 Hz (d) 0.1 Hz

33. A pendulum made of a uniform wire of cross sectional area A has time period T. When an additional mass M is added to its bob, the time period changes to T_M. If the Young's modulus of the material of the wire is Y then $\frac{1}{Y}$ is equal to: (g = *gravitational acceleration*) **[2015]**

(a) $\left[1-\left(\frac{T_M}{T}\right)^2\right]\frac{A}{Mg}$ (b) $\left[1-\left(\frac{T}{T_M}\right)^2\right]\frac{A}{Mg}$

(c) $\left[\left(\frac{T_M}{T}\right)^2-1\right]\frac{A}{Mg}$ (d) $\left[\left(\frac{T_M}{T}\right)^2-1\right]\frac{Mg}{A}$

34. A particle moves with simple harmonic motion in a straight line. In first τ s, after starting from rest it travels a distance a, and in next τ s it travels 2a, in same direction, then: **[2014]**

(a) amplitude of motion is 3a
(b) time period of oscillations is 8τ
(c) amplitude of motion is 4a
(d) time period of oscillations is 6τ

35. In an experiment for determining the gravitational acceleration g of a place with the help of a simple pendulum, the measured time period square is plotted against the string length of the pendulum in the figure. **[Online April 19, 2014]**

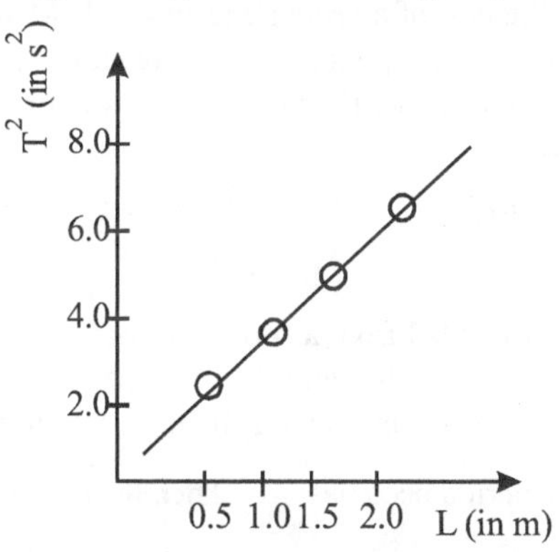

What is the value of g at the place?
(a) 9.81 m/s^2 (b) 9.87 m/s^2
(c) 9.91 m/s^2 (d) 10.0 m/s^2

36. The amplitude of a simple pendulum, oscillating in air with a small spherical bob, decreases from 10 cm to 8 cm in 40 seconds. Assuming that Stokes law is valid, and ratio of the coefficient of viscosity of air to that of carbon dioxide is 1.3. The time in which amplitude of this pendulum will reduce from 10 cm to 5 cm in carbon dioxide will be close to ($ln\,5 = 1.601$, $ln\,2 = 0.693$). **[Online April 9, 2014]**

(a) 231 s (b) 208 s (c) 161 s (d) 142 s

37. Two bodies of masses 1 kg and 4 kg are connected to a vertical spring, as shown in the figure. The smaller mass executes simple harmonic motion of angular frequency 25 rad/s, and amplitude 1.6 cm while the bigger mass remains stationary on the ground. The maximum force exerted by the system on the floor is (take g = 10 ms^{-2}) **[Online April 9, 2014]**

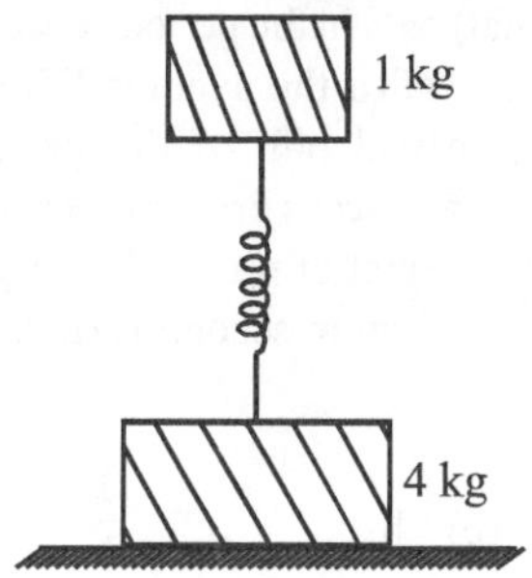

(a) 20 N (b) 10 N (c) 60 N (d) 40 N

38. An ideal gas enclosed in a vertical cylindrical container supports a freely moving piston of mass M. The piston and the cylinder have equal cross sectional area A. When the piston is in equilibrium, the volume of the gas is V_0 and its pressure is P_0. The piston is slightly displaced from the equilibrium position and released. Assuming that the system is completely isolated from its surrounding, the piston executes a simple harmonic motion with frequency **[2013]**

(a) $\frac{1}{2\pi}\frac{A\gamma P_0}{V_0 M}$ (b) $\frac{1}{2\pi}\frac{V_0 M P_0}{A^2\gamma}$

(c) $\frac{1}{2\pi}\sqrt{\frac{A^2\gamma P_0}{MV_0}}$ (d) $\frac{1}{2\pi}\sqrt{\frac{MV_0}{A\gamma P_0}}$

39. A mass $m = 1.0$ kg is put on a flat pan attached to a vertical spring fixed on the ground. The mass of the spring and the pan is negligible. When pressed slightly and released, the mass executes simple harmonic motion. The spring constant is 500 N/m. What is the amplitude A of the motion, so that the mass m tends to get detached from the pan ? (Take $g = 10$ m/s^2).
The spring is stiff enough so that it does not get distorted during the motion. **[Online April 22, 2013]**

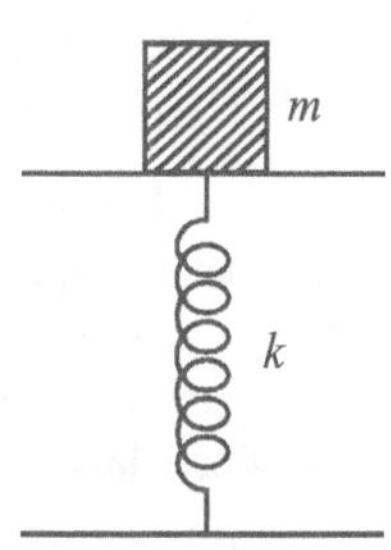

(a) A > 2.0 cm (b) A = 2.0 cm
(c) A < 2.0 cm (d) A = 1.5 cm

40. Two simple pendulums of length 1 m and 4 m respectively are both given small displacement in the same direction at the same instant. They will be again in phase after the shorter pendulum has completed number of oscillations equal to : **[Online April 9, 2013]**

(a) 2 (b) 7 (c) 5 (d) 3

41. If a simple pendulum has significant amplitude (up to a factor of 1/e of original) only in the period between $t = 0s$ to $t = \tau$ s, then τ may be called the average life of the pendulum. When the spherical bob of the pendulum suffers a retardation (due to viscous drag) proportional to its velocity with b as the constant of proportionality, the average life time of the pendulum in second is (assuming damping is small) **[2012]**

(a) $\frac{0.693}{b}$ (b) b (c) $\frac{1}{b}$ (d) $\frac{2}{b}$

42. A ring is suspended from a point S on its rim as shown in the figure. When displaced from equilibrium, it oscillates with time period of 1 second. The radius of the ring is (take $g = \pi^2$) **[Online May 19, 2012]**

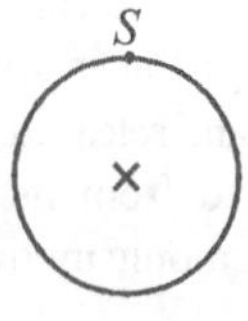

(a) 0.15m (b) 1.5m (c) 1.0m (d) 0.5m

43. A wooden cube (density of wood 'd') of side 'ℓ' floats in a liquid of density 'ρ' with its upper and lower surfaces horizontal. If the cube is pushed slightly down and released, it performs simple harmonic motion of period 'T' **[2011 RS]**

(a) $2\pi\sqrt{\frac{\ell d}{\rho g}}$ (b) $2\pi\sqrt{\frac{\ell \rho}{dg}}$

(c) $2\pi\sqrt{\frac{\ell d}{(\rho - d)g}}$ (d) $2\pi\sqrt{\frac{\ell \rho}{(\rho - d)g}}$

44. If x, v and a denote the displacement, the velocity and the acceleration of a particle executing simple harmonic motion of time period T, then, which of the following does not change with time? **[2009]**

(a) aT/x (b) $aT + 2\pi v$

(c) aT/v (d) $a^2T^2 + 4\pi^2v^2$

45. Two springs, of force constants k_1 and k_2 are connected to a mass m as shown. The frequency of oscillation of the mass is f. If both k_1 and k_2 are made four times their original values, the frequency of oscillation becomes **[2007]**

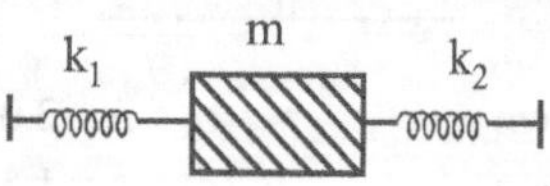

(a) $2f$ (b) $f/2$ (c) $f/4$ (d) $4f$

46. The displacement of an object attached to a spring and executing simple harmonic motion is given by $x = 2 \times 10^{-2} \cos \pi t$ metre. The time at which the maximum speed first occurs is **[2007]**

(a) 0.25 s (b) 0.5 s (c) 0.75 s (d) 0.125 s

47. The bob of a simple pendulum is a spherical hollow ball filled with water. A plugged hole near the bottom of the oscillating bob gets suddenly unplugged. During observation, till water is coming out, the time period of oscillation would **[2005]**

(a) first decrease and then increase to the original value
(b) first increase and then decrease to the original value
(c) increase towards a saturation value
(d) remain unchanged

48. If a simple harmonic motion is represented by $\frac{d^2x}{dt^2} + \alpha x = 0$, its time period is **[2005]**

(a) $\frac{2\pi}{\sqrt{\alpha}}$ (b) $\frac{2\pi}{\alpha}$ (c) $2\pi\sqrt{\alpha}$ (d) $2\pi\alpha$

49. The bob of a simple pendulum executes simple harmonic motion in water with a period t, while the period of oscillation of the bob is t_0 in air. Neglecting frictional force of water and given that the density of the bob is $(4/3) \times 1000$ kg/m^3. Which relationship between t and t_0 is true? **[2004]**

(a) $t = 2t_0$ (b) $t = t_0/2$

(c) $t = t_0$ (d) $t = 4t_0$

50. A particle at the end of a spring executes S.H.M with a period t_1. while the corresponding period for another spring is t_2. If the period of oscillation with the two springs in series is T then **[2004]**

(a) $T^{-1} = t_1^{-1} + t_2^{-1}$ (b) $T^2 = t_1^2 + t_2^2$

(c) $T = t_1 + t_2$ (d) $T^{-2} = t_1^{-2} + t_2^{-2}$

51. A mass M is suspended from a spring of negligible mass. The spring is pulled a little and then released so that the mass executes SHM of time period T. If the mass is increased by m, the time period becomes $\frac{5T}{3}$. Then the ratio of $\frac{m}{M}$ is **[2003]**

(a) $\frac{3}{5}$ (b) $\frac{25}{9}$ (c) $\frac{16}{9}$ (d) $\frac{5}{3}$

52. The length of a simple pendulum executing simple harmonic motion is increased by 21%. The percentage increase in the time period of the pendulum of increased length is **[2003]**

(a) 11% (b) 21% (c) 42% (d) 10%

53. If a spring has time period T, and is cut into n equal parts, then the time period of each part will be **[2002]**

(a) $T\sqrt{n}$ (b) $T/\sqrt{n}$ (c) nT (d) T

54. A child swinging on a swing in sitting position, stands up, then the time period if the swing will **[2002]**

(a) increase
(b) decrease
(c) remains same
(d) increases if the child is long and decreases if the child is short

TOPIC-4 : Damped, Forced Oscillations and Resonance

55. The angular frequency of the damped oscillator is given by,

$\omega = \sqrt{\left(\frac{k}{m} - \frac{r^2}{4m^2}\right)}$ where k is the spring constant, m is the mass of the oscillator and r is the damping constant. If the ratio $\frac{r^2}{mk}$ is 8%, the change in time period compared to the undamped oscillator is approximately as follows: **[Online April 11, 2014]**

(a) increases by 1% (b) increases by 8%
(c) decreases by 1% (d) decreases by 8%

56. The amplitude of a damped oscillator decreases to 0.9 times its original magnitude in 5s. In another 10s it will decrease to α times its original magnitude, where α equals **[2013]**

(a) 0.7 (b) 0.81 (c) 0.729 (d) 0.6

57. A uniform cylinder of length L and mass M having cross-sectional area A is suspended, with its length vertical, from a fixed point by a massless spring, such that it is half submerged in a liquid of density σ at equilibrium position. When the cylinder is given a downward push and released, it starts oscillating vertically with a small amplitude. The time period T of the oscillations of the cylinder will be : **[Online April 25, 2013]**

(a) Smaller than $2\pi\left[\frac{M}{(k + A\sigma g)}\right]^{1/2}$

(b) $2\pi\sqrt{\frac{M}{k}}$

(c) Larger than $2\pi\left[\frac{M}{(k + A\sigma g)}\right]^{1/2}$

(d) $2\pi\left[\frac{M}{(k + A\sigma g)}\right]^{1/2}$

58. Bob of a simple pendulum of length l is made of iron. The pendulum is oscillating over a horizontal coil carrying direct current. If the time period of the pendulum is T then : **[Online April 23, 2013]**

(a) $T < 2\pi\sqrt{\frac{l}{g}}$ and damping is smaller than in air alone.

(b) $T = 2\pi\sqrt{\frac{l}{g}}$ and damping is larger than in air alone.

(c) $T > 2\pi\sqrt{\frac{l}{g}}$ and damping is smaller than in air alone.

(d) $T < 2\pi\sqrt{\frac{l}{g}}$ and damping is larger than in air alone.

59. In forced oscillation of a particle the amplitude is maximum for a frequency ω_1 of the force while the energy is maximum for a frequency ω_2 of the force; then **[2004]**

(a) $\omega_1 < \omega_2$ when damping is small and $\omega_1 > \omega_2$ when damping is large

(b) $\omega_1 > \omega_2$

(c) $\omega_1 = \omega_2$

(d) $\omega_1 < \omega_2$

60. A particle of mass m is attached to a spring (of spring constant k) and has a natural angular frequency ω_0. An external force $F(t)$ proportional to $\cos \omega t (\omega \neq \omega_0)$ is applied to the oscillator. The displacement of the oscillator will be proportional to **[2004]**

(a) $\frac{1}{m(\omega_0^2 + \omega^2)}$ (b) $\frac{1}{m(\omega_0^2 - \omega^2)}$

(c) $\frac{m}{\omega_0^2 - \omega^2}$ (d) $\frac{m}{(\omega_0^2 + \omega^2)}$

Hints & Solutions

TOPIC-1 : Displacement, Phase, Velocity and Acceleration in S.H.M.

1. **(b)** Maximum velocity in SHM, $v_{max} = a\omega$
Maximum acceleration in SHM, $A_{max} = a\omega^2$
where a and ω are maximum amplitude and angular frequency.

Given that, $\frac{A_{max}}{v_{max}} = 10$

i.e., $\omega = 10\ s^{-1}$

Displacement is given by

$x = a \sin(\omega t + \pi/4)$

at $t = 0, x = 5$

$5 = a \sin \pi/4$

$5 = a \sin 45° \Rightarrow a = 5\sqrt{2}$

Maximum acceleration $A_{max} = a\omega^2 = 500\sqrt{2}\ m/s^2$

2. **(b)** We know that $V = \omega\sqrt{A^2 - x^2}$

Initially $V = \omega\sqrt{A^2 - \left(\frac{2A}{3}\right)^2}$

Finally $3v = \omega\sqrt{A'^2 - \left(\frac{2A}{3}\right)^2}$

Where A'= final amplitude (Given at $x = \frac{2A}{3}$, velocity to trebled)

On dividing we get $\frac{3}{1} = \frac{\sqrt{A'^2 - \left(\frac{2A}{3}\right)^2}}{\sqrt{A^2 - \left(\frac{2A}{3}\right)^2}}$

$$9\left[A^2 - \frac{4A^2}{9}\right] = A'^2 - \frac{4A^2}{9} \qquad \therefore A' = \frac{7A}{3}$$

3. **(d)**

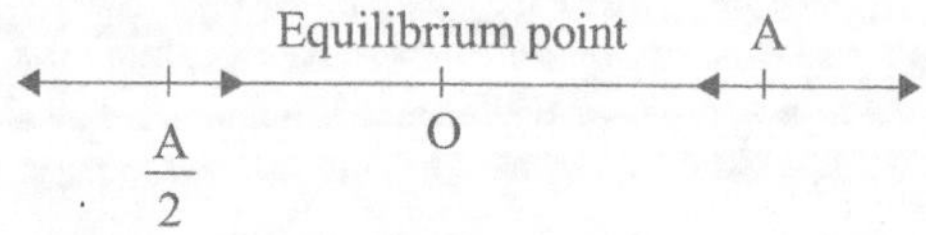

(at time t = 0)

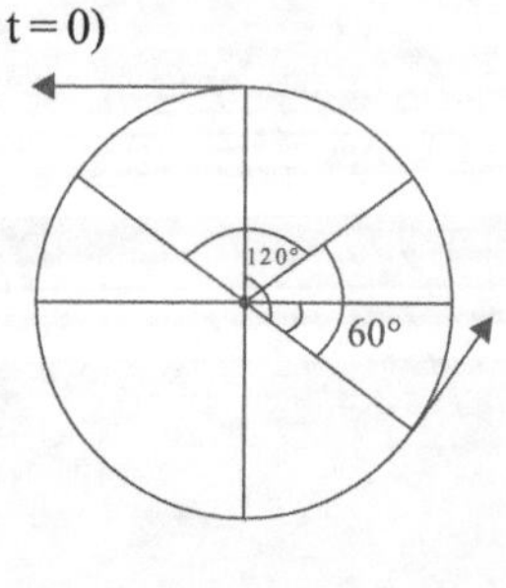

Angle covered to meet $\theta = 60° = \frac{\pi}{3}$ rad.

If they cross each other at time t then

$$t = \frac{\theta}{2\pi} = \frac{\pi}{3 \times 2\pi}T = \frac{T}{6}$$

4. **(c)** As we know,

$F = ma \Rightarrow a \propto F$

or, $a \propto \sin t$

$\Rightarrow \frac{dv}{dt} \propto \sin t$

$\Rightarrow \int_0^0 dV \propto \int_0^t \sin t\, dt$

$V \propto -\cos t + 1$

$\int_0^x dx = \int_0^t (-\cos t + 1)\, dt$

$x = \sin t - \frac{1}{2}\sin 2t$

5. **(c)** At $t = 0$, $x(t) = 0$; $y(t) = 0$

$x(t)$ is a sinusoidal function

At $t = \frac{\pi}{2\omega}$; $x(t) = a$ and $y(t) = 0$

Hence trajectory of particle will look like as (c).

6. **(c)** **Given:** Time period, T = 0.5 sec

Amplitude, A = 1 cm

Average velocity in the interval in which body moves from equilibrium to half of its amplitude, v = ?

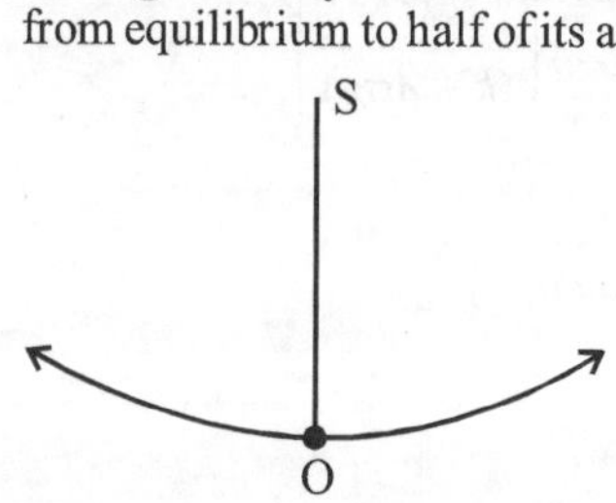

Time taken to a displacement A/2 where A is the amplitude of oscillation from the mean position 'O' is $\frac{T}{12}$

Therefore, time, $t = \frac{0.5}{12}$ sec

Displacement, $s = \frac{A}{2} = \frac{1}{2}$ cm

$\therefore$ Average velocity, $v = \frac{\frac{A}{2}}{t} = \frac{\frac{1}{2}}{\frac{0.5}{12}} = 12\ cm/s$

7. (d) In linear S.H.M., the restoring force acting on particle should always be proportional to the displacement of the particle and directed towards the equilibrium position.

i.e., $F \propto x$

or $F = -bx$ where b is a positive constant.

8. (b) Two perpendicular S.H.Ms are

$x = a_1 \cos \omega t$ ....(1)

and $y = a_2\, 2 \cos \omega t$ ....(2)

From eqn (1)

$$\frac{x}{a_1} = \cos wt$$

and from eqn (2)

$$\frac{y}{a_2} = 2\cos \omega t$$

$$\therefore \quad y = 2\frac{a_2}{a_1}x$$

9. (a) Displacement $y(t) = A \sin(wt + \phi)$[Given]

For $\phi = \frac{2\pi}{3}$

at $t = 0$; $y = A \sin \phi = A \sin \frac{2\pi}{3}$

$= A \sin 120° = 0.87\, A$ [$\because \sin 120° \simeq 0.866$]

Graph (a) depicts $y = 0.87A$ at $t = 0$

10. (a) Let, $x_1 = A \sin \omega t$ and $x^2 = A \sin(\omega t + \phi)$

$$x_2 - x_1 = 2A \cos\left(\omega t + \frac{\phi}{2}\right)\sin\frac{\phi}{2}$$

As the maximum separation between the particles is A,

$$\therefore\ 2A \sin\frac{\phi}{2} = A \qquad \Rightarrow \phi = \frac{\pi}{3}$$

11. (c) The net force becomes zero atthe mean point. Therefore, linear momentum must be conserved.

$\therefore\ Mv_1 = (M+m)v_2$

$$MA_1\sqrt{\frac{k}{M}} = (M+m)A_2\sqrt{\frac{k}{m+M}}$$

$$\therefore\ \left(V = A\sqrt{\frac{k}{M}}\right)$$

$$\because\ A_1\sqrt{M} = A_2\sqrt{M+m}$$

$$\therefore\ \frac{A_1}{A_2} = \sqrt{\frac{m+M}{M}}$$

12. (a) Here,

$x = x_0 \cos(\omega t - \pi/4)$

$\therefore$ Velocity, $v = \frac{dx}{dt} = -x_0\omega \sin\left(\omega t - \frac{\pi}{4}\right)$

Acceleration,

$$a = \frac{dv}{dt} = -x_0\omega^2 \cos\left(\omega t - \frac{\pi}{4}\right)$$

$$= x_0\omega^2 \cos\left[\pi + \left(\omega t - \frac{\pi}{4}\right)\right]$$

$$= x_0\omega^2 \cos\left(\omega t + \frac{3\pi}{4}\right) \quad ...(1)$$

Acceleration, $a = A\cos(\omega t + \delta)$ ...(2)

Comparing the two equations, we get

$A = x_0\omega^2$ and $\delta = \frac{3\pi}{4}$.

13. (b) For block A to move in SHM.

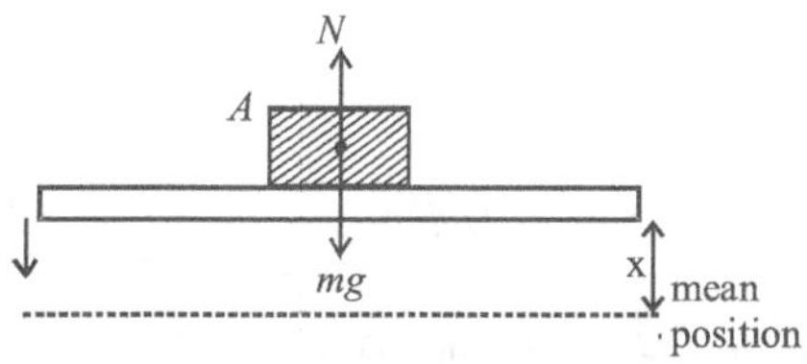

$mg - N = m\omega^2 x$

where x is the distance from mean position

For block to leave contact $N = 0$

$$\Rightarrow mg = m\omega^2 x \Rightarrow x = \frac{g}{\omega^2}$$

14. (a) Maximum velocity,

$$v_{max} = a\omega$$

$$v_{max} = a \times \frac{2\pi}{T}$$

$$\Rightarrow T = \frac{2\pi a}{v_{max}} = \frac{2 \times 3.14 \times 7 \times 10^{-3}}{4.4} \approx 0.01\ s$$

15. (c) Clearly $\sin^2 \omega t$ is a periodic function as $\sin \omega t$ is periodic with period $\frac{\pi}{\omega}$

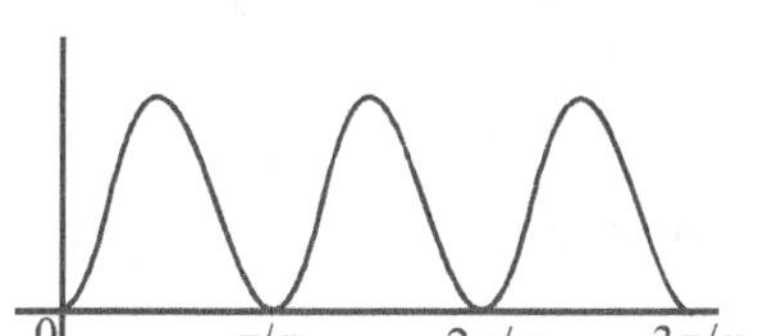

For SHM $\frac{d^2y}{dt^2} \propto -y$

$$\frac{dy}{dt} = 2\omega \sin \omega t \cos \omega t = \omega \sin 2\omega t$$

$$\frac{d^2y}{dt^2} = 2\omega^2 \cos 2\omega t \text{ which is not proportional to } -y.$$

Hence, it is not in SHM.

16. (b) $v_1 = \frac{dy_1}{dt} = 0.1 \times 100\pi \cos\left(100\pi t + \frac{\pi}{3}\right)$

$v_2 = \frac{dy_2}{dt} = -0.1\pi \sin \pi t = 0.1\pi \cos\left(\pi t + \frac{\pi}{2}\right)$

$\therefore$ Phase diff. $= \phi_1 - \phi_2 = \frac{\pi}{3} - \frac{\pi}{2} = \frac{2\pi - 3\pi}{6} = -\frac{\pi}{6}$

17. (c) Maximum velocity during SHM $= A\omega$
But $k = m\omega^2$

$\therefore \omega = \sqrt{\frac{k}{m}}$

$\therefore$ Maximum velocity $= A\sqrt{\frac{k}{m}}$

Here the maximum velocity is same and m is also same

$\therefore A_1\sqrt{k_1} = A_2\sqrt{k_2} \quad \therefore \frac{A_1}{A_2} = \sqrt{\frac{k_2}{k_1}}$

18. (c) $x = 4(\cos \pi t + \sin \pi t)$

$= \sqrt{2} \times 4\left(\frac{\sin \pi t}{\sqrt{2}} + \frac{\cos \pi t}{\sqrt{2}}\right)$

$= 4\sqrt{2}(\sin \pi t \cos 45° + \cos \pi t \sin 45°)$

$x = 4\sqrt{2} \sin(\pi t + 45°)$

on comparing it with $x = A\sin(\omega t + \phi)$

we get $A = 4\sqrt{2}$

TOPIC-2 : Energy in Simple Harmonic Motion

19. (b) For a particle executing SHM
At mean position; $t = 0, \omega t = 0, y = 0, V = V_{max} = a\omega$

$\therefore K.E. = KE_{max} = \frac{1}{2}m\omega^2a^2$

At extreme position : $t = \frac{T}{4}, \omega t = \frac{\pi}{2}, y = A, V = V_{min} = 0$

$\therefore K.E. = KE_{min} = 0$

Kinetic energy in SHM, $KE = \frac{1}{2}m\omega^2(a^2 - y^2)$

$= \frac{1}{2}m\omega^2a^2\cos^2\omega t$

Hence graph (b) correctly depicts kinetic energy time graph.

20. (b) Since system dissipates its energy gradually, and hence amplitude will also decreases with time according to
$a = a_0 e^{-bt/m}$ .... (i)

$\because$ Energy of vibration drop to half of its initial value (E_0), as $E \propto a^2 \Rightarrow a \propto \sqrt{E}$

$a = \frac{a_0}{\sqrt{2}} \Rightarrow \frac{bt}{m} = \frac{10^{-2}t}{0.1} = \frac{t}{10}$

From eq^n (i),

$\frac{a_0}{\sqrt{2}} = a_0 e^{-t/10}$

$\frac{1}{\sqrt{2}} = e^{-t/10}$ or $\sqrt{2} = e^{\frac{t}{10}}$

$\ln\sqrt{2} = \frac{t}{10} \qquad \therefore t = 3.5$ seconds

21. (d) $K.E = \frac{1}{2}k(A^2 - d^2)$

and $P.E. = \frac{1}{2}kd^2$

At mean position $d = 0$. At extrement positions $d = A$

22. (d) As we know, $E = E_0 e^{-\frac{bt}{m}}$

$15 = 45e^{-\frac{b15}{m}}$

[As no. of oscillations = 15 so t = 15sec]

$\frac{1}{3} = e^{-\frac{b15}{m}}$

Taking log on both sides

$\frac{b}{m} = \frac{1}{15}\ell n 3$

23. (b) $\because w = \frac{1}{2}kx^2$

$w_1 = \frac{1}{2}k_1x^2; \quad w_2 = \frac{1}{2}k_2x^2$

Since $w_1 > w_2$ Thus $(k_1 > k_2)$

24. (b) The kinetic energy of a particle executing S.H.M. is given by

$K = \frac{1}{2}ma^2\omega^2\sin^2\omega t$

where, m = mass of particle
a = amplitude
ω = angular frequency
t = time

Now, average K.E. $= \langle K \rangle = \langle \frac{1}{2}m\omega^2a^2\sin^2\omega t \rangle$

$= \frac{1}{2}m\omega^2a^2 \langle \sin^2\omega t \rangle$

$= \frac{1}{2}m\omega^2a^2\left(\frac{1}{2}\right) \quad \left(\because \langle \sin^2\theta \rangle = \frac{1}{2}\right)$

$= \frac{1}{4}m\omega^2a^2 = \frac{1}{4}ma^2(2\pi\nu)^2 \quad (\because \omega = 2\pi\nu)$

or, $\langle K \rangle = \pi^2ma^2\nu^2$

25. (a) K.E. of a body undergoing SHM is given by,

$K.E. = \frac{1}{2}ma^2\omega^2\cos^2\omega t$

$T.E. = \frac{1}{2}ma^2\omega^2$

Given K.E. = 0.75 T.E.

$\Rightarrow 0.75 = \cos^2 \omega t \Rightarrow \omega t = \frac{\pi}{6}$

$\Rightarrow t = \frac{\pi}{6 \times \omega} \Rightarrow t = \frac{\pi \times 2}{6 \times 2\pi} \Rightarrow t = \frac{1}{6} s$

26. (a) At any instant the total energy is

$\frac{1}{2}kA_0^2 = \text{constant}, \text{ where } A_0 = \text{amplitude}$

hence total energy is independent of x.

27. (a) $K.E. = \frac{1}{2}m\omega^2(a^2 - x^2)$

When x = 0, K.E is maximum and is equal to $\frac{1}{2}m\omega^2 a^2$.

28. (c) The kinetic energy (K. E.) and potential energy (U) of a simple harmonic oscillator is given by,

$K.E = \frac{1}{2}k(A^2 - x^2); \quad U = \frac{1}{2}kx^2$

Where A = amplitude and $k = m\omega^2$

x = displacement from the mean position

At the mean position $x = 0$

$\therefore$ K.E. $= \frac{1}{2}kA^2$ = Maximum and U = 0

TOPIC-3 : Time Period, Frequency, Simple Pendulum and Spring Pendulum

29. (b) As we know, Time-period of simple pendulum, $T \propto \sqrt{l}$

differentiating both side, $\frac{\Delta T}{T} = \frac{1}{2}\frac{\Delta l}{l}$

$\because$ change in length $\Delta l = r_1 - r_2$

$5 \times 10^{-4} = \frac{1}{2}\frac{r_1 - r_2}{1}$

$r_1 - r_2 = 10 \times 10^{-4}$

10^{-3} m $= 10^{-1}$ cm $= 0.1$ cm

30. (c) Frequency of spring (f) $= \frac{1}{2\pi}\sqrt{\frac{k}{m}} = 1$ Hz

$\Rightarrow 4\pi^2 = \frac{k}{m}$

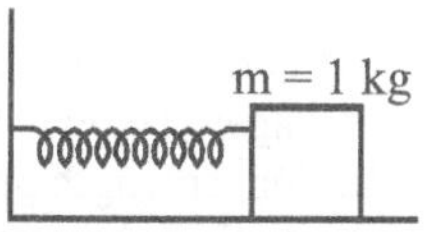

If block of mass m = 1 kg is attached then,

$k = 4\pi^2$

Now, identical springs are attached in parallel with mass m = 8 kg. Hence,

$k_{eq} = 2k$

$F = \frac{1}{2\pi}\sqrt{\frac{k \times 2}{g}} = \frac{1}{2}$Hz

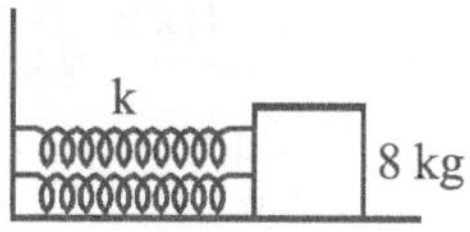

31. (c) Time lost/gained per day $= \frac{1}{2} \propto \Delta\theta \times 86400$ second

$12 = \frac{1}{2}\alpha(40 - \theta) \times 86400$ ....(i)

$4 = \frac{1}{2}\alpha(\theta - 20) \times 86400$ ....(ii)

On dividing we get, $3 = \frac{40 - \theta}{\theta - 20}$

$3\theta - 60 = 40 - \theta$

$4\theta = 100 \Rightarrow \theta = 25°C$

32. (b) Washer contact with piston $\Rightarrow$ N = 0

Given Amplitude A = 7 cm = 0.07 m.

$a_{max} = g = \omega^2 A$

The frequency of piston

$f = \frac{\omega}{2\pi} = \sqrt{\frac{g}{A}}\frac{1}{2\pi} = \sqrt{\frac{1000}{7}}\frac{1}{2\pi} = 1.9$ Hz.

33. (c) As we know, time period, $T = 2\pi\sqrt{\frac{\ell}{g}}$

When additional mass M is added then

$T_M = 2\pi\sqrt{\frac{\ell + \Delta\ell}{g}}$

$\frac{T_M}{T} = \sqrt{\frac{\ell + \Delta\ell}{\ell}}$ or $\left(\frac{T_M}{T}\right)^2 = \frac{\ell + \Delta\ell}{\ell}$

or, $\left(\frac{T_M}{T}\right)^2 = 1 + \frac{Mg}{Ay}$ $\quad \left[\because \Delta\ell = \frac{Mg\ell}{Ay}\right]$

$\therefore \frac{1}{y} = \left[\left(\frac{T_M}{T}\right)^2 - 1\right]\frac{A}{Mg}$

34. (d) In simple harmonic motion, starting from rest,

At $t = 0, x = A$

$x = A\cos\omega t$ ..... (i)

When $t = \tau, x = A - a$

When $t = 2\tau, x = A - 3a$

From equation (i)

$A - a = A\cos\omega\tau$ ......(ii)

$A - 3a = A\cos 2\omega\tau$ ....(iii)

As $\cos 2\omega\tau = 2\cos^2\omega\tau - 1$...(iv)

From equation (ii), (iii) and (iv)

$\frac{A - 3a}{A} = 2\left(\frac{A - a}{A}\right)^2 - 1$

$\Rightarrow \frac{A - 3a}{A} = \frac{2A^2 + 2a^2 - 4Aa - A^2}{A^2}$

$\Rightarrow A^2 - 3aA = A^2 + 2a^2 - 4Aa$

$\Rightarrow 2a^2 = aA$

$\Rightarrow A = 2a$

$\Rightarrow \frac{a}{A} = \frac{1}{2}$

Now, $A - a = A\cos\omega\tau$

$$\Rightarrow \cos\omega\tau = \frac{A-a}{A}$$

$$\Rightarrow \cos\omega\tau = \frac{1}{2} \text{ or } \frac{2\pi}{T}\tau = \frac{\pi}{3}$$

$\Rightarrow T = 6\tau$

35. (b) From graph it is clear that when $L = 1\text{m}, T^2 = 4\text{s}^2$

As we know,

$$T = 2\pi\sqrt{\frac{L}{g}}$$

$$\Rightarrow g = \frac{4\pi^2 L}{T^2}$$

$$= 4\times\left(\frac{22}{7}\right)^2 \times \frac{1}{4} = \left(\frac{22}{7}\right)^2$$

$$\therefore g = \frac{484}{49} = 9.87\text{m/s}^2$$

36. (d) As we know,

$x = x_0 e^{-bt/2m}$

From question,

$$8 = 10e^{-\frac{40b}{2m}} \quad \text{....(i)}$$

$$\text{Similarly, } 5 = 10e^{-\frac{bt}{2m}} \quad \text{....(ii)}$$

Solving eqns (i) and (ii) we get

$t \cong 142$ s

37. (c) Mass of bigger body M = 4 kg

Mass of smaller body m = 1 kg

Smaller mass (m = 1 kg) executes S.H.M of angular frequency $\omega = 25$ rad/s

Amplitude $x = 1.6\text{ cm} = 1.6 \times 10^{-2}$

As we know,

$$T = 2\pi\sqrt{\frac{m}{K}}$$

$$\text{or, } \frac{2\pi}{\omega} = 2\pi\sqrt{\frac{m}{K}}$$

$$\text{or, } \frac{1}{25} = \sqrt{\frac{1}{K}} \; [\because m = 1\text{kg}; \omega = 25 \text{ rad/s}]$$

or, $K = 625\text{ Nm}^{-1}$.

The maximum force exerted by the system on the floor

$= Mg + Kx + mg$

$= 4\times 10 + 625 \times 1.6 \times 10^{-2} + 1 \times 10$

$= 40 + 10 + 10$

$= 60$N

38. (c) $\frac{Mg}{A} = P_0$

$P_0 V_0^\gamma = PV^\gamma$

$Mg = P_0 A \quad \ldots(1)$

$P_0 A x_0^\gamma = PA(x_0 - x)^\gamma$

$$P = \frac{P_0 x_0^\gamma}{(x_0 - x)^\gamma}$$

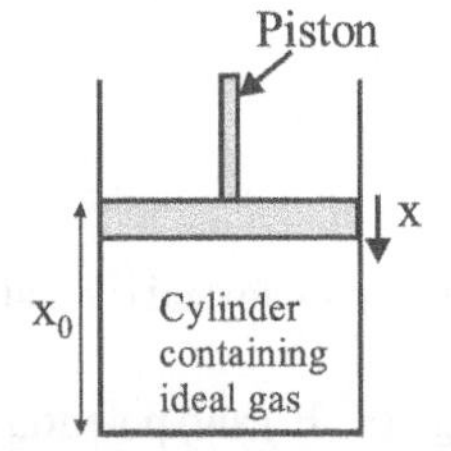

Let piston is displaced by distance x

$$Mg - \left(\frac{P_0 x_0^\gamma}{(x_0 - x)^\gamma}\right)A = F_{\text{restoring}}$$

$$P_0 A\left(1 - \frac{x_0^\gamma}{(x_0 - x)^\gamma}\right) = F_{\text{restoring}} \quad [x_0 - x \approx x_0]$$

$$F = -\frac{\gamma P_0 A x}{x_0}$$

$\therefore$ Frequency with which piston executes SHM.

$$f = \frac{1}{2\pi}\sqrt{\frac{\gamma P_0 A}{x_0 M}} = \frac{1}{2\pi}\sqrt{\frac{\gamma P_0 A^2}{M V_0}}$$

39. (c) As $F = -kx$

40. (a) Let T_1 and T_2 be the time period of the two pendulums

$$T_1 = 2\pi\sqrt{\frac{1}{g}} \text{ and } T_2 = 2\pi\sqrt{\frac{4}{g}}$$

As $\ell_1 < \ell_2$ therefore $T_1 < T_2$

Let at t = 0 they start swinging together. Since their time periods are different, the swinging will not be in unison always. Only when number of completed oscillations differ by an integer, the two pendulums will again begin to swing together

Let longer length pendulum complete n oscillation and shorter length pendulum complete (n + 1) oscillation.

For unison swinging

$(n+1)T_1 = nT_2$

$$(n+1)\times 2\pi\sqrt{\frac{l}{g}} = (n)\times 2\pi\sqrt{\frac{4}{g}}$$

$\Rightarrow n = 1$

$\therefore n + 1 = 1 + 1 = 2$

41. (d) The equation of motion for the pendulum, suffering retardation

$$F = -kx - bv$$

$$\Rightarrow \quad m\frac{d^2x}{dt^2} + kx + b\frac{dk}{dt} = 0$$

$$\Rightarrow \quad \frac{d^2x}{dt^2} + \frac{k}{m}x + \frac{b}{m}\frac{dx}{dt} = 0$$

$$\Rightarrow \quad \frac{d^2x}{dt^2} + \frac{b}{m}\frac{dx}{dt} + \frac{k}{m}x = 0 \qquad \ldots(1)$$

Let $x = e^{\lambda t}$ is the solution of the equation (1)

$$\frac{dx}{dt} = \lambda e^{\lambda t} \Rightarrow \frac{d^2x}{dt^2} = \lambda^2 e^{\lambda t}$$

Substituting in the equation (1)

$$\lambda^2 e^{\lambda t} + \frac{b}{m}\lambda e^{\lambda t} + \frac{k}{m}e^{\lambda t} = 0$$

$$\lambda^2 + \frac{b}{m}\lambda + \frac{k}{m} = 0$$

$$\lambda = \frac{-\frac{b}{m} \pm \sqrt{\frac{b^2}{m^2} - 4\frac{k}{m}}}{2} = \frac{-b \pm \sqrt{b^2 - 4km}}{2m}$$

Solving the equation (1) for x, we have

$$x = e^{\frac{-b}{2m}t}$$

$$\omega = \sqrt{\omega_0^2 - \lambda^2} \text{ where } \omega_0 = \frac{k}{m}, \; \lambda = \frac{+b}{2}$$

The average life $= \frac{1}{\lambda} = \frac{2}{b}$

42. (a)

43. (a)

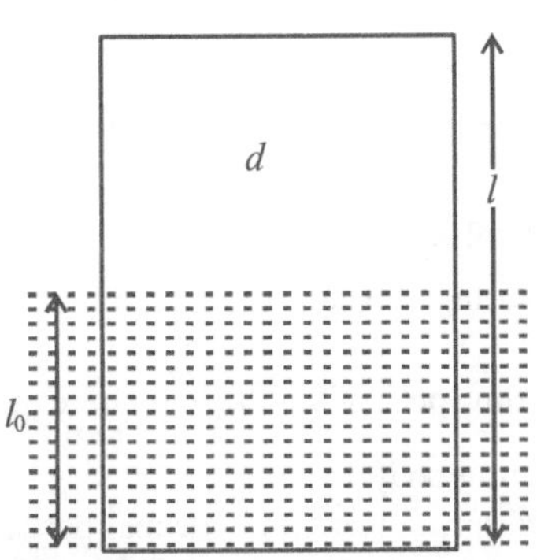

At equilibrium

$$F_b = mg$$

$$\rho A \ell_0 g = dA\ell g \qquad \ldots(i)$$

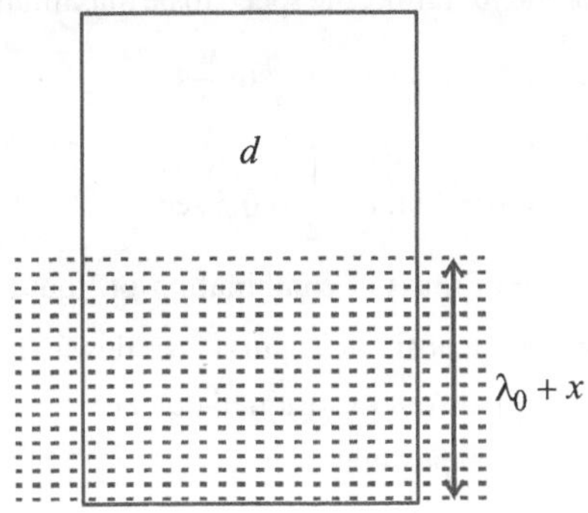

Restoring force,

$$F = mg - F_b'$$

$$F = mg - \rho A(\ell_0 + x)g$$

$$dA\ell a = dA\ell g - \rho A\ell_0 g - \rho gAx$$

$$a = -\frac{\rho g}{d\ell}x$$

Therefore, wooden cube performs S.H.M.

$$\therefore \quad \omega = \sqrt{\frac{\rho g}{d\ell}} \Rightarrow T = 2\pi\sqrt{\frac{\ell d}{\rho g}}$$

44. (a) For an SHM, the acceleration $a = -\omega^2 x$ where ω^2 is a constant. Therefore, $\frac{a}{x}$ is a constant. The time period T is also constant. Therefore, $\frac{aT}{x}$ is a constant.

45. (a) The two springs are in parallel.

$\therefore$ Effective spring constant,

$k = k_1 + k_2$

Now, frequency of oscillation is given by

$$f = \frac{1}{2\pi}\sqrt{\frac{k}{m}}$$

$$\text{or,} \quad f = \frac{1}{2\pi}\sqrt{\frac{k_1 + k_2}{m}} \qquad \ldots(i)$$

When both k_1 and k_2 are made four times their original values, the new frequency is given by

$$f' = \frac{1}{2\pi}\sqrt{\frac{4k_1 + 4k_2}{m}}$$

$$= \frac{1}{2\pi}\sqrt{\frac{4(k_1 + 4k_2)}{m}} = 2\left(\frac{1}{2\pi}\sqrt{\frac{k_1 + k_2}{m}}\right) = 2f$$

46. (b) Here, $x = 2 \times 10^{-2} \cos \pi t$

Speed is given by

$$v = \frac{dx}{dt} = 2 \times 10^{-2} \, \pi \sin \pi t$$

For the first time, the speed to be maximum,

$$\sin \pi t = 1 \text{ or, } \sin \pi t = \sin \frac{\pi}{2}$$

$$\Rightarrow \pi t = \frac{\pi}{2} \text{ or, } t = \frac{1}{2} = 0.5 \text{ sec.}$$

47. **(b)** Centre of mass of combination of liquid and hollow portion (at position ℓ), first goes down (to $\ell + \Delta\ell$) and when total water is drained out, centre of mass regain its original position (to ℓ),

$$T = 2\pi\sqrt{\frac{\ell}{g}}$$

$\therefore$ 'T' first increases and then decreases to original value.

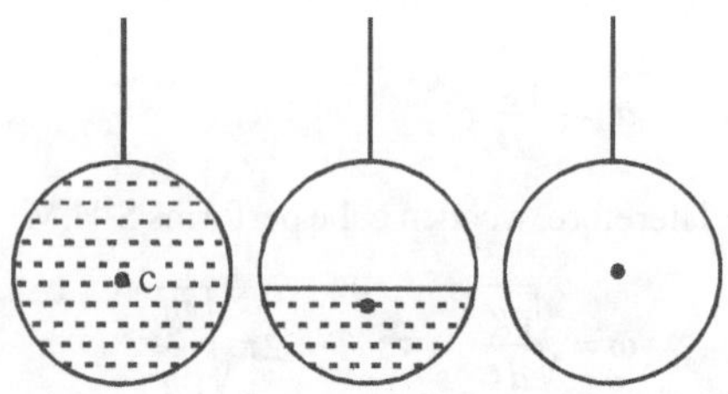

48. **(a)** $\frac{d^2x}{dt^2} = -\alpha x = -\omega^2 x$

$$\Rightarrow \omega = \sqrt{\alpha} \text{ or } T = \frac{2\pi}{\omega} = \frac{2\pi}{\sqrt{\alpha}}$$

49. **(a)** $t = 2\pi\sqrt{\frac{\ell}{g_{eff}}}$; $t_0 = 2\pi\sqrt{\frac{\ell}{g}}$

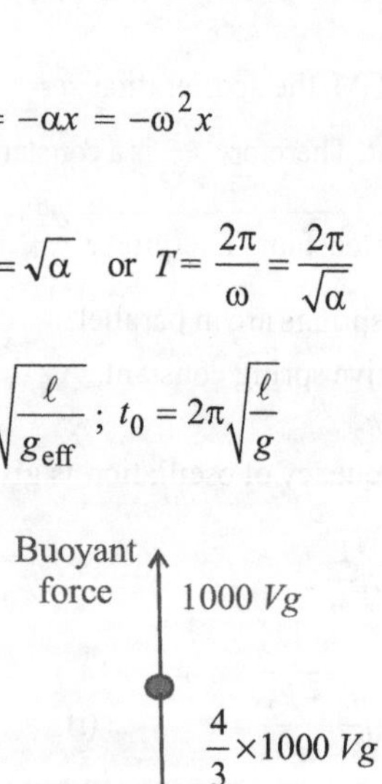

$$\text{Net force} = \left(\frac{4}{3} - 1\right) \times 1000\,Vg = \frac{1000}{3} Vg$$

$$g_{eff} = \frac{1000\,Vg}{3 \times \frac{4}{3} \times 1000V} = \frac{g}{4}$$

$$\therefore t = 2\pi\sqrt{\frac{\ell}{g/4}}$$

$$t = 2t_0$$

50. **(b)** For first spring, $t_1 = 2\pi\sqrt{\frac{m}{k_1}}$,

For second spring, $t_2 = 2\pi\sqrt{\frac{m}{k_2}}$

when springs are in series then, $k_{eff} = \frac{k_1 k_2}{k_l + k_2}$

$$\therefore T = 2\pi\sqrt{\frac{m(k_l + k_2)}{k_1 k_2}}$$

$$\therefore T = 2\pi\sqrt{\frac{m}{k_2} + \frac{m}{k_1}} = 2\pi\sqrt{\frac{t_2^2}{(2\pi)^2} + \frac{t_1^2}{(2\pi)^2}}$$

$$\Rightarrow T^2 = t_1^2 + t_2^2$$

where x is the displacement from the mean position

51. **(c)** $T = 2\pi\sqrt{\frac{M}{k}}$

$$T' = 2\pi\sqrt{\frac{M+m}{k}} = \frac{5T}{3}$$

$$\therefore 2\pi\sqrt{\frac{M+m}{k}} = \frac{5}{3} \times 2\pi\sqrt{\frac{M}{k}}$$

$$M + m = \frac{25}{9} \times M$$

$$1 + \frac{m}{M} = \frac{25}{9} \Rightarrow \frac{m}{M} = \frac{25}{9} - 1 = \frac{16}{9}$$

52. **(d)** $T = 2\pi\sqrt{\frac{\ell}{g}}$ and $T' = 2\pi\sqrt{\frac{1.21\ell}{g}}$

$$(\because \ell' = \ell + 21\% \text{ of } \ell)$$

$$\% \text{ increase} = \frac{T' - T}{T} \times 100$$

$$= \frac{\sqrt{1.21\ell} - \sqrt{\ell}}{\sqrt{\ell}} \times 100 = \left(\sqrt{1.21} - \sqrt{1}\right) \times 100$$

$$= (1.1 - 1) \times 100 = 10\%$$

53. **(b)** Let the spring constant of the original spring be k.

Then its time period T $= 2\pi\sqrt{\frac{m}{k}}$ where m is the mass of oscillating body.

When the spring is cut into n equal parts, the spring constant of one part becomes nk. Therefore the new time period,

$$T' = 2\pi\sqrt{\frac{m}{nk}} = \frac{T}{\sqrt{n}}$$

54. (b) The time period $T = 2\pi\sqrt{\frac{\ell}{g}}$ where ℓ = distance between the point of suspension and the centre of mass of the child.

As shown in the figure, $\ell' < \ell$

$\therefore T' < T$ i.e., the period decreases.

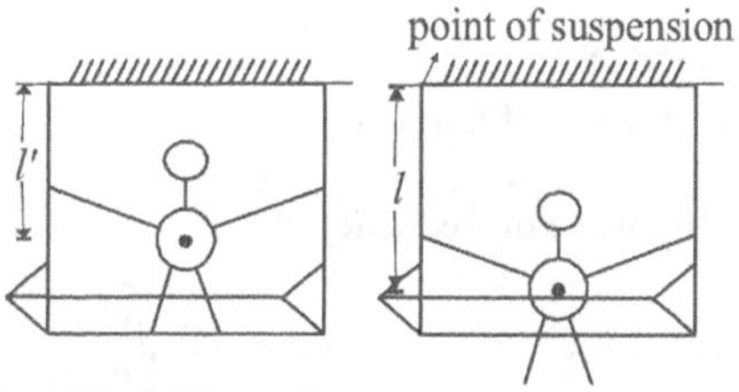

Case (ii) child standing Case (i) child sitting

TOPIC-4 : Damped, Forced Oscillations and Resonance

55. (b) The change in time period compared to the undamped oscillator increases by 8%.

56. (c) $\because A = A_0 e^{-\frac{bt}{2m}}$

(where, A_0 = maximum amplitude)
According to the questions, after 5 second,

$$0.9A_0 = A_0 e^{-\frac{b(5)}{2m}} \quad \ldots(i)$$

After 10 more second,

$$A = A_0 e^{-\frac{b(15)}{2m}} \quad \ldots(ii)$$

From eq^{n}s (i) and (ii)

$A = 0.729 A_0$

$\therefore \alpha = 0.729$

57. (a)

58. (d) When the pendulum is oscillating over a current carrying coil, and when the direction of oscillating pendulum bob is opposite to the direction of current. Its instantaneous acceleration increases.

Hence time period $T < 2\pi\sqrt{\frac{\ell}{g}}$

and damping is larger than in air alone due energy dissipation.

59. (c) Since energy $\propto$ (Amplitude)^2, the maximum for both of them occurs at the same frequency

$\therefore \omega_1 = \omega_2$

60. (b) Equation of displacement is given by

$x = A\sin(\omega t + \phi)$

where $A = \frac{F_0}{m\sqrt{(\omega_0^2 - \omega^2)^2}}$

$= \frac{F_0}{m(\omega_0^2 - \omega^2)}$

Here damping effect is considered to be zero

$\therefore x \propto \frac{1}{m(\omega_0^2 - \omega^2)}$

Chapter 14

Waves

TOPIC-1 : Basic of Mechanical Waves, Progressive and Stationary Waves

1. A transverse wave is represented by

$$y=\frac{10}{\pi}\sin\left(\frac{2\pi}{T}t-\frac{2\pi}{\lambda}x\right)$$

For what value of the wavelength the wave velocity is twice the maximum particle velocity? **[Online April 9, 2014]**

(a) 40 cm (b) 20 cm (c) 10 cm (d) 60 cm

2. In a transverse wave the distance between a crest and neighbouring trough at the same instant is 4.0 cm and the distance between a crest and trough at the same place is 1.0 cm. The next crest appears at the same place after a time interval of 0.4s. The maximum speed of the vibrating particles in the medium is : **[Online April 25, 2013]**

(a) $\frac{3\pi}{2}$ cm/s (b) $\frac{5\pi}{2}$ cm/s

(c) $\frac{\pi}{2}$ cm/s (d) 2π cm/s

3. When two sound waves travel in the same direction in a medium, the displacements of a particle located at 'x' at time 't' is given by :

$y_1 = 0.05\cos(0.50\pi x - 100\pi t)$

$y_2 = 0.05\cos(0.46\pi x - 92\pi t)$

where y_1, y_2 and x are in meters and t in seconds. The speed of sound in the medium is : **[Online April 9, 2013]**

(a) 92 m/s (b) 200 m/s (c) 100 m/s (d) 332 m/s

4. The disturbance $y(x, t)$ of a wave propagating in the positive x-direction is given by $y=\frac{1}{1+x^2}$ at time $t = 0$ and by $y=\frac{1}{\left[1+(x-1)^2\right]}$ at $t = 2$ s, where x and y are in meters. The shape of the wave disturbance does not change during the propagation. The velocity of wave in m/s is **[Online May 26, 2012]**

(a) 2.0 (b) 4.0 (c) 0.5 (d) 1.0

5. The transverse displacement $y(x, t)$ of a wave is given by

$$y(x,t)=e^{-\left(ax^2+bt^2+2\sqrt{ab}\,xt\right)}.$$

This represents a: **[2011]**

(a) wave moving in $-x$ direction with speed $\sqrt{\frac{b}{a}}$

(b) standing wave of frequency $\sqrt{b}$

(c) standing wave of frequency $\frac{1}{\sqrt{b}}$

(d) wave moving in $+x$ direction speed $\sqrt{\frac{a}{b}}$

6. A wave travelling along the x-axis is described by the equation $y(x, t) = 0.005\cos(\alpha x - \beta t)$. If the wavelength and the time period of the wave are 0.08 m and 2.0s, respectively, then α and β in appropriate units are **[2008]**

(a) $\alpha = 25.00\pi, \beta = \pi$

(b) $\alpha = \frac{0.08}{\pi}, \beta = \frac{2.0}{\pi}$

(c) $\alpha = \frac{0.04}{\pi}, \beta = \frac{1.0}{\pi}$

(d) $\alpha = 12.50\pi, \beta = \frac{\pi}{2.0}$

7. A sound absorber attenuates the sound level by 20 dB. The intensity decreases by a factor of **[2007]**

(a) 100 (b) 1000 (c) 10000 (d) 10

8. The displacement y of a particle in a medium can be expressed as, $y=10^{-6}\sin\left(100t+20x+\frac{\pi}{4}\right)m$ where t is in second and x in meter. The speed of the wave is **[2004]**

(a) 20 m/s (b) 5 m/s

(c) 2000 m/s (d) 5π m/s

9. The displacement y of a wave travelling in the x -direction is given by $y=10^{-4}\sin\left(600t-2x+\frac{\pi}{3}\right)$ metres where x is expressed in metres and t in seconds. The speed of the wave - motion, in ms^{-1}, is **[2003]**

(a) 300 (b) 600 (c) 1200 (d) 200

10. When temperature increases, the frequency of a tuning fork **[2002]**

(a) increases

(b) decreases

(c) remains same

(d) increases or decreases depending on the material

TOPIC-2 : Vibration of String and Organ Pipe

11. Two wires W_1 and W_2 have the same radius r and respective densities ρ_1 and ρ_2 such that $\rho_2 = 4\rho_1$. They are joined together at the point O, as shown in the figure. The combination is used as a sonometer wire and kept under tension T. The point O is midway between the two bridges.

When a stationary waves is set up in the composite wire, the joint is found to be a node. The ratio of the number of antinodes formed in W_1 to W_2 is : **[Online April 8, 2017]**

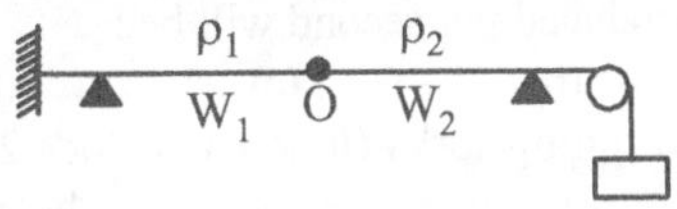

(a) 1 : 1 (b) 1 : 2 (c) 1 : 3 (d) 4 : 1

12. A uniform string of length 20 m is suspended from a rigid support. A short wave pulse is introduced at its lowest end. It starts moving up the string. The time taken to reach the supports is : **[2016]**
(take $g = 10 \text{ ms}^{-2}$)

(a) $2\sqrt{2}$s (b) $\sqrt{2}$ s
(c) $2\pi\sqrt{2}$ s (d) 2 s

13. A pipe open at both ends has a fundamental frequency f in air. The pipe is dipped vertically in water so that half of it is in water. The fundamental frequency of the air column is now : **[2016]**

(a) 2f (b) f
(c) $\frac{f}{2}$ (d) $\frac{3f}{4}$

14. A pipe of length 85 cm is closed from one end. Find the number of possible natural oscillations of air column in the pipe whose frequencies lie below 1250 Hz. The velocity of sound in air is 340 m/s. **[2014]**

(a) 12 (b) 8 (c) 6 (d) 4

15. The total length of a sonometer wire between fixed ends is 110 cm. Two bridges are placed to divide the length of wire in ratio 6 : 3 : 2. The tension in the wire is 400 N and the mass per unit length is 0.01 kg/m. What is the minimum common frequency with which three parts can vibrate? **[Online April 19, 2014]**

(a) 1100 Hz (b) 1000 Hz
(c) 166 Hz (d) 100 Hz

16. A sonometer wire of length 1.5 m is made of steel. The tension in it produces an elastic strain of 1%. What is the fundamental frequency of steel if density and elasticity of steel are 7.7×10^3 kg/m^3 and 2.2×10^{11} N/m^2 respectively? **[2013]**

(a) 188.5 Hz (b) 178.2 Hz
(c) 200.5 Hz (d) 770 Hz

17. A sonometer wire of length 114 cm is fixed at both the ends. Where should the two bridges be placed so as to divide the wire into three segments whose fundamental frequencies are in the ratio 1 : 3 : 4? **[Online April 23, 2013]**

(a) At 36 cm and 84 cm from one end
(b) At 24 cm and 72 cm from one end
(c) At 48 cm and 96 cm from one end
(d) At 72 cm and 96 cm from one end

18. A cylindrical tube, open at both ends, has a fundamental frequency f in air. The tube is dipped vertically in water so that half of it is in water. The fundamental frequency of the air-column is now : **[2012]**

(a) f (b) $f/2$ (c) $3f/4$ (d) $2f$

19. An air column in a pipe, which is closed at one end, will be in resonance wtih a vibrating tuning fork of frequency 264 Hz if the length of the column in cm is (velocity of sound = 330 m/s) **[Online May 26, 2012]**

(a) 125.00 (b) 93.75 (c) 62.50 (d) 187.50

20. A uniform tube of length 60.5 cm is held vertically with its lower end dipped in water. A sound source of frequency 500 Hz sends sound waves into the tube. When the length of tube above water is 16 cm and again when it is 50 cm, the tube resonates with the source of sound. Two lowest frequencies (in Hz), to which tube will resonate when it is taken out of water, are (approximately). **[Online May 19, 2012]**

(a) 281, 562 (b) 281, 843
(c) 276, 552 (d) 272, 544

21. The equation of a wave on a string of linear mass density 0.04 kg m^{-1} is given by

$$y = 0.02(\text{m}) \sin\left[2\pi\left(\frac{t}{0.04(s)} - \frac{x}{0.50(m)}\right)\right].$$

The tension in the string is **[2010]**

(a) 4.0 N (b) 12.5 N (c) 0.5 N (d) 6.25 N

22. While measuring the speed of sound by performing a resonance column experiment, a student gets the first resonance condition at a column length of 18 cm during winter. Repeating the same experiment during summer, she measures the column length to be x cm for the second resonance. Then **[2008]**

(a) 18 > x (b) x > 54
(c) 54 > x > 36 (d) 36 > x > 18

23. A string is stretched between fixed points separated by 75.0 cm. It is observed to have resonant frequencies of 420 Hz and 315 Hz. There are no other resonant frequencies between these two. Then, the lowest resonant frequency for this string is **[2006]**

(a) 105 Hz (b) 1.05 Hz
(c) 1050 Hz (d) 10.5 Hz

24. Tube A has both ends open while tube B has one end closed, otherwise they are identical. The ratio of fundamental frequency of tube A and B is **[2002]**

(a) 1 : 2 (b) 1 : 4 (c) 2 : 1 (d) 4 : 1

25. A wave $y = a \sin(\omega t - kx)$ on a string meets with another wave producing a node at $x = 0$. Then the equation of the unknown wave is **[2002]**

(a) $y = a \sin(\omega t + kx)$
(b) $y = -a \sin(\omega t + kx)$
(c) $y = a \sin(\omega t - kx)$
(d) $y = -a \sin(\omega t - kx)$

TOPIC-3 : Beats, Interference and Superposition of Waves

26. A standing wave is formed by the superposition of two waves travelling in opposite directions. The transverse displacement is given by

$$y(x, t) = 0.5 \sin\left(\frac{5\pi}{4}x\right) \cos(200\,\pi t).$$

What is the speed of the travelling wave moving in the positive x direction ?
(x and t are in meter and second, respectively.) **[Online April 9, 2017]**
(a) 160 m/s (b) 90 m/s (c) 180 m/s (d) 120 m/s

27. A wave represented by the equation $y_1 = a\cos(kx - \omega t)$ is superimposed with another wave to form a stationary wave such that the point $x - 0$ is node. The equation for the other wave is **[Online May 12, 2012]**
(a) $a\cos(kx - \omega t + \pi)$
(b) $a\cos(kx + \omega t + \pi)$
(c) $a\cos\left(kx + \omega t + \frac{\pi}{2}\right)$
(d) $a\cos\left(kx - \omega t + \frac{\pi}{2}\right)$

28. Following are expressions for four plane simple harmonic waves **[Online May 7, 2012]**

(i) $y_1 = A\cos 2\pi\left(n_1 t + \frac{x}{\lambda_1}\right)$

(ii) $y_2 = A\cos 2\pi\left(n_1 t + \frac{x}{\lambda_1} + \pi\right)$

(iii) $y_3 = A\cos 2\pi\left(n_2 t + \frac{x}{\lambda_2}\right)$

(iv) $y_4 = A\cos 2\pi\left(n_2 t - \frac{x}{\lambda_2}\right)$

The pairs of waves which will produce destructive interference and stationary waves respectively in a medium, are
(a) (iii, iv), (i, ii) (b) (i, iii), (ii, iv)
(c) (i, iv), (ii, iii) (d) (i, ii), (iii, iv)

29. A travelling wave represented by $y = A\sin(\omega t - kx)$ is superimposed on another wave represented by $y = A\sin(\omega t + kx)$. The resultant is **[2011 RS]**
(a) A wave travelling along + x direction
(b) A wave travelling along – x direction
(c) A standing wave having nodes at
$x = \frac{n\lambda}{2}, n = 0,1,2....$
(d) A standing wave having nodes at
$x = \left(n + \frac{1}{2}\right)\frac{\lambda}{2};\ n = 0,1,2....$

30. **Statement - 1 :** Two longitudinal waves given by equations : $y_1(x,t) = 2a\sin(\omega t - kx)$ and $y_2(x,t) = a\sin(2\omega t - 2kx)$ will have equal intensity. **[2011 RS]**
Statement - 2 : Intensity of waves of given frequency in same medium is proportional to square of amplitude only.
(a) Statement-1 is true, statement-2 is false.
(b) Statement-1 is true, statement-2 is true, statement-2 is the correct explanation of statement-1
(c) Statement-1 is true, statement-2 is true, statement-2 is not the correct explanation of statement-1
(d) Statement-1 is false, statement-2 is true.

31. Three sound waves of equal amplitudes have frequencies $(\nu - 1)$, ν, $(\nu + 1)$. They superpose to give beats. The number of beats produced per second will be : **[2009]**
(a) 3 (b) 2 (c) 1 (d) 4

32. When two tuning forks (fork 1 and fork 2) are sounded simultaneously, 4 beats per second are heard. Now, some tape is attached on the prong of the fork 2. When the tuning forks are sounded again, 6 beats per second are heard. If the frequency of fork 1 is 200 Hz, then what was the original frequency of fork 2? **[2005]**
(a) 202 Hz (b) 200 Hz (c) 204 Hz (d) 196 Hz

33. A tuning fork of known frequency 256 Hz makes 5 beats per second with the vibrating string of a piano. The beat frequency decreases to 2 beats per second when the tension in the piano string is slightly increased. The frequency of the piano string before increasing the tension was **[2003]**
(a) (256 + 2) Hz (b) (256 – 2) Hz
(c) (256 – 5) Hz (d) (256 + 5) Hz

34. A tuning fork arrangement (pair) produces 4 beats/sec with one fork of frequency 288 cps. A little wax is placed on the unknown fork and it then produces 2 beats/sec. The frequency of the unknown fork is **[2002]**
(a) 286 cps (b) 292 cps (c) 294 cps (d) 288 cps

TOPIC-4 : Musical Sound and Doppler's Effect

35. A toy–car, blowing its horm, is moving with a steady speed of 5 m/s, away from a wall. An observer, towards whom the toy car is moving, is able to hear 5 beats per second. If the velocity of sound in air is 340 m/s, the frequency of the horn of the toy car is close to : **[Online April 10, 2016]**
(a) 680 Hz (b) 510 Hz (c) 340 Hz (d) 170 Hz

36. Two engines pass each other moving in opposite directions with uniform speed of 30 m/s. One of them is blowing a whistle of frequency 540 Hz. Calculate the frequency heard by driver of second engine before they pass each other. Speed of sound is 330 m/sec: **[Online April 9, 2016]**
(a) 450 Hz (b) 540 Hz (c) 270 Hz (d) 648 Hz

37. A train is moving on a straight track with speed 20 ms^{-1}. It is blowing its whistle at the frequency of 1000 Hz. The percentage change in the frequency heard by a person standing near the track as the train passes him is (speed of sound = 320 ms^{-1}) close to : **[2015]**
(a) 18% (b) 24% (c) 6% (d) 12%

38. A source of sound emits sound waves at frequency f_0. It is moving towards an observer with fixed speed v_s ($v_s < v$, where v is the speed of sound in air). If the observer were to move towards the source with speed v_0, one of the following two graphs (A and B) will given the correct variation of the frequency f heard by the observer as v_0 is changed.

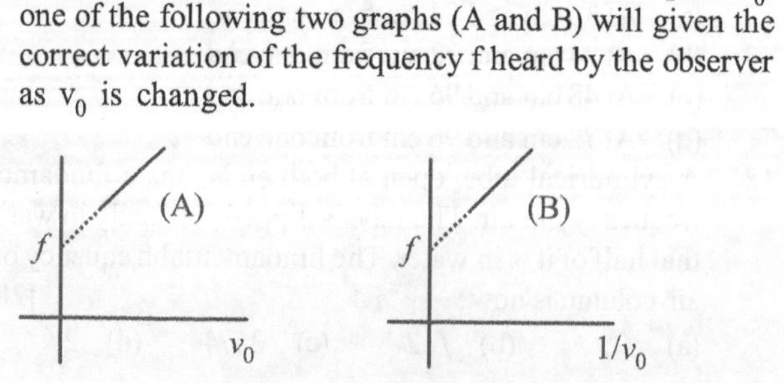

The variation of f with v_0 is given correctly by : **[Online April 11, 2015]**

(a) graph A with slope $= \dfrac{f_0}{(v+v_s)}$

(b) graph B with slope $= \dfrac{f_0}{(v-v_s)}$

(c) graph A with slope $= \dfrac{f_0}{(v-v_s)}$

(d) graph B with slope $= \dfrac{f_0}{(v+v_s)}$

39. A bat moving at 10 ms^{-1} towards a wall sends a sound signal of 8000 Hz towards it. On reflection it hears a sound of frequency *f*. The value of *f* in Hz is close to (speed of sound = 320 ms^{-1}) **[Online April 10, 2015]**

(a) 8516 (b) 8258 (c) 8424 (d) 8000

40. A source of sound A emitting waves of frequency 1800 Hz is falling towards ground with a terminal speed v. The observer B on the ground directly beneath the source receives waves of frequency 2150 Hz. The source A receives waves, reflected from ground of frequency nearly: (Speed of sound = 343 m/s) **[Online April 12, 2014]**

(a) 2150 Hz (b) 2500 Hz (c) 1800 Hz (d) 2400 Hz

41. Two factories are sounding their sirens at 800 Hz. A man goes from one factory to other at a speed of 2m/s. The velocity of sound is 320 m/s. The number of beats heard by the person in one second will be: **[Online April 11, 2014]**

(a) 2 (b) 4 (c) 8 (d) 10

42. A and B are two sources generating sound waves. A listener is situated at C. The frequency of the source at A is 500 Hz. A, now, moves towards C with a speed 4 m/s. The number of beats heard at C is 6. When A moves away from C with speed 4 m/s, the number of beats heard at C is 18. The speed of sound is 340 m/s. The frequency of the source at B is : **[Online April 22, 2013]**

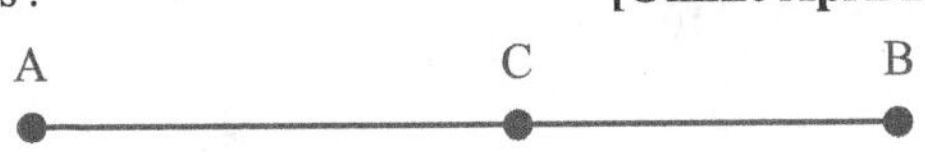

(a) 500 Hz (b) 506 Hz (c) 512 Hz (d) 494 Hz

43. An engine approaches a hill with a constant speed. When it is at a distance of 0.9 km, it blows a whistle whose echo is heard by the driver after 5 seconds. If the speed of sound in air is 330 m/s, then the speed of the engine is : **[Online April 9, 2013]**

(a) 32 m/s (b) 27.5 m/s (c) 60 m/s (d) 30 m/s

44. This question has Statement 1 and Statement 2. Of the four choices given after the Statements, choose the one that best describes the two Statements.

Statement 1: Bats emitting ultrasonic waves can detect the location of a prey by hearing the waves reflected from it.

Statement 2: When the source and the detector are moving, the frequency of reflected waves is changed. **[Online May 12, 2012]**

(a) Statement 1 is false, Statement 2 is true.
(b) Statement 1 is true, Statement 2 is false.
(c) Statement 1 is true, Statement 2 is true, Statement 2 is not the correct explanation of Statement 1.
(d) Statement 1 is true, Statement 2 is true, Statement 2 is the correct explanation of Statement 1.

45. A motor cycle starts from rest and accelerates along a straight path at $2 m/s^2$. At the starting point of the motor cycle there is a stationary electric siren. How far has the motor cycle gone when the driver hears the frequency of the siren at 94% of its value when the motor cycle was at rest? (Speed of sound = 330 ms^{-1}) **[2009]**

(a) 98m (b) 147m (c) 196m (d) 49m

46. A whistle producing sound waves of frequencies 9500 HZ and above is approaching a stationary person with speed v ms^{-1}. The velocity of sound in air is 300 ms^{-1}. If the person can hear frequencies upto a maximum of 10,000 HZ, the maximum value of v upto which he can hear whistle is **[2006]**

(a) $15\sqrt{2}\ ms^{-1}$ (b) $\dfrac{15}{\sqrt{2}}\ ms^{-1}$

(c) $15\ ms^{-1}$ (d) $30\ ms^{-1}$

47. An observer moves towards a stationary source of sound, with a velocity one-fifth of the velocity of sound. What is the percentage increase in the apparent frequency ? **[2005]**

(a) 0.5% (b) zero (c) 20% (d) 5%

Hints & Solutions

TOPIC-1 : Basic of Mechanical Waves, Progressive and Stationary Waves

1. (a) Given, amplitude $a = 10$ cm

wave velocity $= 2 \times$ maximum particle velocity

i.e, $\frac{\omega\lambda}{2\pi} = 2\frac{a\omega}{\pi}$

or, $\lambda = 4a = 4 \times 10 = 40$ cm

2. (b)

3. (b) Standard equation

$$y(x,t) = A\cos\left(\frac{\omega}{V}x - \omega t\right)$$

From any of the displacement equation

Say y_1

$\frac{\omega}{V} = 0.50\pi$ and $\omega = 100\pi$

$\therefore \frac{100\pi}{V} = 0.5\pi$

$\therefore V = \frac{100\pi}{0.5\pi} = 200$ m/s

4. (c) The equation of wave at any time is obtained by putting $X = x - vt$

$$y = \frac{1}{1+x^2} = \frac{1}{1+(x-vt)^2} \quad ...(i)$$

We know at $t = 2$ sec,

$$y = \frac{1}{1+(x-1)^2} \quad ...(ii)$$

On comparing (i) and (ii) we get

$vt = 1$

$V = \frac{1}{t}$

As $t = 2$ sec

$\therefore V = \frac{1}{2} = 0.5$ m/s.

5. (a) Given wave equation is $y(x,t)$

$= e^{\left(-ax^2+bt^2+2\sqrt{ab}\,xt\right)}$

$= e^{-[(\sqrt{a}x)^2+(\sqrt{b}t)^2+2\sqrt{a}x.\sqrt{b}t]}$

$= e^{-(\sqrt{a}x+\sqrt{b}t)^2}$

$= e^{-\left(x+\sqrt{\frac{b}{a}}t\right)^2}$

It is a function of type $y = f(x+vt)$

$\Rightarrow$ Speed of wave $= \sqrt{\frac{b}{a}}$

6. (a) $y(x,t) = 0.005\cos(\alpha x - \beta t)$ (Given)

Comparing it with the standard equation of wave

$y(x,t) = a\cos(kx - \omega t)$ we get

$k = \alpha$ and $\omega = \beta$

But $k = \frac{2\pi}{\lambda}$ and $\omega = \frac{2\pi}{T}$

$\Rightarrow \frac{2\pi}{\lambda} = \alpha$ and $\frac{2\pi}{T} = \beta$

Given that $\lambda = 0.08$ m and $T = 2.0$s

$\therefore \alpha = \frac{2\pi}{0.08} = 25\pi$ and $\beta = \frac{2\pi}{2} = \pi$

7. (a) We have, $L_1 = 10\log\left(\frac{I_1}{I_0}\right)$;

$L_2 = 10\log\left(\frac{I_2}{I_0}\right)$

$\therefore L_1 - L_2 = 10\log\left(\frac{I_1}{I_0}\right) - 10\log\left(\frac{I_2}{I_0}\right)$

or, $\Delta L = 10\log\left(\frac{I_1}{I_0} \times \frac{I_0}{I_2}\right)$

or, $\Delta L = 10\log\left(\frac{I_1}{I_2}\right)$

or, $20 = 10\log\left(\frac{I_1}{I_2}\right)$ or, $2 = \log\left(\frac{I_1}{I_2}\right)$

or, $\frac{I_1}{I_2} = 10^2$ or, $I_2 = \frac{I_1}{100}$.

$\Rightarrow$ Intensity decreases by a factor 100.

8. (b) From equation given,

$\omega = 100$ and $k = 20$

$v = \frac{\omega}{k} = \frac{100}{20} = 5$ m/s

9. (a) $y = 10^{-4}\sin\left(600t - 2x + \frac{\pi}{3}\right)$

But $y = A\sin(\omega t - kx + \phi)$

On comparing we get $\omega = 600$; $k=2$

Also velocity of wave is given by

$v = \frac{\omega}{k} = \frac{600}{2} = 300$ ms^{-1}

10. (b) The frequency of a tuning fork is given by the expression

$$f = \frac{m^2 k}{4\sqrt{3}\pi\ell^2}\sqrt{\frac{Y}{\rho}}$$

As temperature increases, ℓ increases and therefore f decreases.

TOPIC-2 : Vibration of String and Organ Pipe

11. (b) $n_1 = n_2$

$T \rightarrow$ Same

$r \rightarrow$ Same

$l \rightarrow$ Same

Frequency of vibration

$$n = \frac{p}{2l}\sqrt{\frac{T}{\pi r^2 \rho}}$$

As T, r, and l are same for both the wires

$n_1 = n_2$

$$\frac{p_1}{\sqrt{\rho_1}} = \frac{p_2}{\sqrt{\rho_2}}$$

$$\Rightarrow \frac{p_1}{p_2} = \frac{1}{2} \qquad \because \rho_2 = 4\rho_1$$

12. (a) We know that velocity in string is given by

$$v = \sqrt{\frac{T}{\mu}} \qquad ...(I)$$

where $\mu = \frac{m}{l} = \frac{\text{mass of string}}{\text{length of string}}$

The tension $T = \frac{m}{\ell} \times x \times g \qquad ..(II)$

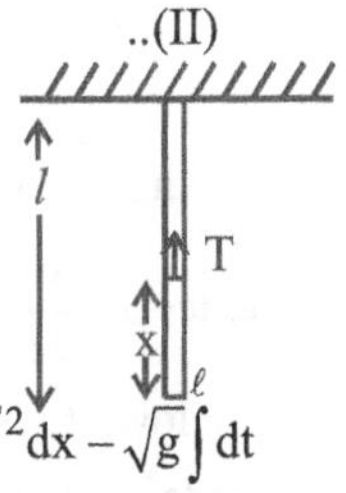

From (1) and (2)

$$\frac{dx}{dt} = \sqrt{gx}$$

$$x^{-1/2}dx = \sqrt{g}\,dt \qquad \therefore \int_0^{\ell} x^{-1/2}dx - \sqrt{g}\int_0^{\ell} dt$$

$$2\sqrt{l} = \sqrt{g} \times t \quad \therefore t = 2\sqrt{\frac{\ell}{g}} = 2\sqrt{\frac{20}{10}} = 2\sqrt{2}$$

13. (b)

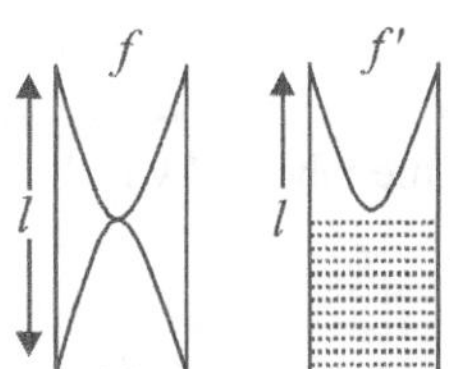

(a) (b)

The fundamental frequency in case (a) is $f = \frac{v}{2\ell}$

The fundamental frequency in case (b) is

$$f' = \frac{v}{4(\ell/2)} = \frac{u}{2\ell} = f$$

14. (c) Length of pipe = 85 cm = 0.85m

Frequency of oscillations of air column in closed organ pipe is given by,

$$f = \frac{(2n-1)v}{4L}$$

$$f = \frac{(2n-1)v}{4L} \leq 1250$$

$$\Rightarrow \frac{(2n-1) \times 340}{0.85 \times 4} \leq 1250$$

$$\Rightarrow 2n - 1 \leq 12.5 \approx 6$$

15. (b) Total length of sonometer wire, l = 110 cm = 1.1 m

Length of wire is in ratio, 6 : 3 : 2 i.e. 60 cm, 30 cm, 20 cm.

Tension in the wire, T = 400 N

Mass per unit length, m = 0.01 kg

Minimum common frequency = ?

As we know,

$$\text{Frequency, } \nu = \frac{1}{2l}\sqrt{\frac{T}{m}} = \frac{1000}{11}\text{Hz}$$

$$\text{Similarly, } \nu_1 = \frac{1000}{6}\text{Hz}$$

$$\nu_2 = \frac{1000}{3}\text{Hz}$$

$$\nu_3 = \frac{1000}{2}\text{Hz}$$

Hence common frequency = 1000 Hz

16. (b) Fundamental frequency,

$$f = \frac{v}{2\ell} = \frac{1}{2\ell}\sqrt{\frac{T}{\mu}} = \frac{1}{2\ell}\sqrt{\frac{T}{A\rho}}$$

$$\left[\because v = \sqrt{\frac{T}{\mu}} \text{ and } \mu = \frac{m}{\ell}\right]$$

$$\text{Also, } Y = \frac{T\ell}{A\Delta\ell} \Rightarrow \frac{T}{A} = \frac{Y\Delta\ell}{\ell}$$

$$\Rightarrow f = \frac{1}{2\ell}\sqrt{\frac{\gamma\Delta\ell}{\ell\rho}} \qquad ....(i)$$

$\ell = 1.5$ m, $\frac{\Delta\ell}{\ell} = 0.01$,

$\rho = 7.7 \times 10^3$ kg/m^3 (given)

$\gamma = 2.2 \times 10^{11}$ N/m^2 (given)

Putting the value of ℓ, $\frac{\Delta\ell}{\ell}$, ρ and γ in eq^n. (i) we get,

$$f = \sqrt{\frac{2}{7}} \times \frac{10^3}{3} \quad \text{or} \quad f \approx 178.2 \text{ Hz}$$

17. (d) Total length of the wire, L = 114 cm

$n_1 : n_2 : n_3 = 1 : 3 : 4$

Let L_1, L_2 and L_3 be the lengths of the three parts

As $n \propto \frac{1}{L}$

$\therefore \quad L_1 : L_2 : L_3 = \frac{1}{1} : \frac{1}{3} : \frac{1}{4} = 12 : 4 : 3$

$\therefore \quad L_1 = \left(\frac{12}{12+4+3} \times 114\right) = 72\,\text{cm}$

$L_2 = \left(\frac{4}{19} \times 114\right) = 24$ cm

and $L_3 = \left(\frac{3}{19} \times 114\right) = 18$ cm

Hence the bridges should be placed at 72 cm and 72 + 24 = 96 cm from one end.

18. **(a)** The fundamental frequency of open tube

$+ \quad \nu_0 = \frac{v}{2l_0} \quad \ldots\text{(i)}$

where l is the length of the tube
v = speed of sound
That of closed tube

$\nu_c = \frac{v}{4l_c} \quad \ldots\text{(ii)}$

According to the problem $l_c = \frac{l_0}{2}$

Thus $\nu_c = \frac{v}{l_0/2} \Rightarrow \nu_c \frac{v}{2l} \quad \ldots\text{(iii)}$

From equations (i) and (iii)

$\nu_0 = \nu_c$

Thus, $\nu_c = f \ (\because \nu_0 = f$ is given)

19. **(b)** Given : Frequency of tuning fork, n = 264 Hz
Length of column L = ?
For closed organ pipe

$n = \frac{v}{4l}$

$\Rightarrow l = \frac{v}{4n} = \frac{330}{4 \times 264} = 0.3125$

or, $l = 0.3125 \times 100 = 31.25$ cm

In case of closed organ pipe only odd harmonics are possible.
Therefore value of l will be $(2n - 1)\ l$
Hence option (b) i.e. 3 × 31.25 = 93.75 cm is correct.

20. **(d)** Two lowest frequencies to which tube will resonates are 272 Hz and 544 Hz.

21. **(d)** $y = 0.02(m)\sin\left[2\pi\left(\frac{t}{0.04(s)}\right) - \frac{x}{0.50(m)}\right]$

Comparing this equation with the standard wave equation

$y = a\sin(\omega t - kx)$

we get

$\omega = \frac{2\pi}{0.04}$

$\Rightarrow \nu = \frac{1}{0.04} = 25\,Hz$

$k = \frac{2\pi}{0.50} \Rightarrow \lambda = 0.5\,\text{m}$

$\therefore$ velocity, $v = \nu\lambda = 25 \times 0.5$ m/s
$= 12.5$ m/s

Velocity on a string is given by

$v = \sqrt{\frac{T}{\mu}}$

$\therefore \ T = v^2 \times \mu = (12.5)^2 \times 0.04 = 6.25\,\text{N}$

22. **(b)** For first resonant length

$\nu = \frac{v}{4\ell_1} = \frac{v}{4 \times 18}$ (in winter)

For second resonant length

$\nu' = \frac{3v'}{4\ell_2} = \frac{3v'}{4x}$ (in summer)

$\therefore \quad \frac{v}{4 \times 18} = \frac{3v'}{4 \times x}$

$\therefore \ x = 3 \times 18 \times \frac{v'}{v} \qquad \therefore \ x = 54 \times \frac{v'}{v}\text{cm}$

$v' > v$ because velocity of light is greater in summer as compared to winter $(v \propto \sqrt{T})$

$\therefore \ x > 54\,\text{cm}$

23. **(a)** Given $\frac{nv}{2\ell} = 315$ and $(n+1)\frac{v}{2\ell} = 420$

$\Rightarrow \frac{n+1}{n} = \frac{420}{315} \Rightarrow n = 3$

Hence $3 \times \frac{v}{2\ell} = 315 \Rightarrow \frac{v}{2\ell} = 105$ Hz

The lowest resonant frequency is when n = 1
Therefore lowest resonant frequency = 105 Hz.

24. **(c)** The fundamental frequency for closed organ pipe is given by

$\upsilon_c = \frac{v}{4\ell} \qquad \left[\because \ell = \frac{\lambda}{4}\right]$

Where ℓ = length of the tube and v is the velocity of sound in air.

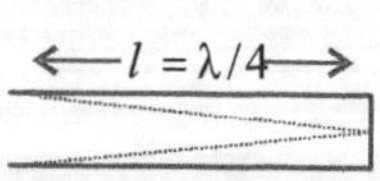

The fundamental frequency for open organ pipe is given by

$\upsilon_0 = \frac{v}{2\ell} \qquad \left[\because \ell = \frac{\lambda}{2}\right]$

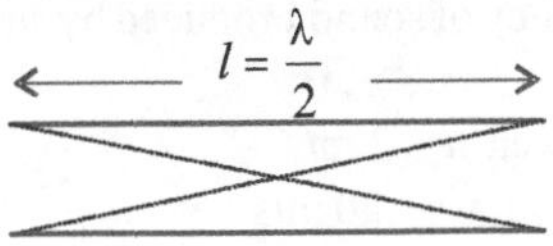

$$\therefore \frac{\upsilon_0}{\upsilon_c} = \frac{v}{2\ell} \times \frac{4\ell}{v} = \frac{2}{1}$$

25. **(b)** To form a node there should be superposition of this wave with the reflected wave. The reflected wave should travel in opposite direction with a phase change of π. The equation of the reflected wave will be

$y = a \sin(\omega t + kx + \pi)$

$\Rightarrow y = -a \sin(\omega t + kx)$

TOPIC-3 : Beats, Interference and Superposition of Waves

26. **(a)** Given, $y(x, t) = 0.5 \sin\left(\frac{5\pi}{4}x\right) \cos(200\pi t)$,

comparing with equation $- y(x, t) = 2a \sin kx \cos \omega t$

$\omega = 200\pi, k = \frac{5\pi}{4}$

speed of travelling wave $v = \frac{\omega}{k} = \frac{200\pi}{5\pi/4} = 160$ m/s

27. **(b)** Since the point $x = 0$ is a node and reflection is taking place from point $x = 0$. This means that reflection must be taking place from the fixed end and hence the reflected ray must suffer an additional phase change of π or a path change of $\frac{\lambda}{2}$.

So, if $y_{incident} = a \cos(kx - \omega t)$

$\Rightarrow y_{incident} = a \cos(-kx - \omega t + \pi)$

$= -a \cos(\omega t + kx)$

Hence equation for the other wave

$y = a \cos(kx + \omega t + \pi)$

28. **(d)** In case of destructive interference

Phase difference $\phi = 180°$ or π

So wave pair (i) and (ii) will produce destructive interference.

Stationary or standing waves will produce by equations (iii) & (iv) as two waves travelling along the same line but in opposite direction.

$n' = n + x$

29. **(d)** $y = A \sin(\omega t - kx) + A \sin(\omega t + kx)$

$y = 2A \sin \omega t \cos kx$

For standing wave nodes

$\cos kx = 0$

$\frac{2\pi}{\lambda} . x = (2n + 1)\frac{\pi}{2}$

$\therefore x = \frac{(2n+1)\lambda}{4}, n = 0, 1, 2, 3, ...$

30. **(a)** Since, $I \propto A^2\omega^2$

$I_1 \propto (2a)^2 \omega^2$

$I_2 \propto a^2 (2\omega)^2$

$I_1 = I_2$

Intensity depends on frequency also.

31. **(b)** Maximum number of beats

$= (v + 1) - (v - 1) = 2$

32. **(d)** Frequency of fork 1 = 200 Hz = n_0

No. of beats heard when fork 2 is sounded with fork 1

$= \Delta n = 4$

Now we know that if on loading (attaching tape) an unknown fork, the beat frequency increases (from 4 to 6 in this case) then the frequency of the unknown fork 2 is given by,

$n = n_0 - \Delta n = 200 - 4 = 196$ Hz

33. **(c)** A tuning fork of frequency 256 Hz makes 5 beats/second with the vibrating string of a piano. Therefore, the frequency of the vibrating string of piano is (256 ± 5) Hz. i.e., either 261Hz or 251 Hz. When the tension in the piano string increases, its frequency will increases. Now since the beat frequency decreases, we can conclude that the frequency of piano string is 251Hz

34. **(b)** A tuning fork produces 4 beats/sec with another tuning fork of frequency 288 cps. From this information we can conclude that the frequency of unknown fork is 288 + 4 cps or 288 – 4 cps i.e. 292 cps or 284 cps. When a little wax is placed on the unknown fork, it produces 2 beats/sec. When a little wax is placed on the unknown fork, its frequency decreases and simultaneously the beat frequency decreases confirming that the frequency of the unknown fork is 292 cps.

NOTE Had the frequency of unknown fork been 284 cps, then on placing wax its frequency would have decreased thereby increasing the gap between its frequency and the frequency of known fork. This would produce high beat frequency.

TOPIC-4 : Musical Sound and Doppler's Effect

35. **(d)** From Doppler's effect

$f(\text{direct}) = f\left(\frac{340}{340-5}\right) = f_1$

$f(\text{by wall}) = f\left(\frac{340}{340+5}\right) = f_2$

Beats = $(f_1 - f_2)$

$5 = f\left(\frac{340}{340-5} - \frac{340}{340+5}\right)$

$\Rightarrow f = 170$ Hz.

36. (d) We know that the apperent frequency

$$f' = \left(\frac{v - v_0}{v - v_s}\right) f \qquad \text{from Doppler's effect}$$

where $v_0 = v_s = 30$ m/s, velocity of observer and source
Speed of sound v = 330 m/s

$$\therefore\ f' = \frac{330+30}{330-30} \times 540 = 648 \text{ Hz.}$$

$\because$ Frequency of whistle (f) = 540 Hz.

37. (d) $f_1 = f\left[\frac{v}{v - v_s}\right] = f \times \frac{320}{300} Hz$

$$f_2 = f\left[\frac{v}{v + v_s}\right] = f \times \frac{320}{340} Hz$$

$$\left(\frac{f_2}{f_1} - 1\right) \times 100 = \left(\frac{300}{340} - 1\right) \times 100 \simeq 12\%$$

38. (c) According to Doppler's effect,

Apparent, frequency $f = \left(\frac{V + V_0}{V - V_S}\right) f_0$

Now, $f = \left(\frac{f_0}{V - V_S}\right) V_0 + \frac{V f_0}{V - V_s}$

So, slope $= \frac{f_0}{V - V_S}$

Hence, option (c) is the correct answer.

39. (a) Reflected frequency of sound reaching bat

$$= \left[\frac{V - (-V_0)}{V - V_s}\right] f = \left[\frac{V + V_0}{V - V_s}\right] f = \frac{V + 10}{V - 10} f$$

$$= \left(\frac{320 + 10}{320 - 10}\right) \times 8000 = 8516 \text{ Hz}$$

40. (b) Given $f_A = 1800$ Hz
$v_t = v$
$f_B = 2150$ Hz
Reflected wave frequency received by A, $f_A' = ?$
Applying doppler's effect of sound,

$$f' = \frac{v_s f}{v_s - v_t}$$

here, $v_t = v_s\left(1 - \frac{f_A}{f_B}\right)$

$$= 343\left(1 - \frac{1800}{2150}\right)$$

$v_t = 55.8372$ m/s
Now, for the reflected wave,

$$\therefore\ f_A' = \left(\frac{v_s + v_t}{v_s - v_t}\right) f_A$$

$$= \left(\frac{343 + 55.83}{343 - 55.83}\right) \times 1800$$

$= 2499.44 \approx 2500$ Hz

41. (d) **Given:** Frequency of sound produced by siren, $f = 800$ Hz
Speed of observer, $u = 2$ m/s
Velocity of sound, $v = 320$ m/s
No. of beats heard per second = ?
No. of extra waves received by the observer per second $= \pm 4\lambda$
$\therefore$ No. of beats/ sec

$$= \frac{2}{\lambda} - \left(-\frac{2}{\lambda}\right) = \frac{4}{\lambda}$$

$$= \frac{2 \times 2}{\frac{320}{800}} \qquad \left(\because \lambda = \frac{V}{f}\right)$$

$$= \frac{2 \times 2 \times 800}{320} = 10$$

42. (c) f = 500 Hz

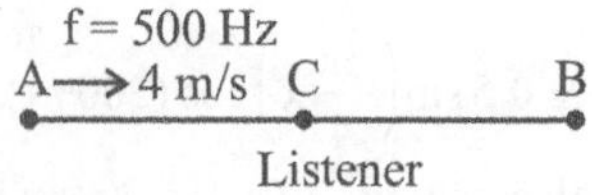

Case 1 : When source is moving towards stationary listener

apparent frequency $\eta' = \eta\left(\frac{v}{v - v_s}\right)$

$$= 500\left(\frac{340}{336}\right) = 506 \text{ Hz}$$

Case 2 : When source is moving away from the stationary listener

$$\eta'' = \eta\left(\frac{v}{v + v_s}\right) = 500\left(\frac{340}{344}\right) = 494 \text{ Hz}$$

In case 1 number of beats heard is 6 and in case 2 number of beats heard is 18 therefore frequency of the source at B = 512 Hz

43. (d)

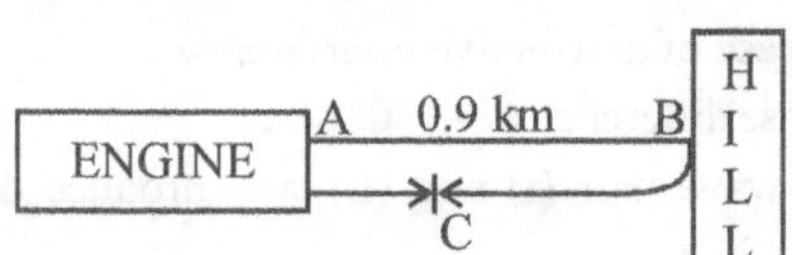

Let after 5 sec engine at point C

$$t = \frac{AB}{330} + \frac{BC}{330}$$

$$5 = \frac{0.9 \times 1000}{330} + \frac{BC}{330}$$

$\therefore$ BC = 750 m
Distance travelled by engine in 5 sec
= 900 m − 750 m = 150 m
Therefore velocity of engine

$$= \frac{150 \text{ m}}{5 \text{ sec}} = 30 \text{ m/s}$$

44. (c) Bats catch the prey by hearing reflected ultrasonic waves.
When the source and the detector (observer) are moving, frequency of reflected waves change. This is according to Doppler's effect.

45. (a)

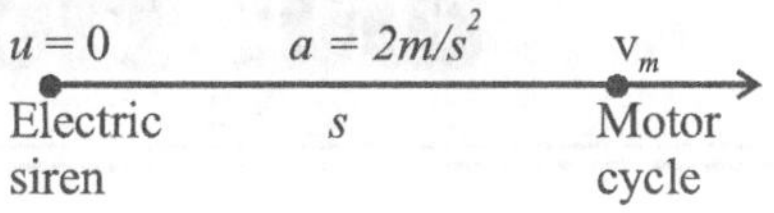

$$v_m^2 - u^2 = 2as$$

$$\therefore\ v_m^2 = 2 \times 2 \times s$$

$$\therefore\ v_m = 2\sqrt{s}$$

According to Doppler's effect

$$v' = v\left[\frac{v - v_m}{v}\right]$$

$$0.94v = v\left[\frac{330 - 2\sqrt{s}}{330}\right]$$

$$\Rightarrow s = 98.01\ m$$

46. (c) $v' = v\left[\frac{v}{v - v_s}\right]$

$$\Rightarrow 10000 = 9500\left[\frac{300}{300 - v}\right]$$

$$\Rightarrow 300 - v = 300 \times 0.95$$

$$\Rightarrow v = 300 - 285 = 15\ ms^{-1}$$

47. (c) $n' = n\left[\frac{v + v_0}{v}\right] = n\left[\frac{v + \frac{v}{5}}{v}\right] = n\left[\frac{6}{5}\right]$

$$\frac{n'}{n} = \frac{6}{5};\ \frac{n' - n}{n} = \frac{6-5}{5} \times 100 = 20\%$$

Chapter 15

Electric Charges and Fields

TOPIC - 1: Electric Charges and Coulomb's Law

1. Shown in the figure are two point charges +Q and –Q inside the cavity of a spherical shell. The charges are kept near the surface of the cavity on opposite sides of the centre of the shell. If σ_1 is the surface charge on the inner surface and Q_1 net charge on it and σ_2 the surface charge on the outer surface and Q_2 net charge on it then : **[Online April 10, 2015]**

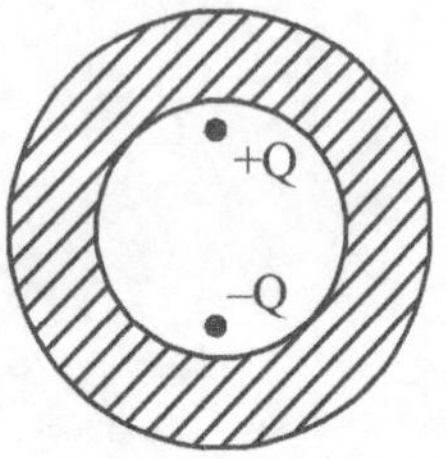

(a) $\sigma_1 \neq 0, Q_1 = 0$; $\sigma_2 = 0, Q_2 = 0$
(b) $\sigma_1 \neq 0, Q_1 = 0$; $\sigma_2 \neq 0, Q_2 = 0$
(c) $\sigma_1 = 0, Q_1 = 0$; $\sigma_2 = 0, Q_2 = 0$
(d) $\sigma_1 \neq 0, Q_1 \neq 0$; $\sigma_2 \neq 0, Q_2 \neq 0$

2. Two charges, each equal to q, are kept at x = – a and x = a on the x-axis. A particle of mass m and charge $q_0 = \frac{q}{2}$ is placed at the origin. If charge q_0 is given a small displacement (y<<a) along the y-axis, the net force acting on the particle is proportional to **[2013]**

(a) y (b) –y (c) $\frac{1}{y}$ (d) $-\frac{1}{y}$

3. Two balls of same mass and carrying equal charge are hung from a fixed support of length l. At electrostatic equilibrium, assuming that angles made by each thread is small, the separation, x between the balls is proportional to : **[Online April 9, 2013]**

(a) l (b) l^2 (c) $l^{2/3}$ (d) $l^{1/3}$

4. Two identical charged spheres suspended from a common point by two massless strings of length l are initially a distance $d(d << l)$ apart because of their mutual repulsion. The charge begins to leak from both the spheres at a constant rate. As a result charges approach each other with a velocity v. Then as a function of distance x between them, **[2011]**

(a) $v \propto x^{-1}$ (b) $v \propto x^{1/2}$ (c) $v \propto x$ (d) $v \propto x^{-1/2}$

5. A charge Q is placed at each of the opposite corners of a square. A charge q is placed at each of the other two corners. If the net electrical force on Q is zero, then Q/q equals: **[2009]**

(a) –1 (b) 1
(c) $-\frac{1}{\sqrt{2}}$ (d) $-2\sqrt{2}$

6. If g_E and g_M are the accelerations due to gravity on the surfaces of the earth and the moon respectively and if Millikan's oil drop experiment could be performed on the two surfaces, one will find the ratio **[2007]**
$\frac{\text{electronic charge on the moon}}{\text{electronic charge on the earth}}$ to be

(a) g_M / g_E (b) 1
(c) 0 (d) g_E / g_M

7. Two spherical conductors B and C having equal radii and carrying equal charges on them repel each other with a force F when kept apart at some distance. A third spherical conductor having same radius as that B but **uncharged** is brought in contact with B, then brought in contact with C and finally removed away from both. The new force of repulsion between B and C is **[2004]**

(a) $F/8$ (b) $3F/4$ (c) $F/4$ (d) $3F/8$

8. Three charges $-q_1$, $+q_2$ and $-q_3$ are place as shown in the figure. The x - component of the force on $-q_1$ is proportional to **[2003]**

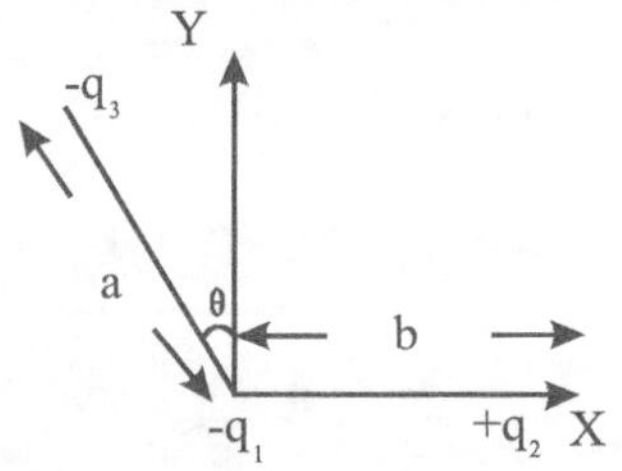

(a) $\frac{q_2}{b^2} - \frac{q_3}{a^2}\cos\theta$ (b) $\frac{q_2}{b^2} + \frac{q_3}{a^2}\sin\theta$

(c) $\frac{q_2}{b^2} + \frac{q_3}{a^2}\cos\theta$ (d) $\frac{q_2}{b^2} - \frac{q_3}{a^2}\sin\theta$

9. If a charge q is placed at the centre of the line joining two equal charges Q such that the system is in equilibrium then the value of q is **[2002]**

(a) $Q/2$ (b) $-Q/2$ (c) $Q/4$ (d) $-Q/4$

TOPIC - 2: Electric Field and Electric Field Lines

10. A long cylindrical shell carries positive surface charge σ in the upper half and negative surface charge - σ in the lower half. The electric field lines around the cylinder will look like figure given in : (*figures are schematic and not drawn to scale*) **[2015]**

(a) 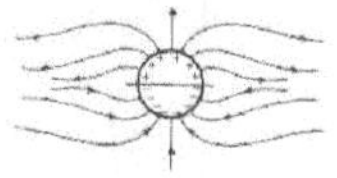 (b) 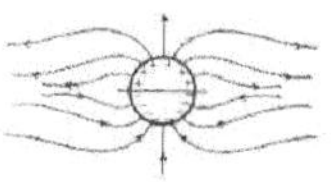

(c) 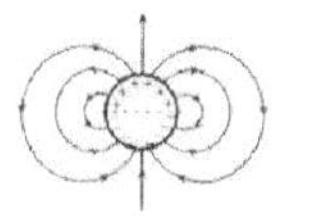 (d) 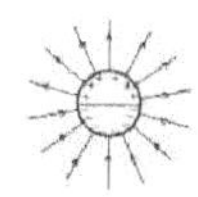

11. A wire of length L (=20 cm), is bent into a semicircular arc. If the two equal halves of the arc were each to be uniformly charged with charges $\pm$ Q, [$|Q| = 10^3\varepsilon_0$ Coulomb where ε_0 is the permittivity (in SI units) of free space] the net electric field at the centre O of the semicircular arc would be : **[Online April 11, 2015]**

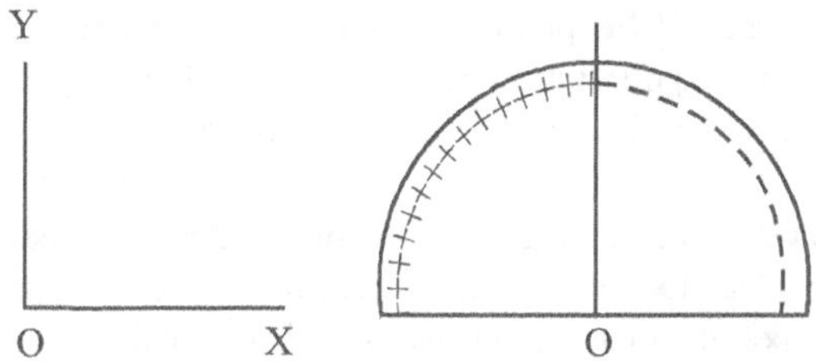

(a) $(50 \times 10^3 \text{N/C})\,\hat{j}$ (b) $(50 \times 10^3 \text{N/C})\,\hat{i}$

(c) $(25 \times 10^3 \text{N/C})\,\hat{j}$ (d) $(25 \times 10^3 \text{N/C})\,\hat{i}$

12. A thin disc of radius $b = 2a$ has a concentric hole of radius 'a' in it (see figure). It carries uniform surface charge 'σ' on it. If the electric field on its axis at height 'h' ($h << a$) from its centre is given as 'Ch' then value of 'C' is : **[Online April 10, 2015]**

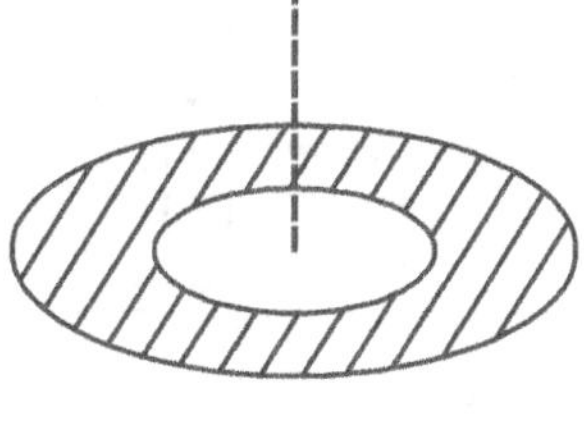

(a) $\dfrac{\sigma}{4a\epsilon_0}$

(b) $\dfrac{\sigma}{8a\epsilon_0}$

(c) $\dfrac{\sigma}{a\epsilon_0}$

(d) $\dfrac{\sigma}{2a\epsilon_0}$

13. A spherically symmetric charge distribution is characterised by a charge density having the following variations:

$$\rho(r) = \rho_0\left(1 - \frac{r}{R}\right) \text{ for } r < R$$

$\rho(r) = 0$ for $r \geq R$

Where r is the distance from the centre of the charge distribution ρ_0 is a constant. The electric field at an internal point (r < R) is: **[Online April 12, 2014]**

(a) $\dfrac{\rho_0}{4\varepsilon_0}\left(\dfrac{r}{3} - \dfrac{r^2}{4R}\right)$ (b) $\dfrac{\rho_0}{\varepsilon_0}\left(\dfrac{r}{3} - \dfrac{r^2}{4R}\right)$

(c) $\dfrac{\rho_0}{3\varepsilon_0}\left(\dfrac{r}{3} - \dfrac{r^2}{4R}\right)$ (d) $\dfrac{\rho_0}{12\varepsilon_0}\left(\dfrac{r}{3} - \dfrac{r^2}{4R}\right)$

14. The magnitude of the average electric field normally present in the atmosphere just above the surface of the Earth is about 150 N/C, directed inward towards the center of the Earth. This gives the total net surface charge carried by the Earth to be: **[Online April 9, 2014]**

[Given $\varepsilon_0 = 8.85 \times 10^{-12}$ C^2/N-m^2, $R_E = 6.37 \times 10^6$ m]

(a) +670 kC (b) −670 kC

(c) −680 kC (d) +680 kC

15. The surface charge density of a thin charged disc of radius R is σ. The value of the electric field at the centre of the disc is $\dfrac{\sigma}{2\epsilon_0}$. With respect to the field at the centre, the electric field along the axis at a distance R from the centre of the disc : **[Online April 25, 2013]**

(a) reduces by 70.7% (b) reduces by 29.3%

(c) reduces by 9.7% (d) reduces by 14.6%

16. A liquid drop having 6 excess electrons is kept stationary under a uniform electric field of 25.5 kVm^{-1}. The density of liquid is 1.26×10^3 kg m^{-3}. The radius of the drop is (neglect buoyancy). **[Online April 23, 2013]**

(a) 4.3×10^{-7}m (b) 7.8×10^{-7}m

(c) 0.078×10^{-7}m (d) 3.4×10^{-7}m

17. In a uniformly charged sphere of total charge Q and radius R, the electric field E is plotted as function of distance from the centre, The graph which would correspond to the above will be: **[2012]**

(a) 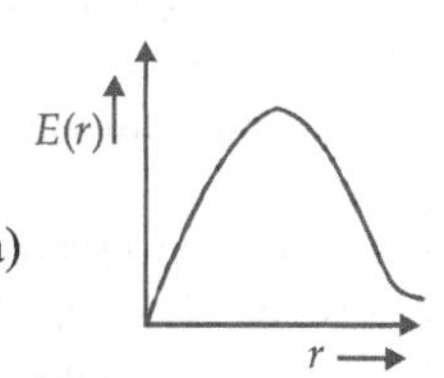

(b) 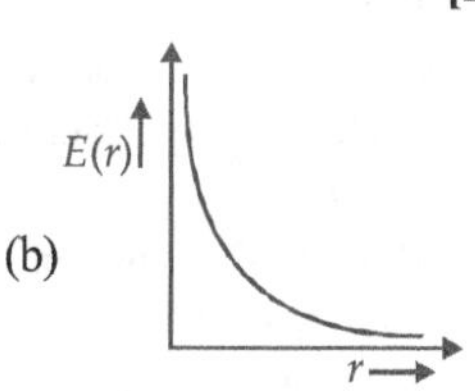

(c) 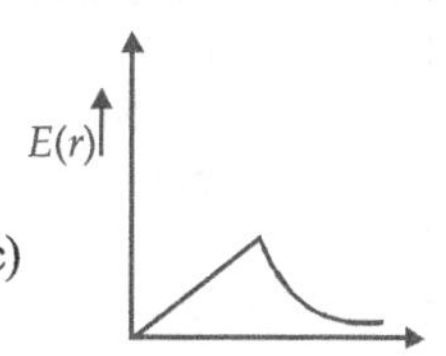

(d) 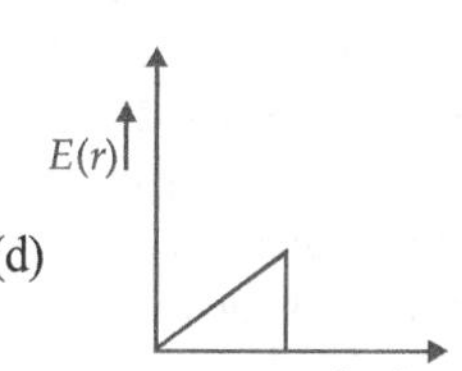

18. Three positive charges of equal value q are placed at vertices of an equilateral triangle. The resulting lines of force should be sketched as in **[Online May 26, 2012]**

(a) 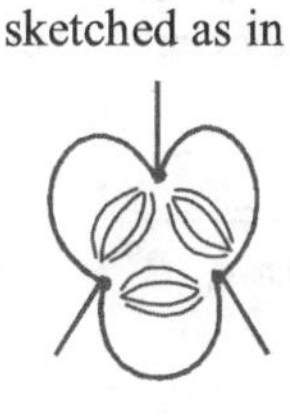 (b) 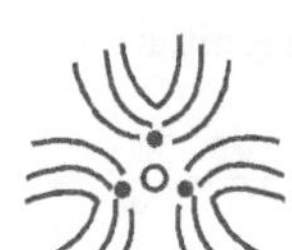

(c) 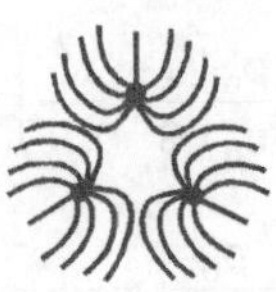 (d) 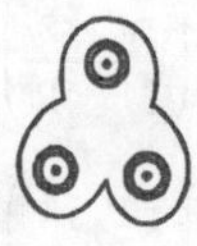

19. A thin semi-circular ring of radius r has a positive charge q distributed uniformly over it. The net field $\vec{E}$ at the centre O is **[2010]**

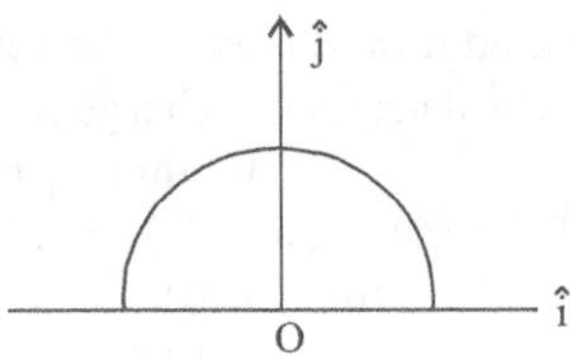

(a) $\frac{q}{4\pi^2\varepsilon_0 r^2}\hat{j}$ (b) $-\frac{q}{4\pi^2\varepsilon_0 r^2}\hat{j}$

(c) $-\frac{q}{2\pi^2\varepsilon_0 r^2}\hat{j}$ (d) $\frac{q}{2\pi^2\varepsilon_0 r^2}\hat{j}$

20. Let there be a spherically symmetric charge distribution with charge density varying as $\rho(r) = \rho_0\left(\frac{5}{4} - \frac{r}{R}\right)$ upto $r = R$, and $\rho(r) = 0$ for $r > R$, where r is the distance from the origin. The electric field at a distance $r(r < R)$ from the origin is given by **[2010]**

(a) $\frac{\rho_0 r}{4\varepsilon_0}\left(\frac{5}{3} - \frac{r}{R}\right)$ (b) $\frac{4\pi\rho_0 r}{3\varepsilon_0}\left(\frac{5}{3} - \frac{r}{R}\right)$

(c) $\frac{\rho_0 r}{4\varepsilon_0}\left(\frac{5}{4} - \frac{r}{R}\right)$ (d) $\frac{\rho_0 r}{3\varepsilon_0}\left(\frac{5}{4} - \frac{r}{R}\right)$

21. This question contains Statement-1 and Statement-2. Of the four choices given after the statements, choose the one that best describes the two statements.

Statement-1 : For a charged particle moving from point P to point Q, the net work done by an electrostatic field on the particle is independent of the path connecting point P to point Q.

Statement-2 : The net work done by a conservative force on an object moving along a closed loop is zero. **[2009]**

(a) Statement-1 is true, Statement-2 is true; Statement-2 is the correct explanation of Statement-1.
(b) Statement-1 is true, Statement-2 is true; Statement-2 is not the correct explanation of Statement-1.
(c) Statement-1 is false, Statement-2 is true.
(d) Statement-1 is true, Statement-2 is false.

22. Let $\rho(r) = \frac{Q}{\pi R^4}r$ be the charge density distribution for a solid sphere of radius R and total charge Q. For a point 'P' inside the sphere at distance r_1 from the centre of the sphere, the magnitude of electric field is : **[2009]**

(a) $\frac{Q}{4\pi\epsilon_0 r_1^2}$ (b) $\frac{Q r_1^2}{4\pi\epsilon_0 R^4}$

(c) $\frac{Q r_1^2}{3\pi\epsilon_0 R^4}$ (d) 0

23. A thin spherical shell of radus R has charge Q spread uniformly over its surface. Which of the following graphs most closely represents the electric field $E(r)$ produced by the shell in the range $0 \le r < \infty$, where r is the distance from the centre of the shell? **[2008]**

(a) 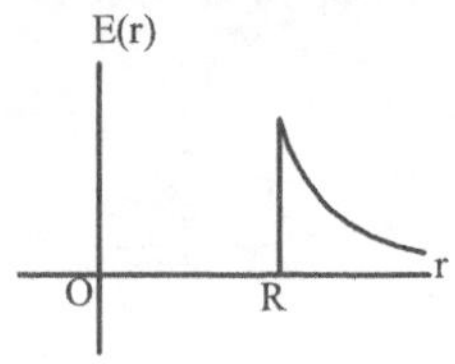

(b) 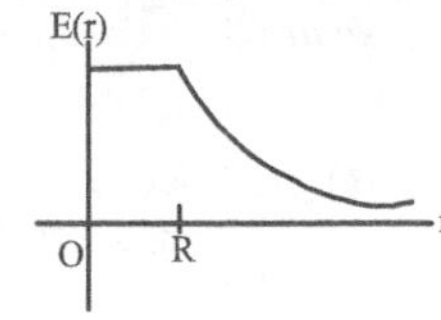

(c) 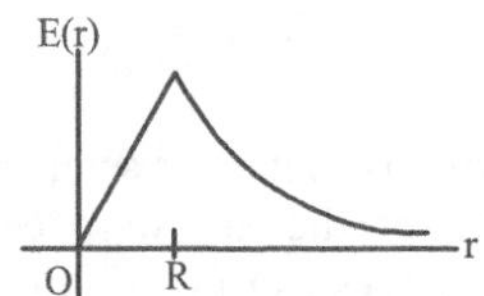

(d) 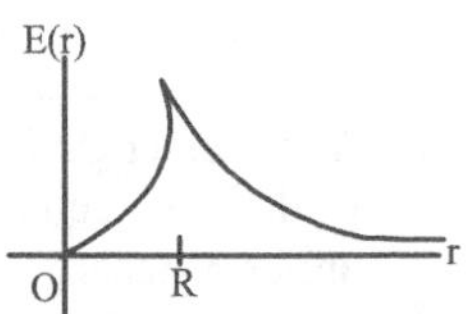

24. Two spherical conductors A and B of radii 1 mm and 2 mm are separated by a distance of 5 cm and are uniformly charged. If the spheres are connected by a conducting wire then in equilibrium condition, the ratio of the magnitude of the electric fields at the surfaces of spheres A and B is **[2006]**

(a) 4 : 1 (b) 1 : 2 (c) 2 : 1 (d) 1 : 4

25. Two point charges + $8q$ and – $2q$ are located at $x = 0$ and $x = L$ respectively. The location of a point on the x axis at which the net electric field due to these two point charges is zero is **[2005]**

(a) $\frac{L}{4}$ (b) $2L$ (c) $4L$ (d) $8L$

26. A charged ball B hangs from a silk thread S, which makes an angle θ with a large charged conducting sheet P, as shown in the figure. The surface charge density σ of the sheet is proportional to **[2005]**

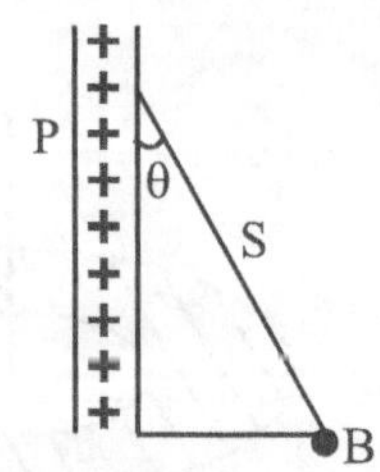

(a) cot θ (b) cos θ (c) tan θ (d) sin θ

27. Four charges equal to -Q are placed at the four corners of a square and a charge q is at its centre. If the system is in equilibrium the value of q is **[2004]**

(a) $-\frac{Q}{2}(1+2\sqrt{2})$ (b) $\frac{Q}{4}(1+2\sqrt{2})$

(c) $-\frac{Q}{4}(1+2\sqrt{2})$ (d) $\frac{Q}{2}(1+2\sqrt{2})$

28. A charged oil drop is suspended in a uniform field of 3×10^4 v/m so that it neither falls nor rises. The charge on the drop will be (Take the mass of the charge = 9.9×10^{-15} kg and $g = 10$ m/s^2) **[2004]**

(a) 1.6×10^{-18}C (b) 3.2×10^{-18}C
(c) 3.3×10^{-18}C (d) 4.8×10^{-18}C

TOPIC - 3 : Electric Dipole, Electric Flux and Gauss's Law

29. An electric dipole has a fixed dipole moment $\vec{p}$, which makes angle θ with respect to x-axis. When subjected to an electric field $\vec{E_1} = E\hat{i}$, it experiences a torque $\vec{T_1} = \tau\hat{i}$. When subjected to another electric field $\vec{E_2} = \sqrt{3}E_1\hat{j}$ it experiences torque $\vec{T_2} = -\vec{T_1}$. The angle θ is : **[2017]**

(a) 60° (b) 90°
(c) 30° (d) 45°

30. Four closed surfaces and corresponding charge distributions are shown below. **[Online April 9, 2017]**

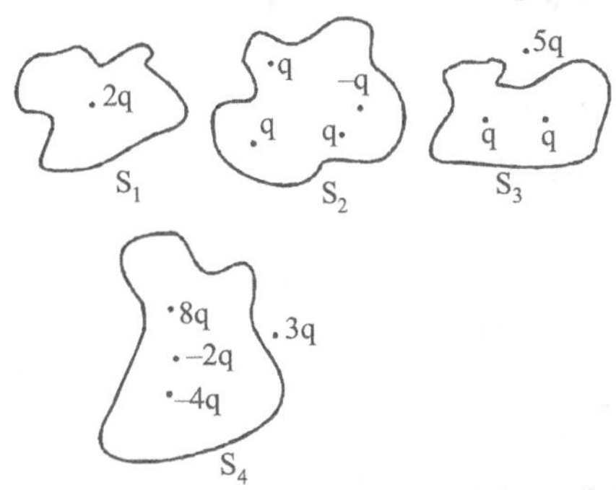

Let the respective electric fluxes through the surfaces be Φ_1, Φ_2, Φ_3, and Φ_4. Then :

(a) $\Phi_1 < \Phi_2 = \Phi_3 > \Phi_4$ (b) $\Phi_1 > \Phi_2 > \Phi_3 > \Phi_4$
(c) $\Phi_1 = \Phi_2 = \Phi_3 = \Phi_4$ (d) $\Phi_1 > \Phi_3 ; \Phi_2 < \Phi_4$

31. The region between two concentric spheres of radii 'a' and 'b', respectively (see figure), have volume charge density $\rho = \frac{A}{r}$, where A is a constant and r is the distance from the centre. At the centre of the spheres is a point charge Q. The value of A such that the electric field in the region between the spheres will be constant, is : **[2016]**

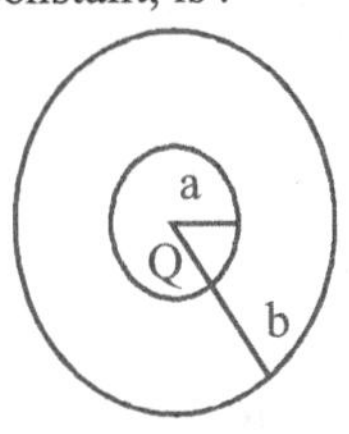

(a) $\frac{2Q}{\pi(a^2 - b^2)}$ (b) $\frac{2Q}{\pi a^2}$

(c) $\frac{Q}{2\pi a^2}$ (d) $\frac{Q}{2\pi(b^2 - a^2)}$

32. The electric field in a region of space is given by, $\vec{E} = E_0\hat{i} + 2E_0\hat{j}$ where E_0 = 100 N/C. The flux of the field through a circular surface of radius 0.02 m parallel to the Y-Z plane is nearly: **[Online April 19, 2014]**

(a) 0.125 Nm²/C (b) 0.02 Nm²/C
(c) 0.005 Nm²/C (d) 3.14 Nm²/C

33. Two point dipoles of dipole moment $\vec{p_1}$ and $\vec{p_2}$ are at a distance x from each other and $\vec{p_1} \parallel \vec{p_2}$. The force between the dipoles is : **[Online April 9, 2013]**

(a) $\frac{1}{4\pi\varepsilon_0}\frac{4p_1p_2}{x^4}$ (b) $\frac{1}{4\pi\varepsilon_0}\frac{3p_1p_2}{x^3}$

(c) $\frac{1}{4\pi\varepsilon_0}\frac{6p_1p_2}{x^4}$ (d) $\frac{1}{4\pi\varepsilon_0}\frac{8p_1p_2}{x^4}$

34. The flat base of a hemisphere of radius a with no charge inside it lies in a horizontal plane. A uniform electric field $\vec{E}$ is applied at an angle $\frac{\pi}{4}$ with the vertical direction. The electric flux through the curved surface of the hemisphere is **[Online May 19, 2012]**

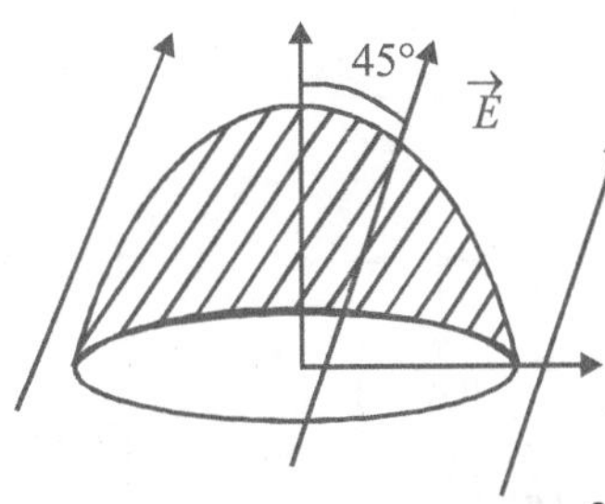

(a) $\pi a^2 E$ (b) $\frac{\pi a^2 E}{\sqrt{2}}$

(c) $\frac{\pi a^2 E}{2\sqrt{2}}$ (d) $\frac{(\pi + 2)\pi a^2 E}{(2\sqrt{2})^2}$

35. An electric dipole is placed at an angle of 30° to a non-uniform electric field. The dipole will experience **[2006]**

(a) a translational force only in the direction of the field
(b) a translational force only in a direction normal to the direction of the field
(c) a torque as well as a translational force
(d) a torque only

36. If the electric flux entering and leaving an enclosed surface respectively is ϕ_1 and ϕ_2, the electric charge inside the surface will be **[2003]**

(a) $(\phi_2 - \phi_1)\varepsilon_0$ (b) $(\phi_1 - \phi_2)/\varepsilon_0$
(c) $(\phi_2 - \phi_1)/\varepsilon_0$ (d) $(\phi_1 - \phi_2)\varepsilon_0$

37. A charged particle q is placed at the centre O of cube of length L ($A\,B\,C\,D\,E\,F\,G\,H$). Another same charge q is placed at a distance L from O. Then the electric flux through $ABCD$ is **[2002]**

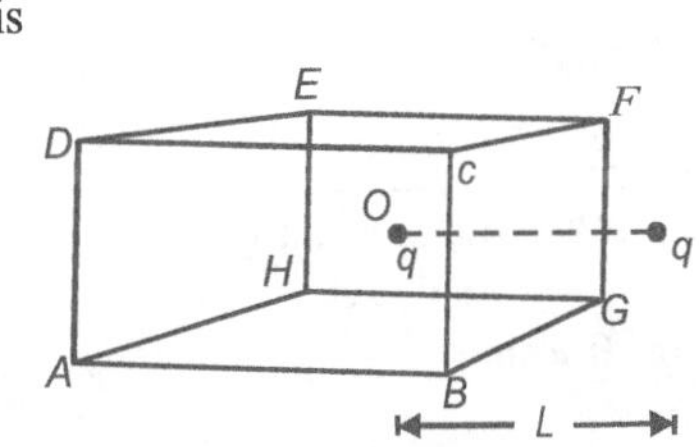

(a) $q/4\pi\epsilon_0 L$ (b) zero
(c) $q/2\pi\epsilon_0 L$ (d) $q/3\pi\epsilon_0 L$

Hints & Solutions

TOPIC - 1: Electric Charges and Coulomb's Law

1. (c) Inside the cavity net charge is zero.

$\therefore \quad Q_1 = 0$ and $\sigma_1 = 0$

There is no effect of point charges $+Q$, $-Q$ and induced charge on inner surface on the outer surface.

$\therefore \quad Q_2 = 0$ and $\sigma_2 = 0$

2. (a)

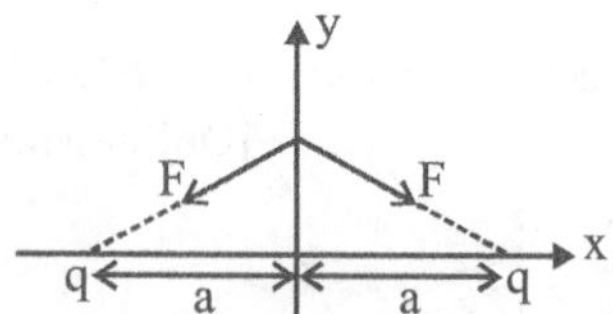

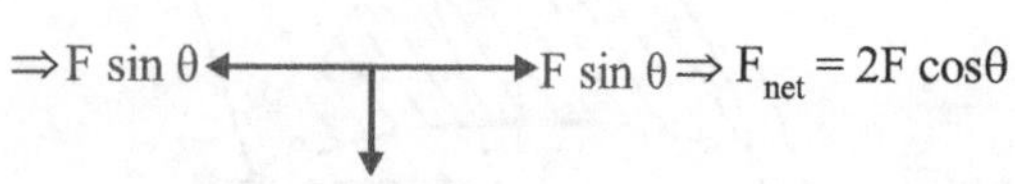

$\Rightarrow F \sin\theta \quad F\sin\theta \Rightarrow F_{net} = 2F\cos\theta$

$2F\cos\theta$

$$F_{net} = \frac{2kq\left(\frac{q}{2}\right)}{\left(\sqrt{y^2+a^2}\right)^2}\cdot\frac{y}{\sqrt{y^2+a^2}}$$

$$F_{net} = \frac{2kq\left(\frac{q}{2}\right)y}{(y^2+a^2)^{3/2}} \Rightarrow \frac{kq^2y}{a^3}$$

So, $F \propto y$

3. (d)

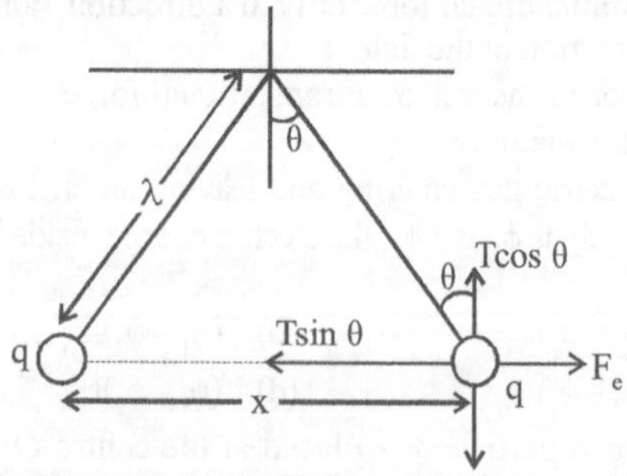

In equilibrium, $F_e = T\sin\theta$

$mg = T\cos\theta$

$$\tan\theta = \frac{F_e}{mg} = \frac{q^2}{4\pi\epsilon_0 x^2 \times mg}$$

also $\tan\theta \approx \sin = \dfrac{x/2}{\ell}$

Hence, $\dfrac{x}{2\ell} = \dfrac{q^2}{4\pi\epsilon_0 x^2 \times mg}$

$$\Rightarrow x^3 = \frac{2q^2\ell}{4\pi\epsilon_0 mg}$$

$$\therefore x = \left(\frac{q^2\ell}{2\pi\epsilon_0 mg}\right)^{1/3}$$

Therefore $x \propto \ell^{1/3}$

4. (d) At any instant

$T\cos\theta = mg$ ....(i)

$T\sin\theta = F_e$ ....(ii)

$$\Rightarrow \frac{\sin\theta}{\cos\theta} = \frac{F_e}{mg}$$

$\Rightarrow F_e = mg\tan\theta$

$$\Rightarrow \frac{kq^2}{x^2} = mg\tan\theta$$

$\Rightarrow q^2 \propto x^2\tan\theta$

$$\sin\theta = \frac{x}{2l}$$

For small θ, $\sin\theta \approx \tan\theta$

$\therefore q^2 \propto x^3$

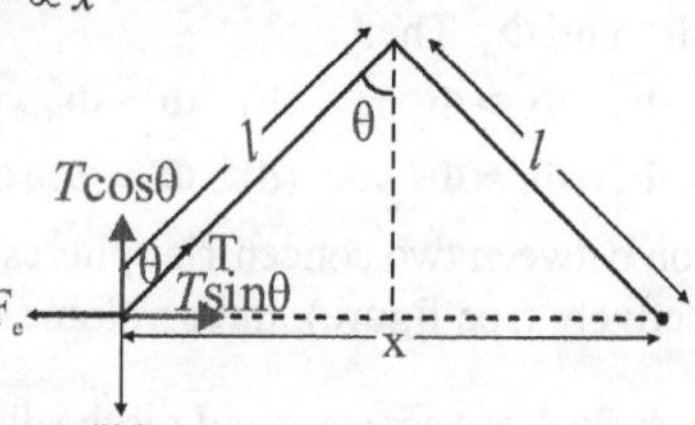

$$\Rightarrow q\frac{dq}{dt} \propto x^2\frac{dx}{dt}$$

$$\therefore \frac{dq}{dt} = \text{const.}$$

$\therefore q \propto x^2.v$

$$\Rightarrow x^{\frac{3}{2}} \propto x^2.v$$

$\Rightarrow v \propto x^{-1/2}$ $\quad [\because q^2 \propto x^3]$

5. (d) Let F be the force between Q and Q. The force between q and Q should be attractive for net force on Q to be zero. Let F' be the force between Q and q. The resultant of F' and F' is R. For equilibrium

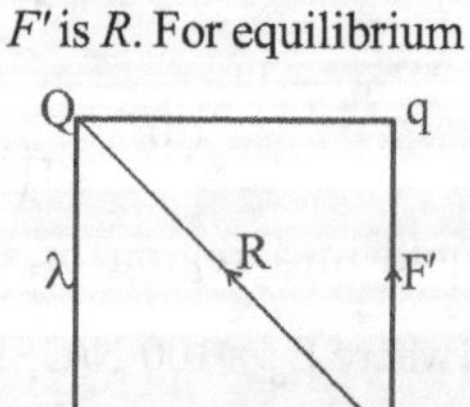

$\vec{R}+\vec{F}=0 \qquad \sqrt{2}\,F'=-F$

$$\sqrt{2}\times k\frac{Qq}{\ell^2}=-k\frac{Q^2}{(\sqrt{2}\,\ell)^2} \Rightarrow \frac{Q}{q}=-2\sqrt{2}$$

6. (b) Electronic charge does not depend on acceleration due to gravity as it is a universal constant.
So, electronic charge on earth
= electronic charge on moon
$\therefore$ Required ratio = 1.

7. (d) 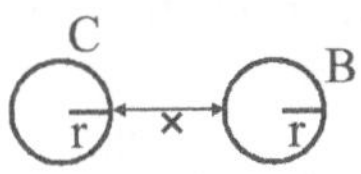

$$F \propto \frac{Q_B Q_C}{x^2}$$

x is distance between the spheres. After first operation charge on B is halved i.e., $\frac{Q}{2}$ and charge on third sphere becomes $\frac{Q}{2}$. Now it is touched to C, charge then equally distributes them selves to make potential same, hence charge on C becomes $\left(Q+\frac{Q}{2}\right)\frac{1}{2}=\frac{3Q}{4}$.

$$\therefore F_{new} \propto \frac{Q_C' Q_B'}{x^2}=\frac{\left(\frac{3Q}{4}\right)\left(\frac{Q}{2}\right)}{x^2}=\frac{3}{8}\frac{Q^2}{x^2}$$

or $F_{new}=\frac{3}{8}F$

8. (b) Force on charge q_1 due to q_2 is

$$F_{12}=k\frac{q_1q_2}{b^2}$$

Force on charge q_1 due to q_3 is

$$F_{13}=k\frac{q_1q_3}{a^2}$$

The X - component of the force (F_x) on q_1 is $F_{12}+F_{13}\sin\theta$

$$\therefore\ F_x=k\frac{q_1q_2}{b^2}+k\frac{q_1q_2}{a^2}\sin\theta$$

$$\therefore\ F_x \propto \frac{q_2}{b^2}+\frac{q_3}{a^2}\sin\theta$$

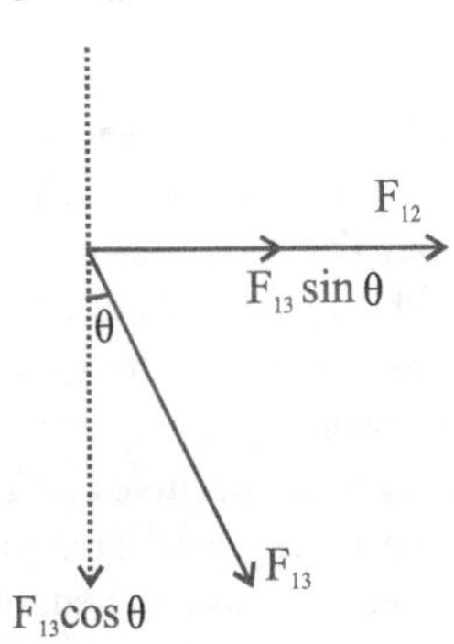

9. (d) For equilibrium of charge Q

$$k\frac{Q\times Q}{(2x)^2}+k\frac{Qq}{x^2}=0$$

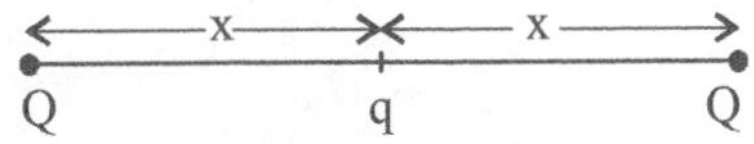

$$\Rightarrow q=-\frac{Q}{4}$$

TOPIC - 2 : Electric Field and Electric Field Lines

10. (c) Field lines originate perpendicular from positive charge and terminate perpendicular at negative charge. Further this system can be treated as an electric dipole.

11. (d) Given: Length of wire L = 20 cm
charge $Q = 10^3\varepsilon_0$
We know, electric field at the centre of the semicircular arc

$$E=\frac{2K\lambda}{r}$$

or, $$E=\frac{2K\left(\frac{2Q}{\pi r}\right)}{r}\left[As\lambda=\frac{2Q}{\pi r}\right]$$

$$=\frac{4KQ}{\pi r^2}=\frac{4KQ\pi^2}{\pi L^2}=\frac{4\pi KQ}{L^2}=25\times10^3\,N/C\hat{i}$$

12. (a) Electric field due to complete disc (R = 2a) at a distance x and on its axis

$$E_1=\frac{\sigma}{2\varepsilon_0}\left[1-\frac{x}{\sqrt{R^2+x^2}}\right]$$

$$E_1=\frac{\sigma}{2\varepsilon_0}\left[1-\frac{h}{\sqrt{4a^2+h^2}}\right]$$

$$=\frac{\sigma}{2\varepsilon_0}\left[1-\frac{h}{2a}\right] \quad \left[\begin{array}{l}\text{here } x=h\\ \text{and, } R=2a\end{array}\right]$$

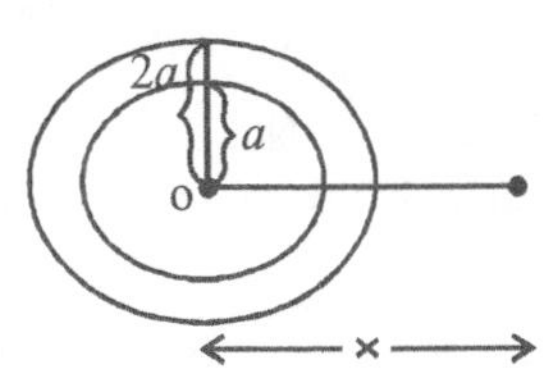

Similarly, electric field due to disc (R = a)

$$E_2=\frac{\sigma}{2\varepsilon_0}\left(1-\frac{h}{a}\right)$$

Electric field due to given disc
$E = E_1 - E_2$

$$\frac{\sigma}{2\varepsilon_0}\left[1-\frac{h}{2a}\right]-\frac{\sigma}{2\varepsilon_0}\left[1-\frac{h}{a}\right]=\frac{\sigma h}{4\varepsilon_0 a}$$

Hence, $c=\frac{\sigma}{4a\varepsilon_0}$

13. (b) Let us consider a spherical shell of radius x and thickness dx.

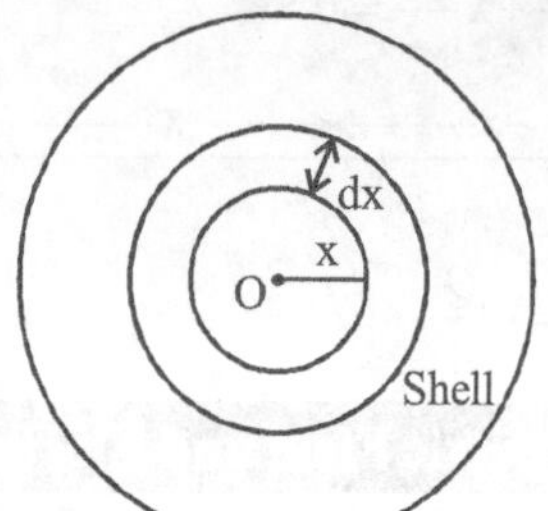

Charge on this shell

$$dq = \rho.4\pi x^2 dx = \rho_0\left(1-\frac{x}{R}\right).4\pi x^2 dx$$

∴ Total charge in the spherical region from centre to r (r < R) is

$$q = \int dq = 4\pi\rho_0\int_0^r\left(1-\frac{x}{R}\right)x^2 dx$$

$$= 4\pi\rho_0\left[\frac{x^3}{3}-\frac{x^4}{4R}\right]_0^r$$

$$= 4\pi\rho_0\left[\frac{r^3}{3}-\frac{r^4}{4R}\right]$$

$$= 4\pi\rho_0 r^3\left[\frac{1}{3}-\frac{r}{4R}\right]$$

∴ Electric field at r, $E = \frac{1}{4\pi\varepsilon_0}.\frac{q}{r^2}$

$$= \frac{1}{4\pi\varepsilon_0}.\frac{4\pi\rho_0 r^3}{r^2}\left[\frac{1}{3}-\frac{r}{4R}\right]$$

$$= \frac{\rho_0}{\varepsilon_0}\left[\frac{r}{3}-\frac{r^2}{4R}\right]$$

14. (c) Given,

Electric field E = 150 N/C

Total surface charge carried by earth q = ?

or, $q = \epsilon_0 E A$

$= \epsilon_0 E \pi r^2$.

$= 8.85 \times 10^{-12} \times 150 \times (6.37 \times 10^6)^2$.

$\simeq$ 680 Kc

As electric field directed inward hence

q = – 680 Kc

15. (a) Electric field intensity at the centre of the disc.

$E = \frac{\sigma}{2\epsilon_0}$ (given)

Electric field along the axis at any distance x from the centre of the disc

$$E' = \frac{\sigma}{2\epsilon_0}\left(1-\frac{x}{\sqrt{x^2+R^2}}\right)$$

From question, x = R (radius of disc)

$$\therefore E' = \frac{\sigma}{2\epsilon_0}\left(1-\frac{R}{\sqrt{R^2+R^2}}\right)$$

$$= \frac{\sigma}{2\epsilon_0}\left(\frac{\sqrt{2}R-R}{\sqrt{2}R}\right)$$

$$= \frac{4}{14}E$$

∴ % reduction in the value of electric field

$$= \frac{\left(E-\frac{4}{14}E\right)\times 100}{E} = \frac{1000}{14}\% \simeq 70.7\%$$

16. (b) $F = qE = mg$ $(q = 6e = 6\times 1.6\times 10^{-19})$

$$\text{Density (d)} = \frac{\text{mass}}{\text{volume}} = \frac{m}{\frac{4}{3}\pi r^3}$$

$$\text{or } r^3 = \frac{m}{\frac{4}{3}\pi d}$$

Putting the value of d and m $\left(=\frac{qE}{g}\right)$ and solving we get $r = 7.8\times 10^{-7}$m

17. (c) $\vec{E}$ inside the charged sphere

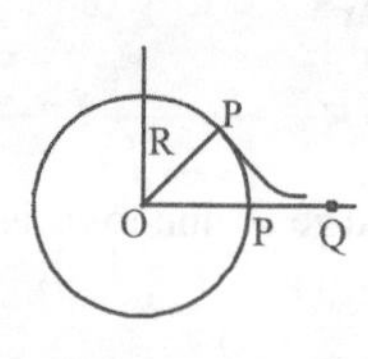

$\vec{E}_{in} = 0$ ...(i)

$\vec{E}$ on the surface of the charged sphere

$$\vec{E}_s = \frac{1}{4\pi\epsilon_0}\frac{q}{R^2} \text{ i.e., } \vec{E}_s \propto \frac{1}{R^2}\hat{n} \quad ...(ii)$$

$\vec{E}$ on any point away from the uniformly charged sphere is given

$$\vec{E} = \frac{1}{4\pi\epsilon_0}\frac{q}{r^2}\hat{n}$$

$$\vec{E} \propto \frac{1}{r^2}\hat{n} \quad ...(iii)$$

∵ R is the radius of the sphere, which is constant, thus $\vec{E}$ is maximum and constant at the surface of the sphere. But decreases on moving away from the surface of the uniformally charged sphere.

18. (c) Electric lines of force due to a positive charge is spherically symmetric.

All the charges are positive and equal in magnitude. So repulsion takes place. Due to which no lines of force are present inside the equilateral triangle and the resulting lines of force obtained as shown:

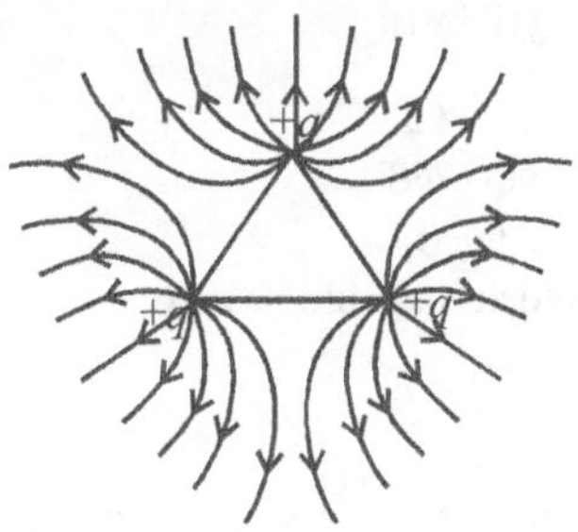

19. **(c)** Let us consider a differential element dl. charge on this element.

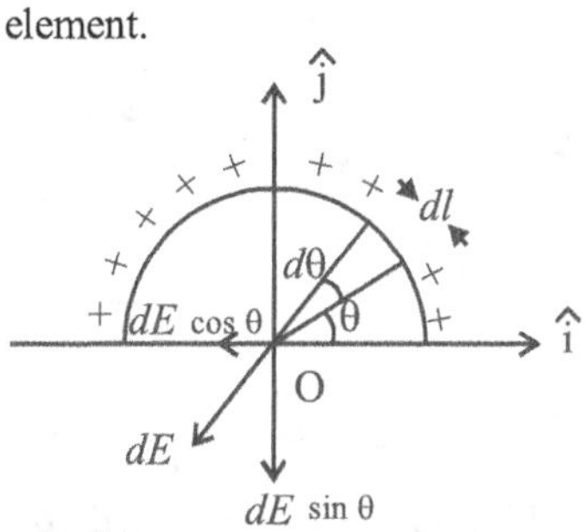

$$dq = \left(\frac{q}{\pi r}\right) dl$$

$$= \frac{q}{\pi r}(r d\theta) \qquad (\because dl = r d\theta)$$

$$= \left(\frac{q}{\pi}\right) d\theta$$

Electric field at O due to dq is

$$dE = \frac{1}{4\pi \epsilon_0} \cdot \frac{dq}{r^2} = \frac{1}{4\pi \epsilon_0} \cdot \frac{q}{\pi r^2} d\theta$$

The component $dE \cos\theta$ will be counter balanced by another element on left portion. Hence resultant field at O is the resultant of the component $dE \sin\theta$ only.

$$\therefore \ E = \int dE \sin\theta = \int_0^{\pi} \frac{q}{4\pi^2 r^2 \epsilon_0} \sin\theta d\theta$$

$$= \frac{q}{4\pi^2 r^2 \epsilon_0} [-\cos\theta]_0^{\pi}$$

$$= \frac{q}{4\pi^2 r^2 \epsilon_0}(+1+1) \quad = \frac{q}{2\pi^2 r^2 \epsilon_0}$$

The direction of E is towards negative y-axis.

$$\therefore \ \vec{E} = -\frac{q}{2\pi^2 r^2 \epsilon_0} \hat{j}$$

20. **(a)** Let us consider a spherical shell of radius x and thickness dx.
Charge on this shell

$$dq = \rho.4\pi x^2 dx = \rho_0 \left(\frac{5}{4} - \frac{x}{R}\right).4\pi x^2 dx$$

$\therefore$ Total charge in the spherical region from centre to r $(r < R)$ is

$$q = \int dq = 4\pi\rho_0 \int_0^r \left(\frac{5}{4} - \frac{x}{R}\right) x^2 dx$$

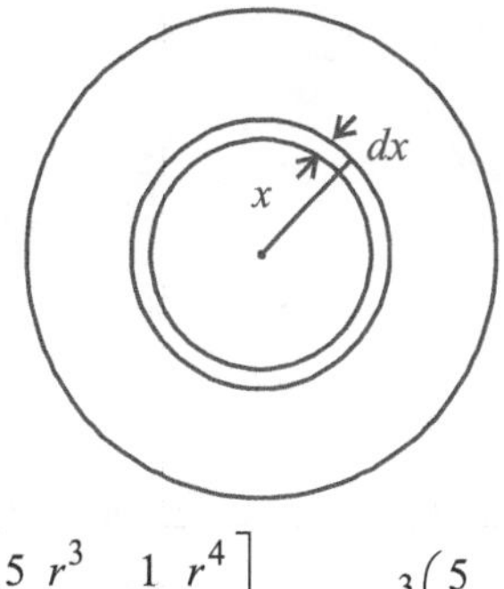

$$= 4\pi\rho_0 \left[\frac{5}{4} \cdot \frac{r^3}{3} - \frac{1}{R} \cdot \frac{r^4}{4}\right] = \pi\rho_0 r^3 \left(\frac{5}{3} - \frac{r}{R}\right)$$

$\therefore$ Electric field at r,

$$E = \frac{1}{4\pi \epsilon_0} \cdot \frac{q}{r^2}$$

$$= \frac{1}{4\pi \epsilon_0} \cdot \frac{\pi\rho_0 r^3}{r^2} \left(\frac{5}{3} - \frac{r}{R}\right)$$

$$= \frac{\rho_0 r}{4 \epsilon_0} \left(\frac{5}{3} - \frac{r}{R}\right)$$

21. **(a)**

22. **(b)**

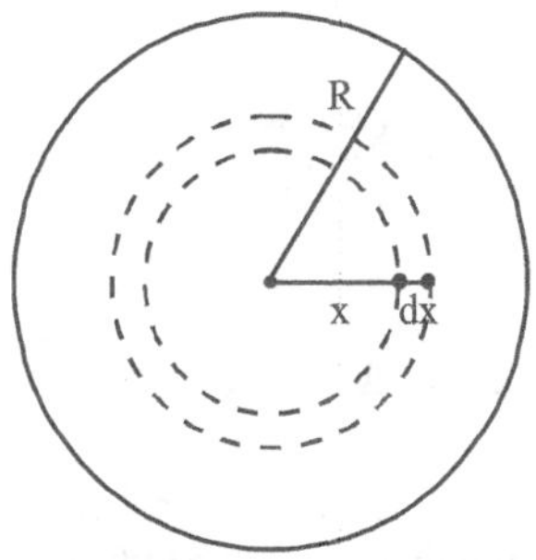

Let us consider a spherical shell of thickness dx and radius x. The volume of this spherical shell $= 4\pi x^2 dx$. The charge enclosed within shell

$$= \left[\frac{Qx}{\pi R^4}\right][4\pi x^2 dx] = \frac{4Q}{R^4} x^3 dx$$

The charge enclosed in a sphere of radius r_1 is

$$= \frac{4Q}{R^4} \int_0^{r_1} x^3 dx = \frac{4Q}{R^4} \left[\frac{x^4}{4}\right]_0^{r_1} = \frac{Q}{R^4} r_1^4$$

$\therefore$ The electric field at point P inside the sphere at a distance r_1 from the centre of the sphere is

$$E = \frac{1}{4\pi \epsilon_0} \frac{\left[\frac{Q}{R^4} r_1^4\right]}{r_1^2}$$

$$= \frac{1}{4\pi \epsilon_0} \frac{Q}{R^4} r_1^2$$

23. (a) The electric field inside a thin spherical shell of radius R has charge Q spread uniformly over its surface is zero.

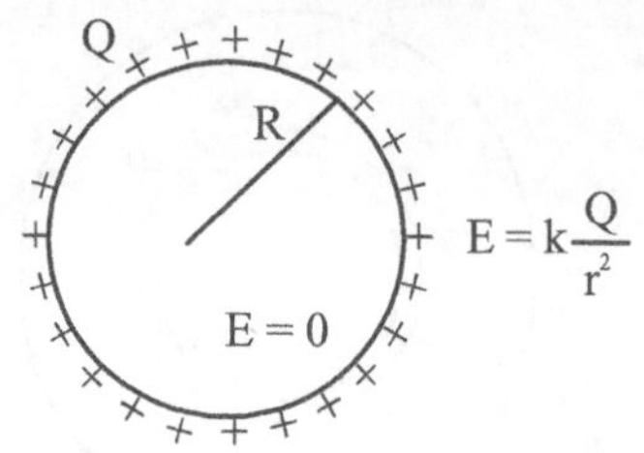

Outside the shell the electric field is $E = k\frac{Q}{r^2}$. These characteristics are represented by graph (a).

24. (c)

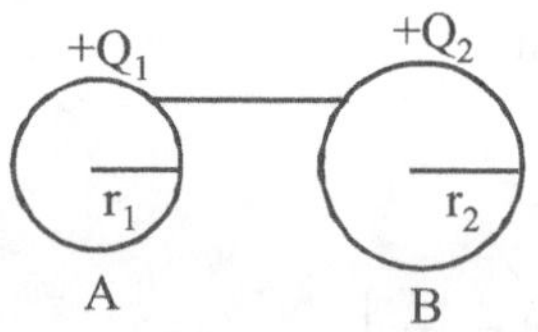

After connection, $V_1 = V_2$

$$\Rightarrow k\frac{Q_1}{r_1} = k\frac{Q_2}{r_2} \Rightarrow \frac{Q_1}{r_1} = \frac{Q_2}{r_2}$$

The ratio of electric fields

$$\frac{E_1}{E_2} = \frac{k\frac{Q_1}{r_1^2}}{k\frac{Q_2}{r_2^2}} \Rightarrow \frac{E_1}{E_2} = \frac{Q_1}{r_1^2} \times \frac{r_2^2}{Q_2}$$

$$\Rightarrow \frac{E_1}{E_2} = \frac{r_1 \times r_2^2}{r_1^2 \times r_2} \Rightarrow \frac{E_1}{E_2} = \frac{r_2}{r_1} = \frac{2}{1}$$

Since the distance between the spheres is large as compared to their diameters, the induced effects may be ignored.

25. (b) $\frac{-K2q}{(x-L)^2} + \frac{K8q}{x^2} = 0 \Rightarrow \frac{1}{(x-L)^2} = \frac{4}{x^2}$

or $\frac{1}{x-L} = \frac{2}{x} \Rightarrow x = 2x - 2L$ or $x = 2L$

26. (c)

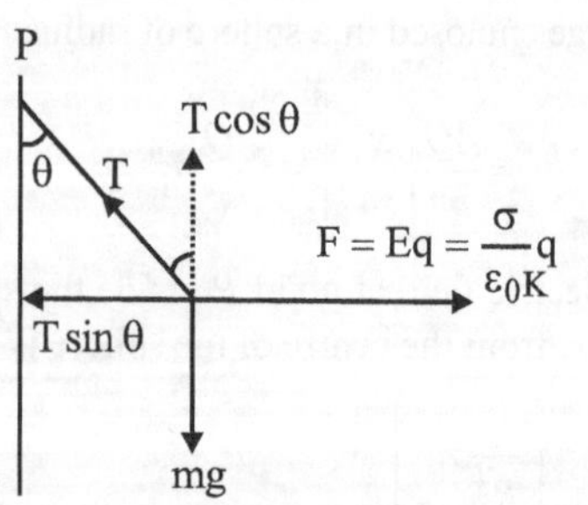

$$T\sin\theta = \frac{\sigma}{\varepsilon_0 K}.q \quad \text{.... (i)}$$

$$T\cos\theta = mg \quad \text{.... (ii)}$$

Dividing (i) by (ii),

$$\tan\theta = \frac{\sigma q}{\varepsilon_0 K.mg}$$

$$\therefore \sigma \propto \tan\theta$$

27. (b) Net field at A should be zero

$$\sqrt{2}\,E_1 + E_2 = E_3$$

$$\therefore \frac{kQ\times\sqrt{2}}{a^2} + \frac{kQ}{(\sqrt{2}\,a)^2} = \frac{kq}{\left(\frac{a}{\sqrt{2}}\right)^2}$$

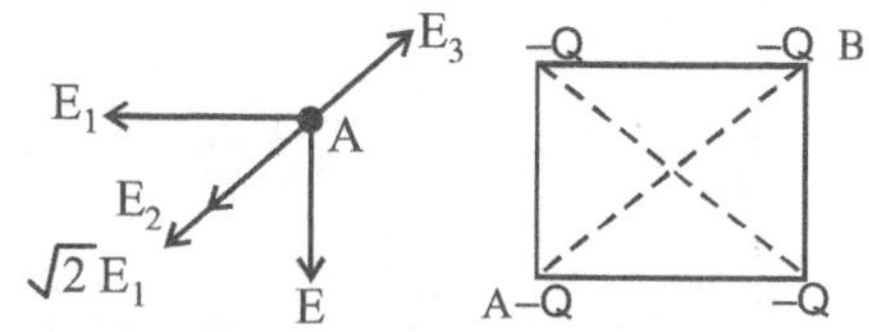

$$\Rightarrow \frac{Q\sqrt{2}}{1} + \frac{Q}{2} = 2q \Rightarrow q = \frac{Q}{4}(2\sqrt{2}+1)$$

28. (c) At equilibrium, electric force on drop balances weight of drop.

$$qE = mg \Rightarrow q = \frac{mg}{E}$$

$$q = \frac{9.9\times10^{-15}\times10}{3\times10^4} = 3.3\times10^{-18}\text{C}$$

TOPIC - 3 : Electric Dipole, Electric Flux and Gauss's Law

29. (a) T = PE sinθ Torque experienced by the dipole in an electric field, $\vec{T} = \vec{P}\times\vec{E}$

$\vec{p} = p\cos\theta\,\hat{i} + p\sin\theta\,\hat{j}$

$\vec{E}_1 = E\hat{i}$

$\vec{T}_1 = \vec{p}\times\vec{E}_1 = (p\cos\theta\,\hat{i} + p\sin\theta\,\hat{j})\times E(\hat{i})$

$\tau\hat{k} = pE\sin\theta(-\hat{k})$ ...(i)

$\vec{E}_2 = \sqrt{3}\,E_1\hat{j}$

$\vec{T}_2 = p\cos\theta\hat{i} + p\sin\theta\hat{j})\times\sqrt{3}\,E_1\hat{j}$

$\tau\hat{k} = \sqrt{3}\,pE_1\cos\theta\hat{k}$ ...(ii)

From eqns. (*i*) and (*ii*)

$pE\sin\theta = \sqrt{3}\,pE\cos\theta$

$\tan\theta = \sqrt{3} \quad \therefore \quad \theta = 60°$

30. (c) The net flux linked with closed surfaces S_1, S_2, S_3 & S_4 are

For surface S_1, $\phi_1 = \frac{1}{\varepsilon_0}(2q)$

For surface S_2, $\phi_2 = \frac{1}{\varepsilon_0}(q+q+q-q) = \frac{1}{\varepsilon_0}2q$

For surface S_3, $\phi_3 = \frac{1}{\varepsilon_0}(q+q) = \frac{1}{\varepsilon_0}(2q)$

For surface S_4, $\phi_4 = \frac{1}{\varepsilon_0}(8q - 2q - 4q) = \frac{1}{\varepsilon_0}(2q)$

Hence, $\phi_1 = \phi_2 = \phi_3 = \phi_4$ i.e. net electric flux is same for all surfaces.

Keep in mind, the electric field due to a charge outside (S_3 and S_4), the Gaussian surface contributes zero net flux through the surface, because as many lines due to that charge enter the surface as leave it.

31. **(c)** Applying Gauss's law

$$\oint_S \vec{E}.\vec{ds} = \frac{Q}{\epsilon_0}$$

$$\therefore E \times 4\pi r^2 = \frac{Q + 2\pi a r^2 - 2\pi A a^2}{\epsilon_0}$$

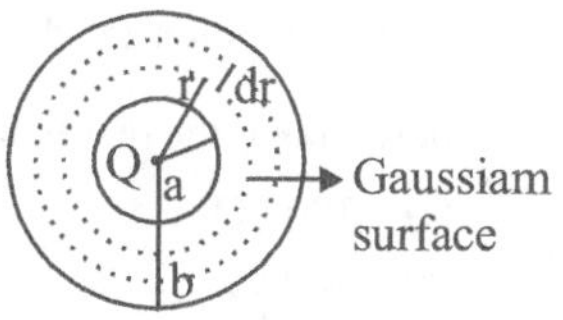

$$\rho = \frac{dr}{dv}$$

$$Q = \rho 4\pi r^2$$

$$Q = \int_a^r \frac{A}{r} 4\pi r^2 dr = 2\pi A\,[r^2 - a^2]$$

$$E = \frac{1}{4\pi \epsilon_0}\left[\frac{Q - 2\pi A a^2}{r^2} + 2\pi A\right]$$

For E to be independent of 'r'

$Q - 2\pi A a^2 = 0$

$$\therefore A = \frac{Q}{2\pi a^2}$$

32. **(a)** $\vec{E} = E_0\hat{i} + 2E_0\hat{j}$

Given, $E_0 = 100 N/c$

So, $\vec{E} = 100\hat{i} + 200\hat{j}$

Radius of circular surface = 0.02 m

$$\text{Area} = \pi r^2 = \frac{22}{7} \times 0.02 \times 0.02$$

$= 1.25 \times 10^{-3}\hat{i}\ m^2$ [Loop is parallel to Y-Z plane]

Now, flux $(\phi) = EA\cos\theta$

$= (100\hat{i} + 200\hat{j}).1.25 \times 10^{-3}\hat{i}\cos 0°$ $[\theta = 0°]$

$= 125 \times 10^{-3}\ Nm^2/c$

$= 0.125\ Nm^2/c$

33. **(c)** Force of interaction

$$F = \frac{1}{4\pi \epsilon_0}.\frac{6p_1p_2}{r^4}$$

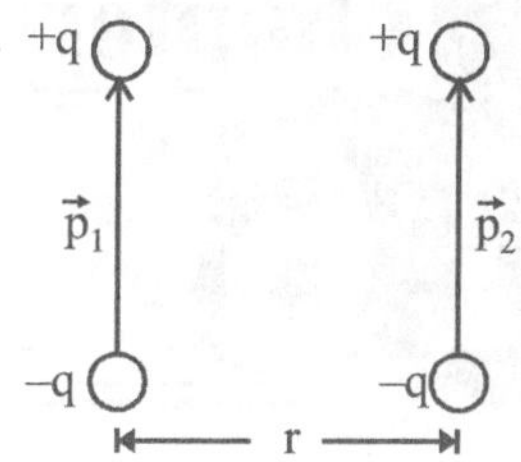

34. **(b)** We know that,

$$\phi = \oint E.dS = E\oint dS \cos 45°$$

In case of hemisphere

$\phi_{curved} = \phi_{circular}$

Therefore, $\phi_{curved} = E\pi a^2.\frac{1}{\sqrt{2}} = \frac{E\pi a^2}{\sqrt{2}}$

35. **(c)**

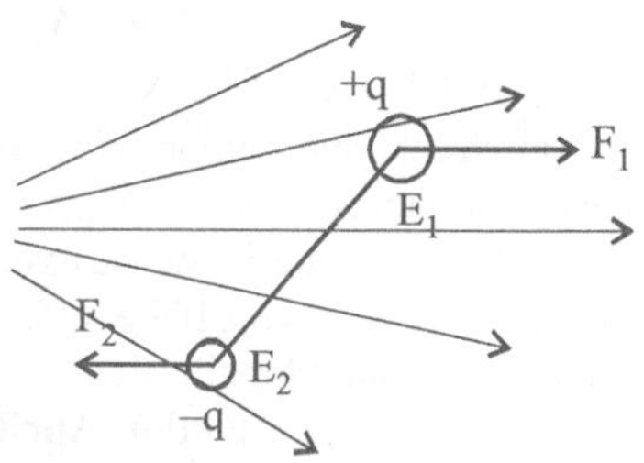

The electric field will be different at the location of the two charges. Therefore the two forces will be unequal. This will result in a force as well as torque.

36. **(a)** The flux entering an enclosed surface is taken as negative and the flux leaving the surface is taken as positive, by convention. Therefore the net flux leaving the enclosed surface = $\phi_2 - \phi_1$

$\therefore$ the charge enclosed in the surface by Gauss's law is $q = \epsilon_0(\phi_2 - \phi_1)$

37. **(b)** Both the charges are identical and placed symmetrically about *ABCD*. The flux crossing *ABCD* due to each charge is $\frac{1}{6}\left[\frac{q}{\epsilon_0}\right]$ but in opposite directions. Therefore the resultant is zero.

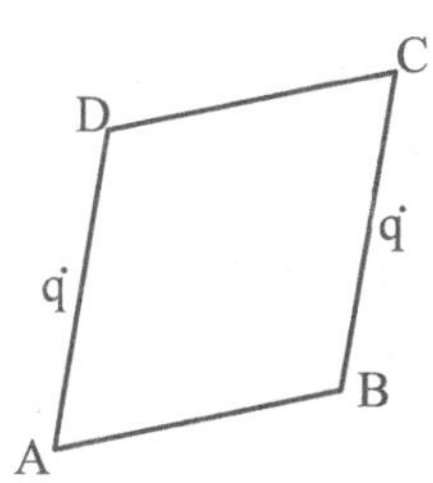

Chapter 16 Electrostatic Potential and Capacitance

TOPIC - 1: Electrostatic Potential and Equipotential Surfaces

1. There is a uniform electrostatic field in a region. The potential at various points on a small sphere centred at P, in the region, is found to vary between in the limits 589.0 V to 589.8 V. What is the potential at a point on the sphere whose radius vector makes an angle of 60° with the direction of the field? **[Online April 8, 2017]**
(a) 589.5 V (b) 589.2 V (c) 589.4 V (d) 589.6 V

2. Within a spherical charge distribution of charge density $\rho(r)$, N equipotential surfaces of potential V_0, $V_0 + \Delta V$, $V_0 + 2\Delta V$, ...$V_0 + N\Delta V$ $(\Delta V > 0)$, are drawn and have increasing radii $r_0, r_1, r_2, \ldots\ldots\ldots r_N$, respectively. If the difference in the radii of the surfaces is constant for all values of V_0 and ΔV then: **[Online April 10, 2016]**
(a) $\rho(r) = \text{constant}$ (b) $\rho(r) \propto \frac{1}{r^2}$
(c) $\rho(r) \propto \frac{1}{r}$ (d) $\rho(r) \propto r$

3. The potential (in volts) of a charge distribution is given by
$V(z) = 30 - 5z^2$ for $|z| \le 1\text{m}$
$V(z) = 35 - 10|z|$ for $|z| \ge 1$ m.
V(z) does not depend on x and y. If this potential is generated by a constant charge per unit volume ρ_0 (in units of ε_0) which is spread over a certain region, then choose the correct statement. **[Online April 9, 2016]**
(a) $\rho_0 = 20\,\varepsilon_0$ in the entire region
(b) $\rho_0 = 10\,\varepsilon_0$ for $|z| \le 1$ m and $\rho_0 = 0$ elsewhere
(c) $\rho_0 = 20\,\varepsilon_0$ for $|z| \le 1$ m and $\rho_0 = 0$ elsewhere
(d) $\rho_0 = 40\,\varepsilon_0$ in the entire region

4. A uniformly charged solid sphere of radius R has potential V_0 (measured with respect to ∞) on its surface. For this sphere the equipotential surfaces with potentials $\frac{3V_0}{2}, \frac{5V_0}{4}, \frac{3V_0}{4}$ and $\frac{V_0}{4}$ have radius R_1, R_2, R_3 and R_4 respectively. Then **[2015]**
(a) $R_1 = 0$ and $R_2 < (R_4 - R_3)$
(b) $2R = R_4$
(c) $R_1 = 0$ and $R_2 > (R_4 - R_3)$
(d) $R_1 \ne 0$ and $(R_2 - R_1) > (R_4 - R_3)$

5. An electric field $\vec{E} = (25\hat{i} + 30\hat{j})\text{NC}^{-1}$ exists in a region of space. If the potential at the origin is taken to be zero then the potential at $x = 2$ *m*, $y = 2$ *m* is : **[Online April 11, 2015]**
(a) –110 J (b) –140 J (c) –120 J (d) –130 J

6. Assume that an electric field $\vec{E} = 30x^2\hat{i}$ exists in space. Then the potential difference $V_A - V_O$, where V_O is the potential at the origin and V_A the potential at x = 2 m is: **[2014]**
(a) 120 J/C (b) –120 J/C
(c) –80 J/C (d) 80 J/C

7. Consider a finite insulated, uncharged conductor placed near a finite positively charged conductor. The uncharged body must have a potential : **[Online April 23, 2013]**
(a) less than the charged conductor and more than at infinity.
(b) more than the charged conductor and less than at infinity.
(c) more than the charged conductor and more than at infinity.
(d) less than the charged conductor and less than at infinity.

8. Two small equal point charges of magnitude *q* are suspended from a common point on the ceiling by insulating mass less strings of equal lengths. They come to equilibrium with each string making angle θ from the vertical. If the mass of each charge is *m*, then the electrostatic potential at the centre of line joining them will be $\left(\frac{1}{4\pi\epsilon_0} = k\right)$. **[Online April 22, 2013]**
(a) $2\sqrt{k\,mg\tan\theta}$ (b) $\sqrt{k\,mg\tan\theta}$
(c) $4\sqrt{k\,mg/\tan\theta}$ (d) $\sqrt{k\,mg/\tan\theta}$

9. A point charge of magnitude + 1 μC is fixed at (0, 0, 0). An isolated uncharged spherical conductor, is fixed with its center at (4, 0, 0). The potential and the induced electric field at the centre of the sphere is : **[Online April 22, 2013]**
(a) 1.8×10^5 V and -5.625×10^6 V/m
(b) 0 V and 0 V/m
(c) 2.25×10^5 V and -5.625×10^6 V/m
(d) 2.25×10^5 V and 0 V/m

10. A charge of total amount Q is distributed over two concentric hollow spheres of radii r and R $(R > r)$ such that the surface charge densities on the two spheres are equal. The electric potential at the common centre is **[Online May 19, 2012]**

(a) $\frac{1}{4\pi\varepsilon_0}\frac{(R-r)Q}{\left(R^2+r^2\right)}$ (b) $\frac{1}{4\pi\varepsilon_0}\frac{(R+r)Q}{2\left(R^2+r^2\right)}$

(c) $\frac{1}{4\pi\varepsilon_0}\frac{(R+r)Q}{\left(R^2+r^2\right)}$ (d) $\frac{1}{4\pi\varepsilon_0}\frac{(R-r)Q}{2\left(R^2+r^2\right)}$

11. The electric potential $V(x)$ in a region around the origin is given by $V(x) = 4x^2$ volts. The electric charge enclosed in a cube of 1 m side with its centre at the origin is (in coulomb) **[Online May 7, 2012]**

(a) $8\varepsilon_0$ (b) $-4\varepsilon_0$ (c) 0 (d) $-8\varepsilon_0$

12. The electrostatic potential inside a charged spherical ball is given by $\phi = ar^2 + b$ where r is the distance from the centre and a, b are constants. Then the charge density inside the ball is: **[2011]**

(a) $-6a\varepsilon_0 r$ (b) $-24\pi a\varepsilon_0$ (c) $-6a\varepsilon_0$ (d) $-24\pi a\varepsilon_0 r$

13. An electric charge $10^{-3}\,\mu$ C is placed at the origin (0, 0) of $X - Y$ co-ordinate system. Two points A and B are situated at $(\sqrt{2}, \sqrt{2})$ and (2, 0) respectively. The potential difference between the points A and B will be **[2007]**

(a) 4.5 volts (b) 9 volts (c) Zero (d) 2 volt

14. Charges are placed on the vertices of a square as shown. Let $\vec{E}$ be the electric field and V the potential at the centre. If the charges on A and B are interchanged with those on D and C respectively, then **[2007]**

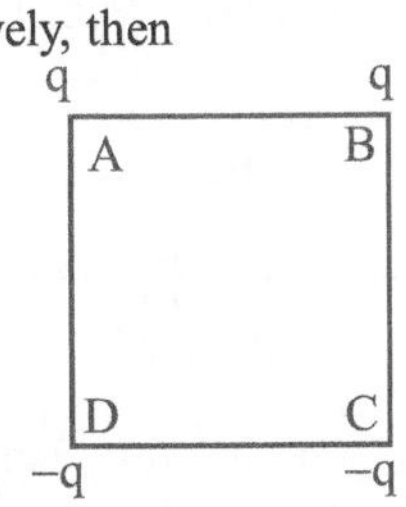

(a) $\vec{E}$ changes, V remains unchanged
(b) $\vec{E}$ remains unchanged, V changes
(c) both $\vec{E}$ and V change
(d) $\vec{E}$ and V remain unchanged

15. The potential at a point x (measured in μ m) due to some charges situated on the x-axis is given by $V(x) = 20/(x^2 - 4)$ volt. The electric field E at $x = 4\ \mu$ m is given by **[2007]**

(a) (10/9) volt/ μ m and in the +ve x direction
(b) (5/3) volt/ μ m and in the –ve x direction
(c) (5/3) volt/ μ m and in the +ve x direction
(d) (10/9) volt/ μ m and in the –ve x direction

16. Two thin wire rings each having a radius R are placed at a distance d apart with their axes coinciding. The charges on the two rings are $+q$ and $-q$. The potential difference between the centres of the two rings is **[2005]**

(a) $\frac{q}{2\pi\epsilon_0}\left[\frac{1}{R}-\frac{1}{\sqrt{R^2+d^2}}\right]$ (b) $\frac{qR}{4\pi\epsilon_0 d^2}$

(c) $\frac{q}{4\pi\epsilon_0}\left[\frac{1}{R}-\frac{1}{\sqrt{R^2+d^2}}\right]$ (d) zero

17. A thin spherical conducting shell of radius R has a charge q. Another charge Q is placed at the centre of the shell. The electrostatic potential at a point P, a distance $\frac{R}{2}$ from the centre of the shell is **[2003]**

(a) $\frac{2Q}{4\pi\varepsilon_o R}$ (b) $\frac{2Q}{4\pi\varepsilon_o R}-\frac{2q}{4\pi\varepsilon_o R}$

(c) $\frac{2Q}{4\pi\varepsilon_o R}+\frac{q}{4\pi\varepsilon_o R}$ (d) $\frac{(q+Q)2}{4\pi\varepsilon_o R}$

TOPIC - 2 : Electric Potential Energy and Work Done in Carrying a Charge

18. This question has Statement-1 and Statement-2. Of the four choices given after the Statements, choose the one that best describes the two Statements.

Statement 1 : No work is required to be done to move a test charge between any two points on an equipotential surface.
Statement 2 : Electric lines of force at the equipotential surfaces are mutually perpendicular to each other. **[Online April 25, 2013]**

(a) Statement 1 is true, Statement 2 is true, Statement 2 is the correct explanation of Statement 1.
(b) Statement 1 is true, Statement 2 is true, Statement 2 is not the correct explanation of Statement 1.
(c) Statement 1 is true, Statement 2 is false.
(d) Statement 1 is false, Statement 2 is true.

19. This questions has statement-1 and statement-2. Of the four choices given after the statements, choose the one that best describes the two statements.

An insulating solid sphere of radius R has a uniformly positive charge density ρ. As a result of this uniform charge distribution there is a finite value of electric potential at the centre of the sphere, at the surface of the sphere and also at a point outside the sphere. The electric potential at infinite is zero. **[2012]**

Statement -1 When a charge q is taken from the centre to the surface of the sphere its potential energy changes by $\frac{q\rho}{3\varepsilon_0}$.

Statement -2 The electric field at a distance r $(r < R)$ from the centre of the sphere is $\frac{\rho r}{3\varepsilon_0}$.

(a) Statement 1 is true, Statement 2 is true; Statement 2 is not the correct explanation of statement 1.
(b) Statement 1 is true Statement 2 is false.
(c) Statement 1 is false Statement 2 is true.
(d) Statement 1 is true, Statement 2 is true, Statement 2 is the correct explanation of Statement 1

20. Two positive charges of magnitude 'q' are placed, at the ends of a side (side 1) of a square of side '$2a$'. Two negative charges of the same magnitude are kept at the other corners. Starting from rest, if a charge Q moves from the middle of side 1 to the centre of square, its kinetic energy at the centre of square is **[2011 RS]**

(a) zero (b) $\frac{1}{4\pi\varepsilon_0}\frac{2qQ}{a}\left(1+\frac{1}{\sqrt{5}}\right)$

(c) $\frac{1}{4\pi\varepsilon_0}\frac{2qQ}{a}\left(1-\frac{2}{\sqrt{5}}\right)$ (d) $\frac{1}{4\pi\varepsilon_0}\frac{2qQ}{a}\left(1-\frac{1}{\sqrt{5}}\right)$

21. Two points P and Q are maintained at the potentials of 10 V and – 4 V, respectively. The work done in moving 100 electrons from P to Q is: **[2009]**

(a) 9.60×10^{-17}J (b) -2.24×10^{-16} J
(c) 2.24×10^{-16} J (d) -9.60×10^{-17} J

22. Two insulating plates are both uniformly charged in such a way that the potential difference between them is $V_2 - V_1 = 20$ V. (i.e., plate 2 is at a higher potential). The plates are separated by $d = 0.1$ m and can be treated as infinitely large. An electron is released from rest on the inner surface of plate 1. What is its speed when it hits plate 2? ($e = 1.6 \times 10^{-19}$ C, $m_e = 9.11 \times 10^{-31}$ kg) **[2006]**

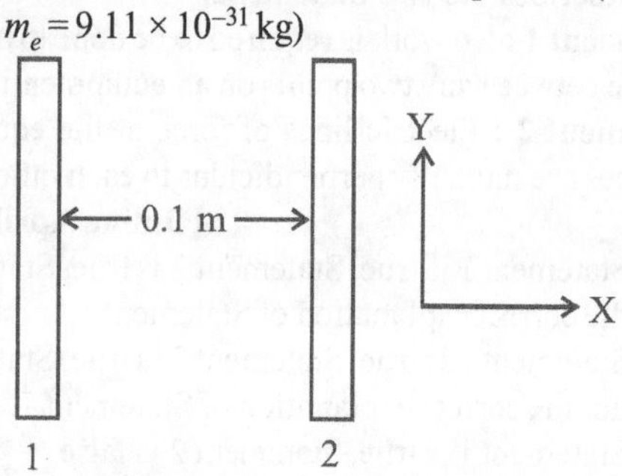

(a) 2.65×10^6 m/s (b) 7.02×10^{12} m/s
(c) 1.87×10^6 m/s (d) 32×10^{-19} m/s

23. A charged particle 'q' is shot towards another charged particle 'Q' which is fixed, with a speed 'v'. It approaches 'Q' upto a closest distance r and then returns. If q were given a speed of '$2v$' the closest distances of approach would be **[2004]**

(a) $r/2$ (b) $2r$ (c) r (d) $r/4$

24. On moving a charge of 20 coulomb by 2 cm, 2 J of work is done, then the potential difference between the points is **[2002]**

(a) 0.1 V (b) 8 V (c) 2 V (d) 0.5 V.

TOPIC - 3: Capacitors, Grouping of Capacitor and Energy Stored in a Capacitor

25. A capacitance of $2\mu F$ is required in an electrical circuit across a potential difference of 1.0 kV. A large number of $1\mu F$ capacitors are available which can withstand a potential difference of not more than 300 V. The minimum number of capacitors required to achieve this is **[2017]**

(a) 24 (b) 32 (c) 2 (d) 16

26. A combination of parallel plate capacitors is maintained at a certain potential difference.

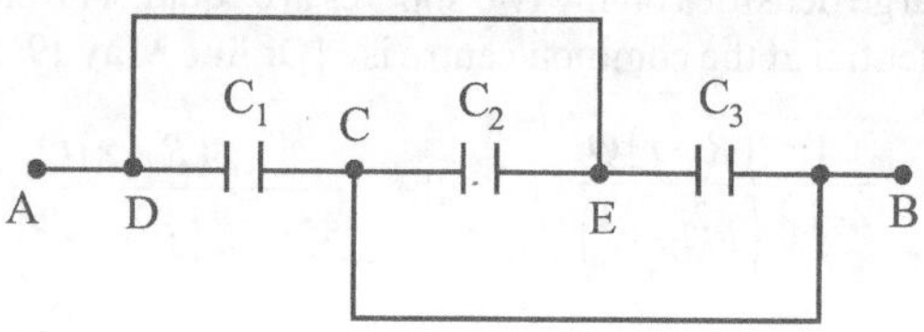

When a 3 mm thick slab is introduced between all the plates, in order to maintain the same potential difference, the distance between the plates is increased by 2.4 mm.
Find the dielectric constant of the slab.
[Online April 9, 2017]

(a) 3 (b) 4 (c) 5 (d) 6

27. The energy stored in the electric field produced by a metal sphere is 4.5 J. If the sphere contains 4 μC charge, its radius will be : [Take : $\frac{1}{4\pi\varepsilon_0} = 9\times10^9 \text{ N} - \text{m}^2/\text{C}^2$]
[Online April 8, 2017]

(a) 20mm (b) 32mm (c) 28mm (d) 16mm

28. A combination of capacitors is set up as shown in the figure. The magnitude of the electric field, due to a point charge Q (having a charge equal to the sum of the charges on the 4 μ F and 9 μ F capacitors), at a point distance 30 m from it, would equal : **[2016]**

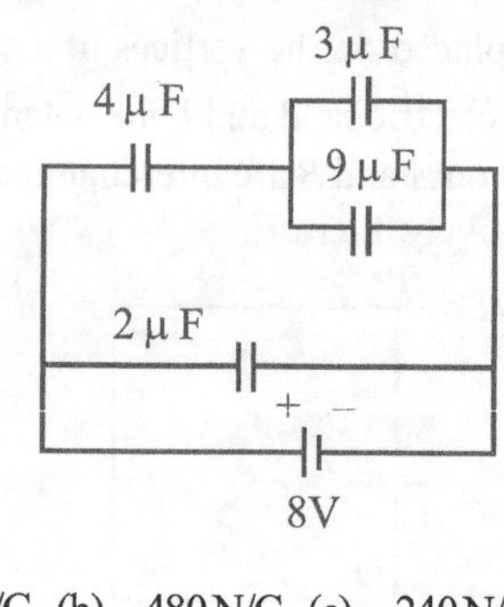

(a) 420N/C (b) 480N/C (c) 240N/C (d) 360N/C

29. Figure shows a network of capacitors where the numbers indicates capacitances in micro Farad. The value of capacitance C if the equivalent capacitance between point A and B is to be 1 μF is : **[Online April 10, 2016]**

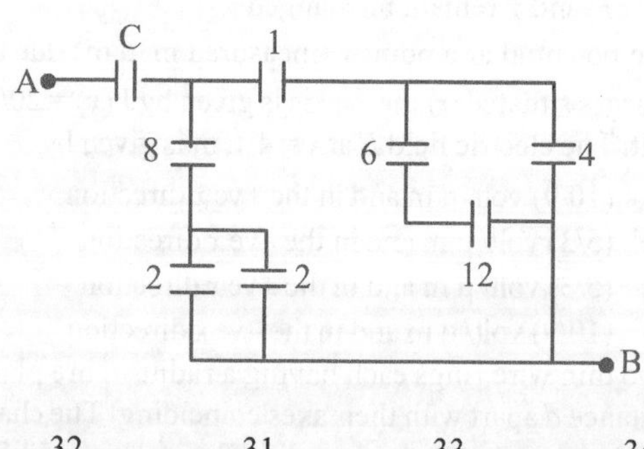

(a) $\frac{32}{23}$μF (b) $\frac{31}{23}$μF (c) $\frac{33}{23}$μF (d) $\frac{34}{23}$μF

30. Three capacitors each of 4 μF are to be connected in such a way that the effective capacitance is 6μF. This can be done by connecting them : **[Online April 9, 2016]**

(a) all in series
(b) all in parallel
(c) two in parallel and one in series
(d) two in series and one in parallel

31. In the given circuit, charge Q_2 on the 2μF capacitor changes as C is varied from 1μF to 3μF. Q_2 as a function of 'C' is given properly by: (*figures are drawn schematically and are not to scale*) **[2015]**

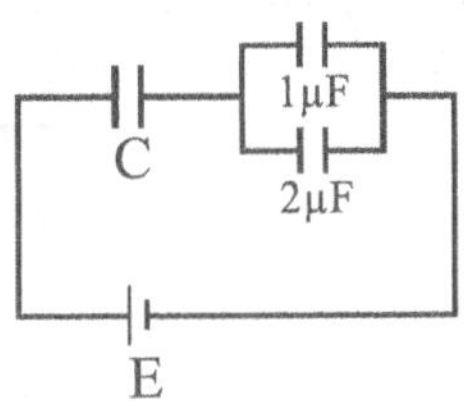

(a)
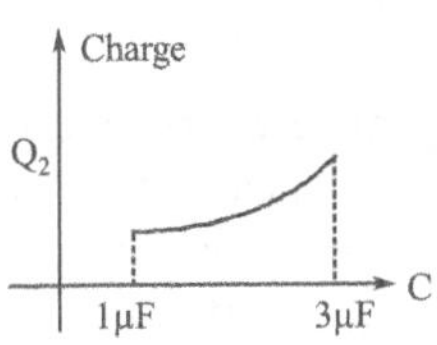

(b)
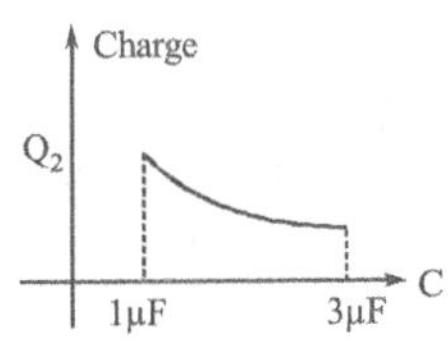

(c)
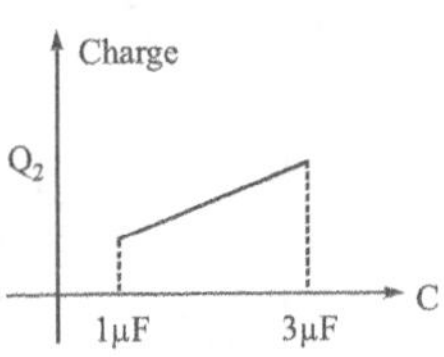

(d)
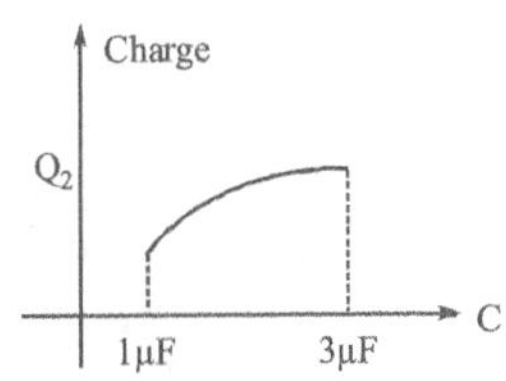

32. In figure a system of four capacitors connected across a 10 V battery is shown. Charge that will flow from switch S when it is closed is : **[Online April 11, 2015]**

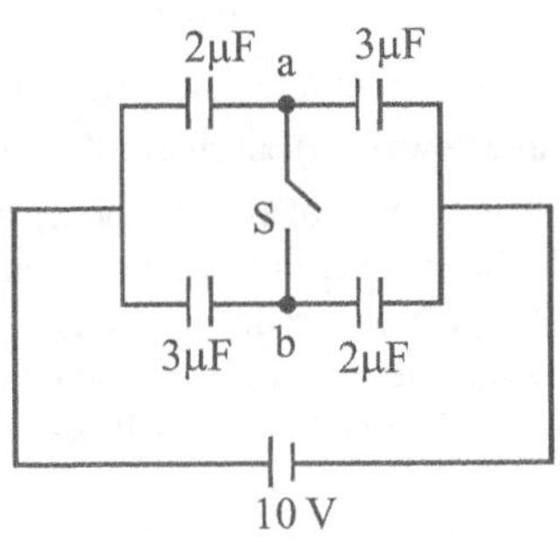

(a) 5 μC from b to a (b) 20 μC from a to b
(c) zero (d) 5 μC from a to b

33. A parallel plate capacitor is made of two circular plates separated by a distance 5 mm and with a dielectric of dialectric constant 2.2 between them. When the electric field in the dielectric is 3×10^4 V/m the charge density of the positive plate will be close to: **[2014]**

(a) $6\times10^{-7}\ C/m^2$ (b) $3\times10^{-7}\ C/m^2$
(c) $3\times10^{4}\ C/m^2$ (d) $6\times10^{4}\ C/m^2$

34. The gap between the plates of a parallel plate capacitor of area A and distance between plates d, is filled with a dielectric whose permittivity varies linearly from ϵ_1 at one plate to ϵ_2 at the other. The capacitance of capacitor is: **[Online April 19, 2014]**

(a) $\epsilon_0(\epsilon_1+\epsilon_2)A/d$
(b) $\epsilon_0(\epsilon_2+\epsilon_1)A/2d$
(c) $\epsilon_0 A/[d\,ln(\epsilon_2/\epsilon_1)]$
(d) $\epsilon_0(\epsilon_2-\epsilon_1)A/[d\,ln(\epsilon_2/\epsilon_1)]$

35. The space between the plates of a parallel plate capacitor is filled with a 'dielectric' whose 'dielectric constant' varies with distance as per the relation:
$K(x)=K_o+\lambda x$ (λ = a constant)
The capacitance C, of the capacitor, would be related to its vacuum capacitance C_o for the relation : **[Online April 12, 2014]**

(a) $C=\dfrac{\lambda d}{ln(1+K_o\lambda d)}C_o$ (b) $C=\dfrac{\lambda}{d.ln(1+K_o\lambda d)}C_o$

(c) $C=\dfrac{\lambda d}{ln(1+\lambda d/K_o)}C_o$ (d) $C=\dfrac{\lambda}{d.ln(1+K_o/\lambda d)}C_o$

36. A parallel plate capacitor is made of two plates of length l, width w and separated by distance d. A dielectric slab (dielectric constant K) that fits exactly between the plates is held near the edge of the plates. It is pulled into the capacitor by a force $F=-\dfrac{\partial U}{\partial x}$ where U is the energy of the capacitor when dielectric is inside the capacitor up to distance x (See figure). If the charge on the capacitor is Q then the force on the dielectric when it is near the edge is: **[Online April 11, 2014]**

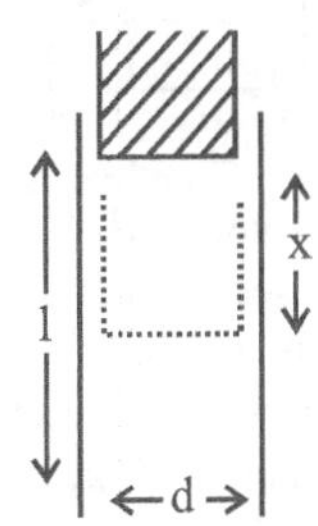

(a) $\dfrac{Q^2 d}{2\omega l^2\varepsilon_0}K$ (b) $\dfrac{Q^2\omega}{2dl^2\varepsilon_0}(K-1)$

(c) $\dfrac{Q^2 d}{2wl^2\varepsilon_0}(K-1)$ (d) $\dfrac{Q^2 w}{2dl^2\varepsilon_0}K$

37. Three capacitors, each of 3 μF, are provided. These cannot be combined to provide the resultant capacitance of: **[Online April 9, 2014]**

(a) 1 μF (b) 2 μF (c) 4.5 μF (d) 6 μF

38. A parallel plate capacitor having a separation between the plates d, plate area A and material with dielectric constant K has capacitance C_0. Now one-third of the material is replaced by another material with dielectric constant 2K, so that effectively there are two capacitors one with area $\frac{1}{3}$ A, dielectric constant 2K and another with area $\frac{2}{3}$ A and dielectric constant K. If the capacitance of this new capacitor is C then $\frac{C}{C_0}$ is **[Online April 25, 2013]**

(a) 1 (b) $\frac{4}{3}$ (c) $\frac{2}{3}$ (d) $\frac{1}{3}$

39. To establish an instantaneous current of 2 A through a 1 μF capacitor ; the potential difference across the capacitor plates should be changed at the rate of : **[Online April 22, 2013]**

(a) 2×10^4 V/s (b) 4×10^6 V/s
(c) 2×10^6 V/s (d) 4×10^4 V/s

40. A uniform electric field $\vec{E}$ exists between the plates of a charged condenser. A charged particle enters the space between the plates and perpendicular to $\vec{E}$. The path of the particle between the plates is a : **[Online April 9, 2013]**

(a) straight line (b) hyperbola
(c) parabola (d) circle

41. The figure shows an experimental plot discharging of a capacitor in an RC circuit. The time constant τ of this circuit lies between : **[2012]**

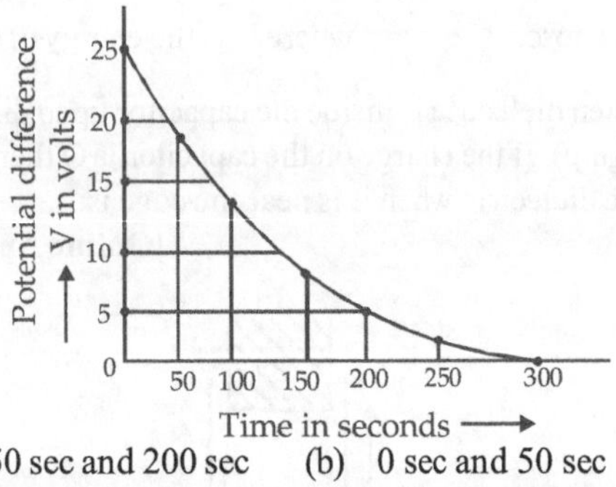

(a) 150 sec and 200 sec (b) 0 sec and 50 sec
(c) 50 sec and 100 sec (d) 100 sec and 150 sec

42. The capacitor of an oscillatory circuit is enclosed in a container. When the container is evacuated, the resonance frequency of the circuit is 10 kHz. When the container is filled with a gas, the resonance frequency changes by 50 Hz. The dielectric constant of the gas is **[Online May 26, 2012]**

(a) 1.001 (b) 2.001 (c) 1.01 (d) 3.01

43. This question has Statement 1 and Statement 2. Of the four choices given after the Statements, choose the one that best describes the two Statements.

Statement 1: It is not possible to make a sphere of capacity 1 farad using a conducting material.

Statement 2: It is possible for earth as its radius is 6.4×10^6 m. **[Online May 26, 2012]**

(a) Statement 1 is true, Statement 2 is true, Statement 2 is the correct explanation of Statement 1.
(b) Statement 1 is false, Statement 2 is true.
(c) Statement 1 is true, Statement 2 is true, Statement 2 is not the correct explanation of Statement 1.
(d) Statement 1 is true, Statement 2 is false.

44. A series combination of n_1 capacitors, each of capacity C_1 is charged by source of potential difference 4 V. When another parallel combination of n_2 capacitors each of capacity C_2 is charged by a source of potential difference V, it has the same total energy stored in it as the first combination has. The value of C_2 in terms of C_1 is then **[Online May 12, 2012]**

(a) $16\frac{n_2}{n_1}C_1$ (b) $\frac{2C_1}{n_1 n_2}$

(c) $2\frac{n_2}{n_1}C_1$ (d) $\frac{16C_1}{n_1 n_2}$

45. Two circuits (a) and (b) have charged capacitors of capacitance C, 2C and 3C with open switches. Charges on each of the capacitor are as shown in the figures. On closing the switches **[Online May 7, 2012]**

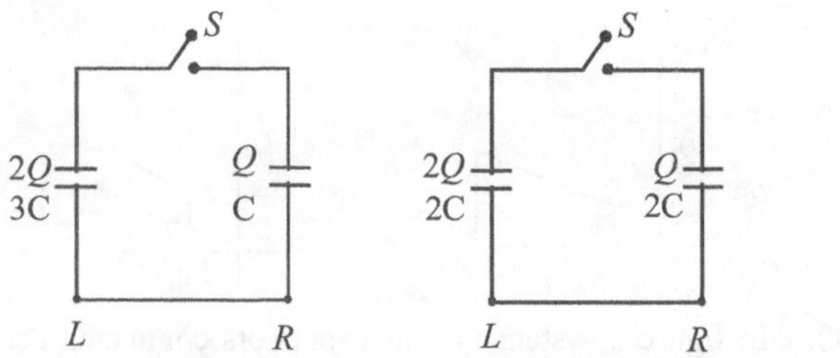

Circuit (a) Circuit (b)

(a) No charge flows in (a) but charge flows from R to L in (b)
(b) Charges flow from L to R in both (a) and (b)
(c) Charges flow from R to L in (a) and from L to R in (b)
(d) No charge flows in (a) but charge flows from L to R in (b)

46. Let C be the capacitance of a capacitor discharging through a resistor R. Suppose t_1 is the time taken for the energy stored in the capacitor to reduce to half its initial value and t_2 is the time taken for the charge to reduce to one-fourth its initial value. Then the ratio t_1/t_2 will be **[2010]**

(a) 1 (b) $\frac{1}{2}$ (c) $\frac{1}{4}$ (d) 2

47. A parallel plate capacitor with air between the plates has capacitance of 9 pF. The separation between its plates is 'd'. The space between the plates is now filled with two dielectrics. One of the dielectrics has dielectric constant $k_1 = 3$ and thickness $\frac{d}{3}$ while the other one has dielectric constant $k_2 = 6$ and thickness $\frac{2d}{3}$. Capacitance of the capacitor is now **[2008]**

(a) 1.8 pF (b) 45 pF (c) 40.5 pF (d) 20.25 pF

48. A parallel plate condenser with a dielectric of dielectric constant K between the plates has a capacity C and is charged to a potential V volt. The dielectric slab is slowly removed from between the plates and then reinserted. The net work done by the system in this process is **[2007]**

(a) zero (b) $\frac{1}{2}(K-1)\,CV^2$

(c) $\frac{CV^2(K-1)}{K}$ (d) $(K-1)\,CV^2$

49. A parallel plate capacitor is made by stacking n equally spaced plates connected alternatively. If the capacitance between any two adjacent plates is 'C' then the resultant capacitance is **[2005]**

(a) $(n+1)C$ (b) $(n-1)C$

(c) nC (d) C

50. A fully charged capacitor has a capacitance 'C'. It is discharged through a small coil of resistance wire embedded in a thermally insulated block of specific heat capacity 's' and mass 'm'. If the temperature of the block is raised by 'ΔT', the potential difference 'V' across the capacitance is **[2005]**

(a) $\frac{mC\Delta T}{s}$ (b) $\sqrt{\frac{2mC\Delta T}{s}}$

(c) $\sqrt{\frac{2ms\Delta T}{C}}$ (d) $\frac{ms\Delta T}{C}$

51. A sheet of aluminium foil of negligible thickness is introduced between the plates of a capacitor. The capacitance of the capacitor **[2003]**

(a) decreases (b) remains unchanged

(c) becomes infinite (d) increases

52. The work done in placing a charge of 8×10^{-18} coulomb on a condenser of capacity 100 micro-farad is **[2003]**

(a) 16×10^{-32} joule (b) 3.1×10^{-26} joule

(c) 4×10^{-10} joule (d) 32×10^{-32} joule

53. If there are n capacitors in parallel connected to V volt source, then the energy stored is equal to **[2002]**

(a) CV (b) $\frac{1}{2}nCV^2$ (c) CV^2 (d) $\frac{1}{2n}CV^2$

54. Capacitance (in F) of a spherical conductor with radius 1 m is **[2002]**

(a) 1.1×10^{-10} (b) 10^{-6}

(c) 9×10^{-9} (d) 10^{-3}

Hints & Solutions

TOPIC - 1: Electrostatic Potential and Equipotential Surfaces

1 (c) Potential gradient is given by,

$\Delta V = E.d$

$0.8 = Ed\,(max)$

$\Delta V = Ed\cos\theta = 0.8 \times \cos 60 = 0.4$

Hence, maximum potential at a point on the sphere $= 589.4\ V$

2. (c) As we know electric field, $E = \frac{-dv}{dr}$

$E =$ constant $\quad \therefore$ dv and dr same

$E = \frac{K\phi}{r^2} = c$

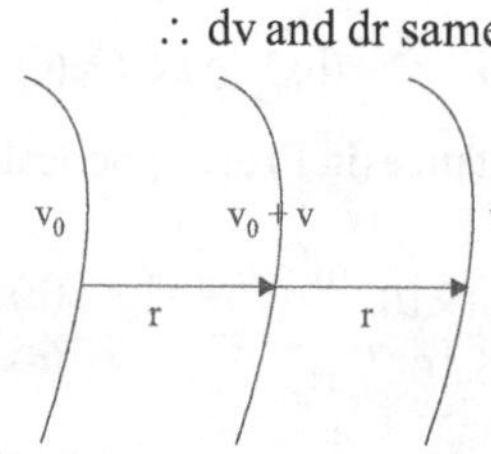

$\Rightarrow \phi \propto r^2$

$\therefore \phi = \int_0^r \rho 4\pi r^2 dr$

$\Rightarrow \rho \propto \frac{1}{r}$

3. (b) $\Sigma_1 = \frac{-dv}{dr} = 10|z|$

$\Sigma_2 = \frac{-dv}{dr} = 10 \qquad$ (constant : E)

$\therefore$ The source is an infinity large non conducting thick plate of thickness 2 m.

$\therefore 10Z \cdot 10A = \frac{\rho \cdot A \propto Z}{\varepsilon_0}$

$\rho_0 = 10e_0$ for $|z| \le 1m$.

4. (a) We know, $V_0 = \frac{Kq}{R} = V$surface

Now, $V_i = \frac{Kq}{2R^3}(3R^2 - r^2)$ [For $r < R$]

At the centre of sphere r = 0. Here

$V = \frac{3}{2}V_0$

Now, $\frac{5}{4}\frac{Kq}{R} = \frac{Kq}{2R^3}(3R^2 - r^2)$

$R_2 = \frac{R}{\sqrt{2}}$

$\frac{3}{4}\frac{Kq}{R} = \frac{Kq}{R^3}$

$\frac{1}{4}\frac{Kq}{R} = \frac{Kq}{R_4}$

$R_4 = 4R$

Also, $R_1 = 0$ and $R_2 < (R_4 - R_3)$

5. (a) As we know, $E = -\frac{dv}{dx}$

Potential at the point x = 2m, y = 2m is given by :

$\int_0^V dV = -\int_0^{2,2} (25dx + 30dy)$

on solving we get,

V = – 110 volt.

6. (c) Potential difference between any two points in an electric field is given by,

$dV = -\vec{E}.\vec{dx}$

$\int_{V_O}^{V_A} dV = -\int_0^2 30x^2 dx$

$V_A - V_O = -[10x^3]_0^2 = -80J/C$

7. (a) The potential of uncharged body is less than that of the charged conductor and more than at infinity.

8. (c)

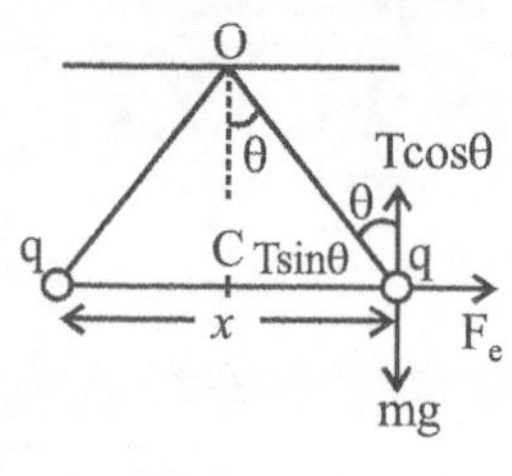

In equilibrium, $F_e = T\sin\theta$

$mg = T\cos\theta$

$\tan\theta = \frac{F_e}{mg} = \frac{q^2}{4\pi\epsilon_0 x^2 \times mg}$

$\therefore x = \sqrt{\frac{q^2}{4\pi\epsilon_0 \tan\theta\, mg}}$

Electric potential at the centre of the line

$V = \frac{kq}{x/2} + \frac{kq}{x/2} = 4\sqrt{kmg/\tan\theta}$

9. (c) $q = 1\mu C = 1 \times 10^{-6} C$

$r = 4\,cm = 4 \times 10^{-2}\,m$

Potential $V = \frac{kq}{r}$

$= \frac{9 \times 10^9 \times 10^{-6}}{4 \times 10^{-2}}$

$= 2.25 \times 10^5\,V.$

Induced electric field $E = -\frac{kq}{r^2}$

$= \frac{9 \times 10^9 \times 1 \times 10^{-6}}{16 \times 10^{-4}} = -5.625 \times 10^6\,V/m$

10. (c) Let q_1 and q_2 be charge on two spheres of radius 'r' and 'R' respectively

As, $q_1 + q_2 = Q$

and $\sigma_1 = \sigma_2$ [Surface charge density are equal]

$\therefore \frac{q_1}{r\pi r^2} = \frac{q_2}{4\pi R^2}$

So, $q_1 = \frac{Qr^2}{R^2 + r^2}$ and $q_2 = \frac{QR^2}{R^2 + r^2}$

Now, potential, $V = \frac{1}{4\pi\varepsilon_0}\left[\frac{q_1}{r} + \frac{q_2}{R}\right]$

$= \frac{1}{4\pi\varepsilon_0}\left[\frac{Qr}{R^2 + r^2} + \frac{QR}{R^2 + r^2}\right]$

$= \frac{Q(R + r)}{R^2 + r^2} \frac{1}{4\pi\varepsilon_0}$

11. (c) Charges reside only on the outer surface of a conductor with cavity.

12. (c) Electric field

$E = -\frac{d\phi}{dr} = -2ar$ ....(i)

By Gauss's theorem

$E = \frac{1}{4\pi\varepsilon_0} \frac{q}{r^2}$ ....(ii)

From (i) and (ii),

$Q = -8\pi\varepsilon_0 ar^3$

$\Rightarrow dq = -24\pi\varepsilon_0 ar^2\,dr$

Charge density, $\rho = \frac{dq}{4\pi r^2 dr} = -6\varepsilon_0 a$

13. (c)

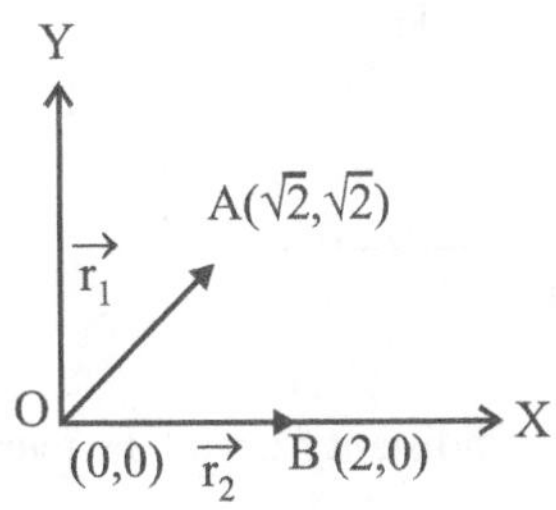

The distance of point $A(\sqrt{2}, \sqrt{2})$ from the origin,

$OA = |\vec{r}_1| = \sqrt{(\sqrt{2})^2 + (\sqrt{2})^2} = \sqrt{4} = 2$ units.

The distance of point $B(2, 0)$ from the origin,

$OB = |\vec{r}_2| = \sqrt{(2)^2 + (0)^2} = 2$ units.

Now, potential at A, $V_A = \frac{1}{4\pi \epsilon_0} \cdot \frac{Q}{(OA)}$

Potential at B, $V_B = \frac{1}{4\pi \epsilon_0} \cdot \frac{Q}{(OB)}$

$\therefore$ Potential difference between the points A and B is given by

$V_A - V_B = \frac{1}{4\pi \epsilon_0} \cdot \frac{Q}{OA} - \frac{1}{4\pi \epsilon_0} \cdot \frac{Q}{OB}$

$= \frac{Q}{4\pi \epsilon_0}\left(\frac{1}{OA} - \frac{1}{OB}\right) = \frac{Q}{4\pi \epsilon_0}\left(\frac{1}{2} - \frac{1}{2}\right)$

$= \frac{Q}{4\pi \epsilon_0} \times 0 = 0.$

14. (a) As shown in the figure, the resultant electric fields before and after interchanging the charges will have the same magnitude, but opposite directions.

Also, the potential will be same in both cases as it is a scalar quantity.

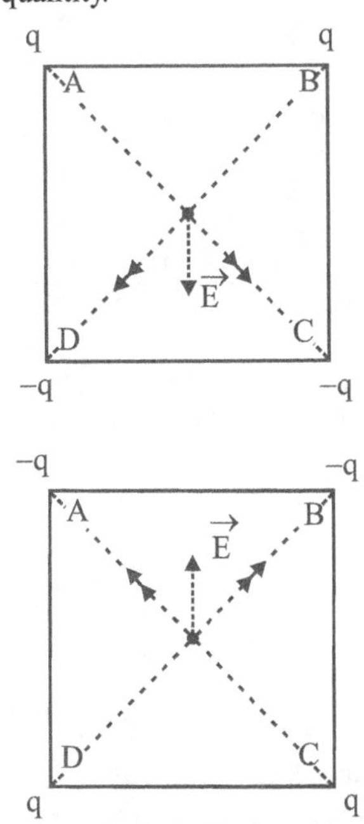

15. (a) Here, $V(x) = \frac{20}{x^2 - 4}$ volt

We know that $E = -\frac{dV}{dx} = -\frac{d}{dx}\left(\frac{20}{x^2-4}\right)$

or, $E = +\frac{40x}{(x^2-4)^2}$

At $x = 4\,\mu m$,

$E = +\frac{40\times 4}{(4^2-4)^2} = +\frac{160}{144} = +\frac{10}{9}$ volt / μm.

Positive sign indicates that $\vec{E}$ is in +ve x-direction.

16. (a)

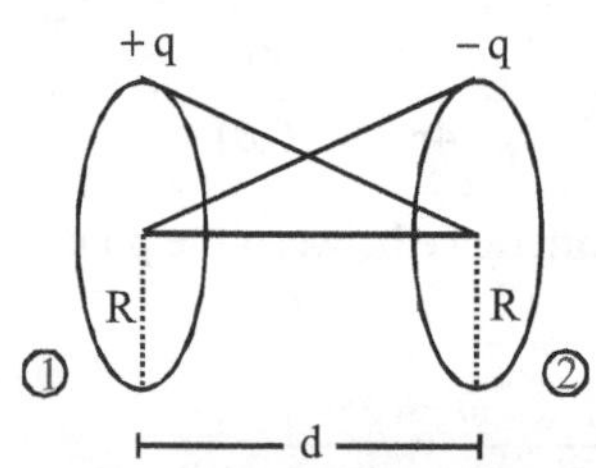

At (1) using, potential $(V_1) = V_{self} + V_{due\ to\ (2)}$

$$\Rightarrow V_1 = \frac{1}{4\pi\varepsilon_0}\left[\frac{q}{R} - \frac{q}{\sqrt{R^2+d^2}}\right]$$

At (2) using potential $(V_2) = V_{self} + V_{due\ to\ (1)}$

$$\Rightarrow V_2 = \frac{1}{4\pi\varepsilon_0}\left[\frac{-q}{R} + \frac{q}{\sqrt{R^2+d^2}}\right]$$

$$\Delta V = V_1 - V_2$$

$$= \frac{1}{4\pi\varepsilon_0}\left[\frac{q}{R} + \frac{q}{R} - \frac{q}{\sqrt{R^2+d^2}} - \frac{q}{\sqrt{R^2+d^2}}\right]$$

$$= \frac{1}{2\pi\varepsilon_0}\left[\frac{q}{R} - \frac{q}{\sqrt{R^2+d^2}}\right]$$

17. (c) Electric potential due to charge Q placed at the centre of the spherical shell at point P is

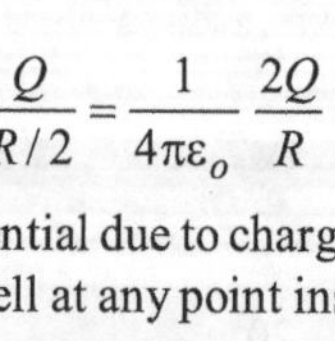

$$V_1 = \frac{1}{4\pi\varepsilon_o}\frac{Q}{R/2} = \frac{1}{4\pi\varepsilon_o}\frac{2Q}{R}$$

Electric potential due to charge q on the surface of the spherical shell at any point inside the shell is

$$V_2 = \frac{1}{4\pi\varepsilon_o}\frac{q}{R}$$

∴ The net electric potential at point P is

$$V = V_1 + V_2 = \frac{1}{4\pi\varepsilon_o}\frac{2Q}{R} + \frac{1}{4\pi\varepsilon_o}\frac{q}{R}$$

TOPIC - 2 : Electric Potential Energy and Work Done in Carrying a Charge

18. (c) The work done is moving a charge along an equipotential surface is always zero.
The direction of electric field is perpendicular to the equipotential surface or lines.

19. (c) The potential energy at the centre of the sphere

$$U_c = \frac{3}{2}\frac{KQq}{R}$$

The potential energy at the surface of the sphere

$$U_s = \frac{KqQ}{R}$$

Now change in the energy

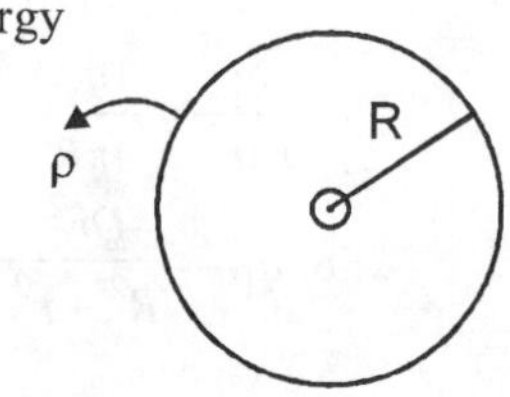

$$\Delta U = U_c - U_s$$

$$= \frac{KQq}{R}\left[\frac{3}{2} - 1\right]$$

$$= \frac{KQq}{2R}$$

Where $Q = \rho.V = \rho.\frac{4}{3}\pi R^3$

$$\Delta U = \frac{2K}{3}\frac{\pi R^3 \rho q}{R}$$

$$\Delta U = \frac{2}{3}\times\frac{1}{4\pi\epsilon_0}\frac{\pi R^3\rho q}{R}$$

$$\Delta U = \frac{R^2\rho q}{6\epsilon_0}$$

20. (d) Potential at point A,

$$V_A = \frac{2kq}{a} - \frac{2kq}{a\sqrt{5}}$$

∴ (potential due to each $q = \frac{kq}{a}$ and potential due to each $-q = \frac{-kq}{a\sqrt{5}}$)

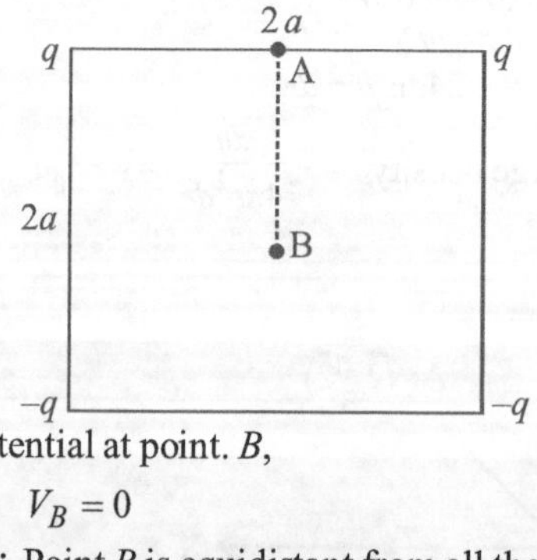

Potential at point. B,

$$V_B = 0$$

(∵ Point B is equidistant from all the four charges)

$\therefore$ Using work energy theorem,

$$(W_{AB})_{electric} = Q(V_A - V_B)$$

$$= \frac{2kqQ}{a}\left[1-\frac{1}{\sqrt{5}}\right]$$

$$= \left(\frac{1}{4\pi\varepsilon_0}\right)\frac{2Qq}{a}\left[1-\frac{1}{\sqrt{5}}\right]$$

21. (c) $\frac{W_{PQ}}{q} = (V_Q - V_P)$

$$\Rightarrow W_{PQ} = q(V_Q - V_P)$$

$$= (-100 \times 1.6 \times 10^{-19})(-4-10)$$

$$= +2.24 \times 10^{-16}\text{J}$$

22. (a) $eV = \frac{1}{2}mv^2$

$$\Rightarrow v = \sqrt{\frac{2eV}{m}} = \sqrt{\frac{2\times 1.6\times 10^{-19}\times 20}{9.1\times 10^{-31}}}$$

$$= 2.65\times 10^6 \text{ m/s}$$

23. (d) $\frac{1}{2}mv^2 = \frac{kQq}{r}$

$$\Rightarrow \frac{1}{2}m(2v)^2 = \frac{kqQ}{r'} \Rightarrow r' = \frac{r}{4}$$

24. (a) We know that $\frac{W_{AB}}{q} = V_B - V_A$

$$\therefore V_B - V_A = \frac{2\text{J}}{20\text{C}} = 0.1\text{J/C} = 0.1\text{V}$$

TOPIC - 3: Capacitors, Grouping of Capacitor and Energy Stored in a Capacitor

25. (b) To get a capacitance of 2 μF arrangement of capacitors of capacitance 1 μF as shown in figure 8 capacitors of 1 μF in parallel with four such branches in series i.e., 32 such capacitors are required.

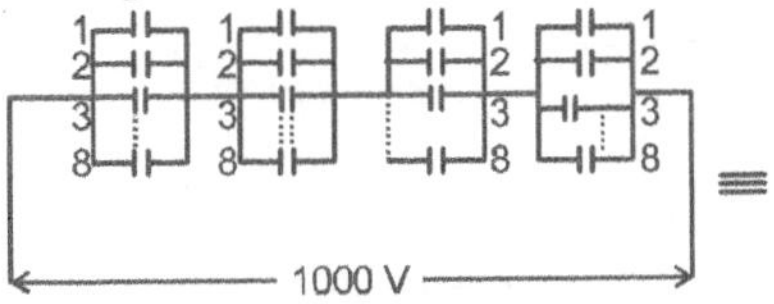

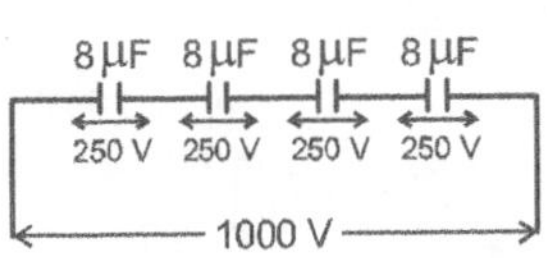

$$\frac{1}{C_{eq}} = \frac{1}{8}+\frac{1}{8}+\frac{1}{8}+\frac{1}{8} \qquad \therefore C_{eq} = 2\ \mu F$$

26. (c) Before introducing a slab capacitance of plates

$$C_1 = \frac{\varepsilon_0 A}{3}$$

If a slab of dielectric constant K is introduced between plates then

$$C = \frac{K\varepsilon_0 A}{d} \text{ then } C_1' = \frac{\varepsilon_0 A}{2.4}$$

C_1 and C_1' are in series hence,

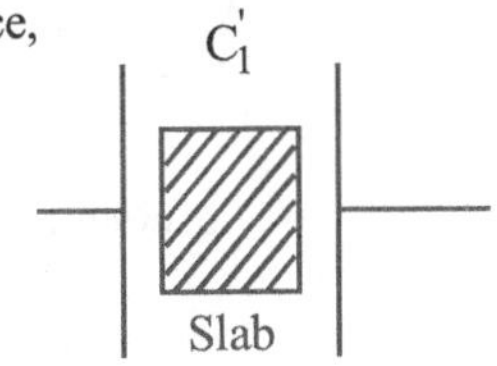

$$\frac{\varepsilon_0 A}{3} = \frac{k\frac{\varepsilon_0 A}{3}\cdot\frac{\varepsilon_0 A}{2.4}}{k\frac{\varepsilon_0 A}{3}+\frac{\varepsilon_0 A}{2.4}}$$

$$3k = 2.4k + 3$$

$$0.6k = 3$$

Hence, the dielectric constant of slap is given by,

$$k = \frac{30}{6} = 5$$

27. (d) Energy of sphere $= \frac{Q^2}{2C}$

$$4.5 = \frac{16\times 10^{-12}}{2C}$$

$$C = \frac{16\times 10^{-12}}{9} = 4\pi\varepsilon_0 R$$

(capacity of spherical conductor)

$$R = \frac{16\times 10^{-12}}{9}\times\frac{1}{4\pi\varepsilon_0} \qquad \because \frac{1}{4\pi\varepsilon_0} = 9\times 10^9$$

$$= 9\times 10^9 \times \frac{16}{9}\times 10^{-12} = 16 \text{ mm}$$

28. (a)

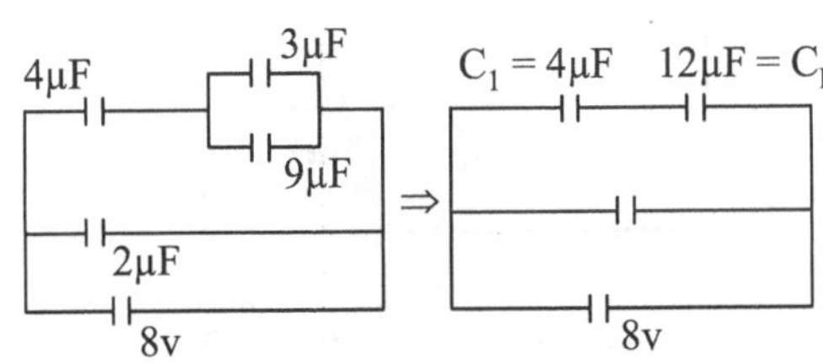

Charge on C_1 is $q_1 = \left[\left(\frac{12}{4+12}\right)\times 8\right]\times 4 = 24\mu c$

The voltage across C_P is $V_P = \frac{4}{4+12}\times 8 = 2v$

$\therefore$ Voltage across 9μF is also 2V

$\therefore$ Charge on 9μF capacitor $= 9\times 2 = 18\mu C$

$\therefore$ Total charge on 4 μF and 9μF = 42μc

$$\therefore E = \frac{KQ}{r^2} = 9\times 10^9 \times \frac{42\times 10^{-6}}{30\times 30} = 420\,\text{Nc}^{-1}$$

29. (a) Capacitors 2μF and 2μF are parallel, their equivalent = 4 μF

6μF and 12 μF are in series, their equivalent = 4 μF

Now 4μF (2 and 2 μF) and 8μF in series = $\frac{3}{8}\mu F$

And 4μF (12 & 6 μF) and 4μF in parallel = 4 + 4 = 8μF

8μF in series with 1 μF = $\frac{1}{8}+1 \Rightarrow \frac{8}{9}\mu F$

Now $C_{eq} = \frac{8}{9}+\frac{8}{3}=\frac{32}{9}$

C_{eq} of circuit = $\frac{32}{9}$

With C - $\frac{1}{C_{eq}} = \frac{1}{C}+\frac{9}{32}=1 \Rightarrow C=\frac{32}{23}$

30. (d) To get effective capacitance of 6 μF two capacitors of 4 μF each connected in sereies and one of 4 μF capacitor in parallel with them.

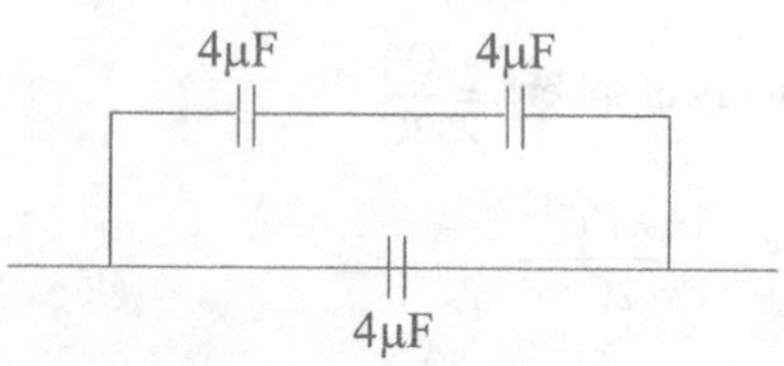

Two capacitances in series

$$\therefore \frac{1}{C}=\frac{1}{C_1}+\frac{1}{C_2}=\frac{1}{4}+\frac{1}{4}=\frac{1}{2}$$

1 capacitor in parallel

$$\therefore C_{eq} = C_3 + C = 4+2 = 6\,\mu F$$

31. (d)

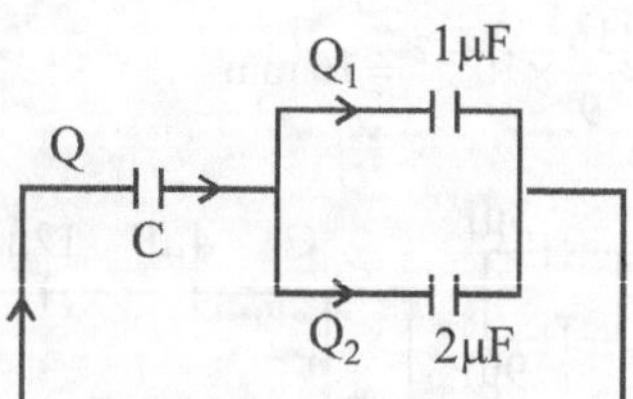

From figure, $Q_2 = \frac{2}{2+1}Q = \frac{2}{3}Q$

$$Q = E\left(\frac{C\times 3}{C+3}\right)$$

$$\therefore Q_2 = \frac{2}{3}\left(\frac{3CE}{C+3}\right) = \frac{2CE}{C+3}$$

Therefore graph d correctly dipicts.

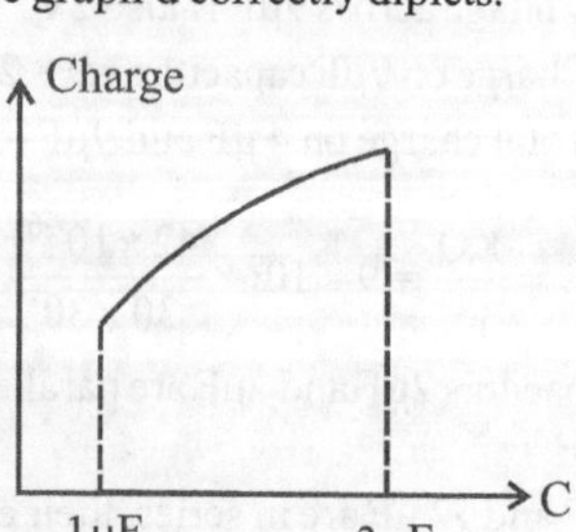

32. (a) when switch is closed

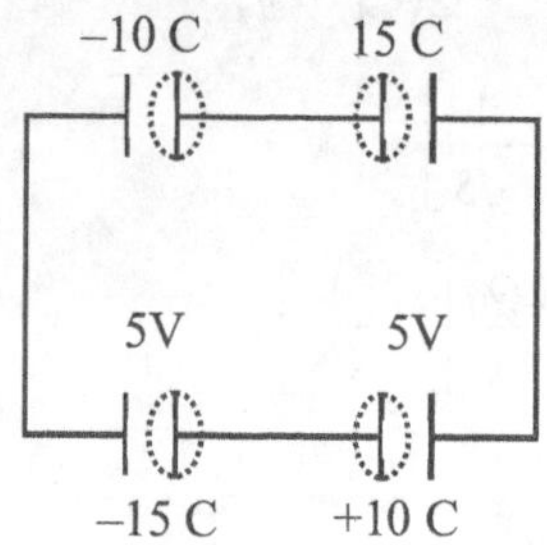

When switch is open

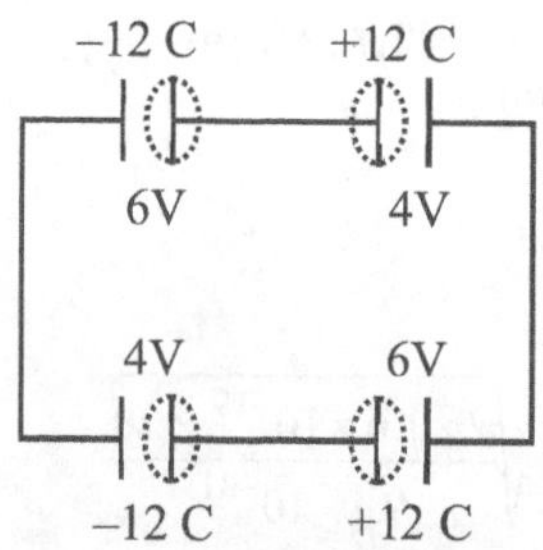

Charge of 5μc flows from *b* to *a*

33. (a) Electric field in presence of dielectric between the two plates of a parallel plate capacitor is given by,

$$E = \frac{\sigma}{K\varepsilon_0}$$

Then, charge density

$$\sigma = K\varepsilon_0 E$$
$$= 2.2 \times 8.85 \times 10^{-12} \times 3 \times 10^4$$
$$\approx 6 \times 10^{-7}\ C/m^2$$

34. (d)

35. (c) The value of dielectric constant is given as,

$$K = K_0 + \lambda x$$

And, $V = \int_0^d E\,dr$

$$V = \int_0^d \frac{\sigma}{K}dx$$

$$= \sigma\int_0^d \frac{1}{(K_0+\lambda x)}dx$$

$$= \frac{\sigma}{\lambda}\left[\ln(K_0+\lambda d) - \ln K_0\right]$$

$$= \frac{\sigma}{\lambda}\ln\left(1+\frac{\lambda d}{K_0}\right)$$

Now it is given that capacitance of vacuum = C_0.

Thus, $C = \frac{Q}{V}$

$= \frac{\sigma.s}{v}$ (Let surface area of plates = s)

$$= \frac{\sigma.s}{\frac{\sigma}{\lambda}\frac{}{d}\ln\left(1+\frac{\lambda d}{K_0}\right)}$$

$$= s\lambda.\frac{}{d}\frac{}{\ln\left(1+\frac{\lambda d}{K_0}\right)} \quad (\because \text{ in vacuum } \varepsilon_0 = 1)$$

$$c = \frac{\lambda d}{\ln\left(1+\frac{\lambda d}{K_0}\right)}\cdot C_0 \quad \left(\text{here, } C_0 = \frac{s}{d}\right)$$

36. (c)

37. (d) Possible combination of capacitors

(i) Three capacitors in series combination

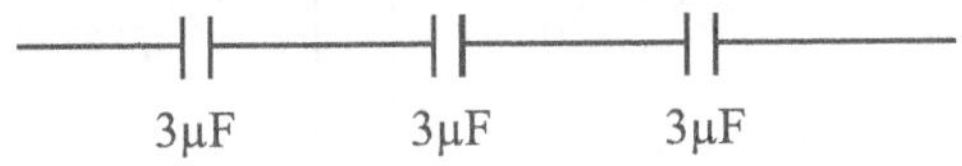

$$\frac{1}{C_{eq}} = \frac{1}{3}+\frac{1}{3}+\frac{1}{3}$$

$$\therefore \quad \frac{1}{C_{eq}} = 1\mu F$$

(ii) Three capacitors in parallel combination

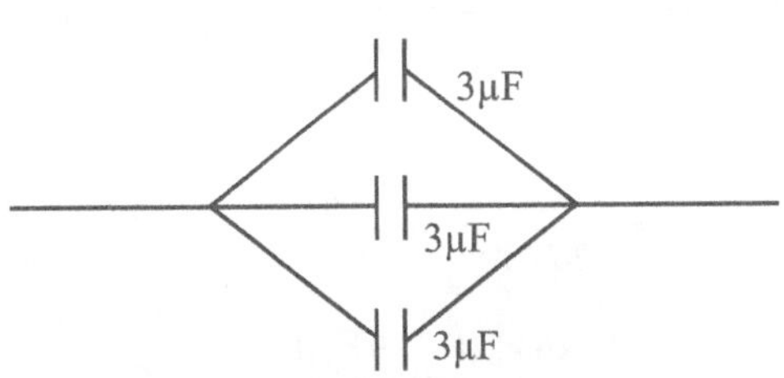

$C_{eq} = 3+3+3 = 9\ \mu F$

(iii) Two capacitors in parallel and one is in series

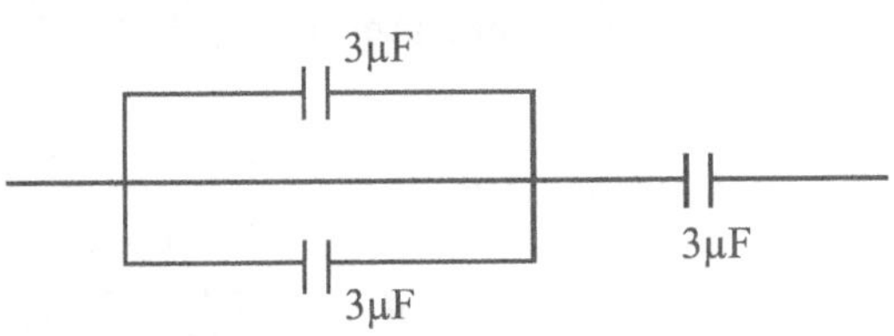

$C_{eq} = 2\mu F$

(iv) Two capacitors in series and one is in parallel

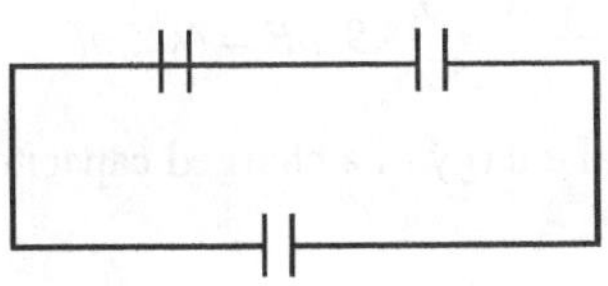

$C_{eq} = 4.5\ \mu F$

38. (b) $C_0 = \frac{k \in_0 A}{d}$

$$C = \frac{k \in_0 2}{3d} + \frac{2k \in_0 A}{3d} = \frac{4}{3}\frac{k \in_0 A}{d}$$

$$\therefore \frac{C}{C_0} = \frac{\frac{4}{3}\frac{k \in_0 A}{d}}{\frac{k \in_0 A}{d}} = \frac{4}{3}$$

39. (c) As, $C = \frac{Q}{V} = \frac{It}{V}$

$$\Rightarrow \frac{V}{t} = \frac{I}{C} = \frac{2}{1\times 10^{-6}}$$

$= 2 \times 10^6$ V/s

40. (c) When charged particle enters perpendicularly in an electric field, it describes a parabolic path

$$y = \frac{1}{2}\left(\frac{QE}{m}\right)\left(\frac{x}{4}\right)^2$$

This is the equation of parabola.

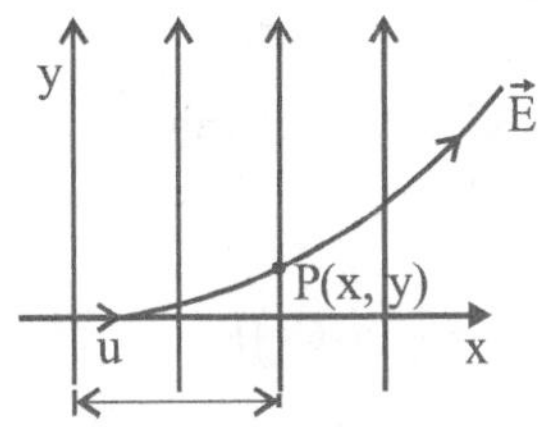

41. (d) The discharging of a capacitor is given as

$q = q_0 \exp[-t/RC]$

RC = time constant = τ

$q = q_0 e^{-t/\tau}$

If e is the capacitance of the capacitor

$q = CV$ and $q = CV_0$

Thus, $CV = CV_0 e^{t/\tau}$

$V = V_0 e^{-t/\tau}$ ...(i)

From the graph (given in the problem when $t = 0.5$, $V = 25$ i.e.,

$V_0 = 25$ volt.

and when $t = 200$, $V = 5$ volt

Thus equation (i) becomes

$5 = 25e^{-200/\tau}$

$\Rightarrow 1/5 = e^{-200/\tau}$

Taking $\log_e$ on both sides

$$\log_e \frac{1}{5} = -200/\tau \Rightarrow -\frac{200}{\tau} = \log e^5$$

$$\tau = \frac{200}{\log_e 5}$$

or $$\tau = \frac{200}{\log_e\left(\frac{10}{2}\right)} = \frac{200}{\log_e 10 - \log_e 2}$$

$$\tau = \frac{200}{2.302-0.693} = \frac{200}{1.609} = 124.300$$

Which lies between 100 s and 1,50 s

42. (c) The dielectric constant of the gas is 1.01

43. (d) Capacitance of sphere is given by :

$C = 4\pi \epsilon_0 r$

If, C = 1F then radius of sphere needed:

$$r = \frac{C}{4\pi \epsilon_0} = \frac{1}{4\pi \times 8.85 \times 10^{-12}}$$

$$\text{or, } r = \frac{10^{12}}{4\pi \times 8.85} = 9 \times 10^9 \text{ m}$$

9×10^9 m is very large, it is not possible to obtain such a large sphere. Infact earth has radius 6.4×10^6 m only and capacitance of earth is 711μF.

44. (d) Equivalent capacitance of n_2 number of capacitors each of capacitance C_2 in parallel $= n_2C_2$

Equivalent capacitance of n_1 number of capacitors each of capacitances C_1 in series.

Capacitance of each is $C_1 = \frac{C_1}{n_1}$

According to question, total energy stored in both the combinations are same

$$\text{i.e., } \frac{1}{2}\left(\frac{C_1}{n_1}\right)(4V)^2 = \frac{1}{2}(n_2C_2)V^2$$

$$\therefore C_2 = \frac{16C_1}{n_1 n_2}$$

45. (c) Charge (or current) always flows from higher potential to lower potential.

$$\text{Potential} = \frac{\text{Charge}}{\text{Capacitance}}$$

46. (c) Initial energy of capacitor, $E_1 = \frac{q_1^2}{2C}$

Final energy of capacitor,

$$E_2 = \frac{1}{2}E_1 = \frac{q_1^2}{4C} = \frac{\left(\frac{q_1}{\sqrt{2}}\right)^2}{2C}$$

$\therefore t_1$ = time for the charge to reduce to $\frac{1}{\sqrt{2}}$ of its initial value

and t_2 = time for the charge to reduce to $\frac{1}{4}$ of its initial value

We have, $q_2 = q_1 e^{-t/CR}$

$$\Rightarrow \ln\left(\frac{q_2}{q_1}\right) = -\frac{t}{CR}$$

$$\therefore \ln\left(\frac{1}{\sqrt{2}}\right) = \frac{-t_1}{CR} \quad ...(1)$$

$$\text{and } \ln\left(\frac{1}{4}\right) = \frac{-t_2}{CR} \quad ...(2)$$

$$\text{By (1) and (2), } \frac{t_1}{t_2} = \frac{\ln\left(\frac{1}{\sqrt{2}}\right)}{\ln\left(\frac{1}{4}\right)}$$

$$= \frac{1}{2}\frac{\ln\left(\frac{1}{2}\right)}{2\ln\left(\frac{1}{2}\right)} = \frac{1}{4}$$

47. (c)

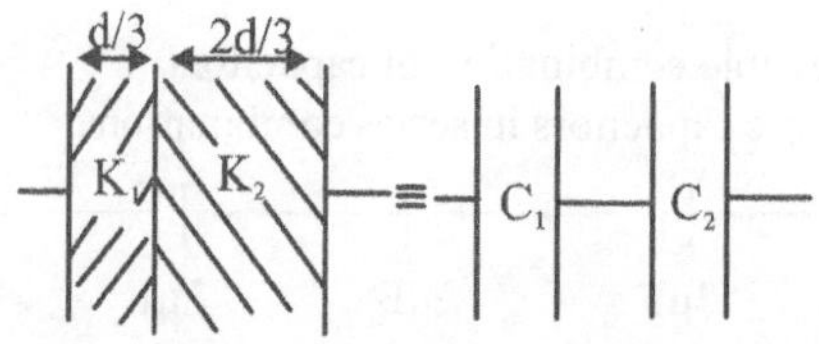

The given capacitance is equal to two capacitances connected in series where

$$C_1 = \frac{k_1 \epsilon_0 A}{d/3} = \frac{3k_1 \epsilon_0 A}{d}$$

$$= \frac{3 \times 3 \epsilon_0 A}{d} = \frac{9 \epsilon_0 A}{d}$$

and

$$C_1 = \frac{k_2 \epsilon_0 A}{2d/3} = \frac{3k_2 \epsilon_0 A}{2d}$$

$$= \frac{3 \times 6 \epsilon_0 A}{2d} = \frac{9 \epsilon_0 A}{d}$$

The equivalent capacitance C_{eq} is

$$\frac{1}{C_{eq}} = \frac{1}{C_1} + \frac{1}{C_2}$$

$$= \frac{d}{9 \epsilon_0 A} + \frac{d}{9 \epsilon_0 A} = \frac{2d}{9 \epsilon_0 A}$$

$$\therefore C_{eq} = \frac{9}{2}\frac{\epsilon_0 A}{d} = \frac{9}{2} \times 9\ pF = 40.5 pF$$

48. (a) The potential energy of a charged capacitor is given by $U = \frac{Q^2}{2C}$.

If a dielectric slab is inserted between the plates, the energy is given by $\frac{Q^2}{2KC}$, where K is the dielectric constant.

Again, when the dielectric slab is removed slowly its energy increases to initial potential energy. Thus, work done is zero.

49. **(b)** As n plates are joined, it means $(n - 1)$ combination joined in parallel.

$\therefore$ resultant capacitance $= (n-1)\,C$

50. **(c)** Applying conservation of energy,

$$\frac{1}{2}CV^2 = m.s\,\Delta t;\ \ V = \sqrt{\frac{2m.s.\Delta t}{C}}$$

51. **(b)** The capacitance of a parallel plate capacitor in which a metal plate of thickness t is inserted is given by

$$C = \frac{\varepsilon_0 A}{d-t}.\ \text{Here } t \to 0\ \therefore C = \frac{\varepsilon_0 A}{d}$$

52. **(d)** The work done is stored as the potential energy. The potential energy stored in a capacitor is given by

$$U = \frac{1}{2}\frac{Q^2}{C} = \frac{1}{2} \times \frac{\left(8\times 10^{-18}\right)^2}{100\times 10^{-6}} = 32\times 10^{-32}\,\text{J}$$

53. **(b)** The equivalent capacitance of n identical capacitors of capacitance C is equal to nC. Energy stored in this capacitor

$$E = \frac{1}{2}(nC)V^2 = \frac{1}{2}nCV^2$$

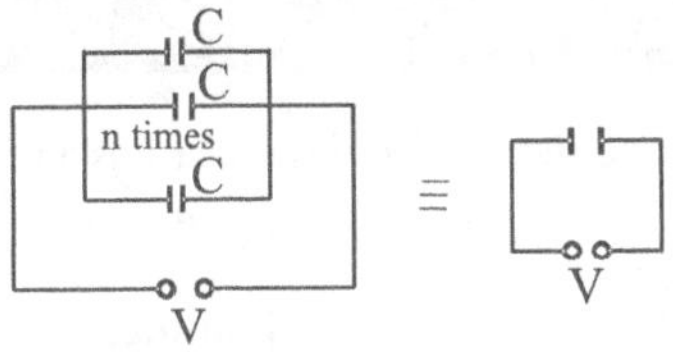

54. **(a)** For an isolated sphere, the capacitance is given by

$$C = 4\pi \in_0 r = \frac{1}{9\times 10^9}\times 1 = 1.1\times 10^{-10}\,\text{F}$$

Chapter 17

Current Electricity

TOPIC - 1: Electric Current, Drift of Electrons, Ohm's Law, Resistance and Resistivity

1. A uniform wire of length l and radius r has a resistance of 100 Ω. It is recast into a wire of radius $\frac{r}{2}$. The resistance of new wire will be : **[Online April 9, 2017]**
(a) 1600 Ω (b) 400 Ω (c) 200 Ω (d) 100 Ω

2. When 5V potential difference is applied across a wire of length 0.1 m, the drift speed of electrons is $2.5 \times 10^{-4}\ ms^{-1}$. If the electron density in the wire is $8 \times 10^{28}\ m^{-3}$, the resistivity of the material is close to : **[2015]**
(a) $1.6 \times 10^{-6}\ \Omega m$ (b) $1.6 \times 10^{-5}\ \Omega m$
(c) $1.6 \times 10^{-8}\ \Omega m$ (d) $1.6 \times 10^{-7}\ \Omega m$

3. Suppose the drift velocity v_d in a material varied with the applied electric field E as $v_d \propto \sqrt{E}$. Then V – I graph for a wire made of such a material is best given by : **[Online April 10, 2015]**

(a) 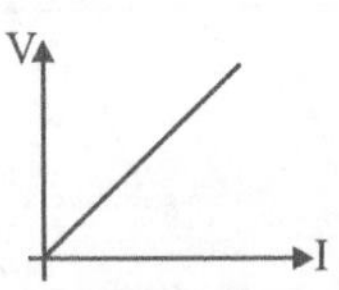

(b) 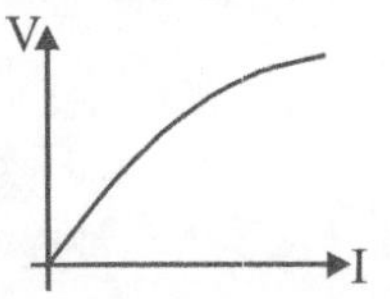

(c) 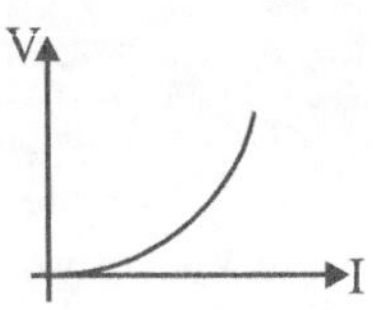

(d) 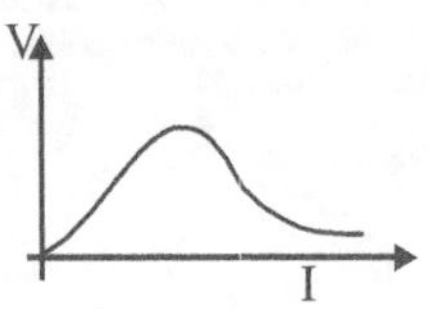

4. Correct set up to verify Ohm's law is : **[Online April 23, 2013]**

(a) 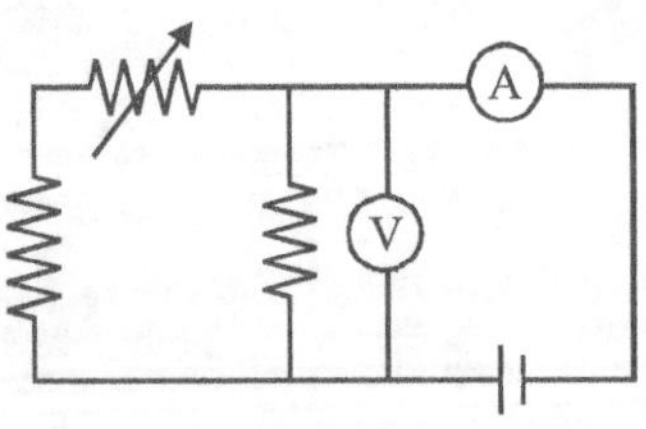

(b) 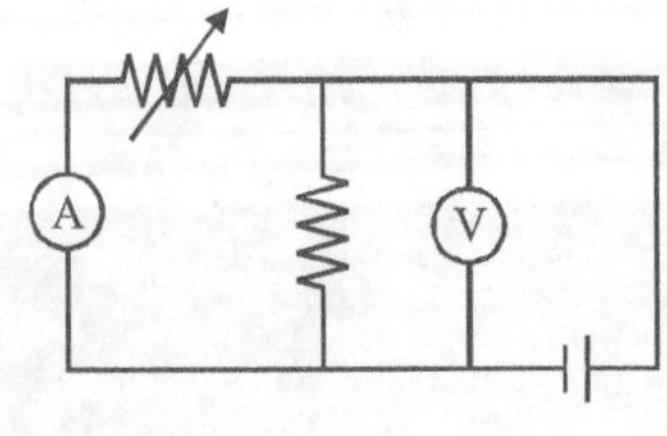

(c) 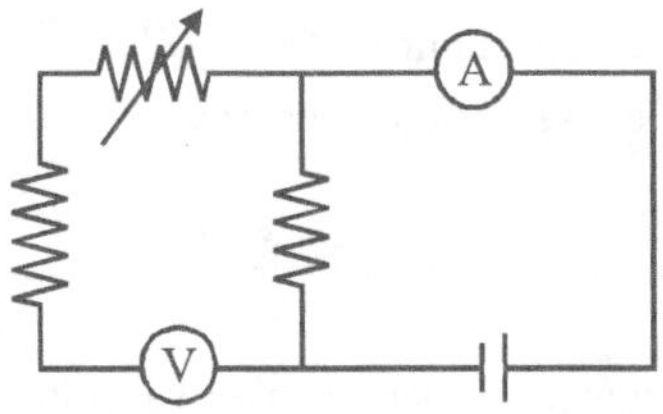

(d) 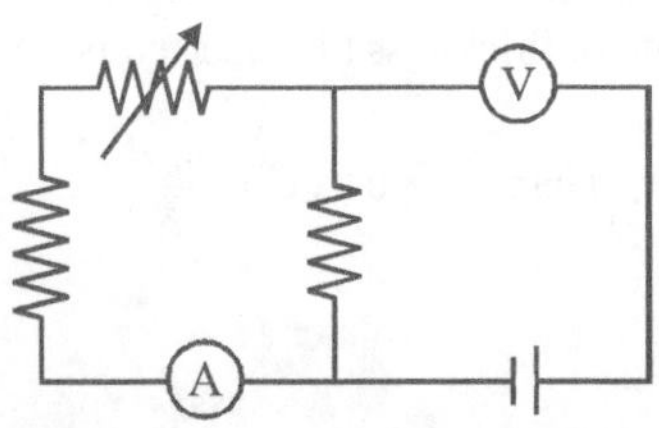

5. The resistance of a wire is R. It is bent at the middle by 180° and both the ends are twisted together to make a shorter wire. The resistance of the new wire is **[Online May 26, 2012]**
(a) $2R$ (b) $R/2$ (c) $R/4$ (d) $R/8$

6. If a wire is stretched to make it 0.1% longer, its resistance will : **[2011]**
(a) increase by 0.2% (b) decrease by 0.2%
(c) decrease by 0.05% (d) increase by 0.05%

DIRECTIONS : Question No. 7 and 8 are based on the following paragraph.

Consider a block of conducting material of resistivity 'ρ' shown in the figure. Current 'I' enters at 'A' and leaves from 'D'. We apply superposition principle to find voltage 'ΔV' developed between 'B' and 'C'. The calculation is done in the following steps:

(i) Take current 'I' entering from 'A' and assume it to spread over a hemispherical surface in the block.
(ii) Calculate field E(r) at distance 'r' from A by using Ohm's law E = ρ j, where j is the current per unit area at 'r'.
(iii) From the 'r' dependence of E(r), obtain the potential V(r) at r.
(iv) Repeat (i), (ii) and (iii) for current 'I' leaving 'D' and superpose results for 'A' and 'D'.

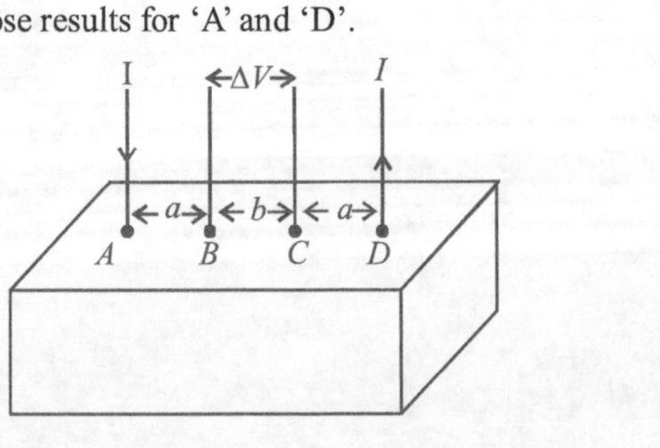

7. ΔV measured between B and C is **[2008]**

(a) $\frac{\rho I}{\pi a}-\frac{\rho I}{\pi(a+b)}$ (b) $\frac{\rho I}{a}-\frac{\rho I}{(a+b)}$

(c) $\frac{\rho I}{2\pi a}-\frac{\rho I}{2\pi(a+b)}$ (d) $\frac{\rho I}{2\pi(a-b)}$

8. For current entering at A, the electric field at a distance 'r' from A is **[2008]**

(a) $\frac{\rho I}{8\pi r^2}$ (b) $\frac{\rho I}{r^2}$ (c) $\frac{\rho I}{2\pi r^2}$ (d) $\frac{\rho I}{4\pi r^2}$

9. The resistance of a wire is 5 ohm at 50°C and 6 ohm at 100°C. The resistance of the wire at 0°C will be **[2007]**

(a) 3 ohm (b) 2 ohm (c) 1 ohm (d) 4 ohm

10. A material 'B' has twice the specific resistance of 'A'. A circular wire made of 'B' has twice the diameter of a wire made of 'A'. then for the two wires to have the same resistance, the ratio l_B/l_A of their respective lengths must be **[2006]**

(a) 1 (b) $\frac{1}{2}$ (c) $\frac{1}{4}$ (d) 2

11. An electric current is passed through a circuit containing two wires of the same material, connected in parallel. If the lengths and radii are in the ratio of $\frac{4}{3}$ and $\frac{2}{3}$, then the ratio of the current passing through the wires will be **[2004]**

(a) 8/9 (b) 1/3 (c) 3 (d) 2

12. The length of a given cylindrical wire is increased by 100%. Due to the consequent decrease in diameter the change in the resistance of the wire will be **[2003]**

(a) 200% (b) 100% (c) 50% (d) 300%

TOPIC - 2: Combination of Resistances

13. In the given circuit diagram when the current reaches steady state in the circuit, the charge on the capacitor of capacitance C will be : **[2017]**

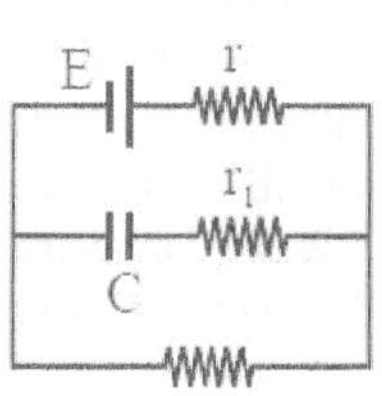

(a) $CE\frac{r_2}{(r+r_2)}$

(b) $CE\frac{r_1}{(r_1+r)}$

(c) CE

(d) $CE\frac{r_1}{(r_2+r)}$

14.

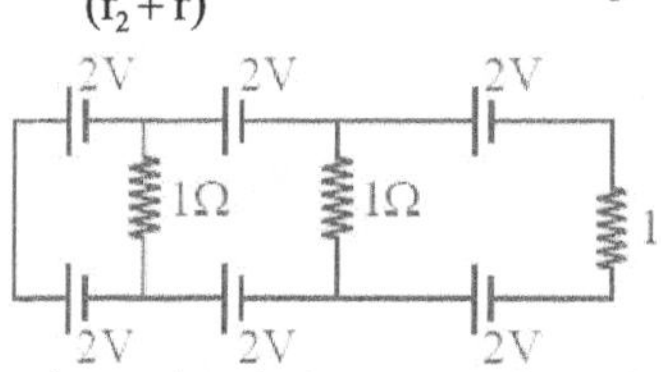

In the above circuit the current in each resistance is **[2017]**

(a) 0.5A (b) 0 A (c) 1 A (d) 0.25 A

15.

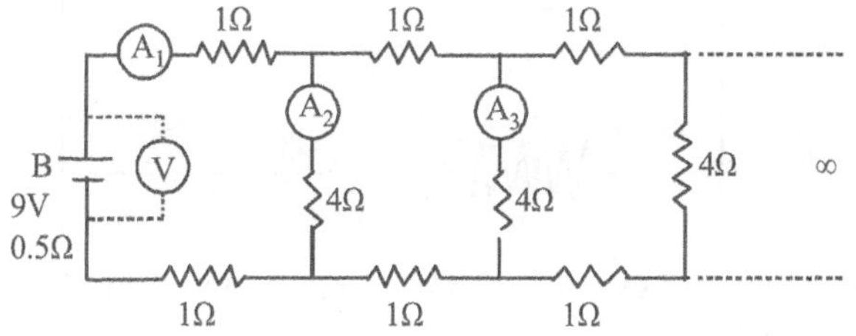

A 9 V battery with internal resistance of 0.5 Ω is connected across an infinite network as shown in the figure. All ammeters A_1, A_2, A_3 and voltmeter V are ideal.

Choose correct statement. **[Online April 8, 2017]**

(a) Reading of A_1 is 2 A (b) Reading of A_1 is 18 A

(c) Reading of V is 9 V (d) Reading of V is 7 V

16. Six equal resistances are connected between points P, Q and R as shown in figure. Then net resistance will be maximum between : **[Online April 25, 2013]**

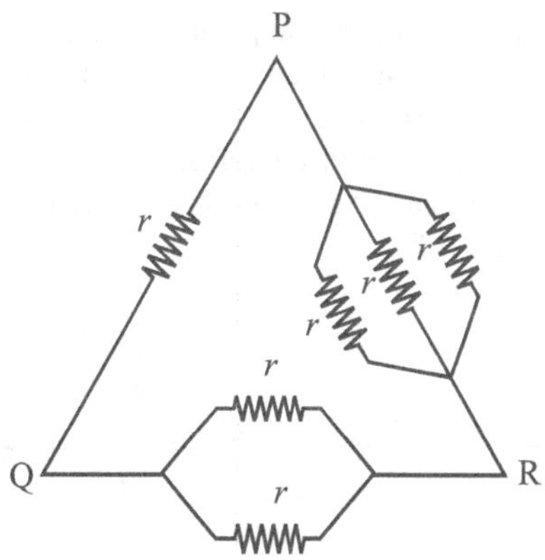

(a) P and R (b) P and Q

(c) Q and R (d) Any two points

17. A letter 'A' is constructed of a uniform wire with resistance 1.0 Ω per cm, The sides of the letter are 20 cm and the cross piece in the middle is 10 cm long. The apex angle is 60 . The resistance between the ends of the legs is close to:

[Online April 9, 2013]

(a) 50.0 Ω (b) 10 Ω (c) 36.7 Ω (d) 26.7 Ω

18. Two conductors have the same resistance at 0°C but their temperature coefficients of resistance are α_1 and α_2. The respective temperature coefficients of their series and parallel combinations are nearly **[2010]**

(a) $\frac{\alpha_1+\alpha_2}{2}, \alpha_1+\alpha_2$ (b) $\alpha_1+\alpha_2, \frac{\alpha_1+\alpha_2}{2}$

(c) $\alpha_1+\alpha_2, \frac{\alpha_1\alpha_2}{\alpha_1+\alpha_2}$ (d) $\frac{\alpha_1+\alpha_2}{2}, \frac{\alpha_1+\alpha_2}{2}$

19. The current I drawn from the 5 volt source will be **[2006]**

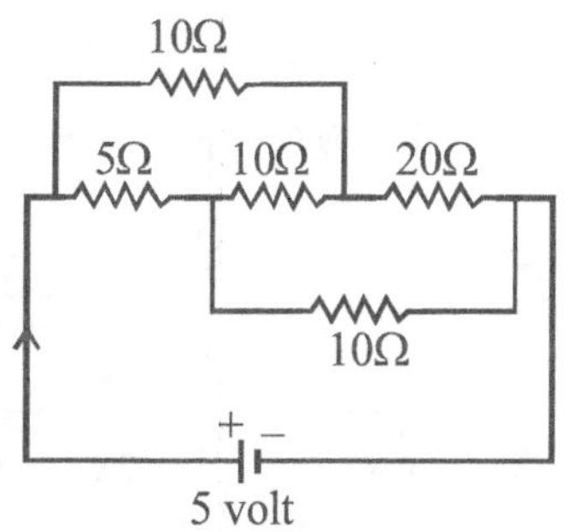

(a) 0.33 A (b) 0.5 A (c) 0.67 A (d) 0.17 A

20. The total current supplied to the circuit by the battery is

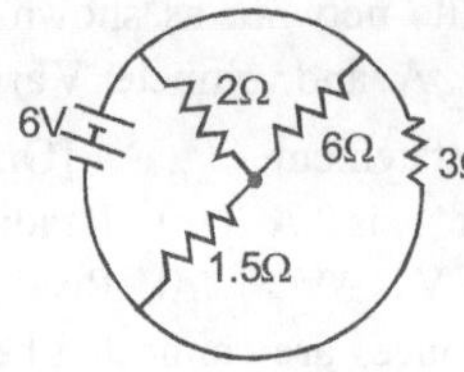

(a) 4 A (b) 2 A **[2004]**
(c) 1 A (d) 6 A

21. The resistance of the series combination of two resistances is S. when they are joined in parallel the total resistance is P. If $S = nP$ then the minimum possible value of n is **[2004]**
(a) 2 (b) 3 (c) 4 (d) 1

22. A 3 volt battery with negligible internal resistance is connected in a circuit as shown in the figure. The current I, in the circuit will be **[2003]**

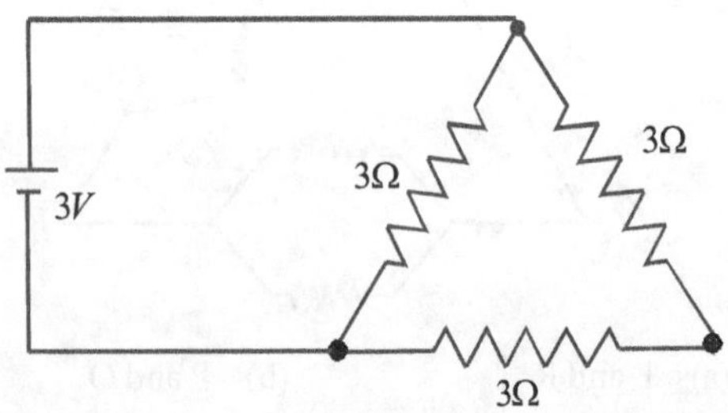

(a) 1 A (b) 1.5 A (c) 2 A (d) 1/3 A

TOPIC - 3: Kirchoff's Laws, Cells, Thermo e.m.f. Electrolysis

23. In the circuit shown, the current in the 1Ω resistor is : **[2015]**

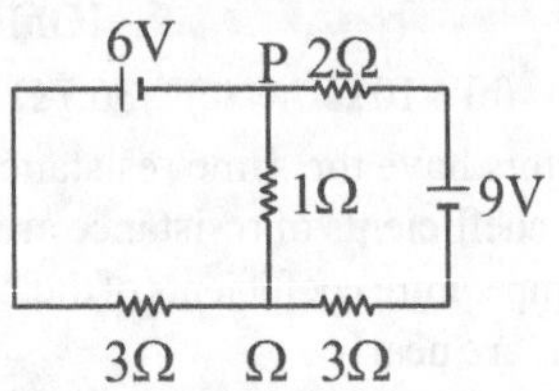

(a) 0.13 A, from Q to P (b) 0.13 A, from P to Q
(c) 1.3A from P to Q (d) 0A

24. In the electric network shown, when no current flows through the 4Ω resistor in the arm EB, the potential difference between the points A and D will be : **[Online April 11, 2015]**

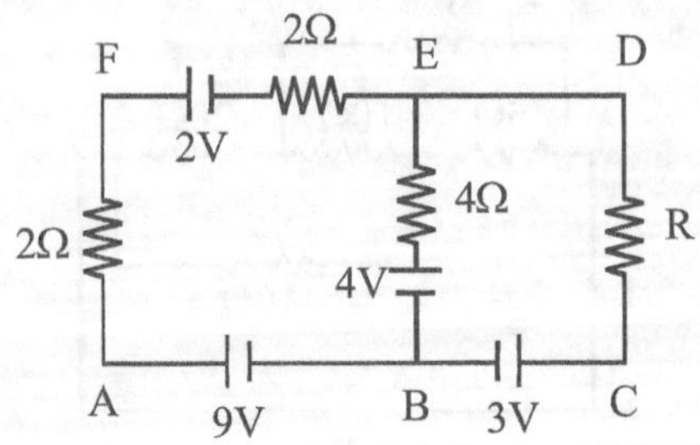

(a) 6 V (b) 3 V
(c) 5 V (d) 4 V

25. The circuit shown here has two batteries of 8.0 V and 16.0 V and three resistors 3 Ω, 9 Ω and 9 Ω and a capacitor of 5.0 μF. **[Online April 12, 2014]**

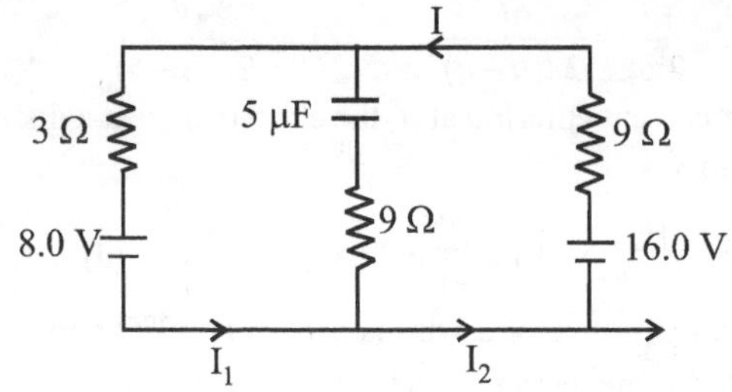

How much is the current I in the circuit in steady state?
(a) 1.6 A (b) 0.67 A (c) 2.5 A (d) 0.25 A

26. In the circuit shown, current (in A) through 50 V and 30 V batteries are, respectively. **[Online April 11, 2014]**

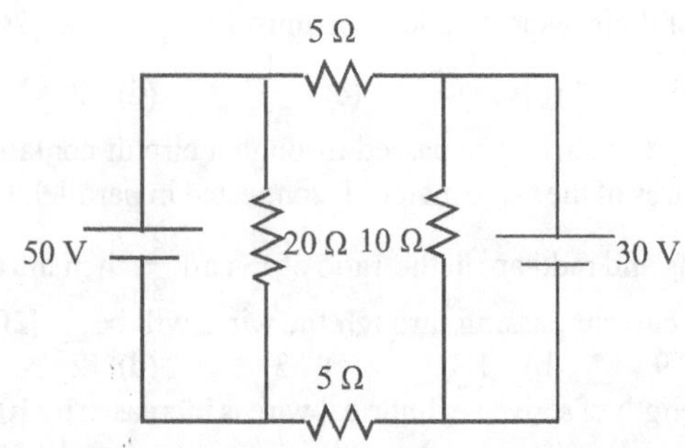

(a) 2.5 and 3 (b) 3.5 and 2
(c) 4.5 and 1 (d) 3 and 2.5

27. A d.c. main supply of e.m.f. 220 V is connected across a storage battery of e.m.f. 200 V through a resistance of 1Ω. The battery terminals are connected to an external resistance 'R'. The minimum value of 'R', so that a current passes through the battery to charge it is: **[Online April 9, 2014]**
(a) 7 Ω (b) 9 Ω (c) 11 Ω (d) Zero

28. A dc source of emf $E_1 = 100$ V and internal resistance $r = 0.5$ Ω, a storage battery of emf $E_2 = 90$ V and an external resistance R are connected as shown in figure. For what value of R no current will pass through the battery ? **[Online April 22, 2013]**

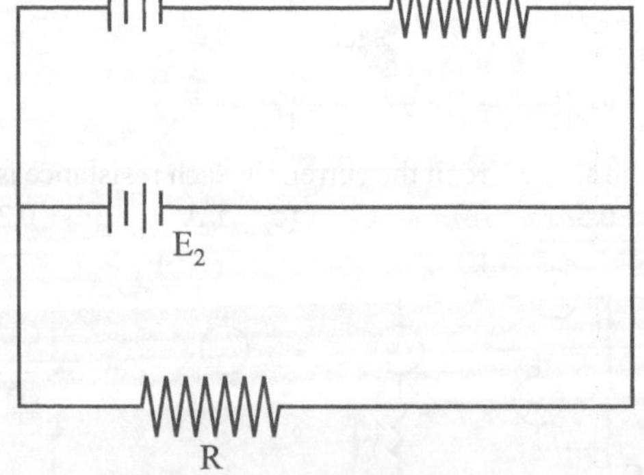

(a) 5.5 Ω (b) 3.5 Ω (c) 4.5 Ω (d) 2.5 Ω

29. A 5V battery with internal resistance 2Ω and a 2V battery with internal resistance 1Ω are connected to a 10Ω resistor as shown in the figure. **[2008]**

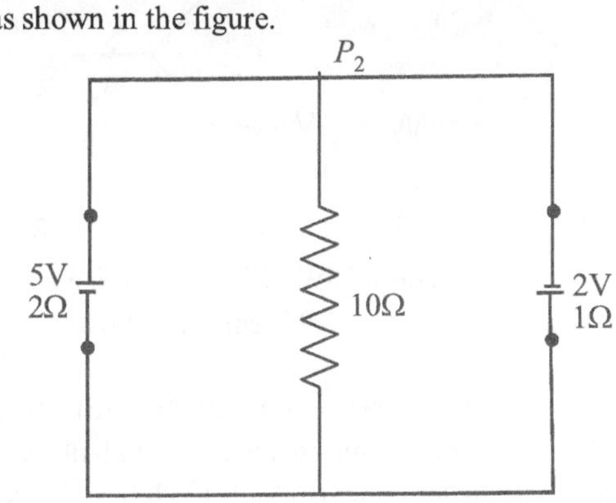

The current in the 10Ω resistor is

(a) 0.27 A P_2 to P_1 (b) 0.03 A P_1 to P_2
(c) 0.03 A P_2 to P_1 (d) 0.27 A P_1 to P_2

30. A battery is used to charge a parallel plate capacitor till the potential difference between the plates becomes equal to the electromotive force of the battery. The ratio of the energy stored in the capacitor and the work done by the battery will be **[2007]**

(a) 1/2 (b) 1 (c) 2 (d) 1/4

31. The Kirchhoff's first law ($\Sigma i = 0$) and second law ($\Sigma iR = \Sigma E$), where the symbols have their usual meanings, are respectively based on **[2006]**

(a) conservation of charge, conservation of momentum
(b) conservation of energy, conservation of charge
(c) conservation of momentum, conservation of charge
(d) conservation of charge, conservatrion of energy

32. A thermocouple is made from two metals, Antimony and Bismuth. If one junction of the couple is kept hot and the other is kept cold, then, an electric current will **[2006]**

(a) flow from Antimony to Bismuth at the hot junction
(b) flow from Bismuth to Antimony at the cold junction
(c) now flow through the thermocouple
(d) flow from Antimony to Bismuth at the cold junction

33. Two sources of equal emf are connected to an external resistance R. The internal resistance of the two sources are R_1 and R_2 ($R_1 > R_1$). If the potential difference across the source having internal resistance R_2 is zero, then **[2005]**

(a) $R = R_2 - R_1$
(b) $R = R_2 \times (R_1 + R_2)/(R_2 - R_1)$
(c) $R = R_1 R_2 /(R_2 - R_1)$
(d) $R = R_1 R_2 /(R_1 - R_2)$

34. Two voltameters, one of copper and another of silver, are joined in parallel. When a total charge q flows through the voltameters, equal amount of metals are deposited. If the electrochemical equivalents of copper and silver are Z_1 and Z_2 respectively the charge which flows through the silver voltameter is **[2005]**

(a) $\dfrac{q}{1+\dfrac{Z_2}{Z_1}}$ `(b) $\dfrac{q}{1+\dfrac{Z_1}{Z_2}}$ (c) $q\dfrac{Z_2}{Z_1}$ (d) $q\dfrac{Z_1}{Z_2}$

35. An energy source will supply a constant current into the load if its internal resistance is **[2005]**

(a) very large as compared to the load resistance
(b) equal to the resistance of the load
(c) non-zero but less than the resistance of the load
(d) zero

36. The thermo emf of a thermocouple varies with the temperature θ of the hot junction as $E = a\theta + b\theta^2$ in volts where the ratio a/b is 700°C. If the cold junction is kept at 0°C, then the neutral temperature is **[2004]**

(a) 1400°C
(b) 350°C
(c) 700°C
(d) No neutral temperature is possible for this termocouple.

37. The electrochemical equivalent of a metal is 3.35×10^{-7} kg per Coulomb. The mass of the metal liberated at the cathode when a 3A current is passed for 2 seconds will be **[2004]**

(a) 6.6×10^{57}kg (b) 9.9×10^{-7} kg
(c) 19.8×10^{-7} kg (d) 1.1×10^{-7} kg

38. The thermo e.m.f. of a thermo-couple is 25 μV/°C at room temperature. A galvanometer of 40 ohm resistance, capable of detecting current as low as 10^{-5} A, is connected with the thermo couple. The smallest temperature difference that can be detected by this system is **[2003]**

(a) 16°C (b) 12°C (c) 8°C (d) 20°C

39. The negative Zn pole of a Daniell cell, sending a constant current through a circuit, decreases in mass by 0.13g in 30 minutes. If the electeochemical equivalent of Zn and Cu are 32.5 and 31.5 respectively, the increase in the mass of the positive Cu pole in this time is **[2003]**

(a) 0.180 g (b) 0.141g (c) 0.126 g (d) 0.242 g

40. The mass of product liberated on anode in an electrochemical cell depends on **[2002]**

(a) $(It)^{1/2}$ (b) It (c) I/t (d) I^2t

(where t is the time period for which the current is passed).

TOPIC - 4: Heating Effect of Current

41. The figure shows three circuits I, II and III which are connected to a 3V battery. If the powers dissipated by the configurations I, II and III are P_1, P_2 and P_3 respectively, then : **[Online April 9, 2017]**

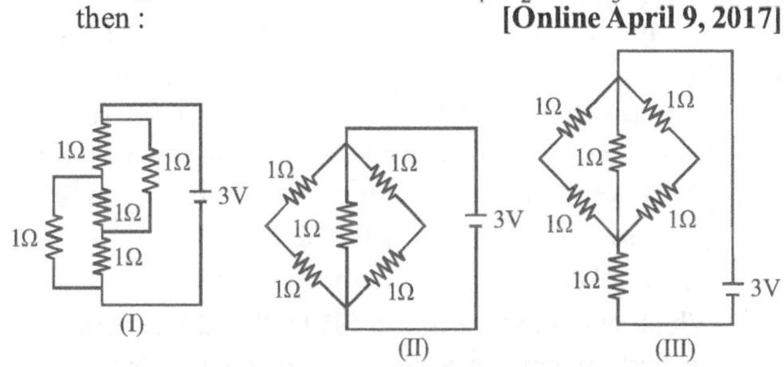

(a) $P_1 > P_2 > P_3$ (b) $P_1 > P_3 > P_2$
(c) $P_2 > P_1 > P_3$ (d) $P_3 > P_2 > P_1$

42. The resistance of an electrical toaster has a temperature dependence given by $R(T) = R_0[1 + \alpha(T - T_0)]$ in its range of operation. At $T_0 = 300K$, $R = 100\ \Omega$ and at $T = 500$ K, $R = 120\ \Omega$. The toaster is connected to a voltage source at 200 V and its temperature is raised at a constant rate from 300 to 500 K in 30 s. The total work done in raising the temperature is : **[Online April 10, 2016]**

(a) $400 \ln\frac{5}{6}$ J (b) $200 \ln\frac{2}{3}$ J

(c) 300 J (d) $400 \ln\frac{1.5}{1.3}$ J

43.

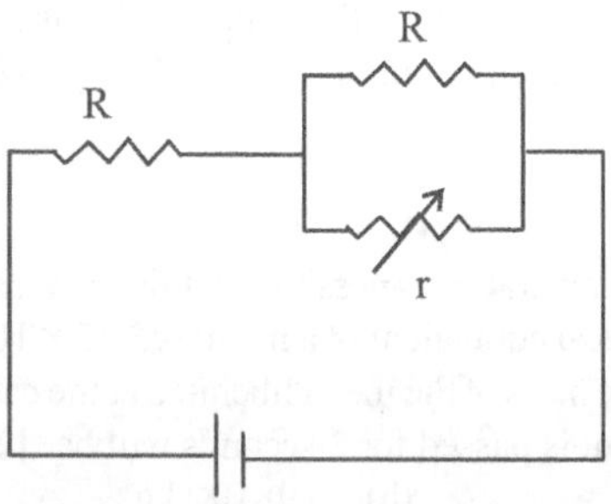

In the circuit shown, the resistance r is a variable resistance. If for r = fR, the heat generation in r is maximum then the value of f is : **[Online April 9, 2016]**

(a) $\frac{1}{2}$ (b) 1

(c) $\frac{1}{4}$ (d) $\frac{3}{4}$

44. In a large building, there are 15 bulbs of 40 W, 5 bulbs of 100 W, 5 fans of 80 W and 1 heater of 1 kW. The voltage of electric mains is 220 V. The minimum capacity of the main fuse of the building will be: **[2014]**

(a) 8 A (b) 10 A (c) 12 A (d) 14 A

45. Four bulbs B_1, B_2, B_3 and B_4 of 100 W each are connected to 220 V main as shown in the figure. **[Online April 19, 2014]**

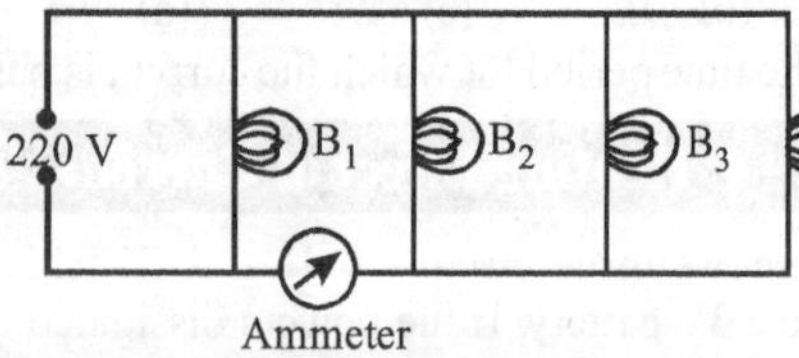

The reading in an ideal ammeter will be:

(a) 0.45 A (b) 0.90 A (c) 1.35 A (d) 1.80 A

46. The supply voltage to room is 120V. The resistance of the lead wires is 6Ω. A 60 W bulb is already switched on. What is the decrease of voltage across the bulb, when a 240 W heater is switched on in parallel to the bulb? **[2013]**

(a) zero (b) 2.9 Volt

(c) 13.3 Volt (d) 10.04 Volt

47. Which of the four resistances P, Q, R and S generate the greatest amount of heat when a current flows from A to B ? **[Online April 23, 2013]**

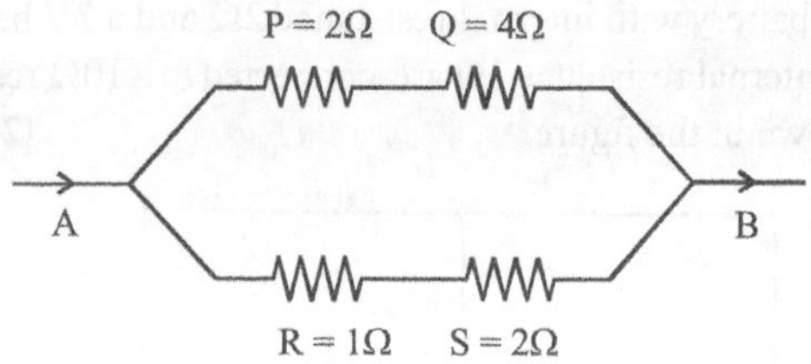

(a) Q (b) S (c) P (d) R

48. Two electric bulbs rated 25W – 220 V and 100W – 220V are connected in series to a 440 V supply. Which of the bulbs will fuse? **[2012]**

(a) Both (b) 100 W (c) 25 W (d) Neither

49. A 6.0 volt battery is connected to two light bulbs as shown in figure. Light bulb 1 has resistance 3 ohm while light bulb 2 has resistance 6 ohm. Battery has negligible internal resistance. Which bulb will glow brighter? **[Online May 19, 2012]**

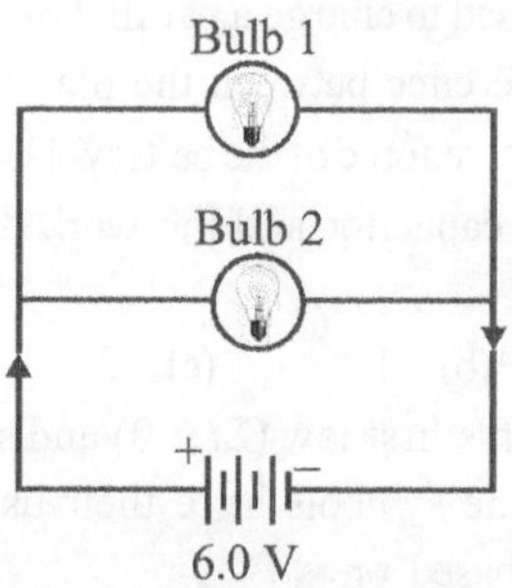

(a) Bulb 1 will glow more first and then its brightness will become less than bulb 2
(b) Bulb 1
(c) Bulb 2
(d) Both glow equally

50. Three resistors of 4 Ω, 6 Ω and 12 Ω are connected in parallel and the combination is connected in series with a 1.5 V battery of 1 Ω internal resistance. The rate of Joule heating in the 4 Ω resistor is **[Online May 12, 2012]**

(a) 0.55 W (b) 0.33 W (c) 0.25 W (d) 0.86 W

51. This question has Statement 1 and Statement 2. Of the four choices given after the Statements, choose the one that best describes the two Statements.

Statement 1: The possibility of an electric bulb fusing is higher at the time of switching ON.

Statement 2: Resistance of an electric bulb when it is not lit up is much smaller than when it is lit up. **[Online May 7, 2012]**

(a) Statement 1 is true, Statement 2 is false
(b) Statement 1 is false, Statement 2 is true, Statement 2 is not a correct explanation of Statement 1.
(c) Statement 1 is true, Statement 2 is true, Statement 2 is a correct explanation of Statement 1.
(d) Statement 1 is false, Statement 2 is true.

52. The resistance of a bulb filmanet is 100Ω at a temperature of 100°C. If its temperature coefficient of resistance be 0.005 per °C, its resistance will become 200 Ω at a temperature of **[2006]**
(a) 300°C (b) 400°C
(c) 500°C (d) 200°C

53. An electric bulb is rated 220 volt - 100 watt. The power consumed by it when operated on 110 volt will be **[2006]**
(a) 75 watt (b) 40 watt (c) 25 watt (d) 50 watt

54. A heater coil is cut into two equal parts and only one part is now used in the heater. The heat generated will now be **[2005]**
(a) four times (b) doubled
(c) halved (d) one fourth

55. The resistance of hot tungsten filament is about 10 times the cold resistance. What will be the resistance of 100 W and 200 V lamp when not in use ? **[2005]**
(a) 20Ω (b) 40Ω (c) 200Ω (d) 400Ω

56. The thermistors are usually made of **[2004]**
(a) metal oxides with high temperature coefficient of resistivity
(b) metals with high temperature coefficient of resistivity
(c) metals with low temperature coefficient of resistivity
(d) semiconducting materials having low temperature coefficient of resistivity

57. Time taken by a 836 W heater to heat one litre of water from 10°C to 40°C is **[2004]**
(a) 150 s (b) 100 s (c) 50 s (d) 200 s

58. A 220 volt, 1000 watt bulb is connected across a 110 volt mains supply. The power consumed will be **[2003]**
(a) 750 watt (b) 500 watt
(c) 250 watt (d) 1000 watt

59. A wire when connected to 220 V mains supply has power dissipation P_1. Now the wire is cut into two equal pieces which are connected in parallel to the same supply. Power dissipation in this case is P_2. Then $P_2 : P_1$ is **[2002]**
(a) 1 (b) 4 (c) 2 (d) 3

60. If in the circuit, power dissipation is 150 W, then R is **[2002]**

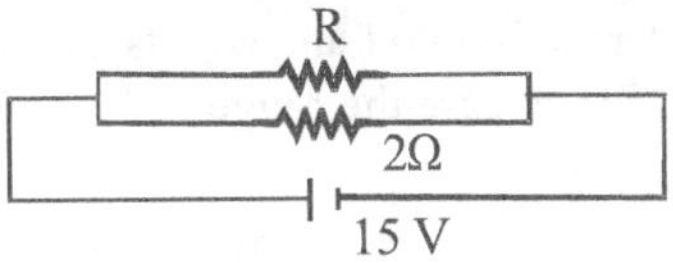

(a) 2Ω (b) 6Ω (c) 5Ω (d) 4Ω

TOPIC - 5: Wheatstone Bridge and Different Measuring Instruments.

61. Which of the following statements is false ? **[2017]**
(a) A rheostat can be used as a potential divider
(b) Kirchhoff's second law represents energy conservation
(c) Wheatstone bridge is the most sensitive when all the four resistances are of the same order of magnitude
(d) In a balanced wheatstone bridge if the cell and the galvanometer are exchanged, the null point is disturbed.

62. In a meter bridge experiment resistances are connected as shown in the figure. Initially resistance P = 4 Ω and the neutral point N is at 60 cm from A. Now an unknown resistance R is connected in series to P and the new position of the neutral point is at 80 cm from A. The value of unknown resistance R is : **[Online April 9, 2017]**

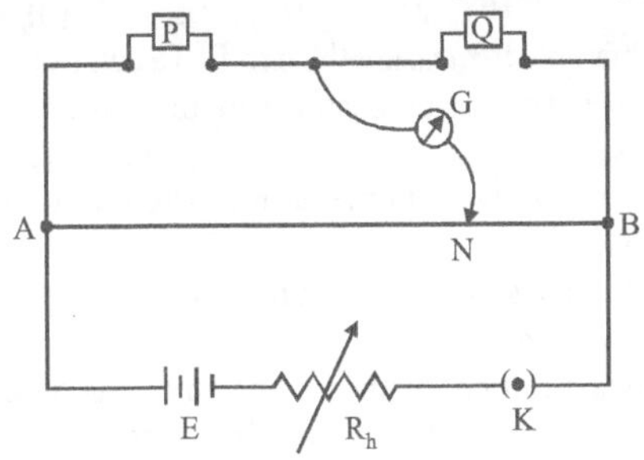

(a) $\frac{33}{5}\Omega$ (b) 6 Ω (c) 7 Ω (d) $\frac{20}{3}\Omega$

63. A potentiometer PQ is set up to compare two resistances as shown in the figure. The ammeter A in the circuit reads 1.0 A when two way key K_3 is open. The balance point is at a length l_1 cm from P when two way key K_3 is plugged in between 2 and 1, while the balance point is at a length l_2 cm from P when key K_3 is plugged in between 3 and 1. The ratio of two resistances $\frac{R_1}{R_2}$, is found to be : **[Online April 8, 2017]**

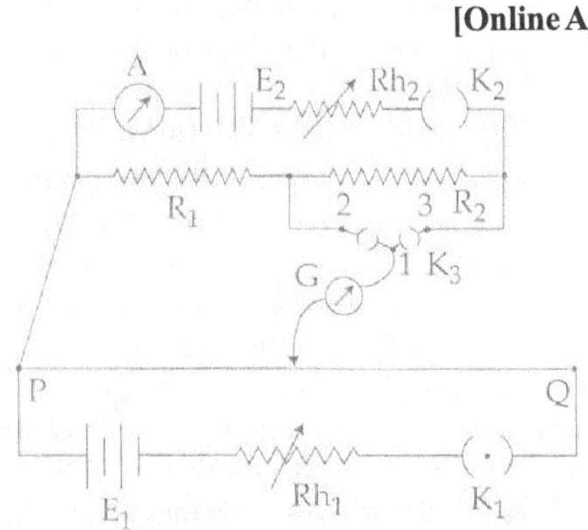

(a) $\frac{l_1}{l_1+l_2}$ (b) $\frac{l_2}{l_2-l_1}$ (c) $\frac{l_1}{l_1-l_2}$ (d) $\frac{l_1}{l_2-l_1}$

64. A 10V battery with internal resistance 1Ω and a 15V battery with internal resistance 0.6 Ω are connected in parallel to a voltmeter (see figure). The reading in the voltmeter will be close to : **[Online April 10, 2015]**

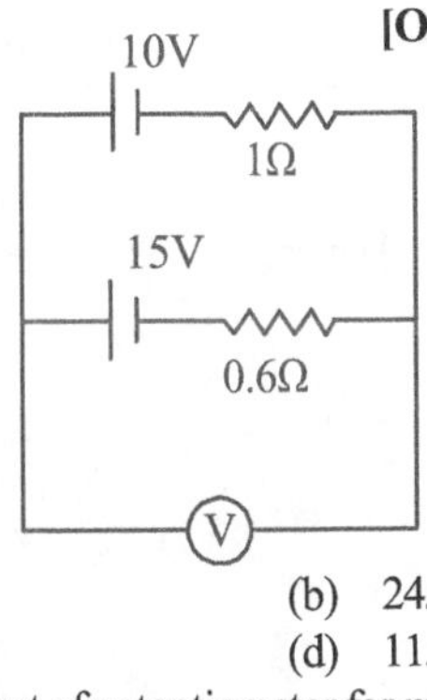

(a) 12.5 V (b) 24.5 V
(c) 13.1 V (d) 11.9 V

65. In an experiment of potentiometer for measuring the internal

resistance of primary cell a balancing length ℓ is obtained on the potentiometer wire when the cell is open circuit. Now the cell is short circuited by a resistance R. If R is to be equal to the internal resistance of the cell the balancing length on the potentiometer wire will be **[Online May 26, 2012]**

(a) ℓ (b) 2ℓ (c) $\ell/2$ (d) $\ell/4$

66. It is preferable to measure the e.m.f. of a cell by potentiometer than by a voltmeter because of the following possible reasons. **[Online May 12, 2012]**

(i) In case of potentiometer, no current flows through the cell.
(ii) The length of the potentiometer allows greater precision.
(iii) Measurement by the potentiometer is quicker.
(iv) The sensitivity of the galvanometer, when using a potentiometer is not relevant.

Which of these reasons are correct?

(a) (i), (iii), (iv) (b) (i), (iii), (iv)
(c) (i), (ii) (d) (i), (ii), (iii), (iv)

67. In a sensitive meter bridge apparatus the bridge wire should possess **[Online May 12, 2012]**

(a) high resistivity and low temperature coefficient.
(b) low resistivity and high temperature coefficient.
(c) low resistivity and low temperature coefficient.
(d) high resistivity and high temperature coefficient.

68. In a metre bridge experiment null point is obtained at 40 cm from one end of the wire when resistance X is balanced against another resistance Y. If X < Y, then the new position of the null point from the same end, if one decides to balance a resistance of 3X against Y, will be close to : **[Online April 9, 2013]**

(a) 80 cm (b) 75 cm (c) 67 cm (d) 50 cm

69. The current in the primary circuit of a potentiometer is 0.2 A. The specific resistance and cross-section of the potentiometer wire are 4×10^{-7} ohm metre and 8×10^{-7} m^2, respectively. The potential gradient will be equal to **[2011 RS]**

(a) 1 V/m (b) 0.5 V/m (c) 0.1 V/m (d) 0.2 V/m

70. Shown in the figure below is a meter-bridge set up with null deflection in the galvanometer.

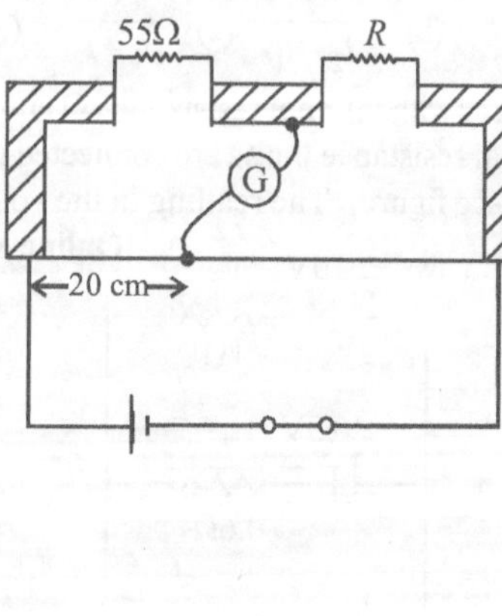

The value of the unknown resistor R is **[2008]**

(a) 13.75 Ω (b) 220 Ω (c) 110 Ω (d) 55 Ω

71. In a Wheatstone's bridge, three resistances P, Q and R connected in the three arms and the fourth arm is formed by two resistances S_1 and S_2 connected in parallel. The condition for the bridge to be balanced will be **[2006]**

(a) $\frac{P}{Q} = \frac{2R}{S_1 + S_2}$ (b) $\frac{P}{Q} = \frac{R(S_1 + S_2)}{S_1 S_2}$

(c) $\frac{P}{Q} = \frac{R(S_1 + S_2)}{2S_1 S_2}$ (d) $\frac{P}{Q} = \frac{R}{S_1 + S_2}$

72. In a potentiometer experiment the balancing with a cell is at length 240 cm. On shunting the cell with a resistance of 2Ω, the balancing length becomes 120 cm. The internal resistance of the cell is **[2005]**

(a) 0.5Ω (b) 1Ω
(c) 2Ω (d) 4Ω

73. In a meter bridge experiment null point is obtained at 20 cm. from one end of the wire when resistance X is balanced against another resistance Y. If $X < Y$, then where will be the new position of the null point from the same end, if one decides to balance a resistance of 4 X against Y **[2004]**

(a) 40 cm (b) 80 cm
(c) 50 cm (d) 70 cm

74. The length of a wire of a potentiometer is 100 cm, and the e. m.f. of its standard cell is E volt. It is employed to measure the e.m.f. of a battery whose internal resistance is 0.5Ω. If the balance point is obtained at $\ell = 30$ cm from the positive end, the e.m.f. of the battery is **[2003]**

(a) $\frac{30E}{100.5}$ (b) $\frac{30E}{(100 - 0.5)}$

(c) $\frac{30(E - 0.5i)}{100}$ (d) $\frac{30E}{100}$

where i is the current in the potentiometer wire.

75. An ammeter reads upto 1 ampere. Its internal resistance is 0.81ohm. To increase the range to 10 A the value of the required shunt is **[2003]**

(a) 0.03 Ω (b) 0.3 Ω
(c) 0.9 Ω (d) 0.09 Ω

76. If an ammeter is to be used in place of a voltmeter, then we must connect with the ammeter a **[2002]**

(a) low resistance in parallel
(b) high resistance in parallel
(c) high resistance in series
(d) low resistance in series.

Hints & Solutions

TOPIC - 1: Electric Current, Drift of Electrons, Ohm's Law, Resistance and Resistivity

1. **(a)** Given, $R_1 = 100\,\Omega$, $r' = r/2$, $R_2 = ?$

Resistivity of wire, $R = \frac{\rho l}{A}$ $\because$ Area × length = volume

Hence, $R = \frac{\rho V}{A^2}$

Since, $\rho \to$ constant, $V \to$ constant

$R \propto \frac{1}{A^2}$

or $R \propto \frac{1}{r^4}$ $\because A = \pi r^2$

$\frac{R_2}{R_1} = 16 \Rightarrow R_2 = 16 \times 100 = 1600\,\Omega$, Resistance of new wire.

2. **(b)** $V = IR = (neAv_d)\rho\frac{\ell}{A}$

$\therefore \quad \rho = \frac{V}{V_d l n e}$

Here V = potential difference

l = length of wire

n = no. of electrons per unit volume of conductor.

e = no. of electrons

Placing the value of above parameters we get resistivity

$$\rho = \frac{5}{8\times10^{28}\times1.6\times10^{-19}\times2.5\times10^{-4}\times0.1}$$

$= 1.6 \times 10^{-5}\,\Omega\text{m}$

3. **(c)** $i = neAV_d$ and $V_d \propto \sqrt{E}$ (Given)

or, $i \propto \sqrt{E}$

$i^2 \propto E$

$i^2 \propto V$

Hence graph (c) correctly dipicts the *V-I* graph for a wire made of such type of material.

4. **(a)** In ohm's law, we check V = IR where I is the correent flowing through a resistor and V is the potential difference across that resistor. Only option (a) fits the above criteria. Remember that ammeter is connected in series with resistance and voltmeter parallel with the resistance.

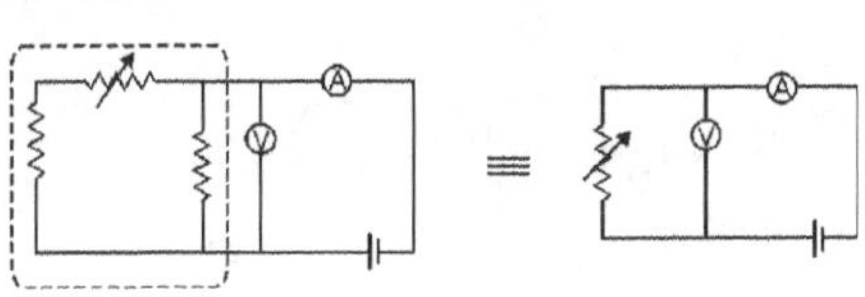

5. **(c)** Resistance of wire $(R) = \rho\frac{l}{A}$

If wire is bent in the middle then

$l' = \frac{l}{2}, A' = 2A$

$\therefore$ New resistance, $R' = \rho\frac{l'}{A'}$

$$= \frac{\rho\frac{l}{2}}{2A} = \frac{\rho l}{4A} = \frac{R}{4}.$$

6. **(a)** Resistance of wire

$R = \frac{\rho l}{A} = \frac{\rho l^2}{C}$ (where $Al = C$)

$\therefore$ Fractional change in resistance

$$\frac{\Delta R}{R} = 2\frac{\Delta l}{l}$$

$\therefore$ Resistance will increase by 0.2%

7. **(a)** Let j be the current density.

Then $j \times 2\pi r^2 = I \Rightarrow j = \frac{I}{2\pi r^2}$

$\therefore \quad E = \rho j = \frac{\rho I}{2\pi r^2}$

Now, $\Delta V'_{BC} = -\int_{a+b}^{a} \vec{E}.\vec{dr} = -\int_{a+b}^{a} \frac{\rho I}{2\pi r^2}dr$

$$= -\frac{\rho I}{2\pi}\left[-\frac{1}{r}\right]_{a+b}^{a} = \frac{\rho I}{2\pi a} - \frac{\rho I}{2\pi\,(a+b)}$$

On applying superposition as mentioned we get

$$\Delta V_{BC} = 2\times\Delta V'_{BC} = \frac{\rho I}{\pi a} - \frac{\rho I}{\pi(a+b)}$$

8. **(c)** As shown in Answer 7 (a) $E = \frac{\rho I}{2\pi r^2}$

9. **(d)** We know that

$R_t = R_0(1 + \alpha t)$,

where R_t is the resistance of the wire at t °C,

R_0 is the resistance of the wire at 0°C

and α is the temperature coefficient of resistance.

$\Rightarrow R_{50} = R_0(1 + 50\,\alpha)$ ... (i)

$R_{100} = R_0(1 + 100\,\alpha)$ ... (ii)

From (i), $R_{50} - R_0 = 50\,\alpha R_0$ ... (iii)

From (ii), $R_{100} - R_0 = 100\,\alpha R_0$ ... (iv)

Dividing (iii) by (iv), we get

$$\frac{R_{50}-R_0}{R_{100}-R_0}=\frac{1}{2}$$

Here, $R_{50}=5\Omega$ and $R_{100}=6\Omega$

$$\therefore \frac{5-R_0}{6-R_0}=\frac{1}{2}$$

or, $6-R_0=10-2R_0$ or, $R_0=4\Omega$.

10. (d) $\rho_B=2\rho_A$

$d_B=2d_A$

$$R_B=R_A \Rightarrow \frac{\rho_B\ell_B}{A_B}=\frac{\rho_A\ell_A}{A_A}$$

$$\therefore \frac{\ell_B}{\ell_A}=\frac{\rho_A}{\rho_B}\times\frac{d_B^2}{d_A^2}=\frac{\rho_A}{2\rho_A}\times\frac{4d_A^2}{d_A^2}=2$$

11. (b)

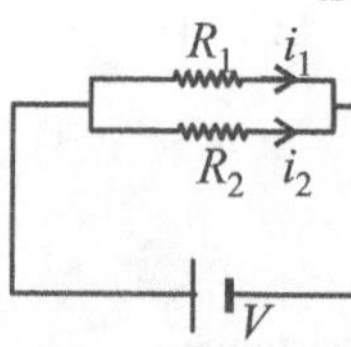

$$R_1=\frac{\rho\ell_1}{\pi r_1^2};\ R_2=\frac{\rho\ell_2}{\pi r_2^2}$$

$i_1R_1=i_2R_2$ (same potential difference)

$$\therefore \frac{i_1}{i_2}=\frac{R_2}{R_1}=\frac{\ell_2}{\ell_1}\times\frac{r_1^2}{r_2^2}=\frac{3}{4}\times\frac{4}{9}=\frac{1}{3}$$

12. (d) The total volume remains the same before and after stretching.

Therefore $A\times\ell=A'\times\ell'$

Here $\ell'=2\ell$

$$\therefore A'=\frac{A\times\ell}{\ell'}=\frac{A\times\ell}{2\ell}=\frac{A}{2}$$

Percentage change in resistance

$$=\frac{R_f-R_i}{R_i}\times100=\frac{\rho\left(\frac{\ell'}{A'}-\frac{\ell}{A}\right)}{\rho\frac{\ell}{A}}\times100$$

$$=\left[\left(\frac{\ell'}{A'}\times\frac{A}{\ell}\right)-1\right]\times100=\left[\left(\frac{2\ell}{A/2}\times\frac{A}{\ell}\right)-1\right]\times100$$

$=300\%$

TOPIC - 2: Combination of Resistances

13. (a) In steady state, flow fo current through capacitor will be zero.

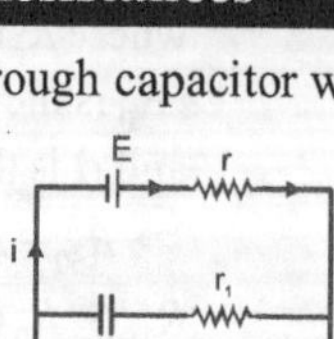

Current through the circuit,

$$i=\frac{E}{r+r_2}$$

Potential difference through capacitor

$$V_c=\frac{Q}{C}=E-ir=E-\left(\frac{E}{r+r_2}\right)r$$

$$\therefore Q=CE\frac{r_2}{r+r_2}$$

14. (b) The potential difference in each loop is zero.

$\therefore$ No current will flow or current in each resistance is Zero.

15. (a) The given circuit can be redrawn as,

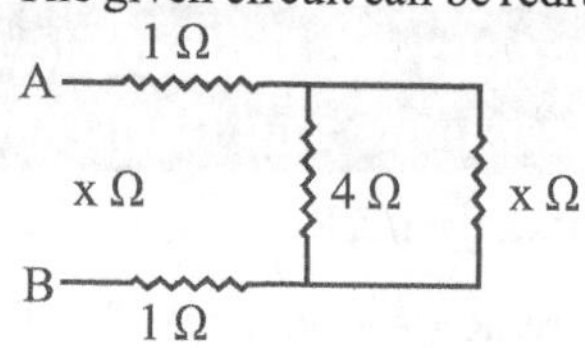

as 4 Ω and x Ω are parallel $x'=\frac{1}{4}+\frac{1}{x}=\frac{(4+x)}{4x}$

$$x'=\frac{4x}{4+x}$$

& 1 Ω and 1 Ω are also parallel x" = 2 Ω

Now equivalent resistance of circuit

$$x=\frac{4x}{4+x}+2=\frac{8+6x}{4+x}$$

$4x+x^2=8+6x$

$x^2-2x-8=0$

$$x=\frac{2\pm\sqrt{4-4(1)(-8)}}{2}=\frac{2\pm\sqrt{36}}{2}=\frac{2\pm6}{2}=4\Omega$$

Reading of Ammeter $A_1=\frac{V}{(R+r)}$

$$A_1=\frac{9}{4+0.5}=2\text{ Ampere}$$

16. (b) Resistance between P and Q

$$r_{PQ}=r\,||\left(\frac{r}{3}+\frac{r}{2}\right)=\frac{r\times\frac{5}{6}r}{r+\frac{5}{6}r}=\frac{5}{11}r$$

Resistance between Q and R

$$r_{QR}=\frac{r}{2}\,||\,(r+\frac{r}{3})=\frac{\frac{r}{2}\times\frac{4}{3}r}{\frac{r}{2}+\frac{4}{3}r}=\frac{4}{11}r$$

Resistance between P and R

$$r_{PR}=\frac{r}{3}\,||\left(\frac{r}{2}+r\right)=\frac{\frac{r}{3}\times\frac{3}{2}r}{\frac{r}{3}+\frac{3}{2}r}=\frac{3}{11}r$$

Hence, it is clear that r_{PQ} is maximum

17. (d)

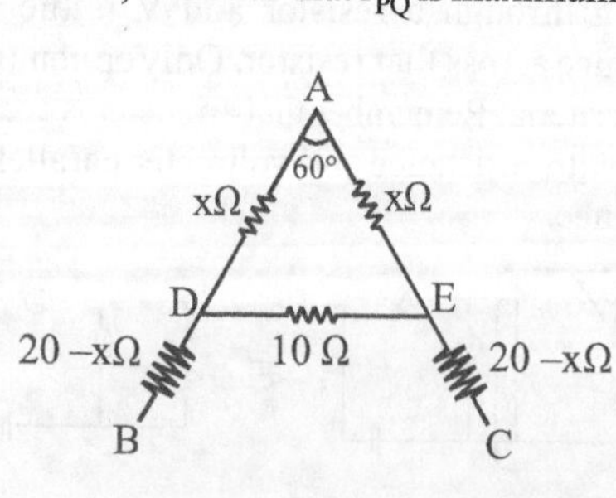

For ADE $\frac{1}{R'} = \frac{1}{2x} + \frac{1}{10}$

or $R' = \frac{20x}{10 + 2x}$

$R_{BC} = \frac{20x}{10 + 2x} + 20 - x + 20 - x$ ...(i)

or $\frac{20x}{10 + 2x} + 40 = 2x$

Solving we get

$x = 10\,\Omega$

Putting the value of $x = 10\,\Omega$ in equation (i)

We get

$R_{BC} = \frac{20 \times 10}{10 + 2 \times 10} + 20 - 10 + 20 - 10$

$= \frac{80}{3} = 26.7\,\Omega$

18. (d) $R_1 = R_0[1 + \alpha_1 \Delta t]$; $R_2 = R_0[1 + \alpha_2 \Delta t]$

In Series, $R = R_1 + R_2$

$= R_0[2 + (\alpha_1 + \alpha_2)\Delta t]$

$= 2R_0\left[1 + \left(\frac{\alpha_1 + \alpha_2}{2}\right)\Delta t\right]$

$\therefore \alpha_{eq} = \frac{\alpha_1 + \alpha_2}{2}$

In Parallel, $\frac{1}{R} = \frac{1}{R_1} + \frac{1}{R_2}$

$= \frac{1}{R_0[1 + \alpha_1 \Delta t]} + \frac{1}{R_0[1 + \alpha_2 \Delta t]}$

$= \alpha_{eq} = \frac{\alpha_1 + \alpha_2}{2}$

19. (b) The network of resistors is a balanced wheatstone bridge. The equivalent circuit is

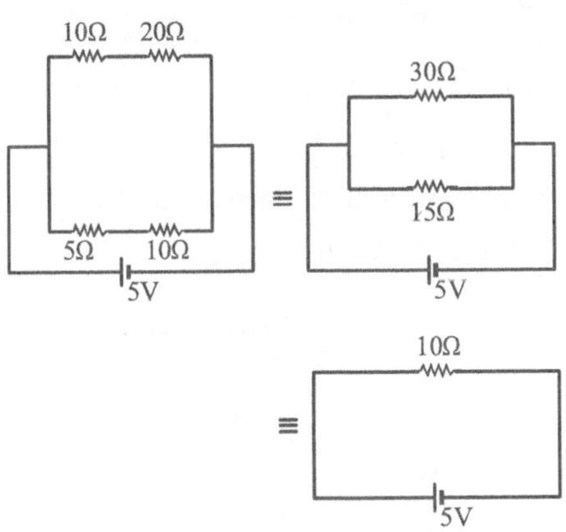

$R_{eq} = \frac{15 \times 30}{15 + 30} = 10\,\Omega$

$\Rightarrow I = \frac{V}{R} = \frac{5}{10} = 0.5$ A

20. (a)

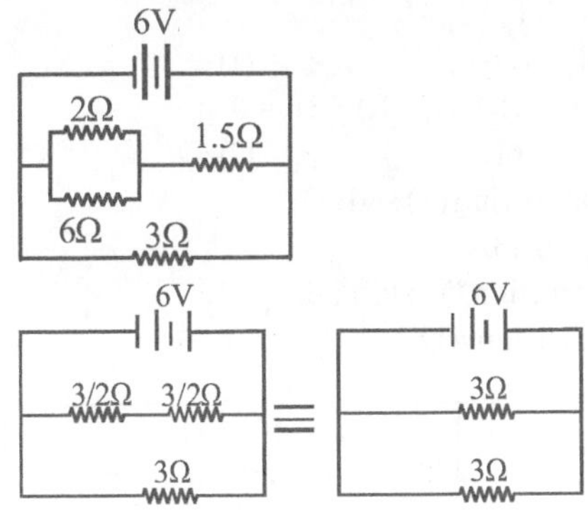

hence $R_{eq} = 3/2$; $\therefore I = \frac{6}{3/2} = 4$A

21. (c)

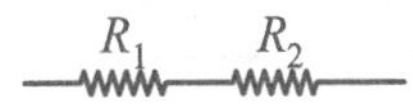

Resistance of the series combination,

$S = R_1 + R_2$

Resistance of the parallel combination,

$P = \frac{R_1 R_2}{R_1 + R_2}$

$S = nP \Rightarrow R_1 + R_2 = \frac{n(R_1 R_2)}{(R_1 + R_2)}$

$\Rightarrow (R_1 + R_2)^2 = nR_1R_2$

Minimum value of n is 4 for that

$(R_1 + R_2)^2 = 4R_1R_2 \Rightarrow (R_1 - R_2)^2 = 0$

22. (b) $R_p = \frac{3 \times 6}{3 + 6} = \frac{18}{9} = 2\Omega$

$\therefore V = IR \Rightarrow I = \frac{V}{R} = \frac{3}{2} = 1.5A$

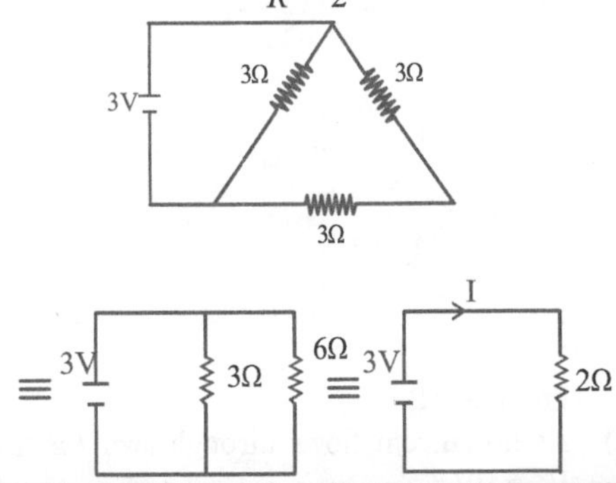

TOPIC - 3: Kirchoff's Laws, Cells, Thermo e.m.f. Electrolysis

23. (a) From KVL

$-6 + 3I_1 + 1(I_i - I_2) = 0$

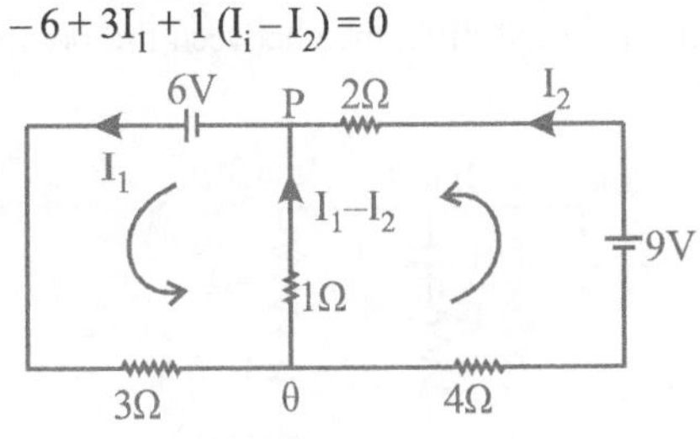

$6 = 3I_1 + I_1 - I_2$

$4I_1 - I_2 = 6$ ...(1)

$-9 + 2I_2 - (I_1 - I_2) + 3I_2 = 0$

$-I_1 + 6I_2 = 9$ ...(2)

On solving (1) and (2)

$I_1 = 0.13A$

Direction Q to P, since $I_1 > I_2$.

Alternatively

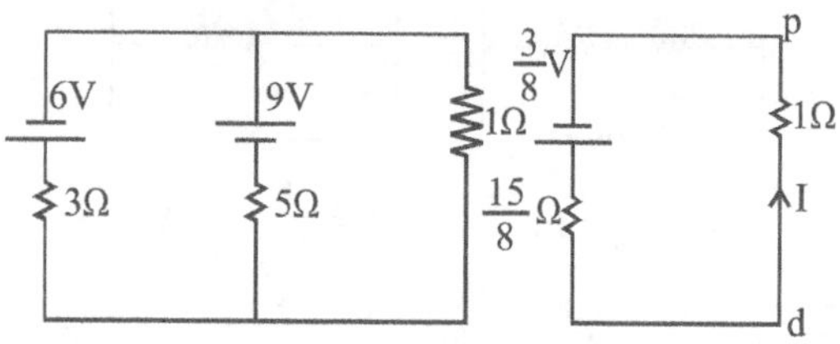

$$Eq = \frac{\frac{E_1}{r_1} + \frac{E_2}{r_2}}{\frac{1}{r_1} + \frac{1}{r_2}} = \frac{\frac{6}{3} - \frac{9}{5}}{\frac{1}{3} + \frac{1}{5}} = \frac{3}{8V}$$

$$\therefore \quad I = \frac{\frac{3}{8}}{\frac{15}{8} + 1} = \frac{3}{23} = 0.13A$$

Considering potential at P as 0V and at Q as x volt, then

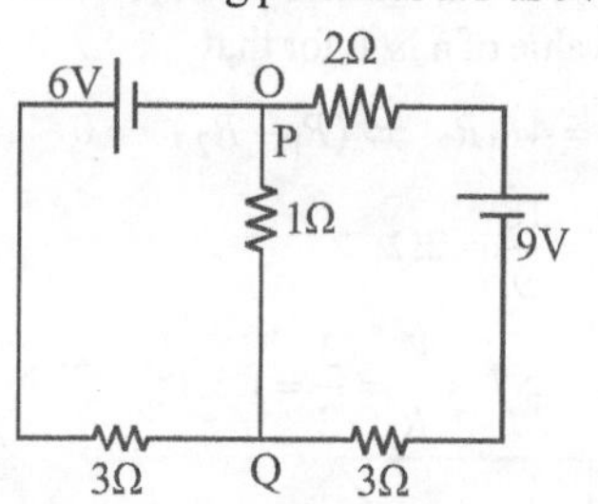

$$\frac{x-6}{3} + \frac{x-0}{1} + \frac{x+9}{5} = 0$$

$$\therefore \quad x = \frac{2}{23}$$

$$\therefore \quad i = \frac{x-0}{1} = \frac{2}{23} = 0.13A$$

From Q to P

24. **(c)** As no current flows through arm *EB* then

$V_D = 0V$

$V_E = 0V$

$V_B = -4V$

$V_A = 5V$

So, potential difference between the points *A* and *D*

$V_A - V_D = 5V$

25. **(b)**

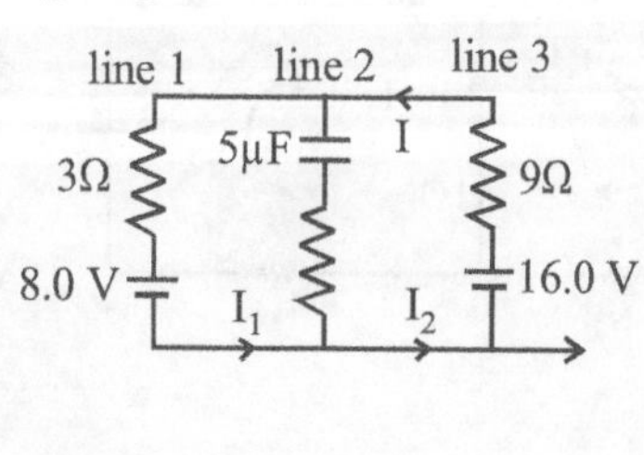

In steady state capacitor is fully charged hence no current will flow through line 2.

By simplyfing the circuit

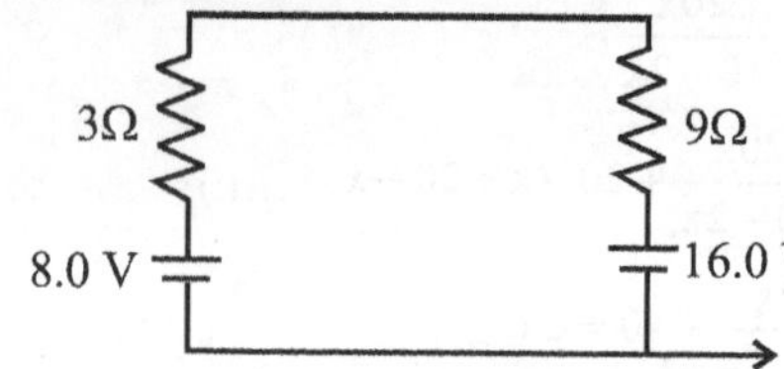

Hence resultant potential difference across resistances will be 8.0 V.

Thus current $I = \frac{V}{R}$

$$= \frac{8.0}{3+9} = \frac{8}{12}$$

or, $\quad I = \frac{2}{3} = 0.67\,A$

26. **(a)** Current through 50 V and 30 V batteries are respectively 2.5 A and 3 A.

27. **(c)** Given, emf of cell E = 200 V

Internal resistance of cells = 1 Ω

D. C. main supply voltage V = 220 V

External resistance R = ?

$$r = \left(\frac{E-V}{V}\right)R$$

$$1 = \left(\frac{20}{220}\right) \times R$$

$\therefore \quad R = 11\,\Omega.$

28. **(c)** $\frac{100}{R+r} = \frac{90}{R}$

$$\Rightarrow \quad \frac{R+r}{R} = \frac{10}{9}$$

$$\Rightarrow \quad 1 + \frac{0.5}{R} = \frac{10}{9}$$

$$\Rightarrow \quad \frac{0.5}{R} = \frac{1}{9}$$

$\therefore \; R = 4.5\,\Omega$

29. **(c)** Applying Kirchoff's loop law in ABP_2P_1A, we get

$-2i + 5 - 10\,i_1 = 0$ .....(i)

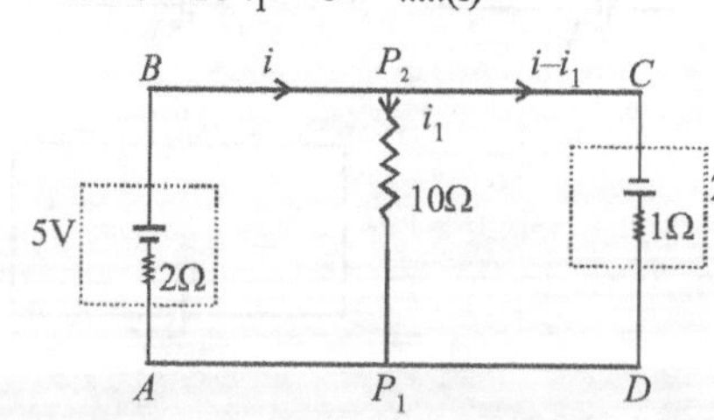

Again applying Kirchoff's loop law in $P_2CDP_1P_2$ we get, $10\,i_1 + 2 - i + i_1 = 0$ ....(ii)

From (i) and (ii) $11\,i_1 + 2 - \left[\frac{5 - 10i_1}{2}\right] = 0$

$\Rightarrow i_1 = \frac{1}{32}$ A from P_2 to P_1

30. (a) Required ratio

$$= \frac{\text{Energy stored in capacitor}}{\text{Workdone by the battery}} = \frac{\frac{1}{2}CV^2}{Ce^2}$$

where C = Capacitance of capacitor
V = Potential difference,
e = emf of battery

$$= \frac{\frac{1}{2}Ce^2}{Ce^2} = \frac{1}{2} \quad (\because V = e)$$

31. (d) **NOTE** Kirchhoff's first law is based on conservation of charge and Kirchhoff's second law is based on conservation of energy.

32. (d) At cold junction, current flows from Antimony to Bismuth (because current flows from metal occurring later in the series to metal occurring earlier in the thermoelectric series).

33. (a)

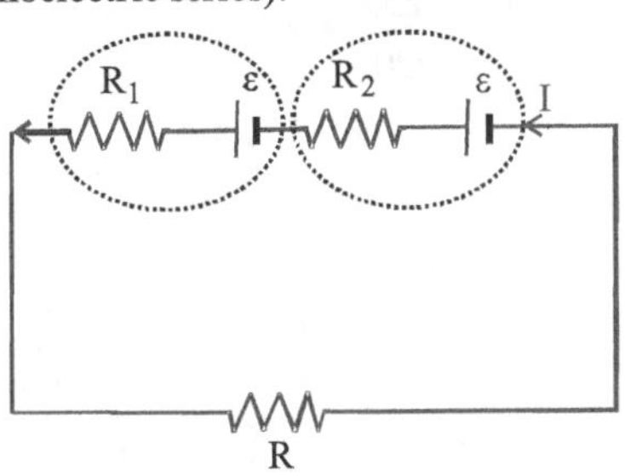

$$I = \frac{2\varepsilon}{R + R_1 + R_2}$$

Potential difference across second cell

$= V = \varepsilon - iR_2 = 0$

$$\varepsilon - \frac{2\varepsilon}{R + R_1 + R_2}.R_2 = 0$$

$R + R_1 + R_2 - 2R_2 = 0$

$R + R_1 - R_2 = 0$

$\therefore R = R_2 - R_1$

34. (a) Mass deposited

$m = Zq$

$$\Rightarrow Z \propto \frac{1}{q} \Rightarrow \frac{Z_1}{Z_2} = \frac{q_2}{q_1} \quad \text{....(i)}$$

Also $q = q_1 + q_2$ ....(ii)

$$\Rightarrow \frac{q}{q_2} = \frac{q_1}{q_2} + 1$$

(Dividing (ii) by q_2)

$$\Rightarrow q_2 = \frac{q}{1 + \frac{q_1}{q_2}} \quad \text{....(iii)}$$

From equation (i) and (iii),

$$q_2 = \frac{q}{1 + \frac{Z_2}{Z_1}}$$

35. (d) $I = \frac{E}{R + r}$, Internal resistance (r) is zero, $I = \frac{E}{R}$ = constant.

36. (d) Neutral temperature is the temperature of a hot junction at which E is maximum.

$$\Rightarrow \frac{dE}{d\theta} = 0 \text{ or } a + 2b\theta = 0 \Rightarrow \theta = \frac{-a}{2b} = -350$$

$$\Rightarrow \frac{d^2E}{d\theta^2} = 2b$$

hence no θ is possible for E to be maximum no neutral temperature is possible.

37. (c) The mass liberated m and electrochemical equivalent of a metal Z, are related as

$m = Zit$

$\Rightarrow m = 3.3 \times 10^{-7} \times 3 \times 2 = 19.8 \times 10^{-7}$ kg

38. (a) Let θ be the smallest temperature difference that can be detected by the thermocouple, then

$I \times R = (25 \times 10^{-6})\,\theta$

where I is the smallest current which can be detected by the galvanometer of resistance R.

Here $I = 10^{-5} A$, $R = 40\,\Omega$

$\therefore 10^{-5} \times 40 = 25 \times 10^{-6} \times \theta$

$\therefore \theta = 16°C$.

39. (c) According to Faraday's first law of electrolysis

$m = Z \times q$

For same q, $m \propto Z$

$$\therefore \frac{m_{Cu}}{m_{Zn}} = \frac{Z_{Cu}}{Z_{Zn}}$$

$$\Rightarrow m_{Cu} = \frac{Z_{Cu}}{Z_{Zn}} \times m_{Zn} = \frac{31.5}{32.5} \times 0.13 = 0.126 \text{ g}$$

40. (b) According to Faraday's first law of electrolysis

$m = ZIt \Rightarrow m \propto It$

TOPIC - 4: Heating Effect of Current

41. (c) From the given circuit, net resistances

$R_I = 1\,\Omega$, $R_{II} = 1/2\,\Omega$, $R_{III} = 3/2\,\Omega$

It is clear that $R_3 > R_1 > R_2$

Hence, $P_3 < P_1 < P_2$

As Power (P) $= \frac{V^2}{R} \Rightarrow P \propto \frac{1}{R}$

42. (None) Work done in 30s, $W = \int_0^{30} \frac{V^2}{R} dt$

$$\text{or,} \quad W = \int_0^{30} \frac{(200)^2}{100(1 + \alpha\frac{20t}{3})} dt = \frac{(200)^2}{100} \int_0^{30} \frac{dt}{1 + \frac{20\alpha}{3}t}$$

$$= \frac{400\times 3}{20\alpha}\,\ell n\left(\frac{\frac{1+20\alpha}{3}\times 30}{1}\right) = 60{,}000\,\ell n\left(\frac{6}{5}\right)$$

$$\because\ 120 = 100\left[1+\alpha(200)\right]$$

$$\therefore\ \alpha = \frac{1}{1000}$$

43. **(c)** Heat energy will be maximum when resistance will be minimum.

44. **(c)** Total power consumed by electrical appliances in the building, $P_{total} = 2500\text{W}$

Watt = Volt × ampere

$\Rightarrow\ 2500 = V\times I \Rightarrow 2500 = 220I$

$\Rightarrow\ I = \frac{2500}{220} = 11.36 \approx 12\text{A}$

(Minimum capacity of main fuse)

45. **(c)** Current in each bulb $= \frac{\text{Power}}{\text{Voltage}}$

$= \frac{100}{220} = 0.45\text{A}$

Current through ammeter = 0.45 × 3 = 1.35 A

46. **(d)**

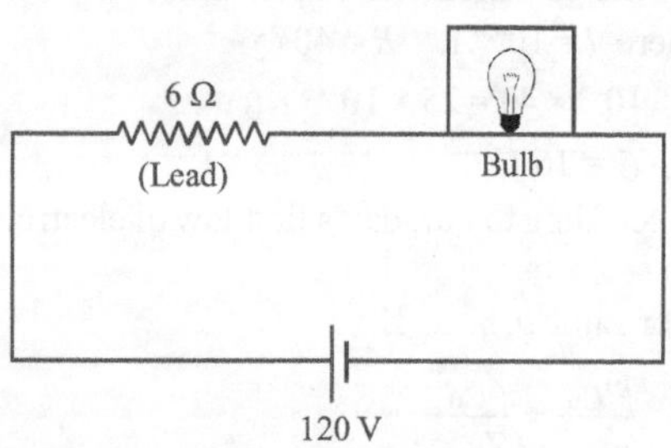

Power of bulb = 60 W (given)

Resistance of bulb $= \frac{120\times 120}{60} = 240\Omega$ $\left[\because P = \frac{V^2}{R}\right]$

Power of heater = 240W (given)

Resistance of heater $= \frac{120\times 120}{240} = 60\Omega$

Voltage across bulb before heater is switched on,

$V_1 = \frac{240}{246}\times 120 = 117.73$ volt

Voltage across bulb after heater is switched on,

$V_2 = \frac{48}{54}\times 120 = 106.66$ volt

Hence decrease in voltage

$V_1 - V_2 = 117.073 - 106.66 = 10.04$ Volt (approximately)

47. **(b)**

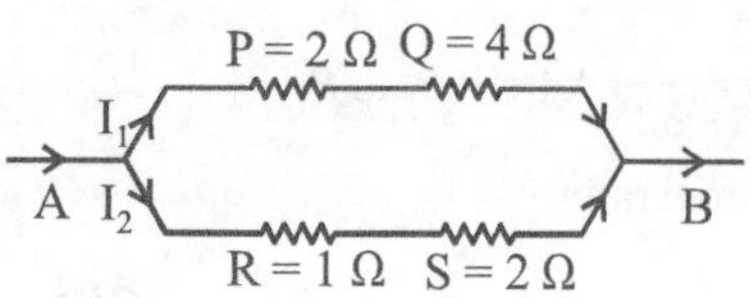

$R_1 = P + Q = 2\,\Omega + 4\,\Omega = 6\,\Omega$

$R_2 = R + S = 1\Omega + 2\,\Omega = 3\,\Omega$

$I_1R_1 = I_2R_2$

$I_1 = \frac{R_2}{R_1}I_2 = \frac{3}{6}I_2 = \frac{I_2}{2}$

or $I_2 = 2I_1$

Heat flow $H = I^2 Rt$

For Q, $H_Q = I_1^2\,Qt = \frac{I_2^2}{4}\times 4t = I_2^2 t$

For S, $H_S = I_2^2\,St = I_2^2\cdot 2t = 2I_2^2 t$

∴ Greatest amount of heat generated by S.

48. **(c)** The current upto which bulb rated 25W – 220V, will not fuse

$I_1 = \frac{W_1}{V_1} = \frac{25}{220}$ Amp

Similarly, $I_2 = \frac{W_2}{V_2} = \frac{100}{220}$ Amp

The current flowing through the circuit

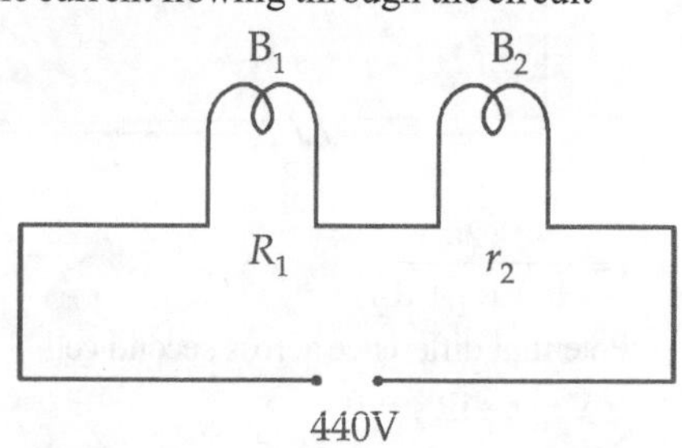

$I = \frac{440}{R_{eff}}$

$R_{eff} = R_1 + R_2$

$R_1 = \frac{V_1^2}{P_1} = \frac{(220)^2}{25}$; $R_2 = \frac{V_2^2}{P} = \frac{(220)^2}{100}$

$$I = \frac{440}{\frac{(220)^2}{25} + \frac{(220)^2}{100}}$$

$$= \frac{440}{(220)^2\left[\frac{1}{25} + \frac{1}{100}\right]}$$

$I = \frac{40}{220}$ Amp

$\because\ I_1\left(= \frac{25}{220}A\right) < I\left(= \frac{40}{220}A\right) < I_2\left(= \frac{100}{200}A\right)$

Thus the bulb rated 25 W–220 will fuse.

49. (b) Total resistance $= \frac{6 \times 3}{6+3} = 2\Omega$

Current in circuit $= \frac{6}{2} = 3A$

Therefore current through bulb 1 is $2A$ and bulb 2 is $1A$. So bulb 1 will glow more

50. (c) Resistors 4 Ω, 6 Ω and 12 Ω are connected in parallel, its equivalent resistance (R) is given by

$$\frac{1}{R} = \frac{1}{4} + \frac{1}{6} + \frac{1}{12} \Rightarrow R = \frac{12}{6} = 2\Omega$$

Again R is connected to 1.5 V battery whose internal resistance $r = 1\ \Omega$.

Equivalent resistance now,

$R' = 2\Omega + 1\Omega = 3\Omega$

Current, $I_{total} = \frac{V}{R'} = \frac{1.5}{3} = \frac{1}{2}$ A

$I_{total} = \frac{1}{2} = 3x + 2x + x = 6x$

$\Rightarrow x = \frac{1}{12}$

$\therefore$ Current through 4Ω resistor $= 3x$

$= 3 \times \frac{1}{12} = \frac{1}{4} A$

Therefore, rate of Joule heating in the 4Ω resistor

$= I^2 R = \left(\frac{1}{4}\right)^2 \times 4 = \frac{1}{4} = 0.25\text{W}$

51. (c)

52. (b) $R_1 = R_0[1 + \alpha \times 100] = 100$ ....(1)

$R_2 = R_0[1 + \alpha \times T] = 200$ ....(2)

On dividing we get

$\frac{200}{100} = \frac{1+\alpha T}{1+100\alpha} \Rightarrow 2 = \frac{1+0.005T}{1+100 \times 0.005}$

$\Rightarrow T = 400°\text{C}$

NOTE We may use this expression as an approximation because the difference in the answers is appreciable. For accurate results one should use $R = R_0 e^{\alpha \Delta T}$

53. (c) The resistance of the bulb is

$R = \frac{V^2}{P} = \frac{(220)^2}{100}$

The power consumed when operated at 110 V is

$P = \frac{(110)^2}{(220)^2/100} = \frac{100}{4} = 25$ W

54. (b) $H = \frac{V^2 t}{R}$

Resistance of half the coil $= \frac{R}{2}$

$\therefore$ As R reduces to half, 'H' will be doubled.

55. (b) $P = Vi = \frac{V^2}{R}$

$R_{hot} = \frac{V^2}{P} = \frac{200 \times 200}{100} = 400\Omega$

$R_{cold} = \frac{400}{10} = 40\Omega$

56. (a) Thermistors are usually made of metal oxides with high temperature coefficient of resistivity.

57. (a) $\Delta Q = mC_p \times \Delta T$

$= 1 \times 4180 \times (40 - 10) = 4180 \times 30$

($\because \Delta Q$ = heat supplied in time t for heating 1L water from 10°C to 40°C)

also $\Delta Q = 836 \times t \Rightarrow t = \frac{4180 \times 30}{836} = 150$ s

58. (c) We know that $R = \frac{V^2_{rated}}{P_{rated}} = \frac{(220)^2}{1000}$

When this bulb is connected to 110 volt mains supply we get

$P = \frac{V^2}{R} = \frac{(110)^2 \times 1000}{(220)^2} = \frac{1000}{4} = 250\text{W}$

59. (b) **Case 1:** $P_1 = \frac{V^2}{R}$

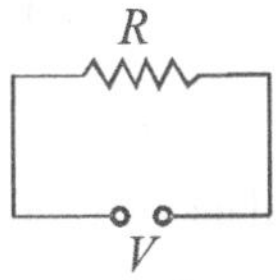

Case 2: The wire is cut into two equal pieces. Therefore, the resistance of the individual wire is $\frac{R}{2}$. These are connected in parallel

$\therefore R_{eq} = \frac{R/2}{2} = \frac{R}{4}$

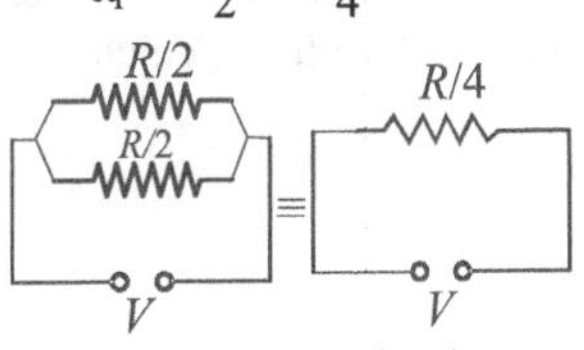

$\therefore P_2 = \frac{V^2}{R/4} = 4\left(\frac{V^2}{R}\right) = 4P_1$

60. (b) The equivalent resistance is $R_{eq} = \frac{2 \times R}{2+R}$

$\therefore$ Power dissipation $P = \frac{V^2}{R_{eq}}$

$\therefore 150 = \frac{15 \times 15}{R_{eq}}$

$\therefore R_{eq} = \frac{15}{10} = \frac{3}{2}$

$\Rightarrow \frac{2R}{2+R} = \frac{3}{2} \Rightarrow 4R = 6 + 3R \Rightarrow R = 6\Omega$

TOPIC - 5: Wheatstone Bridge and Different Measuring Instruments.

61. (d) There is no change in null point, if the cell and the galvanometer are exchanged in a balanced wheatstone bridge.

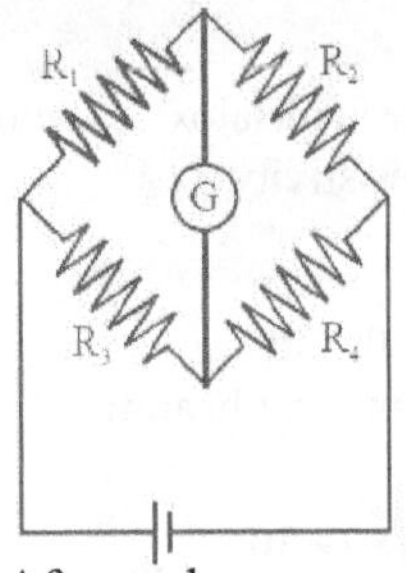

On balancing condition $\frac{R_1}{R_3}=\frac{R_2}{R_4}$

After exchange

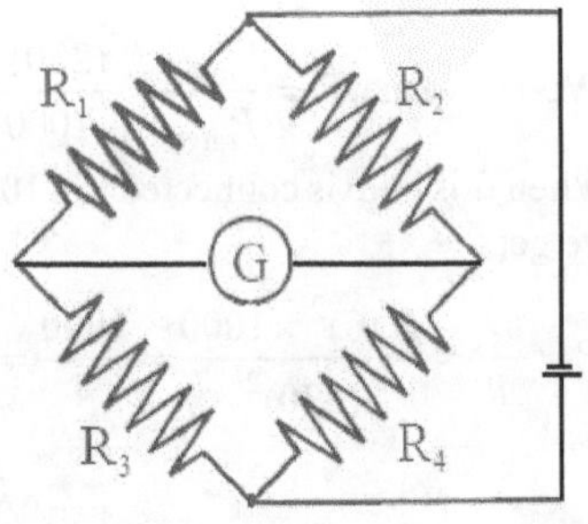

On balancing condition $\frac{R_1}{R_2}=\frac{R_3}{R_4}$

62. (d) In balance position of bridge, $\frac{P}{Q}=\frac{l}{(100-l)}$

Initially neutral position is 60 cm. from A, so

$$\frac{4}{60}=\frac{Q}{40}\Rightarrow Q=\frac{16}{6}=\frac{8}{3}\Omega$$

Now, when unknown resistance R is connected in series to P, neutral point is 80 cm from A then,

$$\frac{4+R}{80}=\frac{Q}{20}$$

$$\frac{4+R}{80}=\frac{8}{60}$$

$$R=\frac{64}{6}-4=\frac{64-24}{6}=\frac{40}{6}\Omega$$

Hence, the value of unknown resistance R is $=\frac{20}{3}\Omega$

63. (d) When key is at point (1)

$V_1=iR_1=xl_1$

When key is at (3)

$V_2=i(R_1+R_2)=xl_2$

$$\frac{R_1}{R_1+R_2}=\frac{l_1}{l_2}\Rightarrow\frac{R_1}{R_2}=\frac{l_1}{l_2-l_1}$$

64. (c) As the two cells oppose each other hence, the effective emf in closed circuit is 15 – 10 = 5 V and net resistance is 1 + 0.6 = 1.6 Ω (because in the closed circuit the internal resistance of two cells are in series.

Current in the circuit,

$$I=\frac{\text{effective emf}}{\text{total resistance}}=\frac{5}{1.6}A$$

The potential difference across voltmeter will be same as the terminal voltage of either cell.

Since the current is drawn from the cell of 15 V

$$\therefore\quad V_1=E_1-Ir_1$$

$$=15-\frac{5}{1.6}\times 0.6=13.1\text{ V}$$

65. (c) Balancing length l will give emf of cell

$\therefore E=Kl$

Here K is potential gradient.

If the cell is short circuited by resistance 'R'

Let balancing length obtained be l' then

$V=kl'$

$$r=\left(\frac{E-V}{V}\right)R$$

$\Rightarrow V=E-V$ $\quad[\because r=R\text{ given}]$

$\Rightarrow 2V=E$

or, $2Kl'=Kl$

$\therefore\quad l'=\frac{l}{2}$

66. (c) To measure the emf of a cell we prefer potentiometer rather than voltmeter because

(i) the length of potentiometer which allows greater precision.

(ii) in case of potentiometer, no current flows through the cell.

(iii) of high sensitivity.

67. (a) Bridge wire in a sensitive meter bridge wire should be of high resistivity and low temperature coefficient.

68. (c) From question, $\frac{x}{y}=\frac{40}{100-40}=\frac{2}{3}$

$$\Rightarrow x=\frac{2}{3}y$$

Again, $\frac{3x}{y}=\frac{Z}{100-Z}$

or $\frac{3\times\frac{2y}{3}}{y}=\frac{Z}{100-Z}$

Solving we get Z = 67 cm

Therefore new position of null point ≅ 67 cm

69. (c) Potential gradient

$$x=\frac{V}{\ell}=\frac{IR}{\ell}=\frac{I}{\ell}\left(\frac{\rho\ell}{A}\right)=\frac{I\rho}{A}$$

$$x=\frac{0.2\times 4\times 10^{-7}}{8\times 10^{-7}}=\frac{0.8}{8}=0.1\text{ V/m}$$

70. (b) According to the condition of balancing

$$\frac{55}{20}=\frac{R}{80}\Rightarrow R=220\Omega$$

71. (b) $\frac{P}{Q} = \frac{R}{S}$ where $S = \frac{S_1 S_2}{S_1 + S_2}$

72. (c) The internal resistance of the cell,

$$r = \left(\frac{\ell_1 - \ell_2}{\ell_2}\right) \times R = \frac{240 - 120}{120} \times 2 = 2\Omega$$

73. (c) $\frac{R_1}{R_2} = \frac{\ell_1}{\ell_2}$ where $\ell_2 = 100 - \ell_1$

In the first case $\frac{X}{Y} = \frac{20}{80}$

In the second case

$$\frac{4X}{Y} = \frac{\ell}{100 - \ell} \Rightarrow \ell = 50$$

74. (d) From the principle of potentiometer, $V \propto l$

$\Rightarrow \frac{V}{E} = \frac{l}{L}$; where

V = emf of battery, E = emf of standard cell.

L = length of potentiometer wire

$$V = \frac{El}{L} = \frac{30E}{100}$$

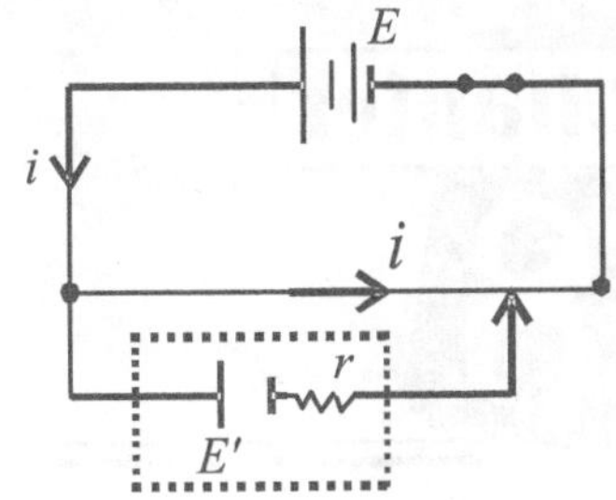

NOTE In this arrangement, the internal resistance of the battery E does not play any role as current is not passing through the battery.

75. (d) $i_g \times G = (i - i_g) S$

$$\therefore\ S = \frac{i_g \times G}{i - i_g} = \frac{1 \times 0.81}{10 - 1} = 0.09\Omega$$

76. (c) To convert a galvanometer into a voltmeter we connect a high resistance in series with the galvanometer. The same procedure needs to be done if ammeter is to be used as a voltmeter.

Chapter 18

Moving Charges and Magnetism

TOPIC - 1: Motion of Charged Particle in Magnetic Field

1. A negative test charge is moving near a long straight wire carrying a current. The force acting on the test charge is parallel to the direction of the current. The motion of the charge is : **[Online April 9, 2017]**
(a) away from the wire
(b) towards the wire
(c) parallel to the wire along the current
(d) parallel to the wire opposite to the current

2. In a certain region static electric and magnetic fields exist. The magnetic field is given by $\vec{B} = B_0(\hat{i} + 2\hat{j} - 4\hat{k})$. If a test charge moving with a velocity $\vec{v} = v_0(3\hat{i} - \hat{j} + 2\hat{k})$ experiences no force in that region, then the electric field in the region, in SI units, is : **[Online April 8, 2017]**
(a) $\vec{E} = -v_0B_0(3\hat{i} - 2\hat{j} - 4\hat{k})$ (b) $\vec{E} = -v_0B_0(\hat{i} + \hat{j} + 7\hat{k})$
(c) $\vec{E} = v_0B_0(14\hat{j} + 7\hat{k})$ (d) $\vec{E} = -v_0B_0(14\hat{j} + 7\hat{k})$

3. Consider a thin metallic sheet perpendicular to the plane of the paper moving with speed 'v' in a uniform magnetic field B going into the plane of the paper (See figure). If charge densities σ_1 and σ_2 are induced on the left and right surfaces, respectively, of the sheet then (ignore fringe effects): **[Online April 10, 2016]**

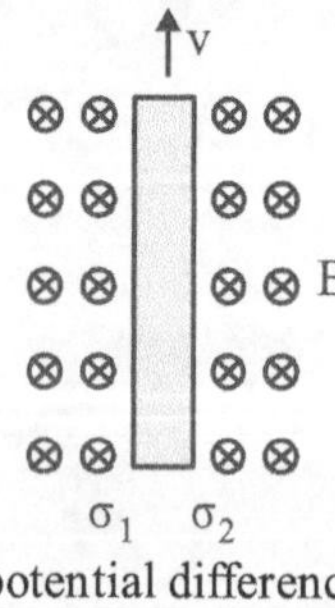

(a) $\sigma_1 = \frac{-\epsilon_0 vB}{2}, \sigma_2 = \frac{\epsilon_0 vB}{2}$
(b) $\sigma_1 = \epsilon_0 vB, \sigma_2 = -\epsilon_0 vB$
(c) $\sigma_1 = \frac{\epsilon_0 vB}{2}, \sigma_2 = \frac{-\epsilon_0 vB}{2}$
(d) $\sigma_1 = \sigma_2 = \epsilon_0 vB$

4. A proton (mass m) accelerated by a potential difference V flies through a uniform transverse magnetic field B. The field occupies a region of space by width '*d*'. If α be the angle of deviation of proton from initial direction of motion (see figure), the value of *sin* α will be : **[Online April 10, 2015]**

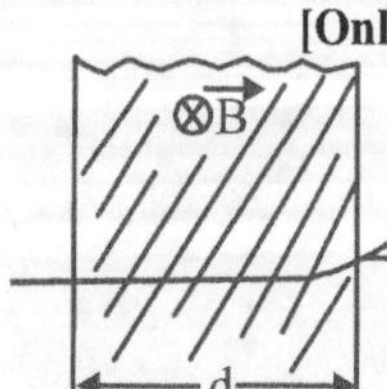

(a) $qV\sqrt{\frac{Bd}{2m}}$
(b) $\frac{B}{2}\sqrt{\frac{qd}{mV}}$
(c) $\frac{B}{d}\sqrt{\frac{q}{2mV}}$ (d) $Bd\sqrt{\frac{q}{2mV}}$

5. A positive charge 'q' of mass 'm' is moving along the + x axis. We wish to apply a uniform magnetic field B for time Δt so that the charge reverses its direction crossing the y axis at a distance d. Then: **[Online April 12, 2014]**
(a) $B = \frac{mv}{qd}$ and $\Delta t = \frac{\pi d}{v}$ (b) $B = \frac{mv}{2qd}$ and $\Delta t = \frac{\pi d}{2v}$
(c) $B = \frac{2mv}{qd}$ and $\Delta t = \frac{\pi d}{2v}$ (d) $B = \frac{2mv}{qd}$ and $\Delta t = \frac{\pi d}{v}$

6. A particle of charge 16×10^{-16} C moving with velocity 10 ms^{-1} along *x*-axis enters a region where magnetic field of induction $\vec{B}$ is along the *y*-axis and an electric field of magnitude 10^4 Vm^{-1} is along the negative *z*-axis. If the charged particle continues moving along *x*-axis, the magnitude of $\vec{B}$ is : **[Online April 23, 2013]**
(a) 16×10^3 Wb m^{-2} (b) 2×10^3 Wb m^{-2}
(c) 1×10^3 Wb m^{-2} (d) 4×10^3 Wb m^{-2}

7. Proton, deuteron and alpha particle of same kinetic energy are moving in circular trajectories in a constant magnetic field. The radii of proton, deuteron and alpha particle are respectively r_p, r_d and r_α. Which one of the following relation is correct? **[2012]**
(a) $r_\alpha = r_p = r_d$ (b) $r_\alpha = r_p < r_d$
(c) $r_\alpha > r_d > r_p$ (d) $r_\alpha = r_d > r_p$

8. This question has Statement 1 and Statement 2. Of the four choices given after the Statements, choose the one that best describes the two Statements.
Statement 1: A charged particle is moving at right angle to a static magnetic field. During the motion the kinetic energy of the charge remains unchanged.
Statement 2: Static magnetic field exert force on a moving charge in the direction perpendicular to the magnetic field. **[Online May 26, 2012]**
(a) Statement 1 is false, Statement 2 is true.
(b) Statement 1 is true, Statement 2 is true, Statement 2 is not the correct explanation of Statement 1.
(c) Statement 1 is true, Statement 2 is false.
(d) Statement 1 is true, Statement 2 is true, Statement 2 is the correct explanation of Statement 1.

9. A proton and a deuteron are both accelerated through the same potential difference and enter in a magnetic field perpendicular to the direction of the field. If the deuteron follows a path of radius R, assuming the neutron and proton masses are nearly equal, the radius of the proton's path will be **[Online May 19, 2012]**

(a) $\sqrt{2}R$ (b) $\frac{R}{\sqrt{2}}$ (c) $\frac{R}{2}$ (d) R

10. The magnetic force acting on charged particle of charge 2 μC in magnetic field of 2 T acting in y-direction, when the particle velocity is $\left(2\hat{i}+3\hat{j}\right)\times10^6\,\text{ms}^{-1}$ is **[Online May 12, 2012]**

(a) 8 N in z-direction (b) 8 N in y-direction
(c) 4 N in y-direction (d) 4 N in z-direction

11. The velocity of certain ions that pass undeflected through crossed electric field $E = 7.7$ k V/m and magnetic field $B = 0.14$ T is **[Online May 7, 2012]**

(a) 18 km/s (b) 77 km/s
(c) 55 km/s (d) 1078 km/s

12. An electric charge $+q$ moves with velocity $\vec{v} = 3\hat{i}+4\hat{j}+\hat{k}$ in an electromagnetic field given by $\vec{E} = 3\hat{i}+\hat{j}+2\hat{k}$ and $\vec{B} = \hat{i}+\hat{j}-3\hat{k}$ The y - component of the force experienced by $+q$ is: **[2011 RS]**

(a) $11q$ (b) $5q$ (c) $3q$ (d) $2q$

13. A charged particle with charge q enters a region of constant, uniform and mutually orthogonal fields $\vec{E}$ and $\vec{B}$ with a velocity $\vec{v}$ perpendicular to both $\vec{E}$ and $\vec{B}$, and comes out without any change in magnitude or direction of $\vec{v}$. Then **[2007]**

(a) $\vec{v} = \vec{B}\times\vec{E}/E^2$ (b) $\vec{v} = \vec{E}\times\vec{B}/B^2$
(c) $\vec{v} = \vec{B}\times\vec{E}/B^2$ (d) $\vec{v} = \vec{E}\times\vec{B}/E^2$

14. A charged particle moves through a magnetic field perpendicular to its direction. Then **[2007]**

(a) kinetic energy changes but the momentum is constant
(b) the momentum changes but the kinetic energy is constant
(c) both momentum and kinetic energy of the particle are not constant
(d) both momentum and kinetic energy of the particle are constant

15. In a region, steady and uniform electric and magnetic fields are present. These two fields are parallel to each other. A charged particle is released from rest in this region. The path of the particle will be a **[2006]**

(a) helix (b) straight line
(c) ellipse (d) circle

16. A charged particle of mass m and charge q travels on a circular path of radius r that is perpendicular to a magnetic field B. The time taken by the particle to complete one revolution is **[2005]**

(a) $\frac{2\pi q^2 B}{m}$ (b) $\frac{2\pi mq}{B}$ (c) $\frac{2\pi m}{qB}$ (d) $\frac{2\pi qB}{m}$

17. A uniform electric field and a uniform magnetic field are acting along the same direction in a certain region. If an electron is projected along the direction of the fields with a certain velocity then **[2005]**

(a) its velocity will increase
(b) Its velocity will decrease
(c) it will turn towards left of direction of motion
(d) it will turn towards right of direction of motion

18. A particle of mass M and charge Q moving with velocity $\vec{v}$ describe a circular path of radius R when subjected to a uniform transverse magnetic field of induction B. The work done by the field when the particle completes one full circle is **[2003]**

(a) $\left(\frac{Mv^2}{R}\right)2\pi R$ (b) zero
(c) $BQ2\pi R$ (d) $BQv2\pi R$

19. If an electron and a proton having same momenta enter perpendicular to a magnetic field, then **[2002]**

(a) curved path of electron and proton will be same (ignoring the sense of revolution)
(b) they will move undeflected
(c) curved path of electron is more curved than that of the proton
(d) path of proton is more curved.

20. The time period of a charged particle undergoing a circular motion in a uniform magnetic field is independent of its

(a) speed (b) mass **[2002]**
(c) charge (d) magnetic induction

TOPIC - 2: Magnetic Field Lines, Biot-Savart's Law and Ampere's Circuital Law

21. Two identical wires A and B, each of length 'l', carry the same current I. Wire A is bent into a circle of radius R and wire B is bent to form a square of side 'a'. If B_A and B_B are the values of magnetic field at the centres of the circle and square respectively, then the ratio $\frac{B_A}{B_B}$ is: **[2016]**

(a) $\frac{\pi^2}{16}$ (b) $\frac{\pi^2}{8\sqrt{2}}$ (c) $\frac{\pi^2}{8}$ (d) $\frac{\pi^2}{16\sqrt{2}}$

22. Two long current carrying thin wires, both with current I, are held by insulating threads of length L and are in equilibrium as shown in the figure, with threads making an angle 'θ' with the vertical. If wires have mass λ per unit length then the value of I is:
(g = *gravitational acceleration*) **[2015]**

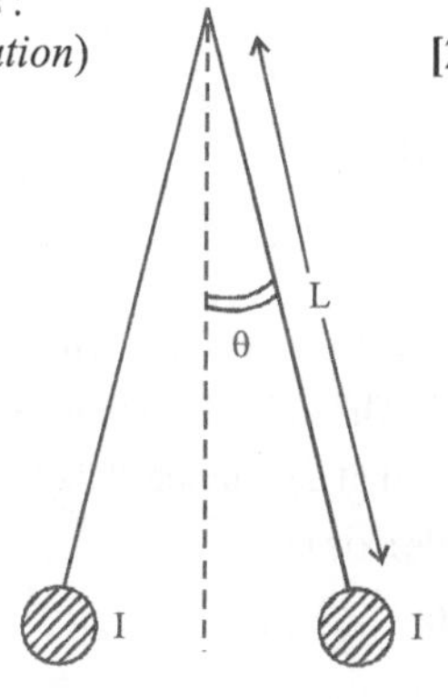

(a) $2\sqrt{\frac{\pi gL}{\mu_0}}\tan\theta$

(b) $\sqrt{\frac{\pi\lambda gL}{\mu_0}}\tan\theta$

(c) $\sin\theta\sqrt{\frac{\pi\lambda gL}{\mu_0\cos\theta}}$

(d) $2\sin\theta\sqrt{\frac{\pi\lambda gL}{\mu_0\cos\theta}}$

23. Consider two thin identical conducting wires covered with very thin insulating material. One of the wires is bent into a loop and produces magnetic field B_1, at its centre when a current I passes through it. The ratio $B_1 : B_2$ is: **[Online April 12, 2014]**

(a) 1 : 1 (b) 1 : 3 (c) 1 : 9 (d) 9 : 1

24. A parallel plate capacitor of area 60 cm^2 and separation 3 mm is charged initially to 90 μC. If the medium between the plate gets slightly conducting and the plate loses the charge initially at the rate of 2.5×10^{-8} C/s, then what is the magnetic field between the plates ? **[Online April 23, 2013]**

(a) 2.5×10^{-8} T (b) 2.0×10^{-7} T
(c) 1.63×10^{-11} T (d) Zero

25. A current i is flowing in a straight conductor of length L. The magnetic induction at a point on its axis at a distance $\frac{L}{4}$ from its centre will be : **[Online April 22, 2013]**

(a) Zero (b) $\frac{\mu_0 i}{2\pi L}$ (c) $\frac{\mu_0 i}{\sqrt{2}L}$ (d) $\frac{4\mu_0 i}{\sqrt{5}\pi L}$

26. Choose the correct sketch of the magnetic field lines of a circular current loop shown by the dot ⊙ and the cross ⊗. **[Online April 22, 2013]**

(a) 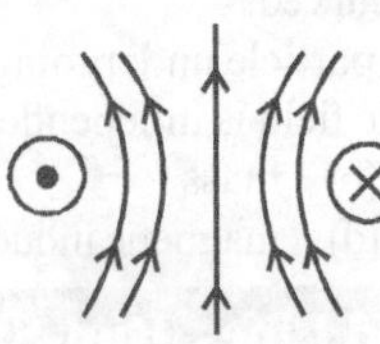

(b) 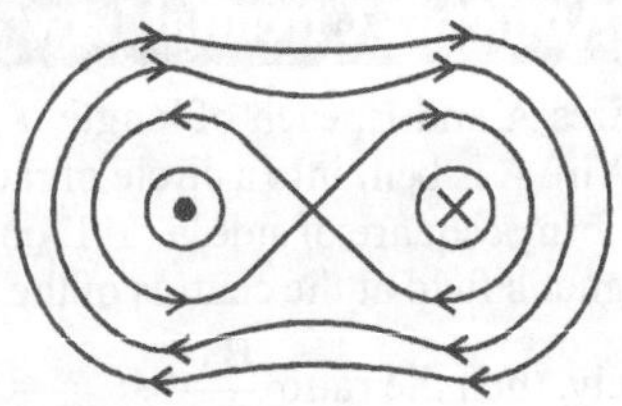

(c) 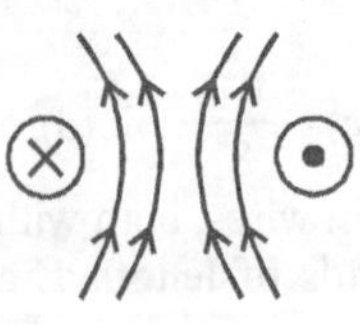

(d) 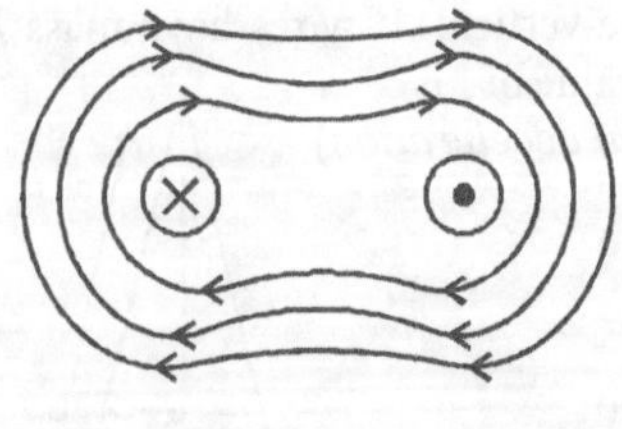

27. An electric current is flowing through a circular coil of radius R. The ratio of the magnetic field at the centre of the coil and that at a distance $2\sqrt{2}R$ from the centre of the coil and on its axis is : **[Online April 9, 2013]**

(a) $2\sqrt{2}$ (b) 27 (c) 36 (d) 8

28. A charge Q is uniformly distributed over the surface of non-conducting disc of radius R. The disc rotates about an axis perpendicular to its plane and passing through its centre with an angular velocity ω. As a result of this rotation a magnetic field of induction B is obtained at the centre of the disc. If we keep both the amount of charge placed on the disc and its angular velocity to be constant and vary the radius of the disc then the variation of the magnetic induction at the centre of the disc will be represented by the figure : **[2012]**

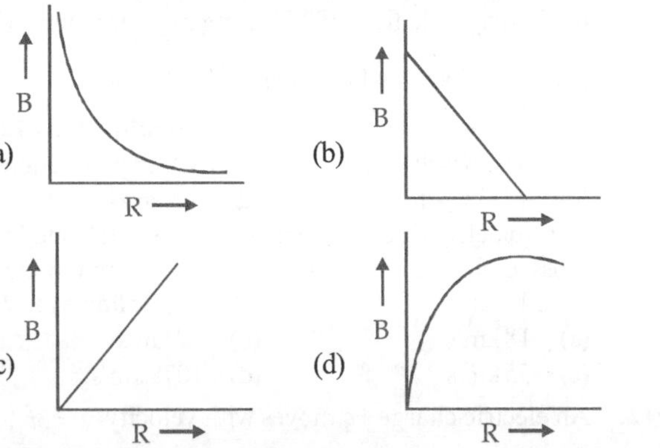

29. A current I flows in an infinitely long wire with cross section in the form of a semi-circular ring of radius R. The magnitude of the magnetic induction along its axis is: **[2011]**

(a) $\frac{\mu_0 I}{2\pi^2 R}$ (b) $\frac{\mu_0 I}{2\pi R}$ (c) $\frac{\mu_0 I}{4\pi R}$ (d) $\frac{\mu_0 I}{\pi^2 R}$

30. Two long parallel wires are at a distance 2d apart. They carry steady equal currents flowing out of the plane of the paper as shown. The variation of the magnetic field B along the line XX' is given by **[2010]**

(a)
(b)
(c)
(d)

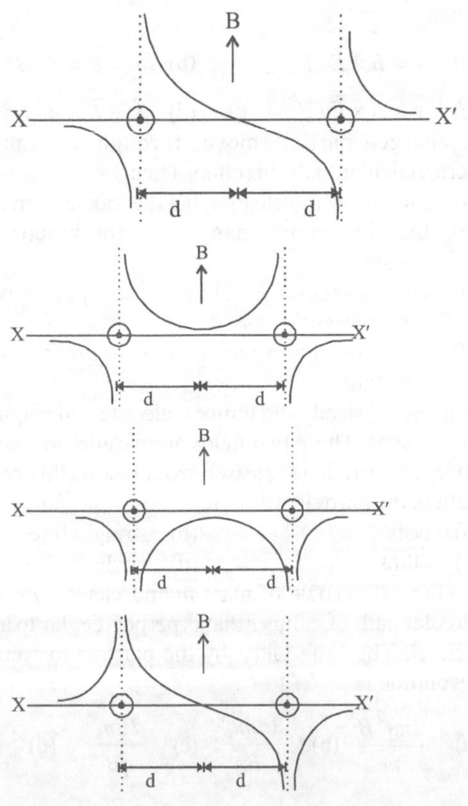

31. A horizontal overhead powerline is at height of 4m from the ground and carries a current of 100A from east to west. The magnetic field directly below it on the ground is ($\mu_0 = 4\pi \times 10^{-7}$ Tm A^{-1}) **[2008]**

(a) 2.5×10^{-7} *T* southward (b) 5×10^{-6} *T* northward

(c) 5×10^{-6} *T* southward (d) 2.5×10^{-7} *T* northward

32. A long straight wire of radius *a* carries a steady current *i*. The current is uniformly distributed across its cross section. The ratio of the magnetic field at *a*/2 and 2*a* is **[2007]**

(a) 1/2 (b) 1/4 (c) 4 (d) 1

33. A current *I* flows along the length of an infinitely long, straight, thin walled pipe. Then **[2007]**

(a) the magnetic field at all points inside the pipe is the same, but not zero

(b) the magnetic field is zero only on the axis of the pipe

(c) the magnetic field is different at different points inside the pipe

(d) the magnetic field at any point inside the pipe is zero

34. Two identical conducting wires *AOB* and *COD* are placed at right angles to each other. The wire *AOB* carries an electric current I_1 and *COD* carries a current I_2. The magnetic field on a point lying at a distance d from *O*, in a direction perpendicular to the plane of the wires *AOB* and *COD*, will be given by **[2007]**

(a) $\frac{\mu_0}{2\pi d}(I_1^2 + I_2^2)$ (b) $\frac{\mu_0}{2\pi}\left(\frac{I_1 + I_2}{d}\right)^{\frac{1}{2}}$

(c) $\frac{\mu_0}{2\pi d}\left(I_1^2 + I_2^2\right)^{\frac{1}{2}}$ (d) $\frac{\mu_0}{2\pi d}(I_1 + I_2)$

35. A long solenoid has 200 turns per cm and carries a current *i*. The magnetic field at its centre is 6.28×10^{-2} Weber/m^2. Another long solenoid has 100 turns per cm and it carries a current $\frac{i}{3}$. The value of the magnetic field at its centre is **[2006]**

(a) 1.05×10^{-2} Weber/m^2 (b) 1.05×10^{-5} Weber/m^2

(c) 1.05×10^{-3} Weber/m^2 (d) 1.05×10^{-4} Weber/m^2

36. Two concentric coils each of radius equal to 2 π cm are placed at right angles to each other. 3 ampere and 4 ampere are the currents flowing in each coil respectively. The magnetic induction in Weber/m^2 at the centre of the coils will be $\left(\mu_0 = 4\pi \times 10^{-7}\ \text{Wb/A.m}\right)$ **[2005]**

(a) 10^{-5} (b) 12×10^{-5}

(c) 7×10^{-5} (d) 5×10^{-5}

37. A current *i* ampere flows along an infinitely long straight thin walled tube, then the magnetic induction at any point inside the tube is **[2004]**

(a) $\frac{\mu_0}{4\pi} \cdot \frac{2i}{r}$ tesla (b) zero

(c) infinite (d) $\frac{2i}{r}$ tesla

38. A long wire carries a steady current. It is bent into a circle of one turn and the magnetic field at the centre of the coil is *B*. It is then bent into a circular loop of n turns. The magnetic field at the centre of the coil will be **[2004]**

(a) $2nB$ (b) $n^2 B$ (c) nB (d) $2n^2 B$

39. The magnetic field due to a current carrying circular loop of radius 3 cm at a point on the axis at a distance of 4 cm from the centre is 54 μT. What will be its value at the centre of loop? **[2004]**

(a) 125 μT (b) 150 μT (c) 250 μT (d) 75 μT

40. If in a circular coil *A* of radius *R*, current *I* is flowing and in another coil *B* of radius 2*R* a current 2*I* is flowing, then the ratio of the magnetic fields B_A and B_B, produced by them will be **[2002]**

(a) 1 (b) 2 (c) 1/2 (d) 4

TOPIC - 3: Force and Torque on Current Carrying Conductor

41. A uniform magnetic field B of 0.3 T is along the positive Z-direction. A rectangular loop (abcd) of sides 10 cm × 5 cm carries a current 1 of 12 A. Out of the following different orientations which one corresponds to stable equilibrium ? **[Online April 9, 2017]**

(a)
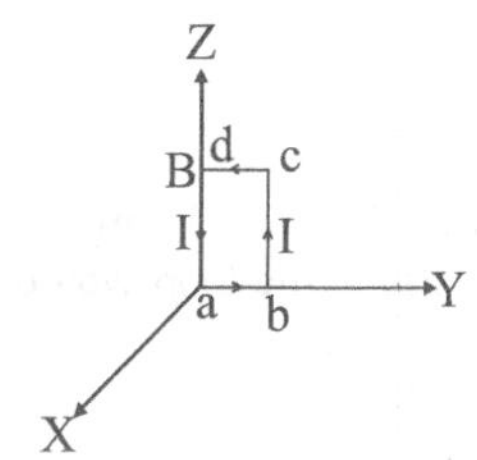

(b)
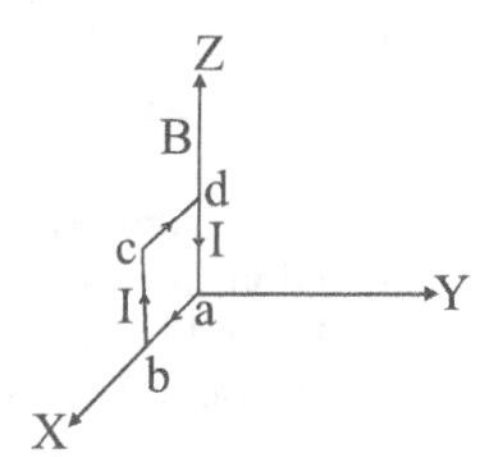

(c)
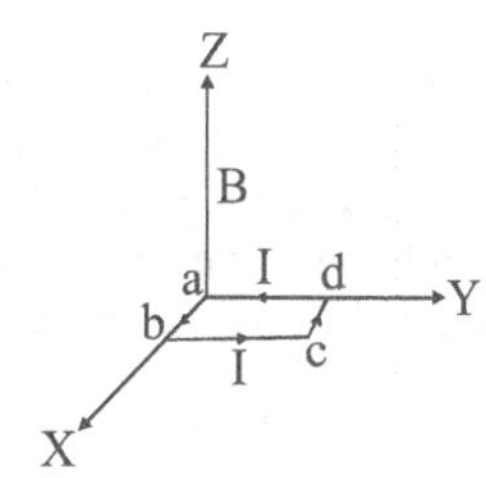

(d)
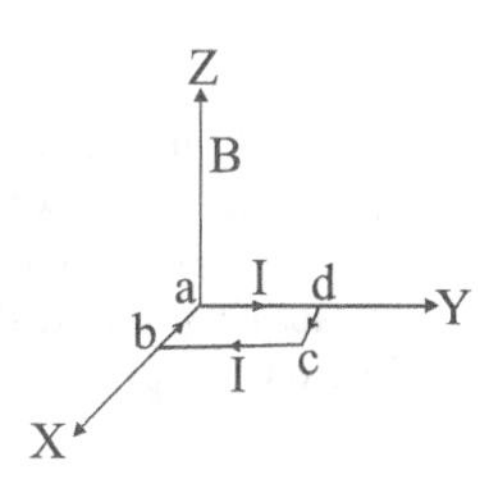

42. Two coaxial solenoids of different radius carry current I in the same direction. $\vec{F_1}$ be the magnetic force on the inner solenoid due to the outer one and $\vec{F_2}$ be the magnetic force on the outer solenoid due to the inner one. Then : **[2015]**

(a) $\vec{F_1}$ is radially inwards and $\vec{F_2} = 0$

(b) $\vec{F_1}$ is radially outwards and $\vec{F_2} = 0$

(c) $\vec{F_1} = \vec{F_2} = 0$

(d) $\vec{F_1}$ is radially inwards and $\vec{F_2}$ is radially outwards

43. A rectangular loop of sides 10 cm and 5 cm carrying a current 1 of 12 A is placed in different orientations as shown in the figures below :

(A)

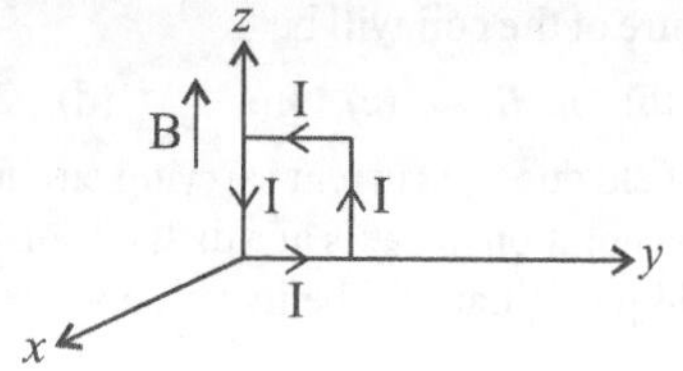

(B)

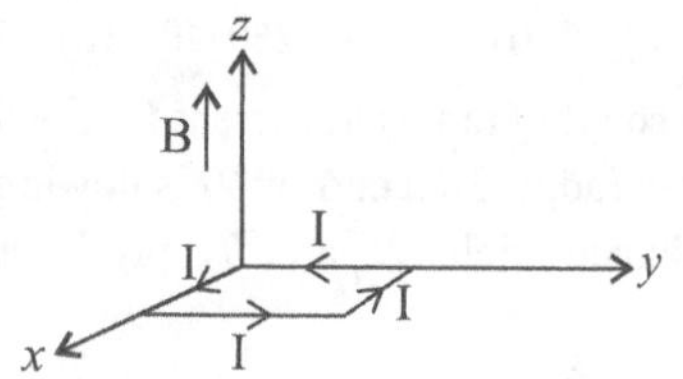

(C)

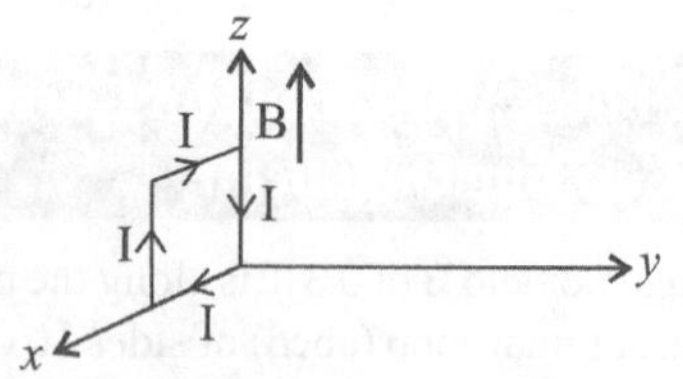

(D)

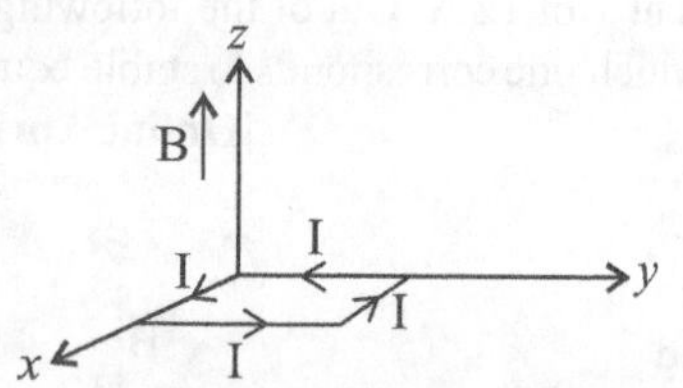

If there is a uniform magnetic field of 0.3 T in the positive z direction, in which orientations the loop would be in (i) stable equilibrium and (ii) unstable equilibrium ? **[2015]**

(a) (B) and (D), respectively
(b) (B) and (C), respectively
(c) (A) and (B), respectively
(d) (A) and (C), respectively

44. Two long straight parallel wires, carrying (adjustable) current I_1 and I_2, are kept at a distance d apart. If the force 'F' between the two wires is taken as 'positive' when the wires repel each other and 'negative' when the wires attract each other, the graph showing the dependence of 'F', on the product $I_1 I_2$, would be : **[Online April 11, 2015]**

(a) 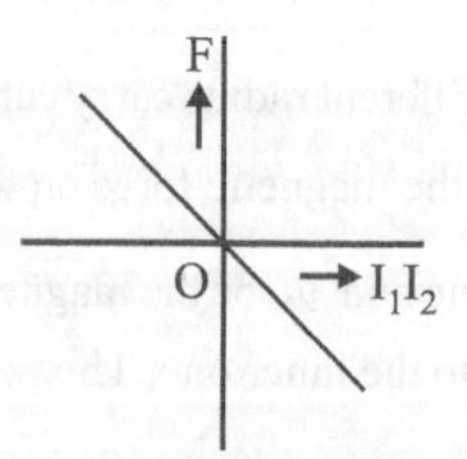

(b) 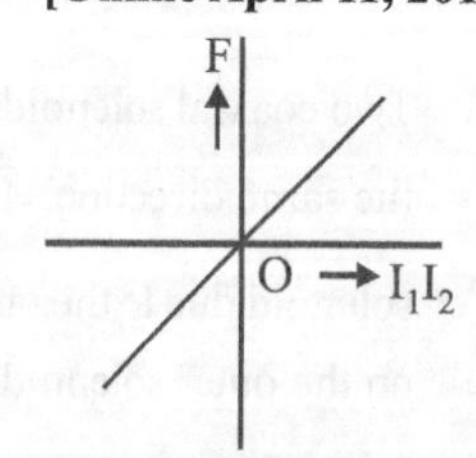

(c) 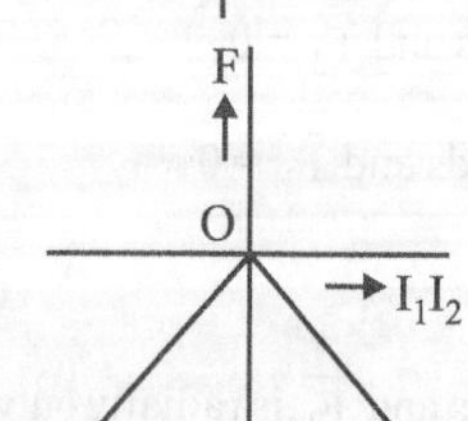

(d) 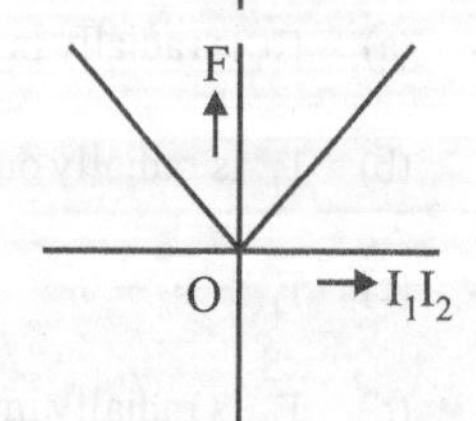

45. A wire carrying current I is tied between points P and Q and is in the shape of a circular arc of radius R due to a uniform magnetic field B (perpendicular to the plane of the paper, shown by xxx) in the vicinity of the wire. If the wire subtends an angle $2\theta_0$ at the centre of the circle (of which it forms an arc) then the tension in the wire is : **[Online April 11, 2015]**

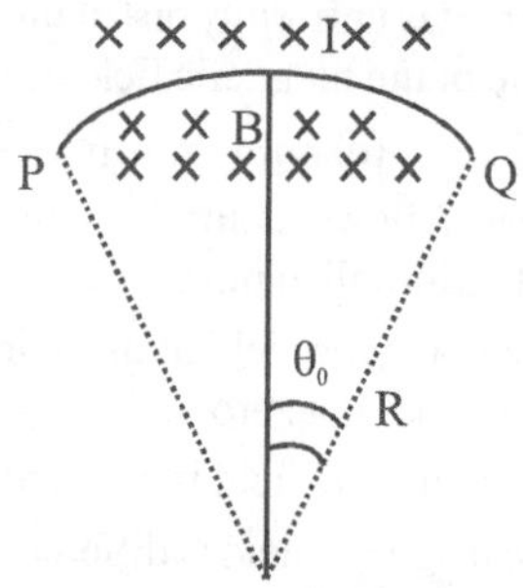

(a) $\frac{IBR}{2\sin\theta_0}$

(b) $\frac{IBR\theta_0}{\sin\theta_0}$

(c) IBR

(d) $\frac{IBR}{\sin\theta_0}$

46. A conductor lies along the z-axis at $-1.5 \le z < 1.5$ m and carries a fixed current of 10.0 A in $-\hat{a}_z$ direction (see figure). For a field $\vec{B} = 3.0\times10^{-4} e^{-0.2x}\ \hat{a}_y$ T, find the power required to move the conductor at constant speed to x = 2.0 m, y = 0 m in 5×10^{-3} s. Assume parallel motion along the x-axis. **[2014]**

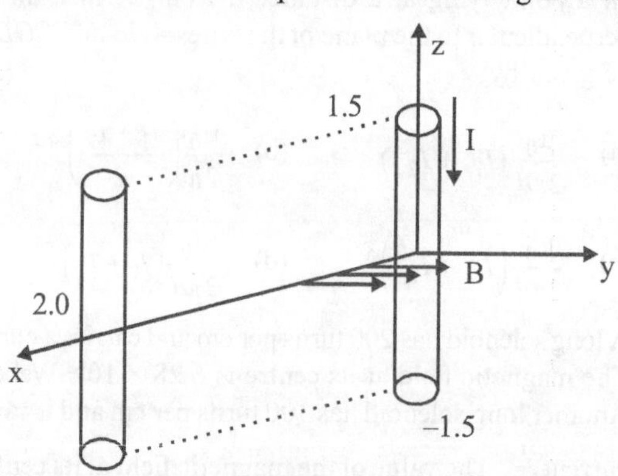

(a) 1.57 W (b) 2.97 W (c) 14.85 W (d) 29.7 W

47. Three straight parallel current carrying conductors are shown in the figure. The force experienced by the middle conductor of length 25 cm is: **[Online April 11, 2014]**

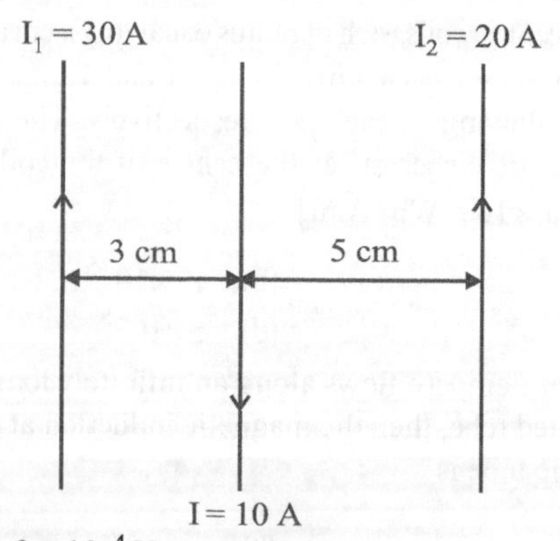

(a) 3×10^{-4} N toward right
(b) 6×10^{-4} N toward right
(c) 9×10^{-4} N toward right
(d) Zero

48. A rectangular loop of wire, supporting a mass m, hangs with one end in a uniform magnetic field $\vec{B}$ pointing out of the plane of the paper. A clockwise current is set up such that $i > mg/Ba$, where a is the width of the loop. Then : **[Online April 23, 2013]**

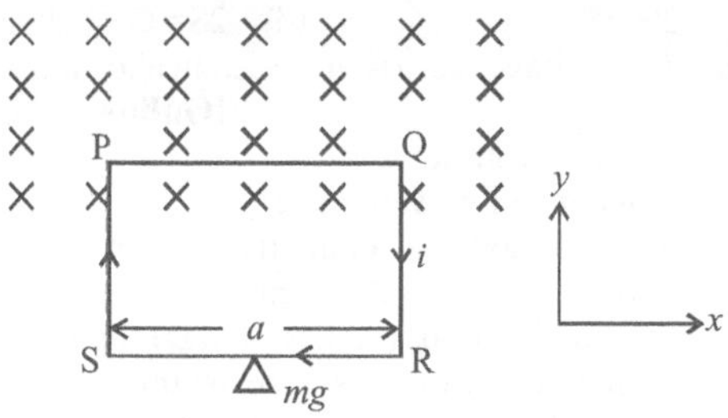

(a) The weight rises due to a vertical force caused by the magnetic field and work is done on the system.
(b) The weight do not rise due to vertical for caused by the magnetic field and work is done on the system.
(c) The weight rises due to a vertical force caused by the magnetic field but no work is done on the system.
(d) The weight rises due to a vertical force caused by the magnetic field and work is extracted from the magnetic field.

49. Currents of a 10 ampere and 2 ampere are passed through two parallel thin wires A and B respectively in opposite directions. Wire A is infinitely long and the length of the wire B is 2 m. The force acting on the conductor B, which is situated at 10 cm distance from A will be **[Online May 26, 2012]**

(a) 8×10^{-5} N (b) 5×10^{-5} N
(c) $8\pi \times 10^{-7}$ N (d) $4\pi \times 10^{-7}$ N

50. The circuit in figure consists of wires at the top and bottom and identical springs as the left and right sides. The wire at the bottom has a mass of 10 g and is 5 cm long. The wire is hanging as shown in the figure. The springs stretch 0.5 cm under the weight of the wire and the circuit has a total resistance of 12 Ω. When the lower wire is subjected to a static magnetic field, the springs, stretch an additional 0.3 cm. The magnetic field is **[Online May 12, 2012]**

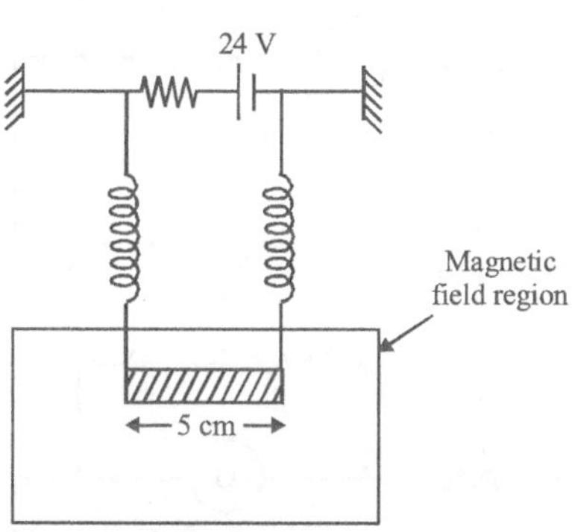

(a) 0.6 T and directed out of page
(b) 1.2 T and directed into the plane of page
(c) 0.6 T and directed into the plane of page
(d) 1.2 T and directed out of page

Directions : Question numbers 51 and 52 are based on the following paragraph.

A current loop $ABCD$ is held fixed on the plane of the paper as shown in the figure. The arcs BC (radius = b) and DA (radius = a) of the loop are joined by two straight wires AB and CD. A steady current I is flowing in the loop. Angle made by AB and CD at the origin O is 30°. Another straight thin wire with steady current I_1 flowing out of the plane of the paper is kept at the origin. **[2009]**

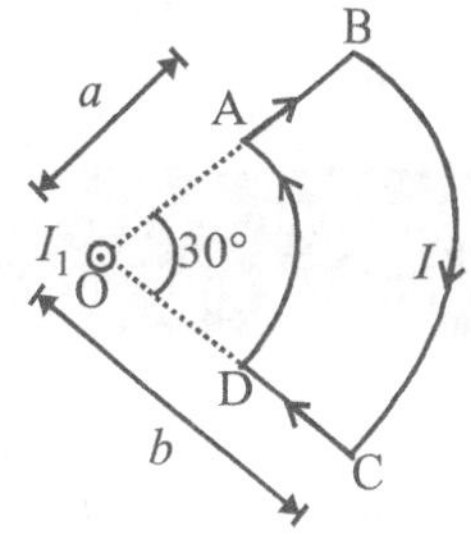

51. The magnitude of the magnetic field (B) due to the loop $ABCD$ at the origin (O) is :

(a) $\dfrac{\mu_o I(b-a)}{24ab}$

(b) $\dfrac{\mu_o I}{4\pi}\left[\dfrac{b-a}{ab}\right]$

(c) $\dfrac{\mu_o I}{4\pi}[2(b-a)+\pi/3(a+b)]$

(d) zero

52. Due to the presence of the current I_1 at the origin:
(a) The forces on AD and BC are zero.
(b) The magnitude of the net force on the loop is given by $\dfrac{I_1 I}{4\pi}\mu_o[2(b-a)+\pi/3(a+b]$.
(c) The magnitude of the net force on the loop is given by $\dfrac{\mu_o I I_1}{24ab}(b-a)$.
(d) The forces on AB and DC are zero.

53. Two long conductors, separated by a distance d carry current I_1 and I_2 in the same direction. They exert a force F on each other. Now the current in one of them is increased to two times and its direction is reversed. The distance is also increased to $3d$. The new value of the force between them is **[2004]**

(a) $-\dfrac{2F}{3}$ (b) $\dfrac{F}{3}$ (c) $-2F$ (d) $-\dfrac{F}{3}$

54. If a current is passed through a spring then the spring will **[2002]**

(a) expand (b) compress
(c) remains same (d) none of these

55. Wires 1 and 2 carrying currents i_1 and i_2 respectively are inclined at an angle θ to each other. What is the force on a small element dl of wire 2 at a distance of r from wire 1 (as shown in figure) due to the magnetic field of wire 1? **[2002]**

(a) $\frac{\mu_0}{2\pi r} i_1 i_2\, dl \tan\theta$

(b) $\frac{\mu_0}{2\pi r} i_1 i_2\, dl \sin\theta$

(c) $\frac{\mu_0}{2\pi r} i_1 i_2\, dl \cos\theta$

(d) $\frac{\mu_0}{4\pi r} i_1 i_2\, dl \sin\theta$

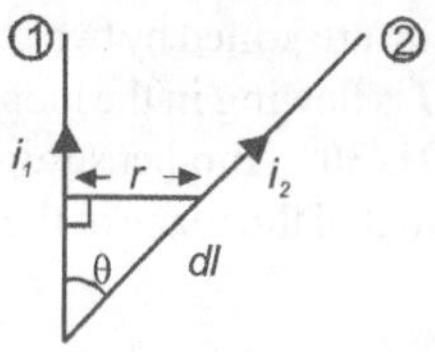

TOPIC - 4: Galvanometer and its Conversion into Ammeter and Voltmeter

56. When a current of 5 mA is passed through a galvanometer having a coil of resistance 15 Ω, it shows full scale deflection. The value of the resistance to be put in series with the galvanometer to convert it into to voltmeter of range 0 – 10 V is **[2017]**

(a) $2.535\times10^3\Omega$ (b) $4.005\times10^3\Omega$

(c) $1.985\times10^3\Omega$ (d) $2.045\times10^3\Omega$

57. A galvanometer having a coil resistance of 100 Ω gives a full scale deflection, when a currect of 1 mA is passed through it. The value of the resistance, which can convert this galvanometer into ammeter giving a full scale deflection for a current of 10 A, is : **[2016]**

(a) 0.1 Ω (b) 3Ω (c) 0.01Ω (d) 2Ω

58. A galvanometer has a 50 division scale. Battery has no internal resistance. It is found that there is deflection of 40 divisions when R = 2400 Ω. Deflection becomes 20 divisions when resistance taken from resistance box is 4900 Ω. Then we can conclude: **[Online April 10, 2016]**

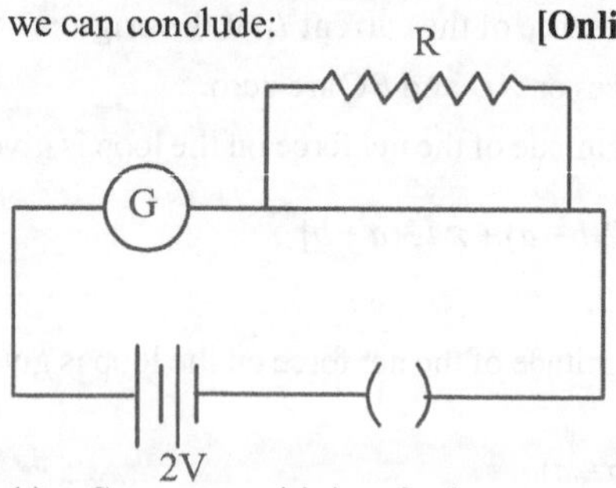

(a) Current sensitivity of galvanometer is 20 μA/ division.
(b) Resistance of galvanometer is 200Ω.
(c) Resistance required on R.B. for a deflection of 10 divisions is 9800Ω.
(d) Full scale deflection current is 2 mA.

59. A 50 Ω resistance is connected to a battery of 5V. A galvanometer of resistance 100 Ω is to be used as an ammeter to measure current through the resistance, for this a resistance r_s is connected to the galvanometer. Which of the following connections should be employed if the measured current is within 1% of the current without the ammeter in the circuit? **[Online April 9, 2016]**

(a) r_s = 0.5 Ω in series with the galvanometer
(b) r_s = 1 Ω in series with galvanometer
(c) r_s = 1Ω in parallel with galvanometer
(d) r_s = 0.5 Ω in parallel with the galvanometer.

60. To know the resistance G of a galvanometer by half deflection method, a battery of emf V_E and resistance R is used to deflect the galvanometer by angle θ. If a shunt of resistance S is needed to get half deflection then G, R and S related by the equation: **[Online April 9, 2016]**

(a) S (R + G) = RG (b) 2S (R + G) = RG
(c) 2G = S (d) 2S = G

61. The AC voltage across a resistance can be measured using a : **[Online April 11, 2015]**

(a) hot wire voltmeter
(b) moving coil galvanometer
(c) potential coil galvanometer
(d) moving magnet galvanometer

62. In the circuit diagrams (A, B, C and D) shown below, R is a high resistance and S is a resistance of the order of galvanometer resistance G. The correct circuit, corresponding to the half deflection method for finding the resistance and figure of merit of the galvanometer, is the circuit labelled as: **[Online April 11, 2014]**

(A)

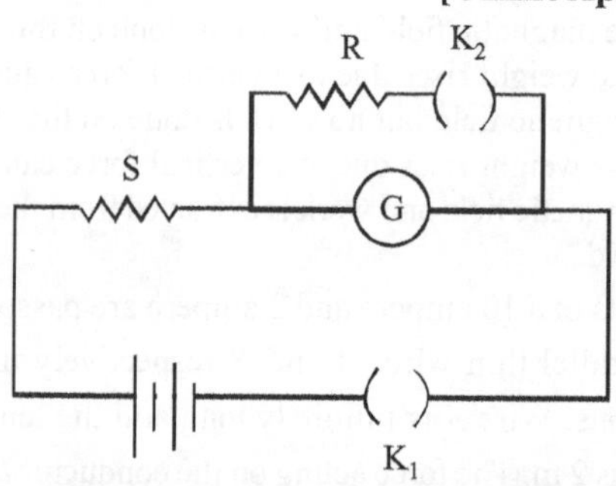

(B)

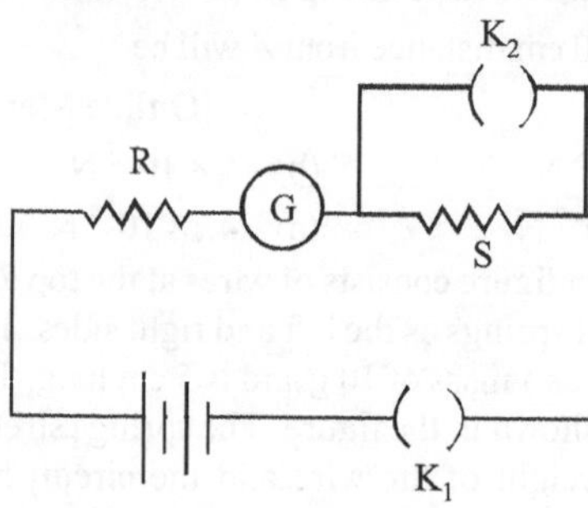

(C)

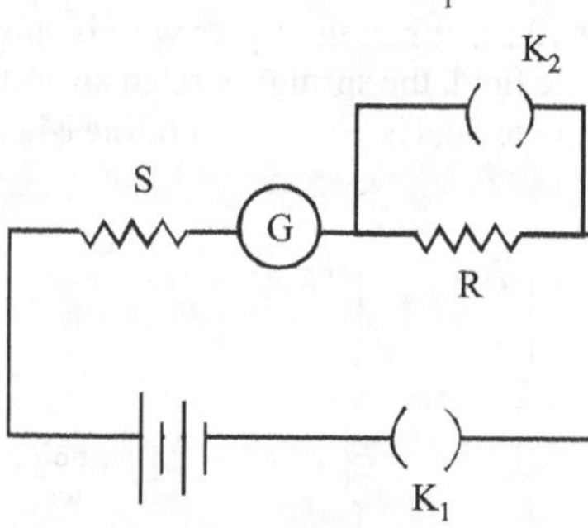

(D)

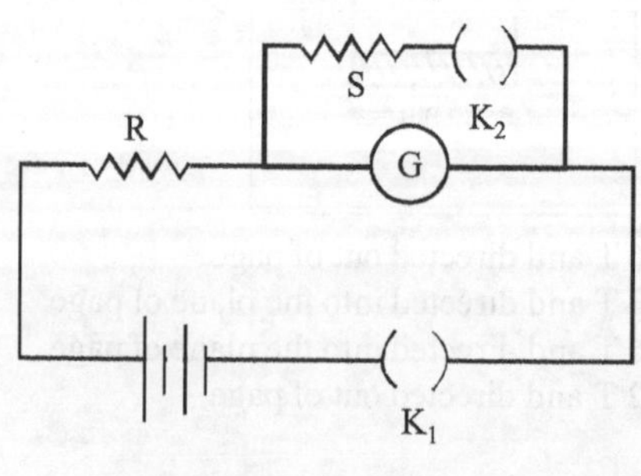

(a) Circuit A with $G = \frac{RS}{(R-S)}$

(b) Circuit B with G = S

(c) Circuit C with G = S

(d) Circuit D with $G = \frac{RS}{(R-S)}$

63. This questions has Statement I and Statement II. Of the four choices given after the Statements, choose the one that best describes into two Statements.

Statement-I : Higher the range, greater is the resistance of ammeter.

Statement-II : To increase the range of ammeter, additional shunt needs to be used across it. **[2013]**

(a) Statement-I is true, Statement-II is true, Statement-II is the correct explanation of Statement-I.

(b) Statement-I is true, Statement-II is true, Statement-II is not the correct explanation of Statement-I.

(c) Statement-I is true, Statement-II is false.

(d) Statement-I is false, Statement-II is true.

64. To find the resistance of a galvanometer by the half deflection method the following circuit is used with resistances $R_1 = 9970$ W, $R_2 = 30$ W and $R_3 = 0$. The deflection in the galvanometer is d. With $R_3 = 107$ W the deflection changed to $\frac{d}{2}$. The galvanometer resistance is approximately: **[Online April 22, 2013]**

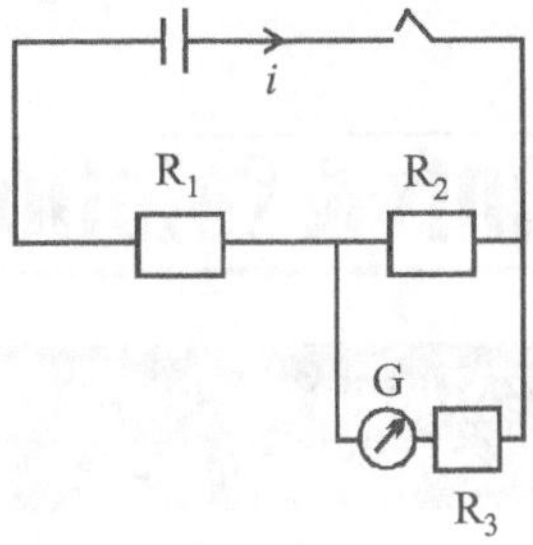

(a) 107 Ω (b) 137Ω (c) 107/2 Ω (d) 77 Ω

65. A shunt of resistance 1 Ω is connected across a galvanometer of 120 Ω resistance. A current of 5.5 ampere gives full scale deflection in the galvanometer. The current that will give full scale deflection in the absence of the shunt is nearly: **[Online April 9, 2013]**

(a) 5.5 ampere (b) 0.5 ampere
(c) 0.004 ampere (d) 0.045 ampere

66. In the circuit, the galvanometer G shows zero deflection. If the batteries A and B have negligible internal resistance, the value of the resistor R will be - **[2005]**

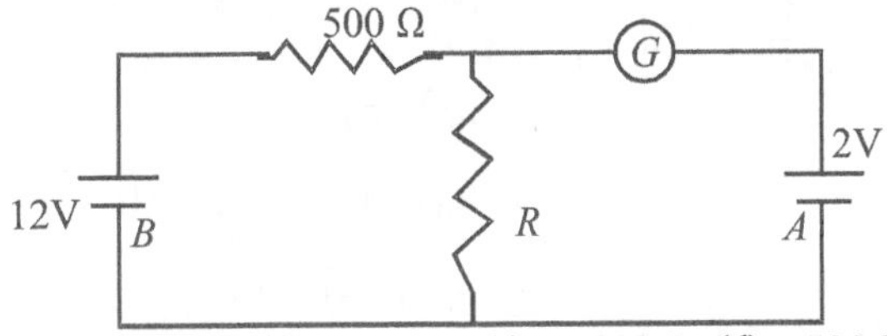

(a) 100Ω (b) 200Ω (c) 1000Ω (d) 500Ω

67. A moving coil galvanometer has 150 equal divisions. Its current sensitivity is 10-divisions per milliampere and voltage sensitivity is 2 divisions per millivolt. In order that each division reads 1 volt, the resistance in ohms needed to be connected in series with the coil will be - **[2005]**

(a) 10^5 (b) 10^3 (c) 9995 (d) 99995

Hints & Solutions

TOPIC - 1: Motion of Charged Particle in Magnetic Field

1. **(b)** The force is parallel to the direction of current in magnetic field,
hence $F = q(v \times \vec{B})$
According to Fleming's left hand rule,

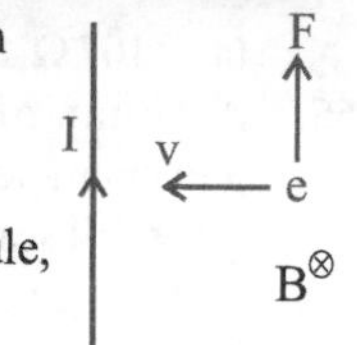

we have, the direction of motion of charge is towards the wire.

2. **(d)** According to question, as the test charge experiences no net force in that region i.e., sum of electric force $(F_e = q\vec{E})$ and magnetic forces $[F_m = q(\vec{v} \times \vec{B})]$ will be zero.
Hence, $F_e + F_m = 0$

$$F_e = -q(\vec{v} \times \vec{B})$$
$$= -B_0 v_0 \left[(3\hat{i} - \hat{j} + 2\hat{k}) \times (\hat{i} + 2\hat{j} - 4\hat{k})\right]$$
$$= -B_0 v_0 (14\hat{j} + 7\hat{k})$$

3. **(b)** $\because F = qE$ and $F = qvB$
$\therefore E = vB$
And Gauss's law in Electrostatics $E = \dfrac{\sigma}{\varepsilon_0}$

$$E = \frac{\sigma}{\varepsilon_0} = vB \Rightarrow \sigma = \varepsilon_0 vB$$
$$\sigma_1 = -\sigma_2$$

4. **(d)** From figure, $\sin\alpha = d/R$

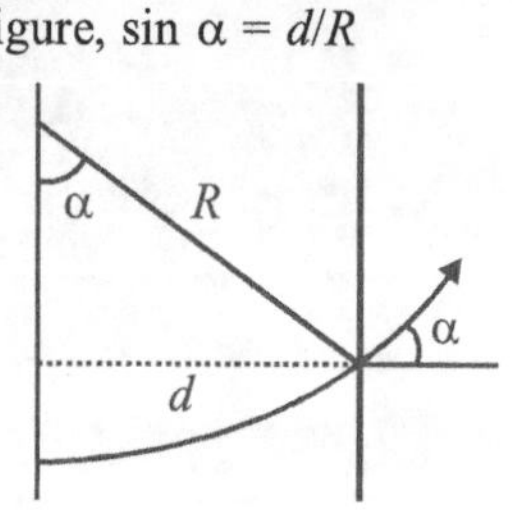

And we know, $\dfrac{mv^2}{R} = qvB$

$$\Rightarrow R = \frac{mv}{qB}$$
$$\therefore \sin\alpha = \frac{dqB}{mv}$$
$$\sin\alpha = Bd\sqrt{\frac{q}{2mV}} \quad \left[\because qV = \frac{1}{2}mv^2\right]$$

5. **(c)** The applied magnetic field provides the required centripetal force to the charge particle, so it can move in circular path of radius $\dfrac{d}{2}$

$$\therefore Bqv = \frac{mv^2}{d/2}$$
$$\text{or,} \quad B = \frac{2mv}{qd}$$

Time interval for which a uniform magnetic field is applied

$$\Delta t = \frac{\pi . \frac{d}{2}}{v}$$

(particle reverses its direction after time Δt by covering semi circle).

$$\Delta t = \frac{\pi d}{2v}$$

6. **(c)** Since particle is moving undeflected
So, $q_E = qvB$
$$\Rightarrow B = \frac{E}{V} = \frac{10^4}{10} = 10^3 \text{ wb/m}^2$$

7. **(b)** $\dfrac{mv^2}{r} = qvB \Rightarrow r = \dfrac{mv}{q_B}$

$$\Rightarrow r_p = \frac{m_p v_p}{q_p B};$$
$$r_d = \frac{m_d v_d}{q_d B}; \quad r_\alpha = \frac{m_\alpha v_\alpha}{q_\alpha B}$$
$$m_\alpha = 4m_p, \; m_d = 2m_p$$
$$q_\alpha = 2q_p, \; q_d = q_p$$

From the problem

$$E_p = E_d = E_\alpha = \frac{1}{2}m_p v_p^2$$
$$= \frac{1}{2}m_d v_d^2 = \frac{1}{2}m_\alpha v_\alpha^2$$
$$\Rightarrow v_p^2 = 2v_d^2 = 4mv_2^2$$

Thus we have, $r_\alpha = r_p < r_d$

8. **(d)** When a charged particle enters the magnetic field in perpendicular direction then it experience a force in perpendicular direction.
i.e. $F = Bqv \sin\theta$
Due to which it moves in a circular path.

9. **(b)** As charge on both proton and deuteron is same i.e. 'e'
Energy acquired by both, $E = eV$

For Deuteron.

Kinetic energy, $\frac{1}{2}mV^2 = eV$

[V is the potential difference]

$$v = \sqrt{\frac{2eV}{m_d}}$$

But $m_d = 2m$

Therefore, $v = \sqrt{\frac{2eV}{2m}} = \sqrt{\frac{eV}{m}}$

Radius of path, $R = \frac{mv}{eB}$

Substituting value of 'v' we get

$$R = \frac{2m\sqrt{\frac{ev}{m}}}{eB}$$

$$\frac{R}{2} = \frac{m\sqrt{\frac{ev}{m}}}{eB} \quad ...(i)$$

For proton :

$$\frac{1}{2}mV^2 = eV$$

$$V = \sqrt{\frac{2eV}{m}}$$

Radius of path, $R' = \frac{mV}{eB} = \frac{m\sqrt{\frac{2eV}{m}}}{eB}$

$R' = \sqrt{2} \times \frac{R}{2}$ [From eq. (i)]

$$R' = \frac{R}{\sqrt{2}}$$

10. (a) $\vec{F} = q\left(\vec{V} \times \vec{B}\right)$

$= 2\times10^{-6}\left[(2\hat{i} + 3\hat{j})\times10^{6}\times2\hat{j}\right]$

$= 2\times4\hat{k} = 8N$ in Z-direction.

11. (c) As velocity $v = \frac{E}{B} = \frac{7.7\times10^{3}}{0.14} = 55$ km/s

12. (a) Lorentz force acting on the particle

$$\vec{F} = q\left[\vec{E} + \vec{v}\times\vec{B}\right]$$

$$= q\left[3\hat{i}+\hat{j}+2\hat{k} + \begin{vmatrix}\hat{i} & \hat{j} & \hat{k}\\ 3 & 4 & 1\\ 1 & 1 & -3\end{vmatrix}\right]$$

$$= q\left[3\hat{i}+\hat{j}+2\hat{k}+\hat{i}(-12-1) - \hat{j}(-9-1) + k(3-4)\right]$$

$$= q\left[3\hat{i}+\hat{j}+2\hat{k}-13\hat{i}+10\hat{j}-\hat{k}\right]$$

$$= q\left[-10\hat{i}+11\hat{j}+\hat{k}\right]$$

$$F_y = 11q\hat{j}$$

Thus, the y component of the force.

13. (b) Here, $\vec{E}$ and $\vec{B}$ are perpendicular to each other and the velocity $\vec{v}$ does not change; therefore

$qE = qvB \Rightarrow v = \frac{E}{B}$

Also,

$$\left|\frac{\vec{E}\times\vec{B}}{B^2}\right| = \frac{E\ B\sin\theta}{B^2} = \frac{E\ B\ \sin 90°}{B^2} = \frac{E}{B} = |\vec{v}| = v$$

14. (b) When a charged particle enters a magnetic field at a direction perpendicular to the direction of motion, the path of the motion is circular. In circular motion the direction of velocity changes at every point (the magnitude remains constant).

Therefore, the tangential momentum will change at every point. But kinetic energy will remain constant as it is given by $\frac{1}{2}mv^2$ and v^2 is the square of the magnitude of velocity which does not change.

15. (b) The charged particle will move along the lines of electric field (and magnetic field). Magnetic field will exert no force. The force by electric field will be along the lines of uniform electric field. Hence the particle will move in a straight line.

16. (c) Equating magnetic force to centripetal force,

$$\frac{mv^2}{r} = qvB\sin 90°$$

Time to complete one revolution,

$$T = \frac{2\pi r}{v} = \frac{2\pi m}{qB}$$

17. (b) Due to electric field, it experiences force and accelerates i.e. its velocity decreases.

18. (b) The workdone, $dW = Fds\cos\theta$

The angle between force and displacement is 90°.

Therefore work done is zero.

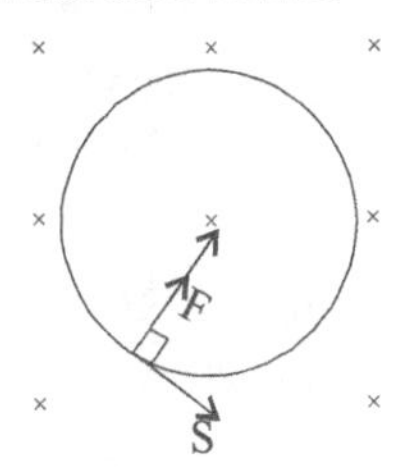

19. (a) When a charged particle enters perpendicular to a magnetic field, then it moves in a circular path of radius.

$$r = \frac{p}{qB}$$

where q = Charge of the particle

p = Momentum of the particle

B = Magnetic field

Here p, q and B are constant for electron and proton, therefore the radius will be same.

20. (a) The time period of a charged particle (m, q) moving in a magnetic field (B) is $T = \frac{2\pi m}{qB}$

The time period does not depend on the speed of the particle.

TOPIC - 2: Magnetic Field Lines, Biot-Savart's Law and Ampere's Circuital Law

21. (b) Case (a) : 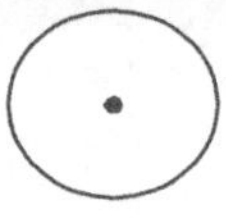

$$\beta_A = \frac{\mu_0}{4\pi}\frac{I}{R} \times 2\pi = \frac{\mu_0}{4\pi}\frac{I}{\ell/2\pi} \times 2\pi \qquad (2\pi R = \ell)$$

$$= \frac{\mu_0}{4\pi}\frac{I}{\ell} \times (2\pi)^2$$

Case (b) :

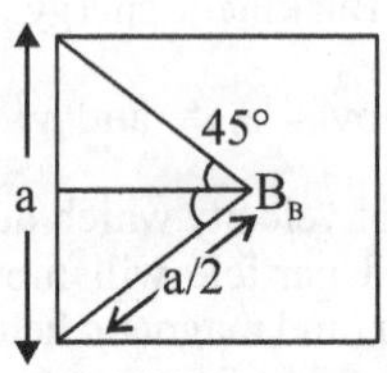

$$B_B = 4 \times \frac{\mu_0}{4\pi}\frac{I}{a/2}[\sin 45° + \sin 45°]$$

$$= 4 \times \frac{\mu_0}{4\pi} \times \frac{I}{\ell/8} \times \frac{2}{\sqrt{2}} = \frac{\mu_0}{4\pi}\frac{I}{\ell} \times 32 \times \sqrt{2} \qquad [4a = 1]$$

22. (d) Let us consider 'ℓ' length of current carrying wire.
At equilibrium
$T\cos\theta = \lambda g \ell$

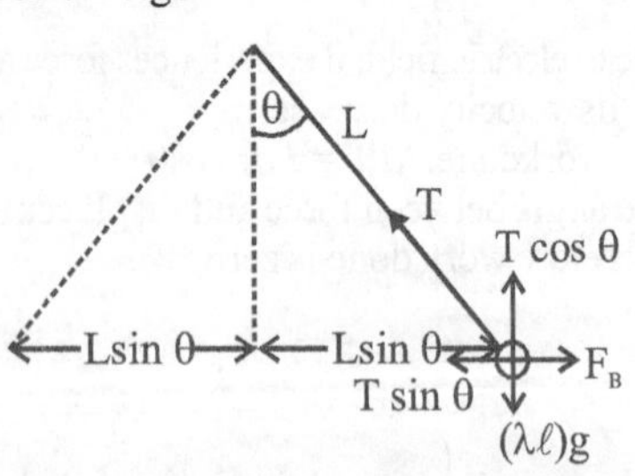

and $T\sin\theta = \frac{\mu_0}{2\pi}\frac{I \times I l}{2L\sin\theta} \quad \left[\because \frac{F_B}{\ell} = \frac{\mu_0}{4\pi}\frac{2I \times I}{2\ell\sin\theta}\right]$

Therefore, $I = 2\sin\theta\sqrt{\frac{\pi\lambda g L}{u_0\cos\theta}}$

23. (b) For loop $B = \frac{\mu_0 n I}{2a}$

where, a is the radius of loop.

Then, $B_1 = \frac{\mu_0 I}{2a}$

Now, for coil $B = \frac{\mu_0 I}{4\pi}.\frac{2nA}{x^3}$

at the centre x = radius of loop

$$B_2 = \frac{\mu_0}{4\pi}.\frac{2\times 3\times (I/3)\times \pi (a/3)^2}{(a/3)^3}$$

$$= \frac{\mu_0.3I}{2a}$$

$$\therefore \frac{B_1}{B_2} = \frac{\mu_0 I/2a}{\mu_0.3I/2a}$$

$$B_1 : B_2 = 1:3$$

24. (d) Magnetic field between the plates in this case is zero.

25. (a) Magnetic field at any point lies on axial position of current carrying conductor $B = 0$

26. (a) If magnetic field is perpendicular and into the plane of the paper, it is represented by cross ⊗ and if the direction of the magnetic field is perpendicular out of the plane of the paper it is represented by dot ⊙.

27. (b) Given : Radius = R

Distance $x = 2\sqrt{2}R$

$$\frac{B_{centre}}{B_{axis}} = \left(1 + \frac{x^2}{R^2}\right)^{3/2} = \left(1 + \frac{(2\sqrt{2}R)^2}{R^2}\right)^{3/2}$$

$$= (9)^{3/2} = 27$$

28. (a) The magnetic field due to a disc is given as

$$B = \frac{\mu_0 \omega Q}{2\pi R} \quad \text{i.e.,} \quad B \propto \frac{1}{R}$$

29. (d) Current in a small element, $dI = \frac{d\theta}{\pi} I$

Magnetic field due to the element

$$dB = \frac{\mu_0}{4\pi}\frac{2dI}{R}$$

The component $dB\cos\theta$, of the field is cancelled by another opposite component.
Therefore,

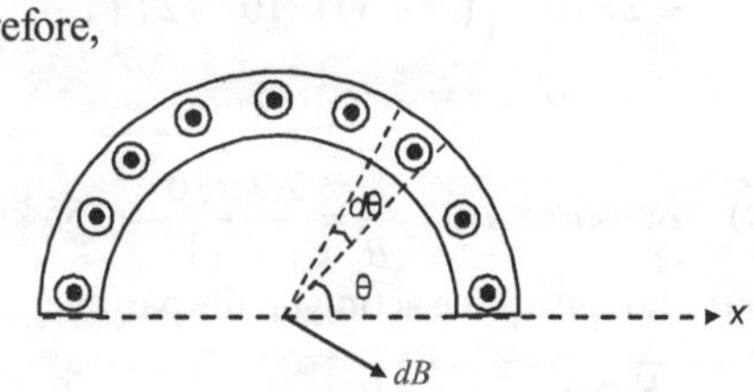

$$B_{net} = \int dB\sin\theta = \frac{\mu_0 I}{2\pi^2 R}\int_0^{\pi}\sin\theta d\theta = \frac{\mu_0 I}{\pi^2 R}$$

30. (a) The magnetic field varies inversely with the distance for a long conductor. That is, $B \propto \frac{1}{d}$

so, graph in option (a) is the correct one.

31. (c) The magnetic field is

$$B = \frac{\mu_0}{4\pi}\frac{2I}{r} = 10^{-7} \times \frac{2 \times 100}{4} = 5 \times 10^{-6}\ T$$

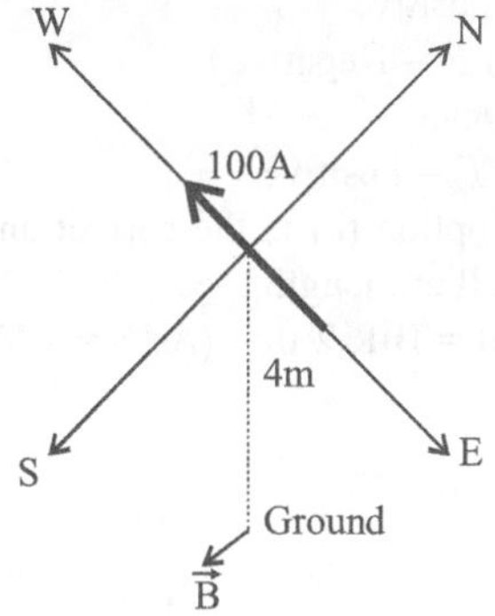

According to right hand palm rule, the magnetic field is directed towards south.

32. **(d)** Here, current is uniformly distributed across the cross-section of the wire, therefore, current enclosed in the amperean path formed at a distance $r_1\left(=\frac{a}{2}\right)$

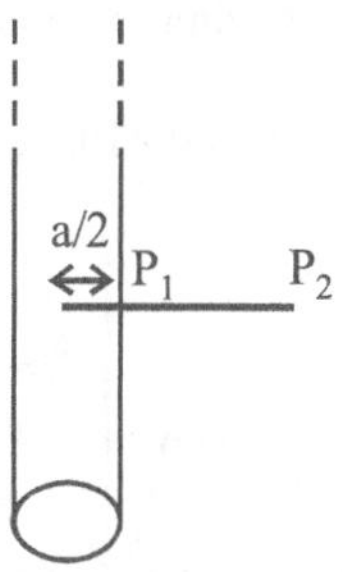

$=\left(\frac{\pi r_1^2}{\pi a^2}\right)\times I$, where I is total current

$\therefore$ Magnetic field at P_1 is

$$B_1=\frac{\mu_0\times\text{current enclosed}}{\text{Path}}$$

$$\Rightarrow B_1=\frac{\mu_0\times\left(\frac{\pi r_1^2}{\pi a^2}\right)\times I}{2\pi r_1}=\frac{\mu_0\times I r_1}{2\pi a^2}$$

Now, magnetic field at point P_2,

$$B_2=\frac{\mu_0}{2\pi}\cdot\frac{I}{(2a)}=\frac{\mu_0 I}{4\pi a}.$$

$$\therefore \text{Required ratio}=\frac{B_1}{B_2}=\frac{\mu_0 I r_1}{2\pi a^2}\times\frac{4\pi a}{\mu_0 I}$$

$$=\frac{2r_1}{a}=\frac{2\times\frac{a}{2}}{a}=1.$$

33. **(d)** There is no current inside the pipe. Therefore

$$\oint\vec{B}.\vec{d\ell}=\mu_o I$$

$I=0$

$\therefore B=0$

34. **(c)** Clearly, the magnetic fields at a point P, equidistant from AOB and COD will have directions perpendicular to each other, as they are placed normal to each other.

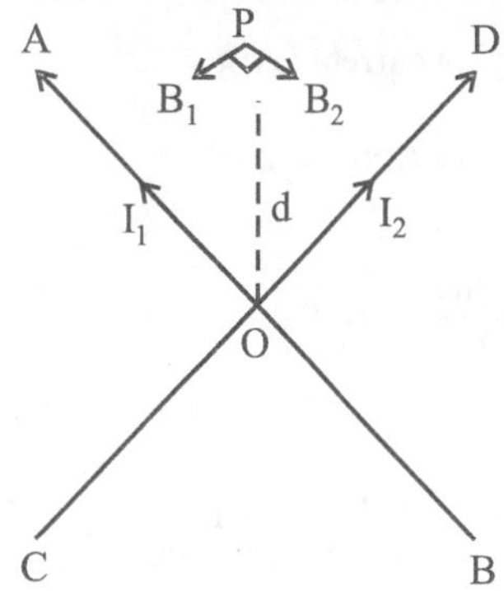

$\therefore$ Resultant field, $B=\sqrt{B_1^2+B_2^2}$

But $B_1=\frac{\mu_0 I_1}{2\pi d}$ and $B_2=\frac{\mu_0 I_2}{2\pi d}$

$$\therefore B=\sqrt{\left(\frac{\mu_0}{2\pi d}\right)^2\left(I_1^2+I_2^2\right)}$$

$$\text{or, } B=\frac{\mu_0}{2\pi d}\left(I_1^2+I_2^2\right)^{1/2}$$

35. **(a)** $\frac{B_2}{B_1}=\frac{\mu_0 n_2 i_2}{\mu_0 n_1 i_1}$

$$\Rightarrow\frac{B_2}{6.28\times10^{-2}}=\frac{100\times\frac{i}{3}}{200\times i}$$

$$\Rightarrow B_2=\frac{6.28\times10^{-2}}{6}=1.05\times10^{-2}\ \text{Wb/m}^2$$

36. **(d)**

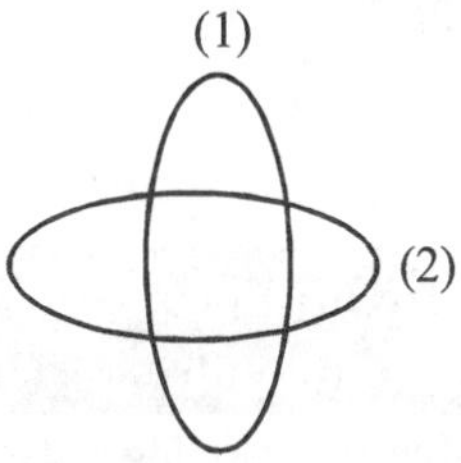

The magnetic field due to circular coil,

$$B_1=\frac{\mu_0 i_1}{2r}=\frac{\mu_0 i_1}{2(2\pi\times10^{-2})}=\frac{\mu_0\times3\times10^2}{4\pi}$$

$$B_2=\frac{\mu_0 i_2}{2(2\pi\times10^{-2})}=\frac{\mu_0\times4\times10^2}{4\pi}$$

$$B=\sqrt{B_1^2+B_2^2}=\frac{\mu_0}{4\pi}.5\times10^2$$

$$\Rightarrow B=10^{-7}\times5\times10^2$$

$$\Rightarrow B=5\times10^{-5}\ \text{Wb/m}^2$$

37. **(b)** Using Ampere's law at a distance r from axis, B is same from symmetry.

$\int\vec{B}.\vec{dl}=\mu_0 i$ i.e., $B\times2\pi r=\mu_0 i$

Here i is zero, for $r<R$, whereas R is the radius

$\therefore B=0$

38. (b) Magentic field at the centre of a circular coil of radius R carrying current i is $B=\frac{\mu_0 i}{2R}$

Given : $n\times(2\pi r')=2\pi R$

$\Rightarrow nr'=R$ ...(1)

$B'=\frac{n.\mu_0 i}{2r'}$ ...(2)

From (1) and (2), $B'=\frac{n\mu_0 i.n}{2\pi R}=n^2 B$

39. (c) The magnetic field at a point on the axis of a circular loop at a distance x from centre is,

$$B=\frac{\mu_0 i\, a^2}{2(x^2+a^2)^{3/2}}$$

$$B'=\frac{\mu_0 i}{2a}$$

$$\therefore\ B'=\frac{B.(x^2+a^2)^{3/2}}{a^3}$$

Put $x=4$ & $a=3\Rightarrow B'=\frac{54(5^3)}{3\times3\times3}=250\ \mu T$

40. (a) We know that the magnetic field produced by a current carrying circular coil of radius r at its centre is

$$B=\frac{\mu_0}{4\pi}\frac{I}{r}\times 2\pi$$

Here $B_A=\frac{\mu_0}{4\pi}\frac{I}{R}\times 2\pi$

and $B_B=\frac{\mu_0}{4\pi}\frac{2I}{2R}\times 2\pi$

$$\Rightarrow \frac{B_A}{B_B}=1$$

TOPIC - 3: Force and Torque on Current Carrying Conductor

41. (c) Magnetic moment of current carrying rectangular loop of area A is given by M = NIA

magnetic moment of current carrying coil is a vector and its direction is given by right hand thumb rule, for rectangular loop, $\vec{B}$ at centre due to current in loop and $\vec{M}$ are always parallel.

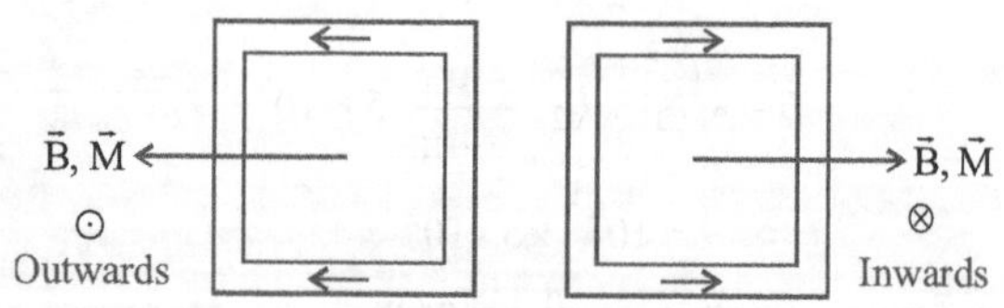

Hence, (c) corresponds to stable equilibrium.

42. (c) $\vec{F}_1=\vec{F}_2=0$

because of action and reaction pair

43. (a) For stable equilibrium $\vec{M}\,||\,\vec{B}$

For unstable equilibrium $\vec{M}\,||\,(-\vec{B})$

44. (a) $I_1 I_2$ = Positive
(attract) F = Negative
$I_1 I_2$= Negative
(repell) F = Positive
Hence, option (a) is the correct answer.

45. (c) For small arc length

$2T\sin\theta$ = BIR 2 θ (As F = BIL and L = RZθ)

T = BIR

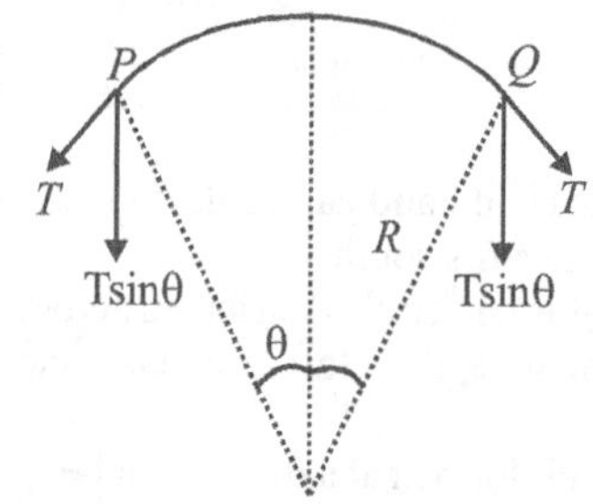

46. (b) Work done in moving the conductor is,

$$W=\int_0^2 F dx=\int_0^2 3.0\times10^{-4}e^{-0.2x}\times10\times3dx$$

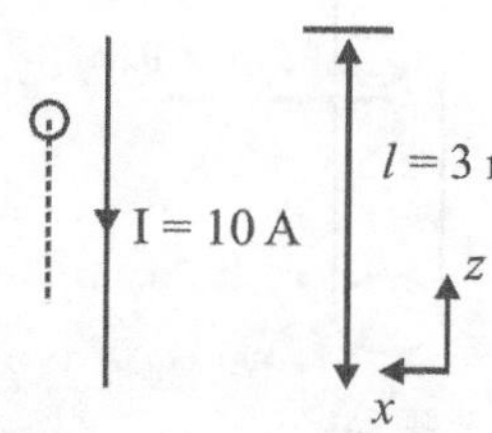

$$=9\times10^{-3}\int_0^2 e^{-0.2x}dx$$

$$=\frac{9\times10^{-3}}{0.2}[-e^{-0.2\times2}+1]$$

$B=3.0\times10^{-4}e^{-0.2x}$ (By exponential function)

$$=\frac{9\times10^{-3}}{0.2}\times[1-e^{-0.4}]$$

$=9\times10^{-3}\times(0.33)=2.97\times10^{-3}$J

Power required to move the conductor is,

$$P=\frac{W}{t}$$

$$P=\frac{2.97\times10^{-3}}{(0.2)\times5\times10^{-3}}=2.97\text{ W}$$

47. (a) I_1 = 30 A I = 10 A I_2 = 20 A

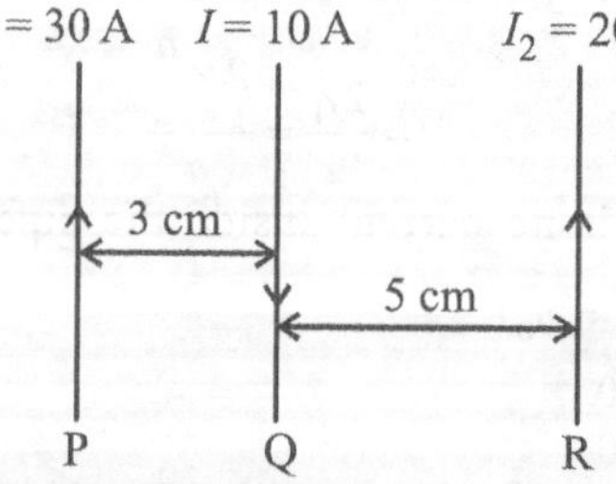

Also given; length of wire Q = 25 cm = 0.25 m

Force on wire Q due to wire R

$$F_{QR} = 10^{-7} \times \frac{2 \times 20 \times 10}{0.05} \times 0.25$$

$= 20 \times 10^{-5}$ N (Towards left)

Force on wire Q due to wire P

$$F_{QP} = 10^{-7} \times \frac{2 \times 30 \times 10}{0.03} \times 0.25$$

$= 50 \times 10^{-5}$ N (Towards right)

Hence, $F_{net} = F_{QP} - F_{QR}$

$= 50 \times 10^{-5}\,N - 20 \times 10^{-5}\,N$

$= 3 \times 10^{-4}$ N towards right

48. (c)

49. (a) Force acting on conductor B due to conductor A is given by relation

$$F = \frac{\mu_0 I_1 I_2 l}{2\pi r}$$

l-length of conductor B

r-distance between two conductors

$$\therefore F = \frac{4\pi \times 10^{-7} \times 10 \times 2 \times 2}{2 \times \pi \times 0.1} = 8 \times 10^{-5}\ N$$

50. (a)

51. (a) The magnetic field at O due to current in DA is

$$B_1 = \frac{\mu_o}{4\pi}\frac{I}{a} \times \frac{\pi}{6} \quad \text{(directed vertically upwards)}$$

The magnetic field at O due to current in BC is

$$B_2 = \frac{\mu_o}{4\pi}\frac{I}{b} \times \frac{\pi}{6} \quad \text{(directed vertically downwards)}$$

The magnetic field due to current AB and CD at O is zero.

Therefore the net magnetic field is

$B = B_1 - B_2$ (directed vertically upwards)

$$= \frac{\mu_o}{4\pi}\frac{I}{a}\frac{\pi}{6} - \frac{\mu_o}{4\pi}\frac{I}{b} \times \frac{\pi}{6}$$

$$= \frac{\mu_o I}{24}\left(\frac{1}{a} - \frac{1}{b}\right) = \frac{\mu_o I}{24ab}(b - a)$$

52. (d) $\vec{F} = I(\vec{\ell} \times \vec{B})$

The force on AD and BC due to current I_1 is zero. This is because the directions of current element $I\,\vec{d\ell}$ and magnetic field $\vec{B}$ are parallel.

53. (a) Force between two long conductor carrying current,

$$F = \frac{\mu_0}{4\pi}\frac{2I_1 I_2}{d} \times \ell$$

$$F' = -\frac{\mu_0}{4\pi}\frac{2(2I_1)I_2}{3d}\ell$$

$$\therefore \frac{F'}{F} = \frac{-2}{3}$$

54. (b) When current is passed through a spring then current flows parallel in the adjacent turns.

When two wires are placed parallel to each other and current flows in the same direction, the wires attract each other.

Similarly, here the various turns attract each other and the spring will compress.

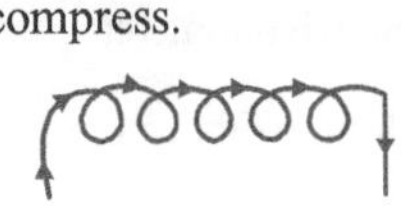

55. (c) Magnetic field due to current in wire 1 at point P distant r from the wire is

$$B = \frac{\mu_0}{4\pi}\frac{i_1}{r}[\cos\theta + \cos\theta]$$

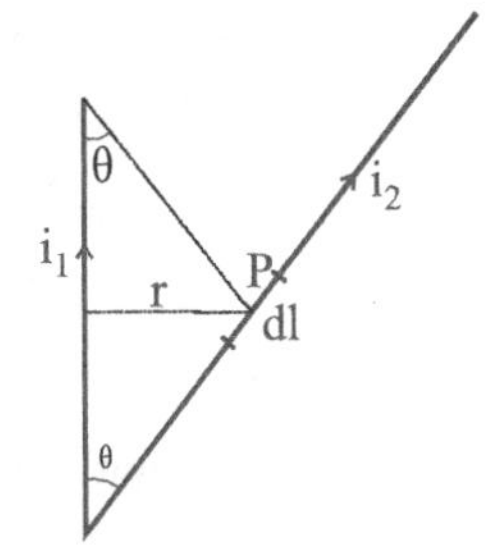

$B = \frac{\mu_0}{2\pi}\frac{i_1 \cos\theta}{r}$ (directed perpendicular to the plane of paper, inwards)

The force exerted due to this magnetic field on current element $i_2\,dl$ is

$dF = i_2\,dl\,B \sin 90°$

$\therefore dF = i_2\,dl$

$$\left[\frac{\mu_0}{2\pi}\frac{i_1 \cos\theta}{r}\right] = \frac{\mu_0}{2\pi r} i_1 i_2\,dl \cos\theta$$

TOPIC - 4: Galvanometer and its Conversion into Ammeter and Voltmeter

56. (c) Given : Current through the galvanometer,

$i_g = 5 \times 10^{-3}\,A$

Galvanometer resistance, $G = 15\,\Omega$

Let resistance R to be put in series with the galvanometer to convert it into a voltmeter.

$V = i_g(R + G)$

$10 = 5 \times 10^{-3}(R + 15)$

$\therefore\ R = 2000 - 15 = 1985$

$= 1.985 \times 10^3\,\Omega$

57. (c) $I_g G = (I - I_g)s$

$\therefore 10^{-3} \times 100 = (10 - 10^{-3}) \times S$

$\therefore S \approx 0.01\,\Omega$

58. (Incomplete question)

59. (d) As we know, $I = \frac{V}{R} = \frac{5}{50} = 0.1$

$I' = 0.099$

When Galvanometer is connected

$$R_{eq} = 50 + \frac{100S}{100 + S} = \frac{V}{I}$$

$$\Rightarrow \frac{100S}{100 + S} = \frac{5}{0.099} - 50$$

$\Rightarrow \frac{100S}{100+S} = 50.50 - 50 \Rightarrow \frac{100S}{100+S} = 0.5$

$\Rightarrow 100S = 50 + 0.5S \Rightarrow 99.5S = 50$

$S = \frac{50}{99.05} = 0.5\Omega$

So, shunt of resistance $= 0.5\Omega$ is connected in parallel with the galvanometer.

60. **(a)** According to Ohm's Law, $I = \frac{V}{R}$

$I_g = \frac{V}{R+G}$

where, I_g-Galvanometer current, G-Galvonometer resistance

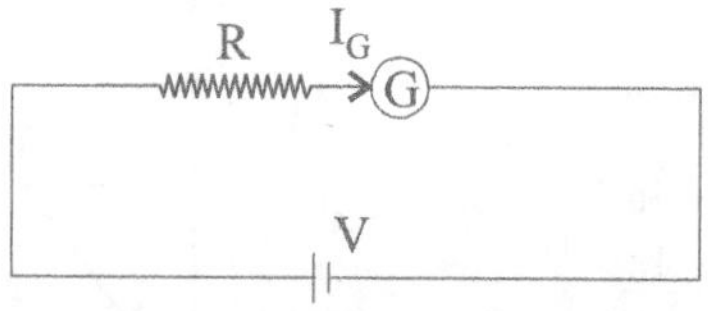

When shunt of resistance S is connected parallel to the Galvanometer then $G = \frac{GS}{G+S}$

$\therefore I = \frac{V}{R + \frac{GS}{G+S}}$

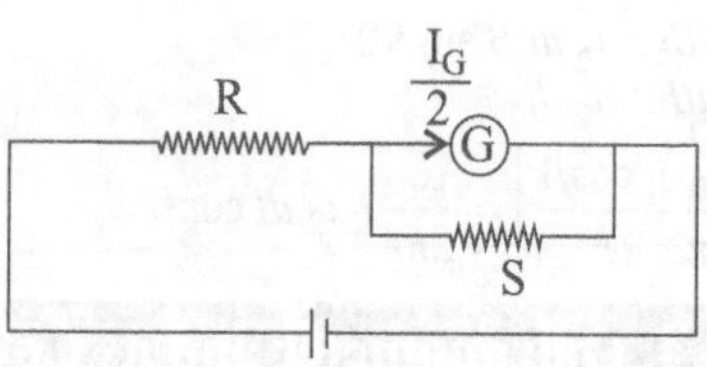

Equal potential difference is given by

$I'_g G = (I - I'_g)S$

$I'_g(G+S) = IS$

$\Rightarrow \frac{I_g}{2} = \frac{IS}{G+S}$

$\Rightarrow \frac{V}{2(R+G)} = \frac{V}{R + \frac{GS}{G+S}} \times \frac{S}{G+S}$

$\Rightarrow \frac{1}{2(R+G)} = \frac{S}{R(G+S)+GS}$

$\Rightarrow R(G+S) + GS = 2S(R+G)$

$\Rightarrow RG + RS + GS = 2S(R+G)$

$\Rightarrow RG = 2S(R+G) - S(R+G)$

$\therefore RG = S(R+G)$

61. **(b)** To measure AC voltage across a resistance a moving coil galvanometer is used.

62. **(d)** The correct circuit diagram is D with galvanometer resistance

$$G = \frac{RS}{R-S}$$

63. **(d)** Statements I is false and Statement II is true

For ammeter, shunt resistance, $S = \frac{IgG}{I - Ig}$

Therefore for I to increase, S should decrease, So additional S can be connected across it.

64. **(d)**

65. **(d)** The current that will given full scale deflection in the absence of the shunt is nearly equal to the current through the galvanometer when shunt is connected i.e. I_g

As $I_g = \frac{IS}{G+S}$

$= \frac{5.5 \times 1}{120+1} = 0.045$ ampere.

66. **(a)**

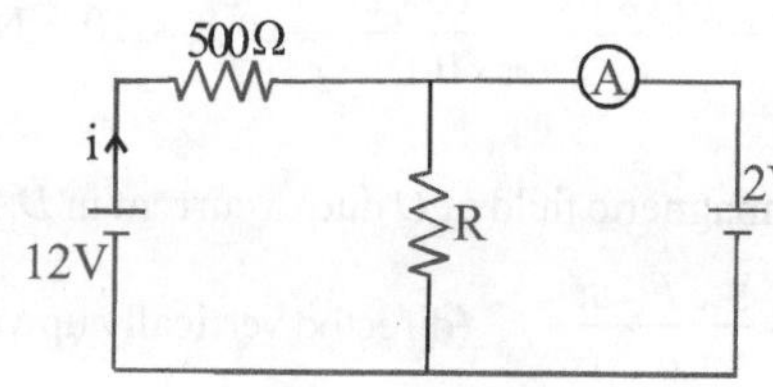

$12 - 2 = (500\Omega)i \Rightarrow i = \frac{10}{500} = \frac{1}{50}$

Again, $i = \frac{12}{500+R} = \frac{1}{50}$

$\Rightarrow 500 + R = 600$

$\Rightarrow R = 100\Omega$

67. **(c)** Resistance of Galvanometer,

$G = \frac{\text{Current sensitivity}}{\text{Voltage sensitivity}} \Rightarrow G = \frac{10}{2} = 5\Omega$

Here i_g = Full scale deflection current $= \frac{150}{10} = 15$ mA

V = voltage to be measured = 150 volts

(such that each division reads 1 volt)

$\Rightarrow R = \frac{150}{15 \times 10^{-3}} - 5 = 9995\Omega$

Chapter 19

Magnetism and Matter

TOPIC - 1: Magnetism, Gauss's Law, Magnetic Moment, Properties of Magnet

1. A magnetic dipole in a constant magnetic field has : **[Online April 8, 2017]**
   (a) maximum potential energy when the torque is maximum.
   (b) zero potential energy when the torque is minimum.
   (c) zero potential energy when the torque is maximum.
   (d) minimum potential energy when the torque is maximum.

2. A magnetic dipole is acted upon by two magnetic fields which are inclined to each other at an angle of 75°. One of the fields has a magnitude of 15 mT. The dipole attains stable equilibrium at an angle of 30° with this field. The magntidue of the other field (in mT) is close to : **[Online April 9, 2016]**
   (a) 1 (b) 11 (c) 36 (d) 1060

3. A 25 cm long solenoid has radius 2 cm and 500 total number of turns. It carries a current of 15 A. If it is equivalent to a magnet of the same size and magnetization $\vec{M}$ (magnetic moment/volume), then $|\vec{M}|$ is : **[Online April 10, 2015]**
   (a) $30000\pi \text{ Am}^{-1}$ (b) $3\pi \text{ Am}^{-1}$
   (c) 30000 Am^{-1} (d) 300 Am^{-1}

4. A bar magnet of length 6 cm has a magnetic moment of 4 J T^{-1}. Find the strength of magnetic field at a distance of 200 cm from the centre of the magnet along its equatorial line. **[Online May 7, 2012]**
   (a) 4×10^{-8} tesla (b) 3.5×10^{-8} tesla
   (c) 5×10^{-8} tesla (d) 3×10^{-8} tesla

5. A thin circular disc of radius R is uniformly charged with density $\sigma > 0$ per unit area. The disc rotates about its axis with a uniform angular speed ω. The magnetic moment of the disc is **[2011 RS]**
   (a) $\pi R^4 \sigma\omega$ (b) $\frac{\pi R^4}{2}\sigma\omega$
   (c) $\frac{\pi R^4}{4}\sigma\omega$ (d) $2\pi R^4 \sigma\omega$

6. A magnetic needle is kept in a non-uniform magnetic field. It experiences **[2005]**
   (a) neither a force nor a torque
   (b) a torque but not a force
   (c) a force but not a torque
   (d) a force and a torque

7. The length of a magnet is large compared to its width and breadth. The time period of its oscillation in a vibration magnetometer is 2s. The magnet is cut along its length into three equal parts and these parts are then placed on each other with their like poles together. The time period of this combination will be **[2004]**
   (a) $2\sqrt{3}$ s (b) $\frac{2}{3}$ s (c) 2 s (d) $\frac{2}{\sqrt{3}}$ s

8. A magnetic needle lying parallel to a magnetic field requiers W units of work to turn it through 60^0. The torque needed to maintain the needle in this position will be **[2003]**
   (a) $\sqrt{3}$W (b) W (c) $\frac{\sqrt{3}}{2}$W (d) 2W

9. The magnetic lines of force inside a bar magnet **[2003]**
   (a) are from north-pole to south-pole of the magnet
   (b) do not exist
   (c) depend upon the area of cross-section of the bar magnet
   (d) are from south-pole to north-pole of the Magnet

TOPIC - 2: The Earth Magnetism, Magnetic Materials and their properties

10. Hysteresis loops for two magnetic materials A and B are given below :

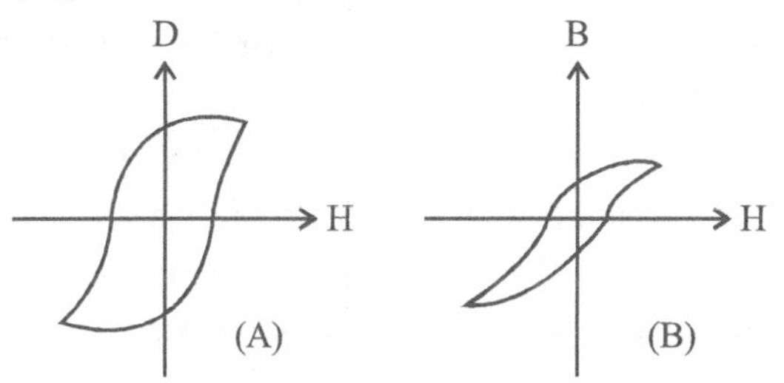

These materials are used to make magnets for elecric generators, transformer core and electromagnet core. Then it is proper to use : **[2016]**
   (a) A for transformers and B for electric generators.
   (b) B for electromagnets and transformers.
   (c) A for electric generators and trasformers.
   (d) A for electromagnets and B for electric generators.

11. A fighter plane of length 20 m, wing span (distance from tip of one wing to the tip of the other wing) of 15m and height 5m is lying towards east over Delhi. Its speed is 240 ms^{-1}. The earth's magnetic field over Delhi is 5×10^{-5}T with the declination angle ~0° and dip of θ such that $\sin\theta = \frac{2}{3}$. If the voltage developed is V_B between the lower and upper side of the plane and V_W between the tips of the wings then V_B and V_W are close to : **[Online April 10, 2016]**
(a) V_B = 40 mV; V_W = 135 mV with left side of pilot at higher voltage
(b) V_B = 45 mV; V_W = 120 mV with right side of pilot at higher voltage
(c) V_B = 40 mV; V_W = 135 mV with right side of pilot at higher voltage
(d) V_B = 45 mV; V_W = 120 mV with left side of pilot at higher voltage

12. A short bar magnet is placed in the magnetic meridian of the earth with north pole pointing north. Neutral points are found at a distance of 30 cm from the magnet on the East – West line, drawn through the middle point of the magnet. The magnetic moment of the magnet in Am^2 is close to: (Given $\frac{\mu_0}{4\pi} = 10^{-7}$ in SI units and B_H =Horizontal component of earth's magnetic field = 3.6×10^{-5} tesla) **[Online April 11, 2015]**
(a) 14.6 (b) 19.4 (c) 9.7 (d) 4.9

13. The coercivity of a small magnet where the ferromagnet gets demagnetized is $3\times10^3 Am^{-1}$. The current required to be passed in a solenoid of length 10 cm and number of turns 100, so that the magnet gets demagnetized when inside the solenoid, is: **[2014]**
(a) 30 mA (b) 60 mA (c) 3 A (d) 6 A

14. An example of a perfect diamagnet is a superconductor. This implies that when a superconductor is put in a magnetic field of intensity B, the magnetic field B_s inside the superconductor will be such that: **[Online April 19, 2014]**
(a) $B_s = -B$ (b) $B_s = 0$
(c) $B_s = B$ (d) $B_s < B$ but $Bs \neq 0$

15. Three identical bars A, B and C are made of different magnetic materials. When kept in a uniform magnetic field, the field lines around them look as follows:

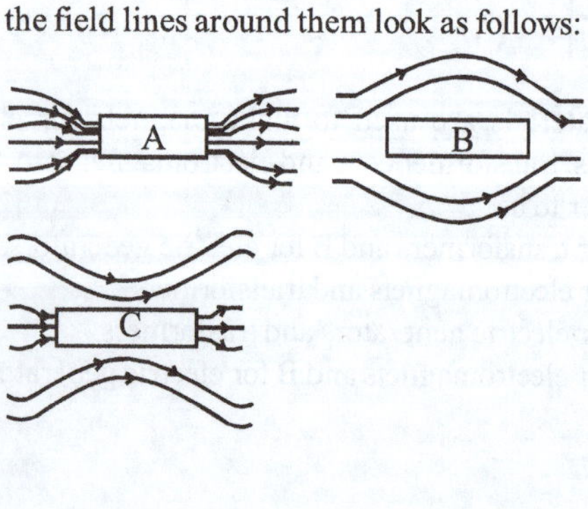

Make the correspondence of these bars with their material being diamagnetic (D), ferromagnetic (F) and paramagnetic (P): **[Online April 11, 2014]**
(a) $A \leftrightarrow D, B \leftrightarrow P, C \leftrightarrow F$
(b) $A \leftrightarrow F, B \leftrightarrow D, C \leftrightarrow P$
(c) $A \leftrightarrow P, B \leftrightarrow F, C \leftrightarrow D$
(d) $A \leftrightarrow F, B \leftrightarrow P, C \leftrightarrow D$

16. The magnetic field of earth at the equator is approximately 4×10^{-5} T. The radius of earth is 6.4×10^6 m. Then the dipole moment of the earth will be nearly of the order of: **[Online April 9, 2014]**
(a) 10^{23} A m^2 (b) 10^{20} A m^2
(c) 10^{16} A m^2 (d) 10^{10} A m^2

17. The mid points of two small magnetic dipoles of length d in end-on positions, are separated by a distance x, (x > > d). The force between them is proportional to x^{-n} where n is: **[Online April 9, 2014]**

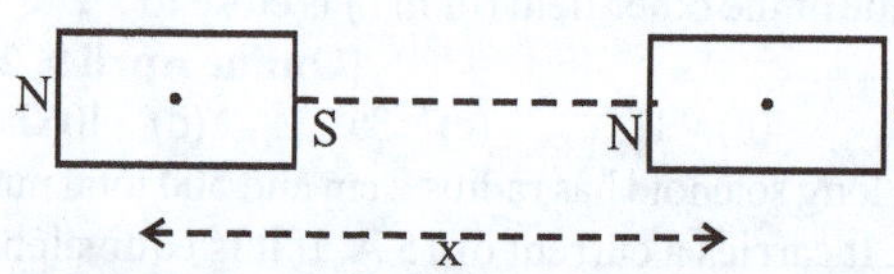

(a) 1 (b) 2 (c) 3 (d) 4

18. Two short bar magnets of length 1 cm each have magnetic moments 1.20 Am^2 and 1.00 Am^2 respectively. They are placed on a horizontal table parallel to each other with their N poles pointing towards the South. They have a common magnetic equator and are separated by a distance of 20.0 cm. The value of the resultand horizontal magnetic induction at the mid-point O of the line joining their centres is close to (Horizontal component of earth.s magnetic induction is 3.6× 10.5Wb/m^2) **[2013]**
(a) 3.6 × 10.5 Wb/m^2 (b) 2.56 × 10.4 Wb/m^2
(c) 3.50 × 10.4 Wb/m^2 (d) 5.80 × 10.4 Wb/m^2

19. The earth's magnetic field lines resemble that of a dipole at the centre of the earth. If the magnetic moment of this dipole is close to 8×10^{22} Am^2, the value of earth's magnetic field near the equator is close to (radius of the earth = 6.4×10^6 m) **[Online April 25, 2013]**
(a) 0.6 Gauss (b) 1.2 Gauss
(c) 1.8 Gauss (d) 0.32 Gauss

20. Relative permittivity and permeability of a material ε_r and μ_r, respectively. Which of the following values of these quantities are allowed for a diamagnetic material? **[2008]**
(a) $\varepsilon_r = 0.5, \mu_r = 1.5$ (b) $\varepsilon_r = 1.5, \mu_r = 0.5$
(c) $\varepsilon_r = 0.5, \mu_r = 0.5$ (d) $\varepsilon_r = 1.5, \mu_r = 1.5$

21. Needles N_1, N_2 and N_3 are made of a ferromagnetic, a paramagnetic and a diamagnetic substance respectively. A magnet when brought close to them will **[2006]**
   (a) attract N_1 and N_2 strongly but repel N_3
   (b) attract N_1 strongly, N_2 weakly and repel N_3 weakly
   (c) attract N_1 strongly, but repel N_2 and N_3 weakly
   (d) attract all three of them

22. The materials suitable for making electromagnets should have **[2004]**
   (a) high retentivity and low coercivity
   (b) low retentivity and low coercivity
   (c) high retentivity and high coercivity
   (d) low retentivity and high coercivity

23. A thin rectangular magnet suspended freely has a period of oscillation equal to T. Now it is broken into two equal halves (each having half of the original length) and one piece is made to oscillate freely in the same field. If its period of oscillation is T', the ratio $\frac{T'}{T}$ is **[2003]**
   (a) $\frac{1}{2\sqrt{2}}$ (b) $\frac{1}{2}$
   (c) 2 (d) $\frac{1}{4}$

24. Curie temperature is the temperature above which **[2003]**
   (a) a ferromagnetic material becomes paramagnetic
   (b) a paramagnetic material becomes diamagnetic
   (c) a ferromagnetic material becomes diamagnetic
   (d) a paramagnetic material becomes ferromagnetic

TOPIC - 3: Magnetic Equipment

25. A magnetic needle of magnetic moment 6.7×10^{-2} Am^2 and moment of inertia 7.5×10^{-6} kg m^2 is performing simple harmonic oscillations in a magnetic field of 0.01 T. Time taken for 10 complete oscillations is : **[2017]**
   (a) 6.98 s (b) 8.76 s
   (c) 6.65 s (d) 8. 89 s

Hints & Solutions

TOPIC - 1: Magnetism, Gauss's Law, Magnetic Moment, Properties of Magnet

1. (c) Potential energy of dipole,
$U = -pE\cos\theta$
Torque experienced by dipole
$\tau = pE\sin\theta$
Torque will be maximum (τ_{max}) when $\theta = 90°$ then potential energy $U = 0$

2. (b) We know that, magnetic dipole moment
$M = NiA\cos\theta$ i.e., $M \propto \cos\theta$
When two magnetic fields are inclined at an angle of 75° the equilibrium will be at 30°, so
$$\cos\theta = \cos(75° - 30°) = \cos 45° = \frac{1}{\sqrt{2}}$$
$$\frac{x}{\sqrt{2}} = \frac{15}{2} \therefore x \approx 11$$

3. (c) $\vec{M}$ (mag. moment/volume) $= \frac{NiA}{A\ell}$
$$= \frac{Ni}{\ell} = \frac{(500)15}{25\times10^{-2}} = 30000\ \text{Am}^{-1}$$

4. (c) Along the equatorial line, magnetic field strength
$$B = \frac{\mu_0}{4\pi}\frac{M}{\left(r^2+\ell^2\right)^{3/2}}$$
Given: $M = 4JT^{-1}$
$r = 200\ \text{cm} = 2\ \text{m}$
$$\ell = \frac{6\text{cm}}{2} = 3\ \text{cm} = 3\times10^{-2}\ \text{m}$$
$$\therefore B = \frac{4\pi\times10^{-7}}{4\pi}\times\frac{4}{\left[2^2+\left(3\times10^{-2}\right)^2\right]^{3/2}}$$
Solving we get, $B = 5\times10^{-8}$ tesla

5. (c) $\frac{q}{2m} = \frac{\text{Magnetic dipole moment}}{\text{Angular momentum}}$

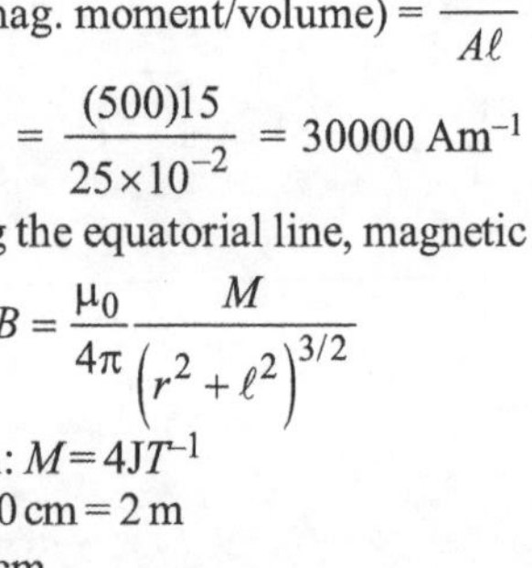

$\therefore$ Magnetic dipole moment (M)
$$M = \frac{q}{2m}\cdot\left(\frac{mR^2}{2}\right).\omega = \frac{1}{4}\sigma.\pi R^4\omega.$$

6. (d) A magnetic needle kept in non uniform magnetic field experience a force and torque due to unequal forces acting on poles.

7. (b) $T = 2\pi\sqrt{\frac{I}{M\times B}} = 2\pi\sqrt{\frac{I}{MB}}$ where $I = \frac{1}{12}m\ell^2$
When the magnet is cut into three pieces the pole strength will remain the same and
$$\text{M.I. } (I') = \frac{1}{12}\left(\frac{m}{3}\right)\left(\frac{\ell}{3}\right)\times 3 = \frac{I}{9}$$
We have, Magnetic moment (M)
= Pole strength (m) × ℓ
$\therefore$ New magnetic moment,
$$M' = m\times\left(\frac{\ell}{3}\right)\times 3 = m\ell = M$$
$$\therefore T' = \frac{T}{\sqrt{9}} = \frac{2}{3}s.$$

8. (a) $W = MB(\cos\theta_1 - \cos\theta_2)$
$= MB(\cos 0° - \cos 60°)$
$= MB(1 - \frac{1}{2}) = \frac{MB}{2}$
$$\therefore \tau = MB\sin\theta = MB\sin 60° = \sqrt{3}\frac{MB}{2} = \sqrt{3}W$$

9. (d) As shown in the figure, the magnetic lines of force are directed from south to north inside a bar magnet.

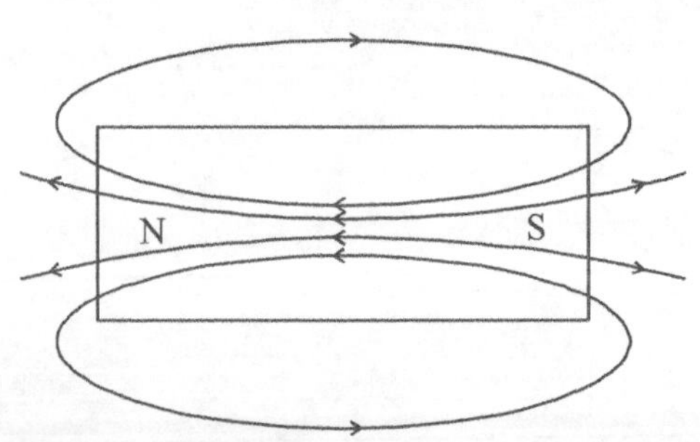

TOPIC - 2: The Earth Magnetism, Magnetic Materials and their properties

10. (b) Graph [A] is for material used for making permanent magnets (high coercivity)
Graph [B] is for making electromagnets and transformers.

11. (d) $V_B = VB_H l = 240\times5\times10^{-5}\cos(\theta)\times5 = 44.7$ mv
By right hand rule, the charge moves to the left of pilot.

12. (c) Here, r = 30cm = 0.3cm

we know $\frac{\mu_0 M}{4\pi r^3} = B_H = 3.6\times10^{-5}$

$\Rightarrow M = \frac{3.6\times10^{-5}}{10^{-7}}(0.3)^3$

Hence, M = 9.7 Am^2

13. (c) Magnetic field in solenoid $B = \mu_0 n\, i$

$\Rightarrow \frac{B}{\mu_0} = ni$

(Where n = number of turns per unit length)

$\Rightarrow \frac{B}{\mu_0} = \frac{Ni}{L}$

$\Rightarrow 3\times10^3 = \frac{100i}{10\times10^{-2}}$

$\Rightarrow i = 3A$

14. (b) Magnetic field inside the superconductor is zero. Diamagnetic substances are repelled in external magnetic field.

15. (b) Diamagnetic materials are repelled in an external magnetic field.
Bar B represents diamagnetic materials.

16. (a) Given, $B = 4\times10^{-5}$ T
$R_E = 6.4\times10^6$ m
Dipole moment of the earth M = ?

$B = \frac{\mu_0}{4\pi}\frac{M}{d^3}$

$4\times10^{-5} = \frac{4\pi\times10^{-7}\times M}{4\pi\times\left(6.4\times10^6\right)^3}$

$\therefore$ $M \cong 10^{23}$ Am^2

17. (d) In magnetic dipole

Force $\propto \frac{1}{r^4}$

In the given question,
Force $\propto x^{-n}$
Hence, n = 4

18. (b) **Given :** $M_1 = 1.20 Am^2$

$M_2 = 1.00 Am^2$

$r = \frac{20}{2} cm = 0.1$ m

$B_{net} = B_1 + B_2 + B_H$

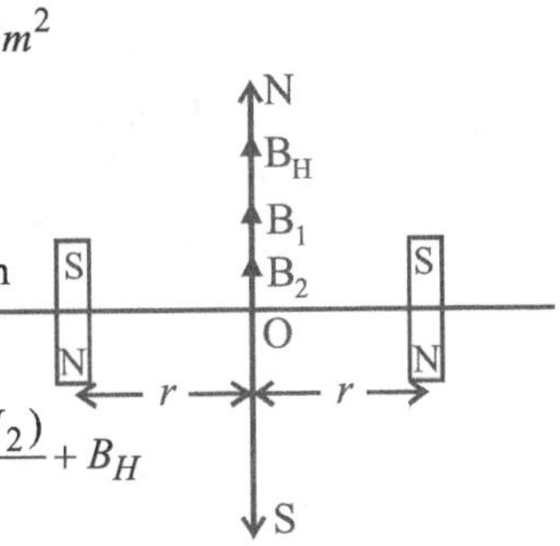

$B_{net} = \frac{\mu_0}{4\pi}\frac{(M_1 + M_2)}{r^3} + B_H$

$= \frac{10^{-7}(1.2+1)}{(0.1)^3} + 3.6\times10^{-5} = 2.56\times10^{-4}$ wb/m^2

19. (a) Given $M = 8\times10^{22}$ Am^2
$d = R_e = 6.4\times10^6$m

Earth's magnetic field, $B = \frac{\mu_0}{4\pi}\cdot\frac{2M}{d^3}$

$= \frac{4\pi\times10^{-7}}{4\pi}\times\frac{2\times8\times10^{22}}{(6.4\times10^6)^3} \cong 0.6$ Gauss

20. (b) For a diamagnetic material, the value of μ_r is less than one. For any material, the value of ϵ_r is always greater than 1.

21. (b) Ferromagnetic substance has magnetic domains whereas paramagnetic substances have magnetic dipoles which get attracted to a magnetic field. Diamagnetic substances do not have magnetic dipole but in the presence of external magnetic field due to their orbital motion of electrons these substances are repelled.

22. (b) Electromagnet should be amenable to magnetisation & demagnetization.
$\therefore$ retentivity & coercivity should be low.

23. (b) The time period of a rectangular magnet oscillating in earth's magnetic field is given by $T = 2\pi\sqrt{\frac{I}{\mu B_H}}$

where I = Moment of inertia of the rectangular magnet
μ = Magnetic moment
B_H = Horizontal component of the earth's magnetic field

Case 1

$T = 2\pi\sqrt{\frac{I}{\mu B_H}}$ where $I = \frac{1}{12}M\ell^2$

Case 2

Magnet is cut into two identical pieces such that each piece has half the original length. Then

$T' = 2\pi\sqrt{\frac{I'}{\mu' B_H}}$

where $I' = \frac{1}{12}\left(\frac{M}{2}\right)\left(\frac{\ell}{2}\right)^2 = \frac{I}{8}$ and $\mu' = \frac{\mu}{2}$

$\therefore \frac{T'}{T} = \sqrt{\frac{I'}{\mu'}\times\frac{\mu}{I}}$

$= \sqrt{\frac{I/8}{\mu/2}\times\frac{\mu}{I}} = \sqrt{\frac{1}{4}} = \frac{1}{2}$

24. (a) The temperature above which a ferromagnetic substance becomes paramagnetic is called Curie's temperature.

TOPIC - 3: Magnetic Equipment

25. (c) Given : Magnetic moment, $M = 6.7\times10^{-2}$ Am^2
Magnetic field, B = 0.01 T
Moment of inertia, $I = 7.5\times10^{-6}$ Kgm^2

Using, $T = 2\pi\sqrt{\frac{I}{MB}}$

$= 2\pi\sqrt{\frac{7.5\times10^{-6}}{6.7\times10^{-2}\times0.01}} = \frac{2\pi}{10}\times1.06 s$

Time taken for 10 complete oscillations
$t = 10T = 2\pi\times1.06$
$= 6.6568 \approx 6.65$ s

Chapter 20

Electromagnetic Induction

TOPIC - 1: Magnetic Flux, Faraday's and Lenz's Law

1. In a coil of resistance $100\,\Omega$, a current is induced by changing the magnetic flux through it as shown in the figure. The magnitude of change in flux through the coil is **[2017]**

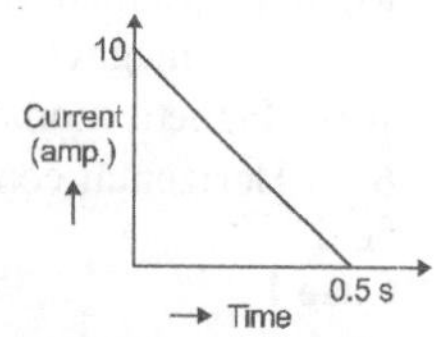

(a) 250 Wb
(b) 275 Wb
(c) 200 Wb
(d) 225 Wb

2. A conducting metal circular–wire–loop of radius r is placed perpendicular to a magnetic field which varies with time as $B = B_0 e^{-t/\tau}$, where B_0 and τ are constants, at time t = 0. If the resistance of the loop is R then the heat generated in the loop after a long time $(t \to \infty)$ is;

[Online April 10, 2016]

(a) $\dfrac{\pi^2 r^4 B_0^4}{2\tau R}$ (b) $\dfrac{\pi^2 r^4 B_0^2}{2\tau R}$

(c) $\dfrac{\pi^2 r^4 B_0^2 R}{\tau}$ (d) $\dfrac{\pi^2 r^4 B_0^2}{\tau R}$

3. When current in a coil changes from 5 A to 2 A in 0.1 s, average voltage of 50 V is produced. The self - inductance of the coil is : **[Online April 10, 2015]**

(a) 6 H (b) 0.67 H
(c) 3 H (d) 1.67 H

4. Figure shows a circular area of radius R where a uniform magnetic field $\vec{B}$ is going into the plane of paper and increasing in magnitude at a constant rate.

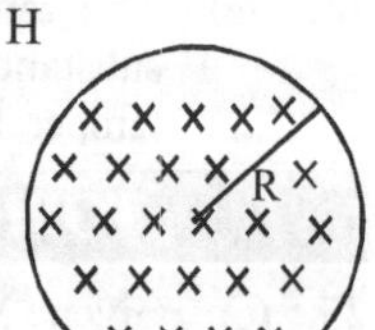

In that case, which of the following graphs, drawn schematically, correctly shows the variation of the induced electric field E(r)? **[Online April 19, 2014]**

(a)
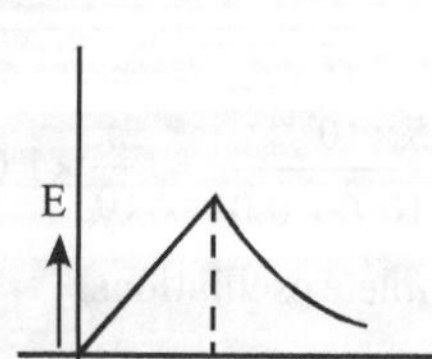

(b)
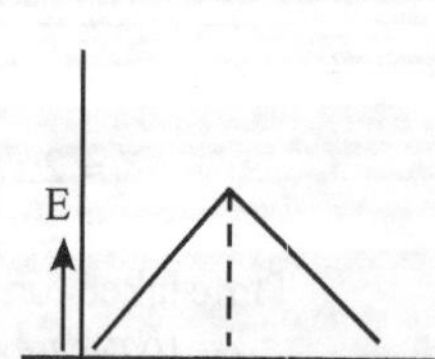

(c)
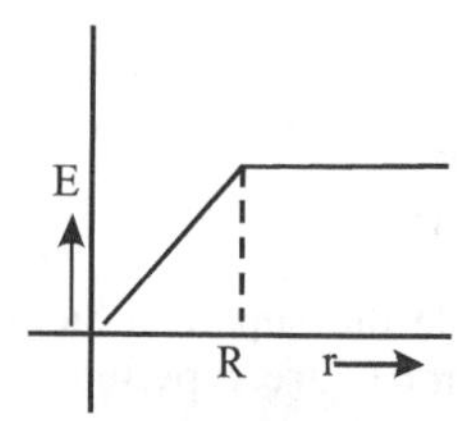

(d)
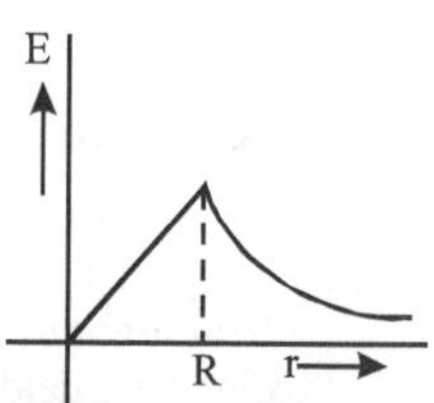

5. A coil of circular cross-section having 1000 turns and 4 cm^2 face area is placed with its axis parallel to a magnetic field which decreases by 10^{-2} Wb m^{-2} in 0.01 s. The e.m.f. induced in the coil is: **[Online April 11, 2014]**

(a) 400mV (b) 200mV
(c) 4mV (d) 0.4mV

6. A circular loop of radius 0.3 cm lies parallel to amuch bigger circular loop of radius 20 cm. The centre of the small loop is on the axis of the bigger loop. The distance between their centres is 15 cm. If a current of 2.0 A flows through the smaller loop, then the flux linked with bigger loop is **[2013]**

(a) 9.1×10^{-11} weber (b) 6×10^{-11} weber
(c) 3.3×10^{-11} weber (d) 6.6×10^{-9} weber

7. Two coils, X and Y, are kept in close vicinity of each other. When a varying current, $I(t)$, flows through coil X, the induced emf ($V(t)$) in coil Y, varies in the manner shown here. The variation of $I(t)$, with time, can then be represented by the graph labelled as graph : **[Online April 9, 2013]**

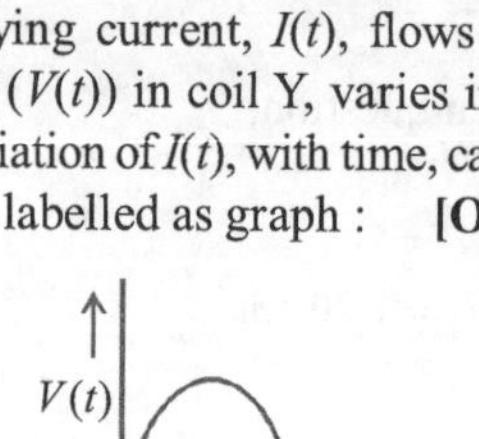

(A)
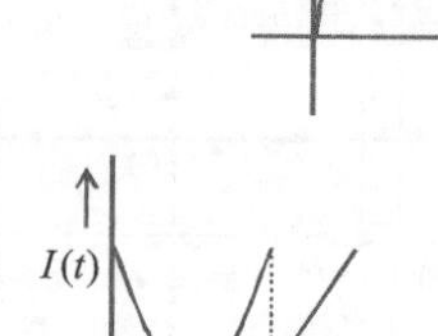

(B)
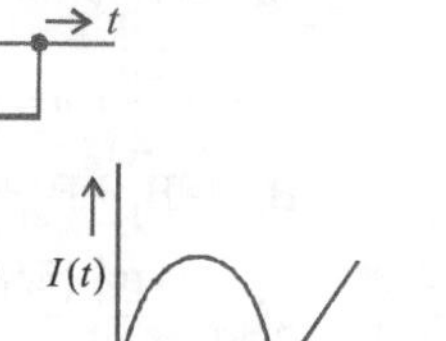

(C)
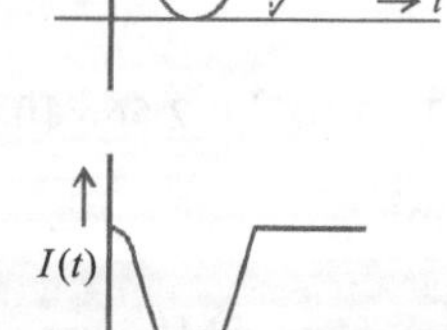

(D)
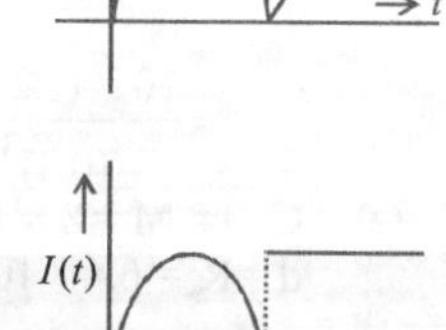

(a) A (b) C
(c) B (d) D

8. A coil is suspended in a uniform magnetic field, with the plane of the coil parallel to the magnetic lines of force. When a current is passed through the coil it starts oscillating; It is very difficult to stop. But if an aluminium plate is placed near to the coil, it stops. This is due to : **[2012]**
   (a) developement of air current when the plate is placed
   (b) induction of electrical charge on the plate
   (c) shielding of magnetic lines of force as aluminium is a paramagnetic material.
   (d) electromagnetic induction in the aluminium plate giving rise to electromagnetic damping.

9. Magnetic flux through a coil of resistance 10 Ω is changed by $\Delta\phi$ in 0.1 s. The resulting current in the coil varies with time as shown in the figure. Then $|\Delta\phi|$ is equal to (in weber) **[Online May 12, 2012]**

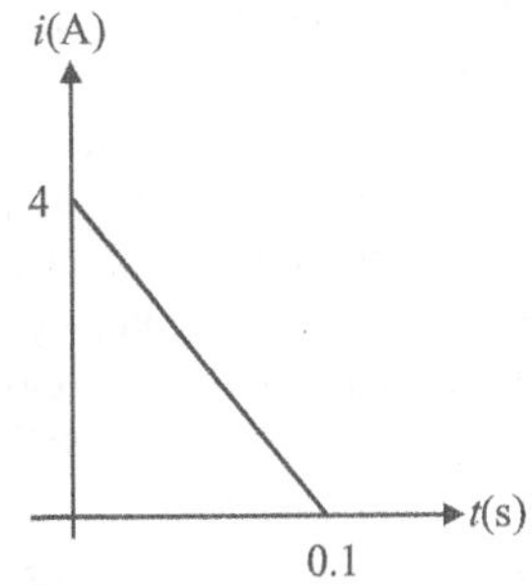

   (a) 6 (b) 4
   (c) 2 (d) 8

10. The flux linked with a coil at any instant 't' is given by $\phi = 10t^2 - 50t + 250$. The induced emf at $t = 3s$ is **[2006]**
   (a) –190 V (b) –10 V
   (c) 10 V (d) 190 V

TOPIC - 2: Motional and Static EMI and Application of EMI

11. A square frame of side 10 cm and a long straight wire carrying current 1 A are in the plate of the paper. Starting from close to the wire, the frame moves towards the right with a constant speed of 10 ms^{-1} (see figure).

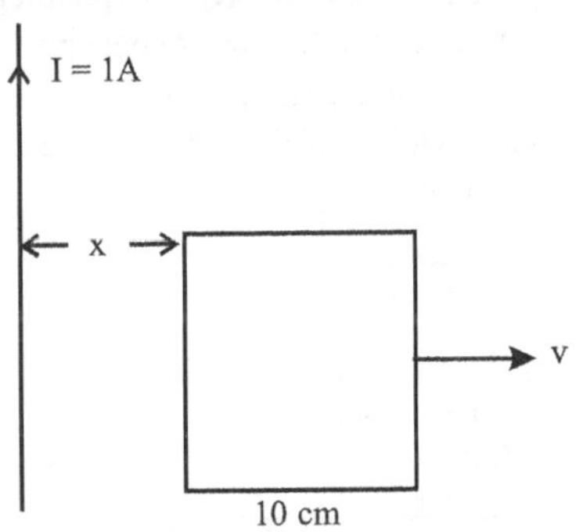

The e.m.f induced at the time the left arm of the frame is at x = 10 cm from the wire is: **[Online April 19, 2014]**
   (a) 2 μV (b) 1 μV
   (c) 0.75 μV (d) 0.5 μV

12. A metallic rod of length 'ℓ' is tied to a string of length 2ℓ and made to rotate with angular speed ω on a horizontal table with one end of the string fixed. If there is a vertical magnetic field 'B' in the region, the e.m.f. induced across the ends of the rod is **[2013]**

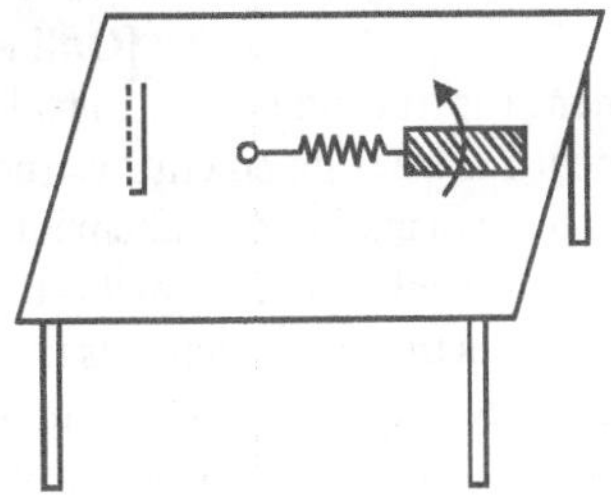

   (a) $\frac{2B\omega\ell^2}{2}$ (b) $\frac{3B\omega\ell^2}{2}$
   (c) $\frac{4B\omega\ell^2}{2}$ (d) $\frac{5B\omega\ell^2}{2}$

13. A coil of self inductance L is connected at one end of two rails as shown in figure. A connector of length l, mass m can slide freely over the two parallel rails. The entire set up is placed in a magnetic field of induction B going into the page. At an instant $t = 0$ an initial velocity v_0 is imparted to it and as a result of that it starts moving along x-axis. The displacement of the connector is represented by the figure. **[Online May 19, 2012]**

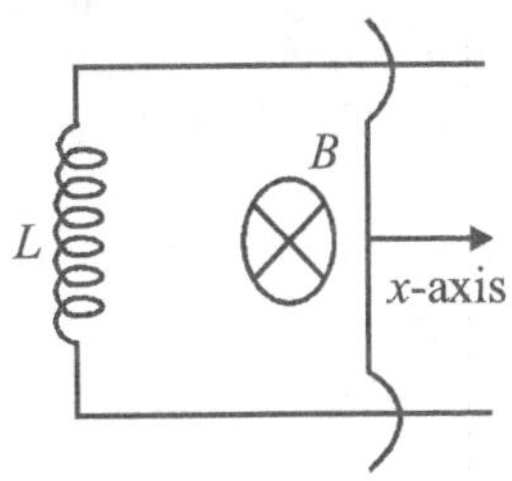

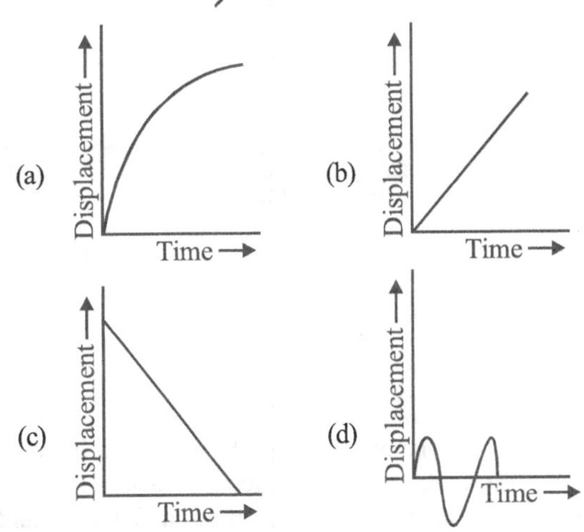

14. This question has Statement 1 and Statement 2. Of the four choices given after the Statements, choose the one that best describes the two Statements.
Statement 1: Self inductance of a long solenoid of length L, total number of turns N and radius r is less than $\frac{\pi\mu_0 N^2 r^2}{L}$.
Statement 2: The magnetic induction in the solenoid in

Statement 1 carrying current I is $\frac{\mu_0 NI}{L}$ in the middle of the solenoid but becomes less as we move towards its ends. **[Online May 19, 2012]**

(a) Statement 1 is true, Statement 2 is false.
(b) Statement 1 is true, Statement 2 is true, Statement 2 is the correct explanation of Statement 1.
(c) Statement 1 is false, Statement 2 is true.
(d) Statement 1 is true, Statement 2 is true, Statement 2 is not the correct explanation of Statement 1.

15. A boat is moving due east in a region where the earth's magnetic field is 5.0×10^{-5} NA^{-1} m^{-1} due north and horizontal. The boat carries a vertical aerial 2 m long. If the speed of the boat is $1.50\ ms^{-1}$, the magnitude of the induced emf in the wire of aerial is: **[2011]**

(a) 0.75 mV (b) 0.50 mV
(c) 0.15 mV (d) 1 mV

16. A horizontal straight wire 20 m long extending from east to west falling with a speed of 5.0 m/s, at right angles to the horizontal component of the earth's magnetic field 0.30×10^{-4} Wb/m^2. The instantaneous value of the e.m.f. induced in the wire will be **[2011 RS]**

(a) 3mV (b) 4.5mV (c) 1.5mV (d) 6.0mV

17. A rectangular loop has a sliding connector PQ of length l and resistance R Ω and it is moving with a speed v as shown. The set-up is placed in a uniform magnetic field going into the plane of the paper. The three currents I_1, I_2 and I are **[2010]**

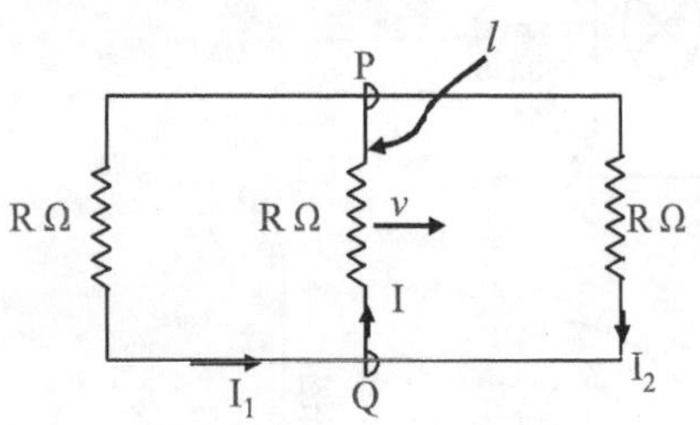

(a) $I_1 = -I_2 = \frac{Blv}{6R}, I = \frac{2Blv}{6R}$

(b) $I_1 = I_2 = \frac{Blv}{3R}, I = \frac{2Blv}{3R}$

(c) $I_1 = I_2 = I = \frac{Blv}{R}$

(d) $I_1 = I_2 = \frac{Blv}{6R}, \ I = \frac{Blv}{3R}$

18. Two coaxial solenoids are made by winding thin insulated wire over a pipe of cross-sectional area $A = 10\ cm^2$ and length = 20 cm. If one of the solenoid has 300 turns and the other 400 turns, their mutual inductance is **[2008]**
$(\mu_0 = 4\pi \times 10^{-7}\ TmA^{-1})$

(a) $2.4\pi \times 10^{-5}$ H (b) $4.8\pi \times 10^{-4}$ H
(c) $4.8\pi \times 10^{-5}$ H (d) $2.4\pi \times 10^{-4}$ H

19. One conducting U tube can slide inside another as shown in figure, maintaining electrical contacts between the tubes. The magnetic field B is perpendicular to the plane of the figure. If each tube moves towards the other at a constant speed v, then the emf induced in the circuit in terms of B, l and v where l is the width of each tube, will be **[2005]**

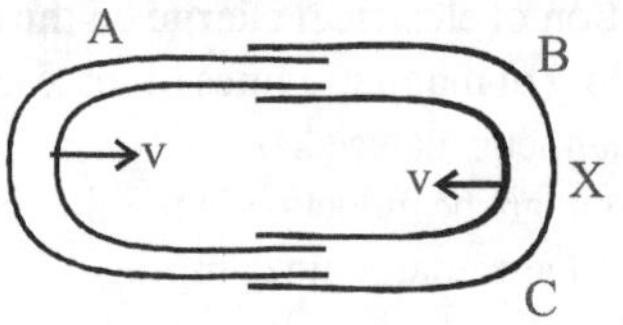

(a) $-Blv$ (b) Blv (c) $2\ Blv$ (d) zero

20. A metal conductor of length 1 m rotates vertically about one of its ends at angular velocity 5 radians per second. If the horizontal component of earth's magnetic field is 0.2×10^{-4}T, then the e.m.f. developed between the two ends of the conductor is **[2004]**

(a) 5mV (b) 50μV (c) 5μV (d) 50mV

21. A coil having n turns and resistance $R\Omega$ is connected with a galvanometer of resistance $4R\Omega$. This combination is moved in time t seconds from a magnetic field W_1 weber to W_2 weber. The induced current in the circuit is **[2004]**

(a) $-\frac{(W_2 - W_1)}{Rnt}$ (b) $-\frac{n(W_2 - W_1)}{5\ Rt}$

(c) $-\frac{(W_2 - W_1)}{5\ Rnt}$ (d) $-\frac{n(W_2 - W_1)}{Rt}$

22. Two coils are placed close to each other. The mutual inductance of the pair of coils depends upon **[2003]**

(a) the rates at which currents are changing in the two coils
(b) relative position and orientation of the two coils
(c) the materials of the wires of the coils
(d) the currents in the two coils

23. When the current changes from +2 A to –2A in 0.05 second, an e.m.f. of 8 V is induced in a coil. The coefficient of self-induction of the coil is **[2003]**

(a) 0.2 H (b) 0.4 H (c) 0.8 H (d) 0.1 H

24. A conducting square loop of side L and resistance R moves in its plane with a uniform velocity v perpendicular to one of its sides. A magnetic induction B constant in time and space, pointing perpendicular and into the plane at the loop exists everywhere with half the loop outside the field, as shown in figure. The induced emf is **[2002]**

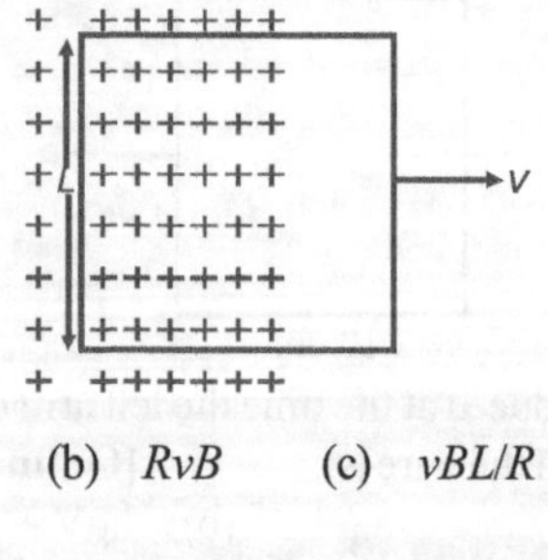

(a) zero (b) RvB (c) vBL/R (d) vBL

Hints & Solutions

TOPIC - 1: Magnetic Flux, Faraday's and Lenz's Law

1. (a) According to Faraday's law of electromagnetic induction, $\varepsilon = \frac{d\phi}{dt}$

Also, $\varepsilon = iR$

$\therefore \quad iR = \frac{d\phi}{dt} \quad \Rightarrow \int d\phi = R\int idt$

Magnitude of change in flux $(d\phi) = R \times$ area under current vs time graph

or, $d\phi = 100 \times \frac{1}{2} \times \frac{1}{2} \times 10 = 250$ Wb

2. (b) Electric flux is given by

$\phi = B.A$

$\phi = B_0 \pi r^2 e^{-t/\tau} \qquad \left(\because B = B_0 e^{-t/\tau}\right)$

Induced E.m.f. $\varepsilon = \frac{d\phi}{dt} = \frac{B_0 \pi r^2}{\tau^2} e^{-t/\tau}$

Heat $= \int_0^\infty \frac{\varepsilon^2}{R} = \frac{\pi^2 r^4 B_0^2}{2\tau R}$

3. (d) According to Faraday's law of electromagnetic induction,

Induced emf, $e = \frac{Ldi}{dt}$

$50 = L\left(\frac{5-2}{0.1\text{sec}}\right)$

$\Rightarrow \quad L = \frac{50 \times 0.1}{3} = \frac{5}{3} = 1.67$ H

4. (a) Inside the sphere field varies linearly i.e., $E \propto r$ with distance and outside varies according to $E \propto \frac{1}{r^2}$

Hence the variation is shown by curve (a)

5. (a) **Given:** No. of turns $N = 1000$

Face area, $A = 4\text{ cm}^2 = 4 \times 10^{-4}\text{ m}^2$

Change in magnetic field,

$\Delta B = 10^{-2}\text{ wbm}^{-2}$

Time taken, $t = 0.01\text{s} = 10^{-2}$ sec

Emf induced in the coil $e = ?$

Applying formula,

Induced emf, $e = \frac{-d\phi}{dt}$

$= N\left(\frac{\Delta B}{\Delta t}\right) A\cos\theta$

$= \frac{1000 \times 10^{-2} \times 4 \times 10^{-4}}{10^{-2}} = 400\text{ mV}$

6. (a) As we know, Magnetic flux, $\phi = B.A$

$\frac{\mu_0 (2)(20 \times 10^{-2})^2}{2[(0.2)^2 + (0.15)^2]} \times \pi(0.3 \times 10^{-2})^2$

On solving

$= 9.216 \times 10^{-11} = 9.2 \times 10^{-11}$ weber

7. (a) Induced emf

$\varepsilon \propto \frac{-di}{dt}$

8. (d) Because of the Lenz's law of conservation of energy

9. (c) As $e = \frac{\Delta\phi}{\Delta t}$ or $Ri = \frac{\Delta\phi}{\Delta t} \quad (\because e = Ri)$

$\Rightarrow \Delta\phi = R(i.\Delta t)$

$= R \times$ area under $i - t$ graph

$= 10 \times \frac{1}{2} \times 4 \times 0.1 = 2$ weber

10. (b) $\phi = 10t^2 - 50t + 250$

$e = -\frac{d\phi}{dt} = -(20t - 50)$

$e_{t=3} = -10\ V$

TOPIC - 2: Motional and Static EMI and Application of EMI

11. (b) In the given question,

Current flowing through the wire, I = 1A

Speed of the frame, $v = 10\text{ ms}^{-1}$

Side of square loop, $l = 10$ cm

Distance of square frame from current carrying wires $x = 10$ cm.

We have to find, e.m.f induced e = ?

According to Biot-Savart's law

$B = \frac{\mu_0}{4\pi} \frac{Idl\sin\theta}{x^2}$

$= \frac{4\pi \times 10^{-7}}{4\pi} \times \frac{1 \times 10^{-1}}{\left(10^{-1}\right)^2}$

$= 10^{-6}$

Induced e.m.f. e = Blv

$= 10^{-6} \times 10^{-1} \times 10$

$= 1\ \mu v$

12. (d) Here, induced e.m.f.

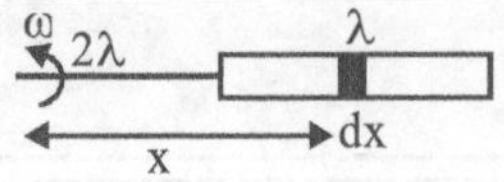

$$e = \int_{2\ell}^{3\ell} (\omega x) B dx = B\omega \frac{[(3\ell)^2 - (2\ell)^2]}{2}$$

$$= \frac{5B\ell^2\omega}{2}$$

13. (d)

14. (b) Self inductance of a long solenoid is given by

$$L = \frac{\mu_0 N^2 A}{l}$$

Magnetic field at the centre of solenoid

$$B = \frac{\mu_0 NI}{l}$$

So both the statements are correct and statement 2 is correct explanation of statement 1

15. (c) Induced emf $= vB_H l = 1.5 \times 5 \times 10^{-5} \times 2$

$= 15 \times 10^{-5}$

$= 0.15\,\text{mV}$

16. (a)

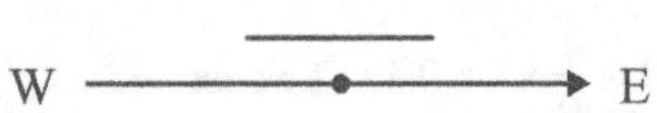

$\varepsilon_{ind} = Bv\ell$

$= 0.3 \times 10^{-4} \times 5 \times 20$

$= 3 \times 10^{-3}\,\text{V} = 3\,\text{mV}.$

17. (b) Due to the movement of resistor R, an emf equal to Blv will be induced in it as shown in figure clearly,

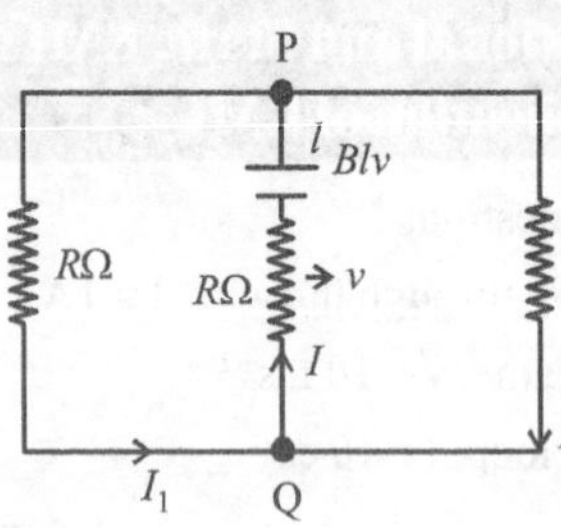

$I = I_1 + I_2$ Also, $I_1 = I_2$

Solving the circuit,

we get $I_1 = I_2 = \dfrac{Blv}{3R}$

and $I = 2I_1 = \dfrac{2Blv}{3R}$

18. (d) $M = \dfrac{\mu_0 N_1 N_2 A}{\ell}$

$$= \frac{4\pi \times 10^{-7} \times 300 \times 400 \times 100 \times 10^{-4}}{0.2}$$

$$M = \frac{\mu_0 N_1 N_2 A}{\ell}$$

$= 2.4\pi \times 10^{-4}\,\text{H}$

19. (c) Relative velocity $= v + v = 2v$

$\therefore$ emf. $= B.l(2v)$

20. (b) $\ell = 1\text{m}, \omega = 5\text{ rad/s}, B = 0.2 \times 10^{-4} T$

$$\varepsilon = \frac{B\omega\ell}{2} = \frac{0.2 \times 10^{-4} \times 5 \times 1}{2} = 50\mu V$$

21. (b) $\dfrac{\Delta\phi}{\Delta t} = \dfrac{(W_2 - W_1)}{t}$

$R_{tot} = (R + 4R)\Omega = 5R\Omega$

$$i = \frac{nd\phi}{R_{tot}dt} = \frac{-n(W_2 - W_1)}{5Rt}$$

($\because W_2$ & W_1 are magnetic flux)

22. (b) Mutual inductance depends on the relative position and orientation of the two coils.

23. (d) $e = -\dfrac{\Delta\phi}{\Delta t} = \dfrac{-\Delta(LI)}{\Delta t} = -L\dfrac{\Delta I}{\Delta t}$

$\therefore |e| = L\dfrac{\Delta I}{\Delta t} \Rightarrow 8 = L \times \dfrac{4}{0.05}$

$\Rightarrow L = \dfrac{8 \times 0.05}{4} = 0.1\text{H}$

24. (d) The induced emf is

$$e = \frac{-d\phi}{dt} = -\frac{d(\vec{B}.\vec{A})}{dt} = \frac{-d(BA\cos 0^\circ)}{dt}$$

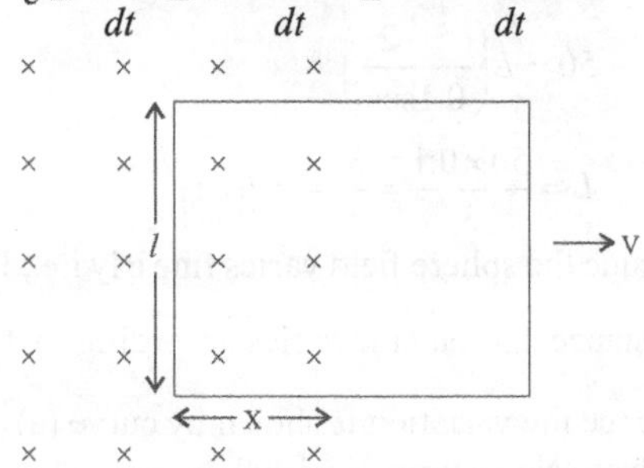

$$\therefore e = -B\frac{dA}{dt} = -B\frac{d(\ell \times x)}{dt}$$

$$\therefore e = -B\ell\frac{dx}{dt} = -B\ell v$$

Chapter 21

Alternating Current

TOPIC - 1: Alternating Current, Voltage and Power

1. A small circular loop of wire of radius a is located at the centre of a much larger circular wire loop of radius b. The two loops are in the same plane. The outer loop of radius b carries an alternating current $I = I_0 \cos(\omega t)$. The emf induced in the smaller inner loop is nearly: **[Online April 8, 2017]**

(a) $\frac{\pi\mu_0 I_0}{2}.\frac{a^2}{b}\omega\sin(\omega t)$ (b) $\frac{\pi\mu_0 I_0}{2}.\frac{a^2}{b}\omega\cos(\omega t)$

(c) $\pi\mu_0 I_0 \frac{a^2}{b}\omega\sin(\omega t)$ (d) $\frac{\pi\mu_0 I_0 b^2}{a}\omega\cos(\omega t)$

2. A sinusoidal voltage $V(t) = 100 \sin(500t)$ is applied across a pure inductance of $L = 0.02$ H. The current through the coil is: **[Online April 12, 2014]**

(a) $10 \cos(500t)$ (b) $-10 \cos(500t)$
(c) $10 \sin(500t)$ (d) $-10 \sin(500t)$

3. In an a.c. circuit the voltage applied is $E = E_0 \sin \omega t$. The resulting current in the circuit is $I = I_0 \sin\left(\omega t - \frac{\pi}{2}\right)$. The power consumption in the circuit is given by **[2007]**

(a) $P = \sqrt{2}E_0 I_0$ (b) $P = \frac{E_0 I_0}{\sqrt{2}}$

(c) $P =$ zero (d) $P = \frac{E_0 I_0}{2}$

4. In a uniform magnetic field of induction B a wire in the form of a semicircle of radius r rotates about the diameter of the circle with an angular frequency ω. The axis of rotation is perpendicular to the field. If the total resistance of the circuit is R, the mean power generated per period of rotation is **[2004]**

(a) $\frac{(B\pi r\omega)^2}{2R}$ (b) $\frac{(B\pi r^2\omega)^2}{8R}$

(c) $\frac{B\pi r^2\omega}{2R}$ (d) $\frac{(B\pi r\omega^2)^2}{8R}$

5. Alternating current can not be measured by D.C. ammeter because **[2004]**

(a) Average value of current for complete cycle is zero
(b) A.C. Changes direction
(c) A.C. can not pass through D.C. Ammeter
(d) D.C. Ammeter will get damaged.

TOPIC - 2: AC Circuit, LCR Circuit, Quality and Power Factor

6. A sinusoidal voltage of peak value 283 V and angular frequency 320/s is applied to a series LCR circuit. Given that $R = 5\,\Omega$, $L = 25$ mH and $C = 1000\,\mu F$. The total impedance, and phase difference between the voltage across the source and the current will respectively be: **[Online April 9, 2017]**

(a) $10\,\Omega$ and $\tan^{-1}\left(\frac{5}{3}\right)$ (b) $7\,\Omega$ and $45°$

(c) $10\,\Omega$ and $\tan^{-1}\left(\frac{8}{3}\right)$ (d) $7\,\Omega$ and $\tan^{-1}\left(\frac{5}{3}\right)$

7. An arc lamp requires a direct current of 10 A at 80 V to function. If it is connected to a 220 V (rms), 50 Hz AC supply, the series inductor needed for it to work is close to: **[2016]**

(a) 0.044 H (b) 0.065 H
(c) 80 H (d) 0.08 H

8. A series LR circuit is connected to a voltage source with $V(t) = V_0 \sin\omega t$. After very large time, current I(t) behaves as $\left(t_0 >> \frac{L}{R}\right)$: **[Online April 9, 2016]**

(a) 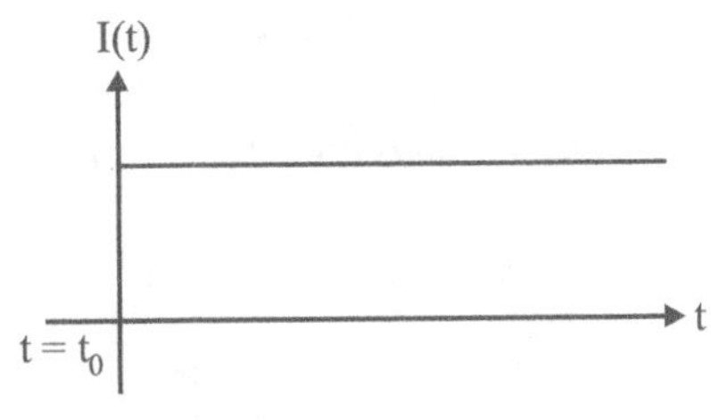

(b) 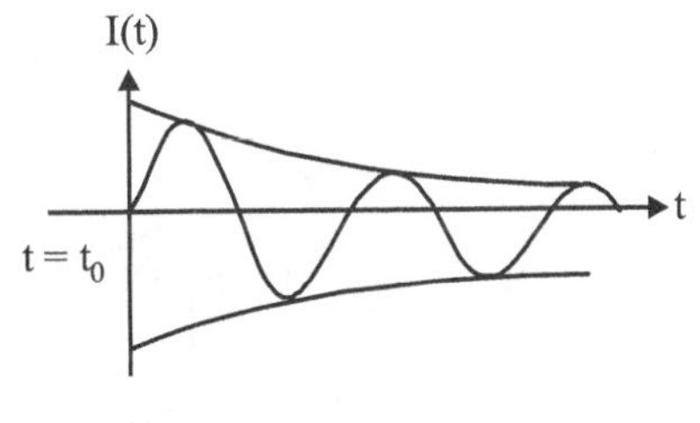

(c) 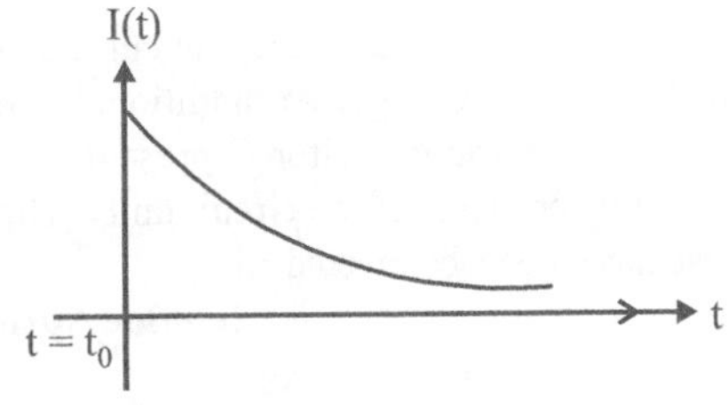

(d) 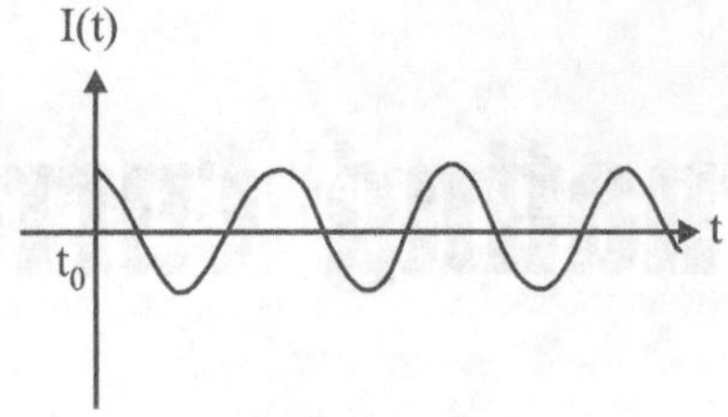

9. An inductor (L = 0.03 H) and a resistor (R = 0.15 kΩ) are connected in series to a battery of 15V emf in a circuit shown below. The key K_1 has been kept closed for a long time. Then at t = 0, K_1 is opened and key K_2 is closed simultaneously. At t = 1 ms, the current in the circuit will be : $(e^5 \cong 150)$ **[2015]**

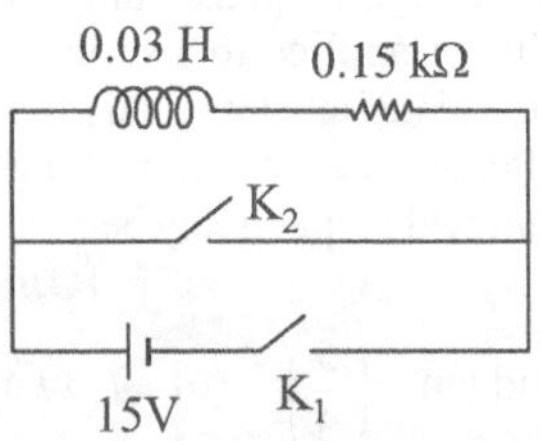

(a) 6.7 mA (b) 0.67 mA
(c) 100 mA (d) 67 mA

10. An LCR circuit is equivalent to a damped pendulum. In an LCR circuit the capacitor is charged to Q_0 and then connected to the L and R as shown below :

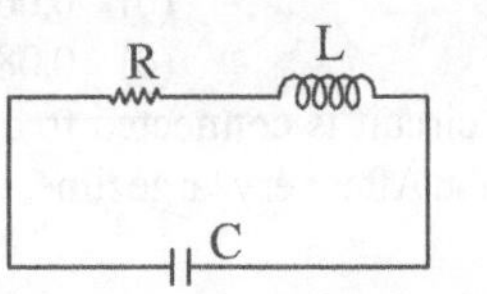

If a student plots graphs of the square of maximum charge (Q^2_{Max}) on the capacitor with time(t) for two different values L_1 and L_2 $(L_1 > L_2)$ of L then which of the following represents this graph correctly ? (*plots are schematic and not drawn to scale*) **[2015]**

(a) 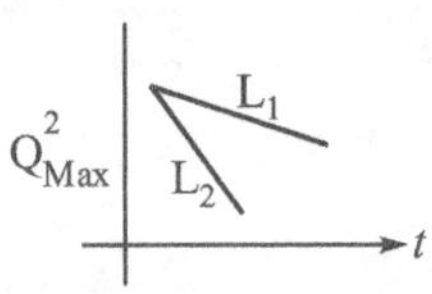

(b) 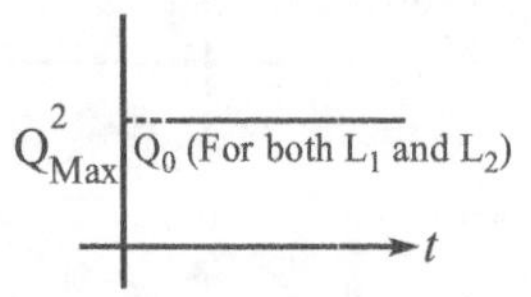

(c) 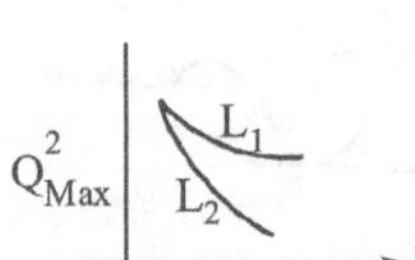

(d) 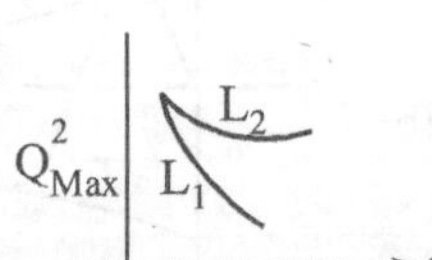

11. For the LCR circuit, shown here, the current is observed to lead the applied voltage. An additional capacitor C', when joined with the capacitor C present in the circuit, makes the power factor of the circuit unity. The capacitor C', must have been connected in : **[Online April 11, 2015]**

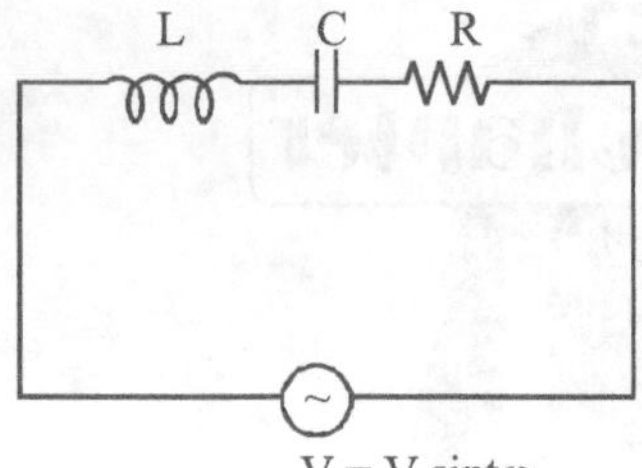

$V = V_0 \sin \omega t$

(a) series with C and has a magnitude $\frac{C}{(\omega^2 LC - 1)}$

(b) series with C and has a magnitude $\frac{1 - \omega^2 LC}{\omega^2 L}$

(c) parallel with C and has a magnitude $\frac{1 - \omega^2 LC}{\omega^2 L}$

(d) parallel with C and has a magnitude $\frac{C}{(\omega^2 LC - 1)}$

12. In the circuits (a) and (b) switches S_1 and S_2 are closed at t = 0 and are kept closed for a long time. The variation of current in the two circuits for t ≥ 0 are roughly shown by figure (figures are schematic and not drawn to scale) : **[Online April 10, 2015]**

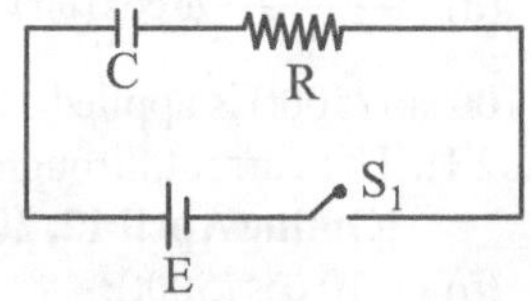

(a)

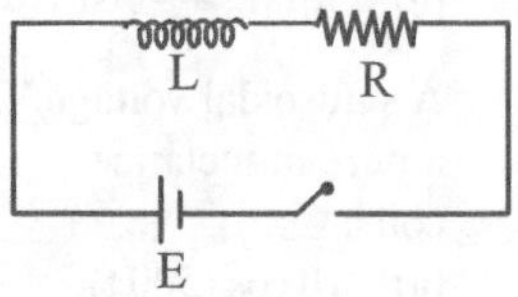

(b)

(a) 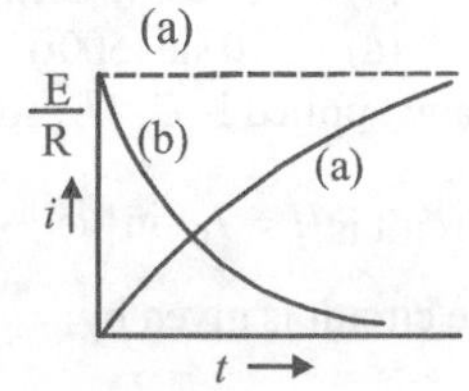

(b) 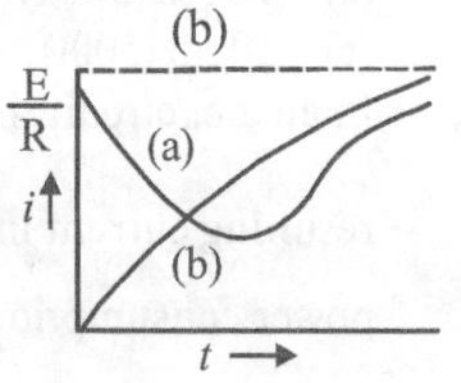

(c) 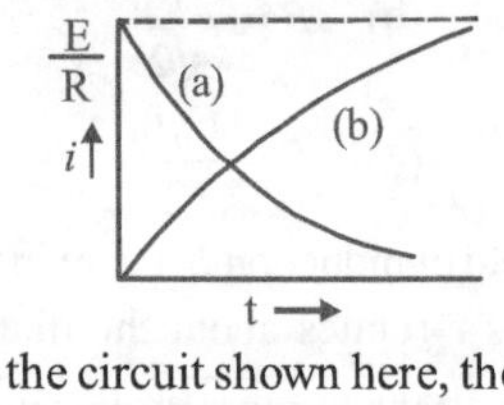

(d) 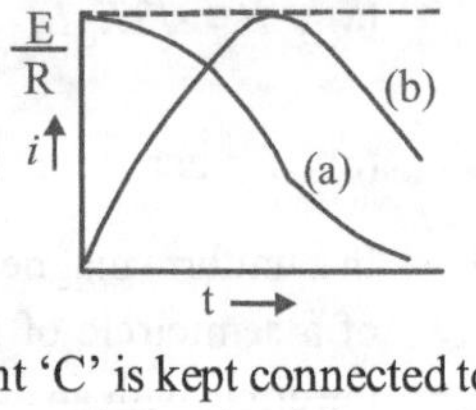

13. In the circuit shown here, the point 'C' is kept connected to point 'A' till the current flowing through the circuit becomes constant. Afterward, suddenly, point 'C' is disconnected from point 'A' and connected to point 'B' at time t = 0. Ratio of the voltage across resistance and the inductor at t = L/R will be equal to: **[2014]**

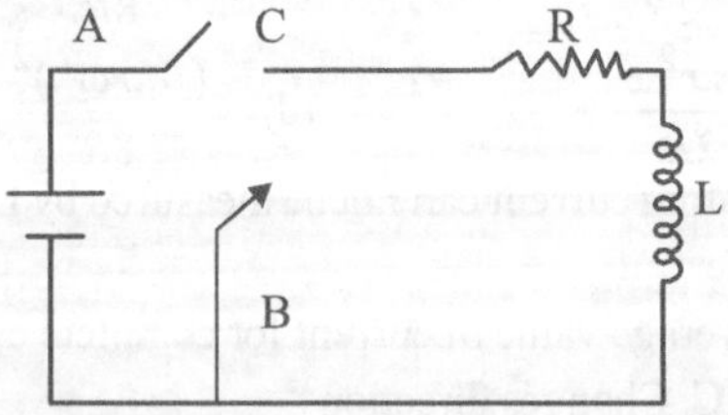

(a) $\frac{e}{1-e}$ (b) 1 (c) –1 (d) $\frac{1-e}{e}$

14. When the rms voltages V_L, V_C and V_R are measured respectively across the inductor L, the capacitor C and the resistor R in a series LCR circuit connected to an AC source, it is found that the ratio $V_L : V_C : V_R = 1 : 2 : 3$. If the rms voltage of the AC sources is 100 V, the V_R is close to: **[Online April 9, 2014]**

(a) 50 V (b) 70 V (c) 90 V (d) 100 V

15. In an LCR circuit as shown below both switches are open initially. Now switch S_1 is closed, S_2 kept open. (q is charge on the capacitor and $\tau = RC$ is Capacitive time constant). Which of the following statement is correct ? **[2013]**

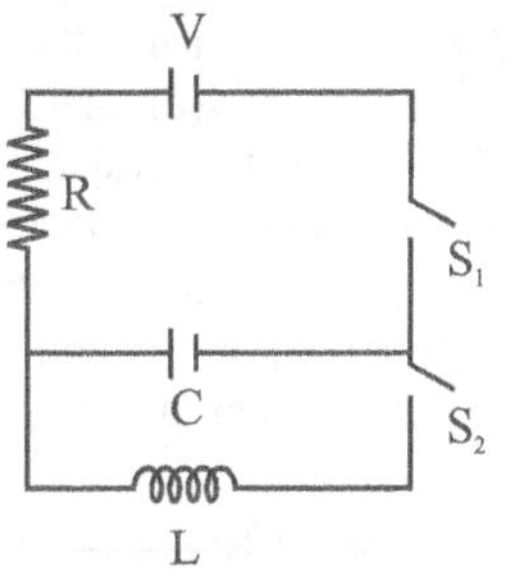

(a) Work done by the battery is half of the energy dissipated in the resistor
(b) At, $t = \tau$, $q = CV/2$
(c) At, $t = 2\tau$, $q = CV(1 - e^{-2})$
(d) At, $t = 2\tau$, $q = CV(1 - e^{-1})$

16. A series LR circuit is connected to an ac source of frequency ω and the inductive reactance is equal to 2R. A capacitance of capacitive reactance equal to R is added in series with L and R. The ratio of the new power factor to the old one is : **[Online April 25, 2013]**

(a) $\sqrt{\frac{2}{3}}$ (b) $\sqrt{\frac{2}{5}}$ (c) $\sqrt{\frac{3}{2}}$ (d) $\sqrt{\frac{5}{2}}$

17. When resonance is produced in a series LCR circuit, then which of the following is not correct ? **[Online April 25, 2013]**
(a) Current in the circuit is in phase with the applied voltage.
(b) Inductive and capacitive reactances are equal.
(c) If R is reduced, the voltage across capacitor will increase.
(d) Impedance of the circuit is maximum.

18. The plot given below is of the average power delivered to an LRC circuit versus frequency. The quality factor of the circuit is : **[Online April 23, 2013]**

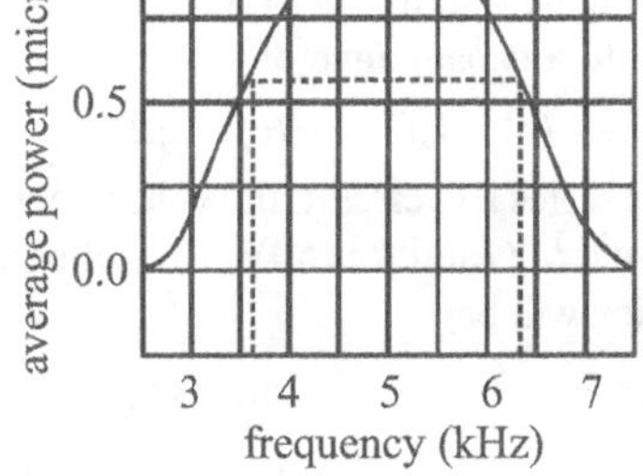

(a) 5.0 (b) 2.0 (c) 2.5 (d) 0.4

19. In a series L-C-R circuit, $C = 10^{-11}$ Farad, $L = 10^{-5}$ Henry and $R = 100$ Ohm, when a constant D.C. voltage E is applied to the circuit, the capacitor acquires a charge 10^{-9} C. The D.C. source is replaced by a sinusoidal voltage source in which the peak voltage E_0 is equal to the constant D.C. voltage E. At resonance the peak value of the charge acquired by the capacitor will be : **[Online April 22, 2013]**

(a) 10^{-15} C (b) 10^{-6} C (c) 10^{-10} C (d) 10^{-8} C

20. An LCR circuit as shown in the figure is connected to a voltage source V_{ac} whose frequency can be varied.

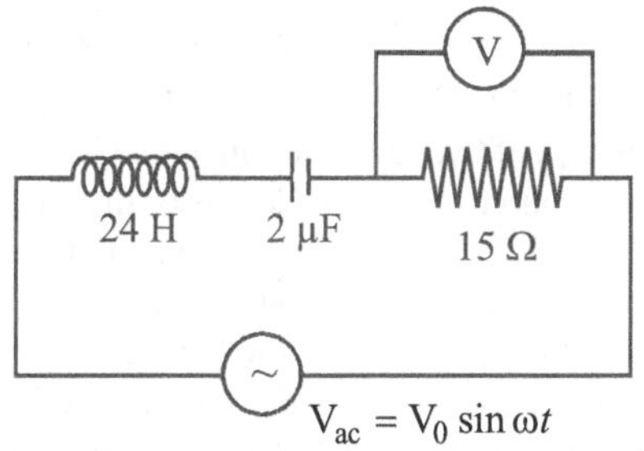

The frequency, at which the voltage across the resistor is maximum, is : **[Online April 22, 2013]**

(a) 902 Hz (b) 143 Hz (c) 23 Hz (d) 345 Hz

21. In the circuit shown here, the voltage across E and C are respectively 300 V and 400 V. The voltage E of the ac source is : **[Online April 9, 2013]**

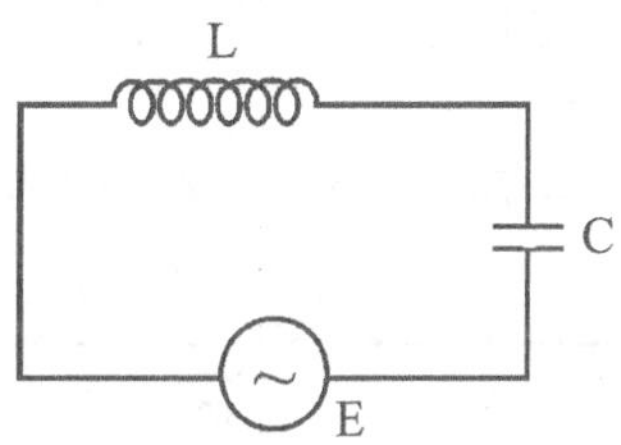

(a) 400 Volt (b) 500 Volt (c) 100 Volt (d) 700 Volt

22. A resistance *R* and a capacitance *C* are connected in series to a battery of negligible internal resistance through a key. The key is closed at $t = 0$. If after *t* sec the voltage across the capacitance was seven times the voltage across R, the value of t is **[Online May 12, 2012]**

(a) $3RC\ \ell n\, 2$ (b) $2RC\ \ell n\, 2$
(c) $2RC\ \ell n\, 7$ (d) $3RC\ \ell n\, 7$

23. In an *LCR* circuit shown in the following figure, what will be the readings of the voltmeter across the resistor and ammeter if an *a.c.* source of 220V and 100 Hz is connected to it as shown? **[Online May 7, 2012]**

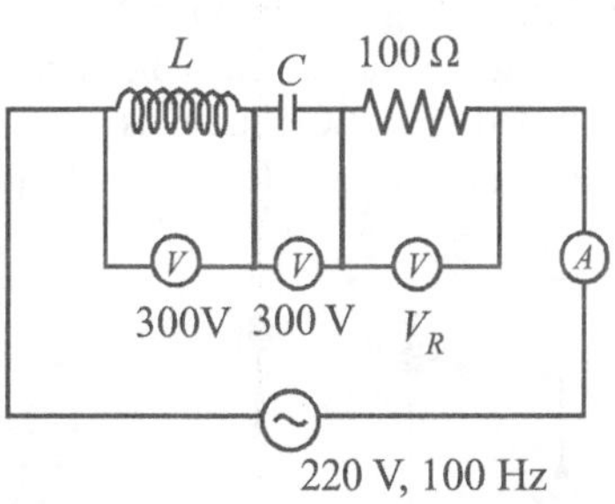

(a) 800 V, 8 A (b) 110 V, 1.1 A
(c) 300 V, 3 A (d) 220V, 2.2 A

24. A fully charged capacitor C with initial charge q_0 is connected to a coil of self inductance L at $t = 0$. The time at which the energy is stored equally between the electric and the magnetic fields is: **[2011]**

(a) $\frac{\pi}{4}\sqrt{LC}$ (b) $2\pi\sqrt{LC}$ (c) $\sqrt{LC}$ (d) $\pi\sqrt{LC}$

25. A resistor 'R' and $2\mu F$ capacitor in series is connected through a switch to 200 V direct supply. Across the capacitor is a neon bulb that lights up at 120 V. Calculate the value of R to make the bulb light up 5 s after the switch has been closed. $(\log_{10} 2.5 = 0.4)$ **[2011]**

(a) $1.7 \times 10^5 \Omega$ (b) $2.7 \times 10^6 \Omega$
(c) $3.3 \times 10^7 \Omega$ (d) $1.3 \times 10^4 \Omega$

26. Combination of two identical capacitors, *a* resistor R and *a* *dc* voltage source of voltage 6V is used in an experiment on a (*C-R*) circuit. It is found that for a parallel combination of the capacitor the time in which the voltage of the fully charged combination reduces to half its original voltage is 10 second. For series combination the time for needed for reducing the voltage of the fully charged series combination by half is **[2011 RS]**

(a) 10 second (b) 5 second
(c) 2.5 second (d) 20 second

27. In the circuit shown below, the key K is closed at $t = 0$. The current through the battery is **[2010]**

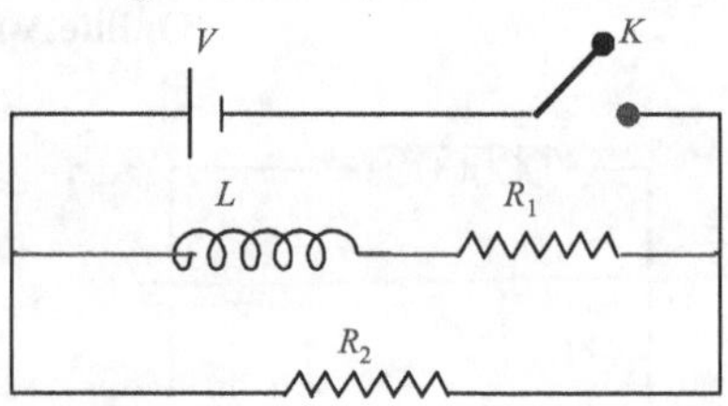

(a) $\frac{VR_1R_2}{\sqrt{R_1^2 + R_2^2}}$ at $t = 0$ and $\frac{V}{R_2}$ at $t = \infty$

(b) $\frac{V}{R_2}$ at $t = 0$ and $\frac{V(R_1 + R_2)}{R_1R_2}$ at $t = \infty$

(c) $\frac{V}{R_2}$ at $t = 0$ and $\frac{VR_1R_2}{\sqrt{R_1^2 + R_2^2}}$ at $t = \infty$

(d) $\frac{V(R_1 + R_2)}{R_1R_2}$ at $t = 0$ and $\frac{V}{R_2}$ at $t = \infty$

28. In a series LCR circuit $R = 200\Omega$ and the voltage and the frequency of the main supply is 220V and 50 Hz respectively. On taking out the capacitance from the circuit the current lags behind the voltage by 30°. On taking out the inductor from the circuit the current leads the voltage by 30°. The power dissipated in the LCR circuit is **[2010]**

(a) 305 W (b) 210 W (c) Zero W (d) 242 W

29.

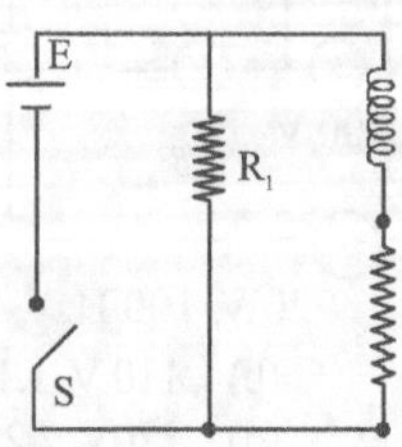

An inductor of inductance $L = 400$ mH and resistors of resistance $R_1 = 2\Omega$ and $R_2 = 2\Omega$ are connected to a battery of emf 12 V as shown in the figure. The internal resistance of the battery is negligible. The switch S is closed at $t = 0$. The potential drop across L as a function of time is **[2009]**

(a) $\frac{12}{t}e^{-3t}$ V (b) $6\left(1 - e^{-t/0.2}\right)$ V
(c) $12e^{-5t}$ V (d) $6e^{-5t}$ V

30. In a series resonant LCR circuit, the voltage across R is 100 volts and $R = 1$ kΩ with $C = 2\mu$F. The resonant frequency ω is 200 rad/s. At resonance the voltage across L is **[2006]**

(a) 2.5×10^{-2} V (b) 40 V
(c) 250 V (d) 4×10^{-3} V

31. An inductor ($L = 100$ mH), a resistor ($R = 100\ \Omega$) and a battery ($E = 100$ V) are initially connected in series as shown in the figure. After a long time the battery is disconnected after short circuiting the points A and B. The current in the circuit 1 ms after the short circuit is **[2006]**

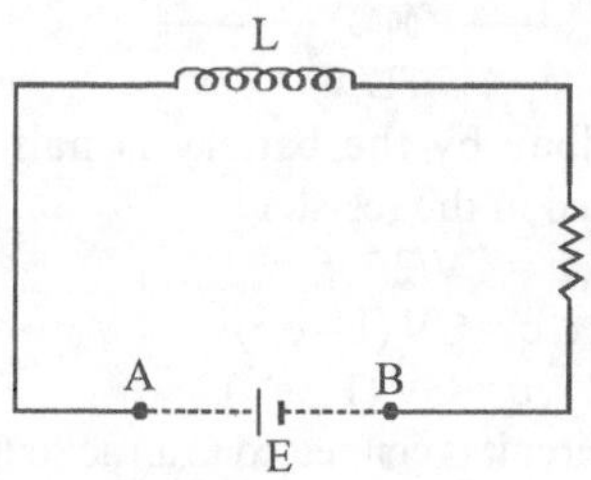

(a) 1/eA (b) eA (c) 0.1 A (d) 1 A

32. In an AC generator, a coil with N turns, all of the same area A and total resistance R, rotates with frequency ω in a magnetic field B. The maximum value of emf generated in the coil is **[2006]**

(a) N.A.B.R.ω (b) N.A.B
(c) N.A.B.R. (d) N.A.B.ω

33. The phase difference between the alternating current and emf is $\frac{\pi}{2}$. Which of the following cannot be the constituent of the circuit? **[2005]**

(a) R, L (b) C alone (c) L alone (d) L, C

34. A circuit has a resistance of 12 ohm and an impedance of 15 ohm. The power factor of the circuit will be **[2005]**

(a) 0.4 (b) 0.8 (c) 0.125 (d) 1.25

35. A coil of inductance 300 mH and resistance 2 Ω is connected to a source of voltage 2V. The current reaches half of its steady state value in **[2005]**

(a) 0.1 s (b) 0.05 s (c) 0.3 s (d) 0.15 s

36. The self inductance of the motor of an electric fan is 10 H. In order to impart maximum power at 50 Hz, it should be connected to a capacitance of **[2005]**

(a) 8μF (b) 4μF (c) 2μF (d) 1μF

37. In an LCR series a.c. circuit, the voltage across each of the components, L, C and R is 50V. The voltage across the LC combination will be **[2004]**

(a) 100 V (b) $50\sqrt{2}$ V
(c) 50 V (d) 0 V (zero)

38. In a LCR circuit capacitance is changed from C to 2 C. For the resonant frequency to remain unchanged, the inductance should be changed from L to [2004]
(a) $L/2$ (b) $2L$ (c) $4L$ (d) $L/4$

39. The power factor of an AC circuit having resistance (R) and inductance (L) connected in series and an angular velocity ω is [2002]
(a) $R/\omega L$ (b) $R/(R^2+\omega^2L^2)^{1/2}$
(c) $\omega L/R$ (d) $R/(R^2-\omega^2L^2)^{1/2}$

40. The inductance between A and D is [2002]

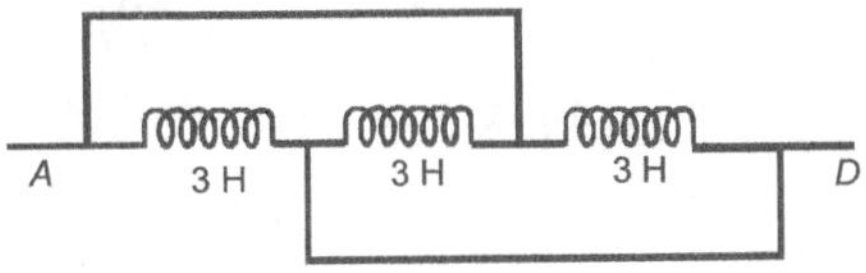

(a) 3.66 H (b) 9 H
(c) 0.66 H (d) 1 H

TOPIC - 3: Transformers and LC Oscillations

41. In an oscillating LC circuit the maximum charge on the capacitor is Q. The charge on the capacitor when the energy is stored equally between the electric and magnetic field is [2003]
(a) $\frac{Q}{2}$ (b) $\frac{Q}{\sqrt{3}}$ (c) $\frac{Q}{\sqrt{2}}$ (d) Q

42. The core of any transformer is laminated so as to [2003]
(a) reduce the energy loss due to eddy currents
(b) make it light weight
(c) make it robust and strong
(d) increase the secondary voltage

43. In a transformer, number of turns in the primary coil are 140 and that in the secondary coil are 280. If current in primary coil is 4 A, then that in the secondary coil is [2002]
(a) 4 A (b) 2 A (c) 6 A (d) 10 A.

Hints & Solutions

TOPIC - 1: Alternating Current, Voltage and Power

1. **(a)** For two concentric circular coil,

Mutual Inductance $M = \frac{\mu_0 \pi N_1 N_2 a^2}{2b}$

here, $N_1 = N_2 = 1$

Hence, $M = \frac{\mu_0 \pi a^2}{2b}$ ..... (i)

and given $I = I_0 \cos \omega t$ ..... (ii)

Now according to Faraday's second law induced emf

$e = -M\frac{dI}{dt}$

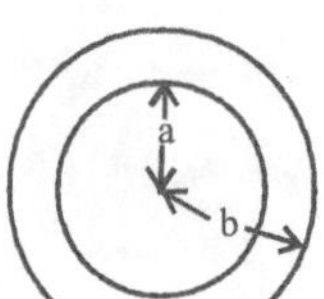

From eq. (ii),

$e = \frac{-\mu_0 \pi a^2}{2b}\frac{d}{dt}(I_0 \cos \omega t)$

$e = \frac{\mu_0 \pi a^2}{2b} I_0 \sin \omega t\,(\omega)$

$e = \frac{\pi \mu_0 I_0}{2} . \frac{a^2}{b} \omega \sin \omega t$

2. **(b)** In a pure inductive circuit current always lags behind the emf by $\frac{\pi}{2}$.

If $v(t) = v_0 \sin \omega t$

then $I = I_0 \sin\left(\omega t - \frac{\pi}{2}\right)$

Now, given $v(t) = 100 \sin(500\,t)$

and $I_0 = \frac{E_0}{\omega L} = \frac{100}{500 \times 0.02}$ $[\because L = 0.02H]$

$I_0 = 10 \sin\left(500t - \frac{\pi}{2}\right)$

$I_0 = -10 \cos(500t)$

3. **(c)** We know that power consumed in a.c. circuit is given by, $P = E_{rms}.I_{rms} \cos\phi$

Here, $E = E_0 \sin\omega t$

$I = I_0 \sin\left(\omega t - \frac{\pi}{2}\right)$

which implies that the phase difference,

$\phi = \frac{\pi}{2}$

$\therefore P = E_{rms}.I_{rms}.\cos\frac{\pi}{2} = 0$

$\left(\because \cos\frac{\pi}{2} = 0\right)$

4. **(b)** $\phi = \vec{B}.\vec{A}$; $\phi = BA\cos\omega t$

$\varepsilon = -\frac{d\phi}{dt} = \omega BA \sin\omega t$; $i = \frac{\omega BA}{R}\sin\omega t$

$P_{inst} = i^2 R = \left(\frac{\omega BA}{R}\right)^2 \times R\sin^2\omega t$

$$P_{avg} = \frac{\int_0^T P_{inst} \times dt}{\int_0^T dt} = \frac{(\omega BA)^2}{R}\frac{\int_0^T \sin^2 \omega t dt}{\int_0^T dt} = \frac{1}{2}\frac{(\omega BA)^2}{R}$$

$\therefore P_{avg} = \frac{(\omega B \pi r^2)^2}{8R}$ $\left[A = \frac{\pi r^2}{2}\right]$

5. **(a)** D.C. ammeter measure average current in AC current, average current is zero for complete cycle. Hence reading will be zero.

TOPIC - 2: AC Circuit, LCR Circuit, Quality and Power Factor

6. **(b)** Given,

$V_0 = 283$ volt, $\omega = 320$, $R = 5\,\Omega$, $L = 25$ mH, $C = 1000\,\mu F$

$X_L = \omega L = 320 \times 25 \times 10^{-3} = 8\,\Omega$

$X_C = \frac{1}{\omega C} = \frac{1}{320 \times 1000 \times 10^{-6}} = 3.1\,\Omega$

Total impedance of the circuit :

$Z = \sqrt{R^2 + (X_L - X_C)^2} = \sqrt{25 + (4.9)^2} = 7\,\Omega$

Phase difference between the voltage and current

$\tan\phi = \frac{X_L - X_C}{R}$

$\tan\phi = \frac{4.9}{5} \approx 1 \Rightarrow \phi = 45°$

7. **(b)** Here

$i = \frac{e}{\sqrt{R^2 + X_L^2}} = \frac{e}{\sqrt{R^2 + \omega^2 L^2}} = \frac{e}{\sqrt{R^2 + 4\pi^2 v^2 L^2}}$

$10 = \frac{220}{\sqrt{64 + 4\pi^2 (50)^2 L}}$ $[\because R = \frac{V}{I} = \frac{80}{10} = 8]$

On solving we get

$L = 0.065\,H$

8. (d)

9. (b) $I(0) = \frac{15\times100}{0.15\times10^3} = 0.1A$

$I(\infty) = 0$

$I(t) = [I(0) - I(\infty)]\, e^{\frac{-t}{L/R}} + i(\infty)$

$I(t) = 0.1\, e^{\frac{-t}{L/R}} = 0.1\, e^{\frac{R}{L}}$

$I(t) = 0.1\, e^{\frac{0.15\times1000}{0.03}} = 0.67mA$

10. (c) From KVL at any time t

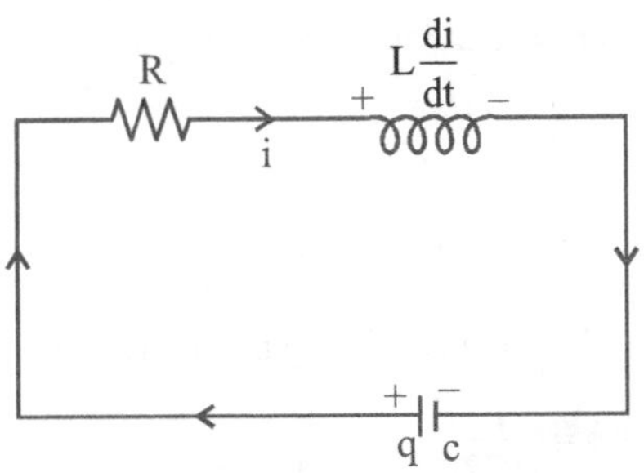

$\frac{q}{c} - iR - L\frac{di}{dt} = 0$

$i = -\frac{dq}{dt} \Rightarrow \frac{q}{c} + \frac{dq}{dt}R + \frac{Ld^2q}{dt^2} = 0$

$\frac{d^2q}{dt^2} + \frac{R}{L}\frac{dq}{dt} + \frac{q}{Lc} = 0$

From damped harmonic oscillator, the amplitude is given by $A = A_o e - \frac{dt}{2m}$

Double differential equation $\frac{d^2x}{dt^2} + \frac{b}{m}\frac{dx}{dt} + \frac{k}{m}x = 0$

$Q_{max} = Q_o e - \frac{Rt}{2L} \Rightarrow Q^2_{max} = Q^2_o e - \frac{Rt}{L}$

Hence damping will be faster for lesser self inductance.

11. (c) Power factor

$$\cos\phi = \frac{R}{\sqrt{R^2 + \left[\omega L - \frac{1}{\omega(C+C')}\right]^2}} = 1$$

On solving we get,

$\omega L = \frac{1}{\omega(C+C')}$

$C' = \frac{1-\omega^2 LC}{\omega^2 L}$

Hence option (c) is the correct answer.

12. (c) For capacitor circuit, $i = i_0 e^{-t/RC}$

For inductor circuit, $i = i_0\left(1 - e^{-\frac{Rt}{L}}\right)$

Hence graph (c) correctly depicts i versus t graph.

13. (c) Applying Kirchhoff's law of voltage in closed loop

$-V_R - V_C = 0 \Rightarrow \frac{V_R}{V_C} = -1$

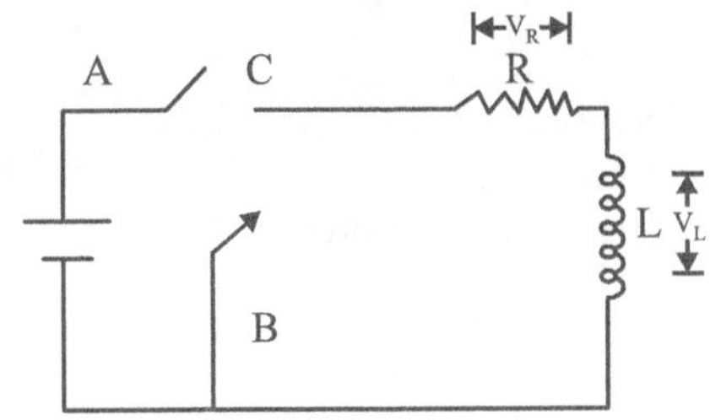

14. (c) Given, $V_L : V_C : V_R = 1:2:3$

$V = 100V$

$V_R = ?$

As we know,

$V = \sqrt{V_R^2 + (V_L - V_C)^2}$

Solving we get, $V_R \simeq 90V$

15. (c) Charge on he capacitor at any time t is given by $q = CV(1-e^{t/\tau})$

at $t = 2\tau$

$q = CV(1 - e^{-2})$

16. (d) Power factor $_{(old)}$

$= \frac{R}{\sqrt{R^2 + X_L^2}} = \frac{R}{\sqrt{R^2 + (2R)^2}} = \frac{R}{\sqrt{5}R}$

Power factor$_{(new)}$

$= \frac{R}{\sqrt{R^2 + (X_L - X_C)^2}} = \frac{R}{\sqrt{R^2 + (2R - R)^2}} = \frac{R}{\sqrt{2}R}$

$\therefore \frac{\text{New power factor}}{\text{Old power factor}} = \frac{\frac{R}{\sqrt{2}R}}{\frac{R}{\sqrt{5}R}} = \sqrt{\frac{5}{2}}$

17. (d) Impedance (Z) of the series LCR circuit is

$Z = \sqrt{R^2 + (X_L - X_C)^2}$

At resonance, $X_L = X_C$

Therefore, $Z_{minimum} = R$

18. (b)

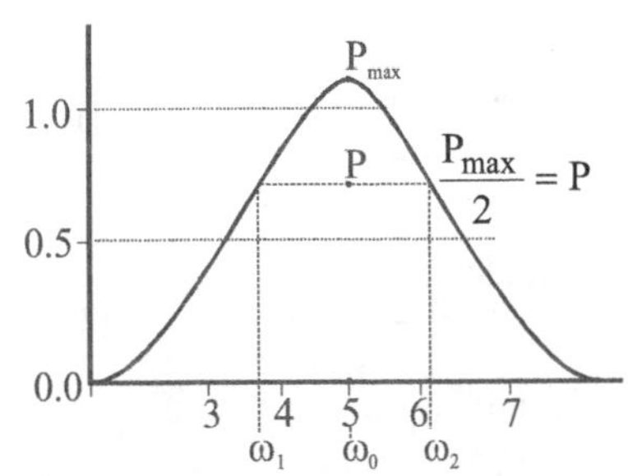

Quality factor of the circuit

$= \frac{\omega_0}{\omega_2 - \omega_1} = \frac{5}{2.5} = 2.0$

19. (d)

20. (c) Frequency $f = \frac{1}{2\pi\sqrt{LC}}$

$= \frac{1}{2\times3.4\sqrt{24\times2\times10^{-6}}}$

$\simeq 23Hz$

21. (c) Voltage E of the ac source
$E = V_C - V_L$
$= 400\,V - 300\,V = 100\,V$

22. (a) $t = 3\,RC\,ln\,2$

23. (d) In case of series RLC circuit,
Equation of voltage is given by

$V^2 = V_R^2 + (V_L - V_C)^2$

Here, $V = 220\,V$; $V_L = V_C = 300\,V$

$\therefore V_R = \sqrt{V^2} = 220V$

Current $i = \frac{V}{R} = \frac{220}{100} = 2.2A$

24. (a) Energy stored in magnetic field $= \frac{1}{2}Li^2$

Energy stored in electric field $= \frac{1}{2}\frac{q^2}{C}$

$\therefore \frac{1}{2}Li^2 = \frac{1}{2}\frac{q^2}{C}$

Also $q = q_0\cos\omega t$ and $\omega = \frac{1}{\sqrt{LC}}$

On solving $t = \frac{\pi}{4}\sqrt{LC}$

25. (b) We have, $V = V_0(1 - e^{-t/RC})$

$\Rightarrow 120 = 200\left(1 - e^{-t/RC}\right)$

$\Rightarrow t = RC\,in\,(2.5)$

$\Rightarrow R = 2.71\times10^6\,\Omega$

26. (c) Time constant for parallel combination $= 2RC$

Time constant for series combination

$= \frac{RC}{2}$

In first case :

$V = V_0 e^{-\frac{t_1}{2RC}} = \frac{V_0}{2}$ ...(1)

In second case :

$V = V_0 e^{-\frac{t_2}{(RC/2)}} = \frac{V_0}{2}$ ....(2)

From (1) and (2)

$\frac{t_1}{2RC} = \frac{t_2}{(RC/2)}$

$\Rightarrow t_2 = \frac{t_1}{4} = \frac{10}{4} = 2.5$ sec.

27. (b) At $t = 0$, no current will flow through L and R_1

$\therefore$ Current through battery $= \frac{V}{R_2}$

At $t = \infty$,

effective resistance, $R_{eff} = \frac{R_1R_2}{R_1 + R_2}$

$\therefore$ Current through battery $= \frac{V}{R_{eff}}$

$= \frac{V(R_1 + R_2)}{R_1R_2}$

28. (d) When capacitance is taken out, the circuit is LR.

$\therefore \tan\phi = \frac{\omega L}{R}$

$\Rightarrow \omega L = R\tan\phi = 200\times\frac{1}{\sqrt{3}} = \frac{200}{\sqrt{3}}$

Again, when inductor is taken out, the circuit is CR.

$\therefore \tan\phi = \frac{1}{\omega CR}$

$\Rightarrow \frac{1}{\omega c} = R\tan\phi = 200\times\frac{1}{\sqrt{3}} = \frac{200}{\sqrt{3}}$

Now, $Z = \sqrt{R^2 + \left(\frac{1}{\omega C} - \omega L\right)^2}$

$= \sqrt{(200)^2 + \left(\frac{200}{\sqrt{3}} - \frac{200}{\sqrt{3}}\right)^2} = 200\,\Omega$

Power dissipated $= V_{rms}I_{rms}\cos\phi$

$= V_{rms}\cdot\frac{V_{rms}}{Z}\cdot\frac{R}{Z}\left(\because \cos\phi = \frac{R}{Z}\right)$

$= \frac{V_{rms}^2 R}{Z^2} = \frac{(220)^2\times200}{(200)^2}$

$= \frac{220\times220}{200} = 242\,W$

29. (c) Growth in current in LR_2 branch when switch is closed is given by

$i = \frac{E}{R_2}[1 - e^{-R_2t/L}]$

$\Rightarrow \frac{di}{dt} = \frac{E}{R_2}\cdot\frac{R_2}{L}\cdot e^{-R_2t/L} = \frac{E}{L}e^{-\frac{R_2t}{L}}$

Hence, potential drop across

$L = \left(\frac{E}{L}e^{-R_2t/L}\right)L = Ee^{-R_2t/L}$

$= 12e^{-\frac{2t}{400\times10^{-3}}} = 12e^{-5t}V$

30. (c) Across resistor, $I = \frac{V}{R} = \frac{100}{1000} = 0.1\,A$

At resonance,

$$X_L = X_C = \frac{1}{\omega C} = \frac{1}{200 \times 2 \times 10^{-6}} = 2500$$

Voltage across L is

$$I X_L = 0.1 \times 2500 = 250\text{V}$$

31. (a) Initially, when steady state is achieved,

$$i = \frac{E}{R}$$

Let E is short circuited at $t = 0$. Then

At $t = 0$, $i_0 = \dfrac{E}{R}$

Let during decay of current at any time the current flowing is $-L\dfrac{di}{dt} - iR = 0$

$$\Rightarrow \frac{di}{i} = -\frac{R}{L}dt \Rightarrow \int_{i_0}^{i}\frac{di}{i} = \int_0^t -\frac{R}{L}dt$$

$$\Rightarrow \log_e \frac{i}{i_0} = -\frac{R}{L}t \Rightarrow i = i_0\, e^{-\frac{R}{L}t}$$

$$\Rightarrow i = \frac{E}{R}e^{-\frac{R}{L}t} = \frac{100}{100}e^{\frac{-100\times10^{-3}}{100\times10^{-3}}} = \frac{1}{e}$$

32. (d) $e = -\dfrac{d\phi}{dt} = -\dfrac{d(N\vec{B}.\vec{A})}{dt}$

$$= -N\frac{d}{dt}(BA\cos\omega t) = NBA\omega\sin\omega t$$

$$\Rightarrow e_{max} = NBA\omega$$

33. (a) Phase difference for R–L circuit lies between $\left(0, \dfrac{\pi}{2}\right)$

34. (b) Power factor $= \cos\phi = \dfrac{R}{Z} = \dfrac{12}{15} = \dfrac{4}{5} = 0.8$

35. (a) The charging of inductance given by,

$$i = i_0\left(1 - e^{-\frac{Rt}{L}}\right)$$

$$\frac{i_0}{2} = i_0(1 - e^{-\frac{Rt}{L}}) \Rightarrow e^{-\frac{Rt}{L}} = \frac{1}{2}$$

Taking log on both the sides,

$$-\frac{Rt}{L} = \log 1 - \log 2$$

$$\Rightarrow t = \frac{L}{R}\log 2 = \frac{300 \times 10^{-3}}{2} \times 0.69$$

$$\Rightarrow t = 0.1 \text{ sec.}$$

36. (d) For maximum power, $X_L = X_C$, which yields

$$C = \frac{1}{(2\pi n)^2 L} = \frac{1}{4\pi^2 \times 50 \times 50 \times 10}$$

$$\therefore C = 0.1 \times 10^{-5} F = 1\mu F$$

37. (d) Since the phase difference between L & C is π,
$\therefore$ net voltage difference across LC
$= 50 - 50 = 0$

38. (a) For resonant frequency to remain same LC should be const. LC = const

$$\Rightarrow LC = L' \times 2C \Rightarrow L' = \frac{L}{2}$$

39. (b) The impedance triangle for resistance (R) and inductor (L) connected in series is shown in the figure.

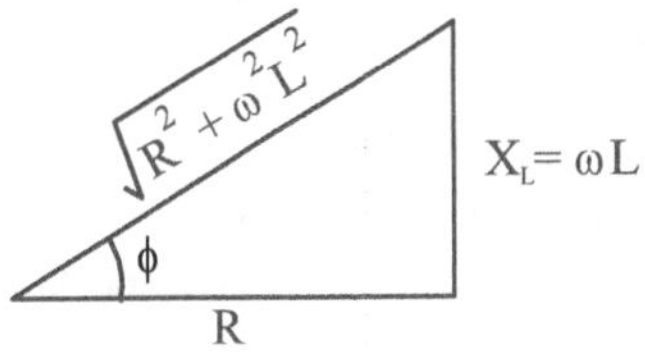

Power factor $\cos\phi = \dfrac{R}{\sqrt{R^2 + \omega^2 L^2}}$

40. (d) These three inductors are connected in parallel. The equivalent inductance L_p is given by

$$\frac{1}{L_p} = \frac{1}{L_1} + \frac{1}{L_2} + \frac{1}{L_3} = \frac{1}{3} + \frac{1}{3} + \frac{1}{3} = \frac{3}{3} = 1$$

$$\therefore L_p = 1$$

TOPIC - 3: Transformers and LC Oscillations

41. (c) When the capacitor is completely charged, the total energy in the LC circuit is with the capacitor and that energy is

$$E = \frac{1}{2}\frac{Q^2}{C}$$

When half energy is with the capacitor in the form of electric field between the plates of the capacitor we get

$\dfrac{E}{2} = \dfrac{1}{2}\dfrac{Q'^2}{C}$ where Q' is the charge on one plate of the capacitor

$$\therefore \frac{1}{2} \times \frac{1}{2}\frac{Q^2}{C} = \frac{1}{2}\frac{Q'^2}{C} \Rightarrow Q' = \frac{Q}{\sqrt{2}}$$

42. (a) Laminated core provide less area of cross-section for the current to flow. Because of this, resistance of the core increases and current decreases thereby decreasing the eddy current losses.

43. (b) $N_p = 140, N_s = 280, I_p = 4A, I_s = ?$

For a transformer $\dfrac{I_s}{I_p} = \dfrac{N_p}{N_s}$

$$\Rightarrow \frac{I_s}{4} = \frac{140}{280} \Rightarrow I_s = 2A$$

Chapter 22

Electromagnetic Waves

TOPIC-1 : Electromagnetic Waves, Conduction and Displacement Current

1. The electric field component of a monochromatic radiation is given by

$$\vec{E} = 2E_0\,\hat{i}\,\cos kz \cos \omega t$$

Its magnetic field $\vec{B}$ is then given by : **[Online April 9, 2017]**

(a) $\frac{2E_0}{c}\hat{j}\sin kz \cos \omega t$ (b) $-\frac{2E_0}{c}\hat{j}\sin kz \sin \omega t$

(c) $\frac{2E_0}{c}\hat{j}\sin kz \sin \omega t$ (d) $\frac{2E_0}{c}\hat{j}\cos kz \cos \omega t$

2. Magnetic field in a plane electromagnetic wave is given by $\vec{B} = B_0 \sin(kx + \omega t)\hat{j}T$
Expression for corresponding electric field will be :
Where c is speed of light. **[Online April 8, 2017]**

(a) $\vec{E} = B_0 c \sin(kx + \omega t)\hat{k}V/m$

(b) $\vec{E} = \frac{B_0}{c}\sin(kx + \omega t)\hat{k}V/m$

(c) $\vec{E} = -B_0 c \sin(kx + \omega t)\hat{k}V/m$

(d) $\vec{E} = B_0 c \sin(kx - \omega t)\hat{k}V/m$

3. Consider an electromagnetic wave propagating in vacuum. Choose the correct statement : **[Online April 10, 2016]**

(a) For an electromagnetic wave propagating in +y direction the electric field is $\vec{E} = \frac{1}{\sqrt{2}}E_{yz}(x,t)\hat{z}$ and the magnetic field is $\vec{B} = \frac{1}{\sqrt{2}}B_z(x,t)\hat{y}$

(b) For an electromagnetic wave propagating in +y direction the electric field is $\vec{E} = \frac{1}{\sqrt{2}}E_{yz}(x,t)\hat{y}$ and the magnetic field is $\vec{B} = \frac{1}{\sqrt{2}}B_{yz}(x,t)\hat{z}$

(c) For an electromagnetic wave propagating in +x direction the electric field is $\vec{E} = \frac{1}{\sqrt{2}}E_{yz}(y,z,t)$ $(\hat{y}+\hat{z})$ and the magnetic field is $\vec{B} = \frac{1}{\sqrt{2}}B_{yz}(y,z,t)(\hat{y}+\hat{z})$

(d) For an electromagnetic wave propagating in +x direction the electric field is $\vec{E} = \frac{1}{\sqrt{2}}E_{yz}(x,t)(\hat{y}-\hat{z})$ and the magnetic field is $\vec{B} = \frac{1}{\sqrt{2}}B_{yz}(x,t)(\hat{y}+\hat{z})$

4. For plane electromagnetic waves propagating in the z-direction, which one of the following combination gives the correct possible direction for $\vec{E}$ and $\vec{B}$ field respectively? **[Online April 11, 2015]**

(a) $(2\hat{i}+3\hat{j})$ and $(\hat{i}+2\hat{j})$ (b) $(-2\hat{i}-3\hat{j})$ and $(3\hat{i}-2\hat{j})$

(c) $(3\hat{i}+4\hat{j})$ and $(4\hat{i}-3\hat{j})$ (d) $(\hat{i}+2\hat{j})$ and $(2\hat{i}-\hat{j})$

5. An electromagnetic wave travelling in the x-direction has frequency of 2×10^{14} Hz and electric field amplitude of 27 Vm^{-1}. From the options given below, which one describes the magnetic field for this wave? **[Online April 10, 2015]**

(a) $\vec{B}(x,t) = (3\times10^{-8}T)\hat{j}$
$\sin[2\pi(1.5 \times 10^{-8}x - 2 \times 10^{14}t)]$

(b) $\vec{B}(x,t) = (9\times10^{-8}T)\hat{i}$
$\sin[2\pi(1.5 \times 10^{-8}x - 2 \times 1014\,t)]$

(c) $\vec{B}(x,t) = (9\times10^{-8}T)\hat{j}$
$\sin[1.5 \times 10^{-6}x - 2 \times 10^{14}t]$

(d) $\vec{B}(x,t) = (9\times10^{-8}T)\hat{k}$
$\sin[2\pi(1.5 \times 10^{-6}x - 2 \times 10^{14}t)]$

6. During the propagation of electromagnetic waves in a medium: **[2014]**

(a) Electric energy density is double of the magnetic energy density.

(b) Electric energy density is half of the magnetic energy density.

(c) Electric energy density is equal to the magnetic energy density.

(d) Both electric and magnetic energy densities are zero.

7. A lamp emits monochromatic green light uniformly in all directions. The lamp is 3% efficient in converting electrical power to electromagnetic waves and consumes 100 W of power. The amplitude of the electric field associated with the electromagnetic radiation at a distance of 5 m from the lamp will be nearly: **[Online April 12, 2014]**
(a) 1.34 V/m (b) 2.68 V/m
(c) 4.02 V/m (d) 5.36 V/m
8. An electromagnetic wave of frequency 1×10^{14} hertz is propagating along z-axis. The amplitude of electric field is 4 V/m. If $\varepsilon_0 = 8.8 \times 10^{-12}$ $C^2/N\text{-}m^2$, then average energy density of electric field will be: **[Online April 11, 2014]**
(a) 35.2×10^{-10} J/m^3 (b) 35.2×10^{-11} J/m^3
(c) 35.2×10^{-12} J/m^3 (d) 35.2×10^{-13} J/m^3
9. The magnetic field in a travelling electromagnetic wave has a peak value of 20 nT. The peak value of electric field strength is: **[2013]**
(a) 3 V/m (b) 6 V/m (c) 9 V/m (d) 12 V/m
10. A plane electromagnetic wave in a non-magnetic dielectric medium is given by $\vec{E} = \vec{E}_0 (4\times10^{-7} x - 50t)$ with distance being in meter and time in seconds. The dielectric constant of the medium is: **[Online April 22, 2013]**
(a) 2.4 (b) 5.8 (c) 8.2 (d) 4.8
11. Select the correct statement from the following: **[Online April 9, 2013]**
(a) Electromagnetic waves cannot travel in vacuum.
(b) Electromagnetic waves are longitudinal waves.
(c) Electromagnetic waves are produced by charges moving with uniform velocity.
(d) Electromagnetic waves carry both energy and momentum as they propagate through space.
12. An electromagnetic wave in vacuum has the electric and magnetic field $\vec{E}$ and $\vec{B}$, which are always perpendicular to each other. The direction of polarization is given by $\vec{X}$ and that of wave propagation by $\vec{k}$. Then **[2012]**
(a) $\vec{X} \parallel \vec{B}$ and $\vec{k} \parallel \vec{B}\times\vec{E}$
(b) $\vec{X} \parallel \vec{E}$ and $\vec{k} \parallel \vec{E}\times\vec{B}$
(c) $\vec{X} \parallel \vec{B}$ and $\vec{k} \parallel \vec{E}\times\vec{B}$
(d) $\vec{X} \parallel \vec{E}$ and $\vec{k} \parallel \vec{B}\times\vec{E}$
13. An electromagnetic wave with frequency ω and wavelength λ travels in the $+y$ direction. Its magnetic field is along $+x$-axis. The vector equation for the associated electric field (of amplitude E_0) is **[Online May 19, 2012]**
(a) $\vec{E} = -E_0 \cos\left(\omega t + \frac{2\pi}{\lambda} y\right)\hat{x}$
(b) $\vec{E} = E_0 \cos\left(\omega t - \frac{2\pi}{\lambda} y\right)\hat{x}$
(c) $\vec{E} = E_0 \cos\left(\omega t - \frac{2\pi}{\lambda} y\right)\hat{z}$
(d) $\vec{E} = -E_0 \cos\left(\omega t + \frac{2\pi}{\lambda} y\right)\hat{z}$
14. An electromagnetic wave of frequency $\nu = 3.0$ MHz passes from vacuum into a dielectric medium with permittivity $\in = 4.0$. Then **[2004]**
(a) wave length is halved and frequency remains unchanged
(b) wave length is doubled and frequency becomes half
(c) wave length is doubled and the frequency remains unchanged
(d) wave length and frequency both remain unchanged.
15. *Electromagnetic waves are transverse in nature* is evident by **[2002]**
(a) polarization (b) interference
(c) reflection (d) diffraction

TOPIC-2 : Electromagnetic Spectrum

16. Arrange the following electromagnetic radiations per quantum in the order of increasing energy: **[2016]**
A : Blue light B : Yellow light
C : X-ray D : Radiowave.
(a) C, A, B, D (b) B, A, D, C
(c) D, B, A, C (d) A, B, D, C
17. Microwave oven acts on the principle of: **[Online April 9, 2016]**
(a) giving rotational energy to water molecules
(b) giving translational energy to water molecules
(c) giving vibrational energy to water molecules
(d) transferring electrons from lower to higher energy levels in water molecule
18. Match List - I (Electromagnetic wave type) with List - II (Its association/application) and select the correct option from the choices given below the lists: **[2014]**

	List 1		List 2
1.	Infrared waves	(i)	To treat muscular strain
2.	Radio waves	(ii)	For broadcasting
3.	X-rays	(iii)	To detect fracture of bones
4.	Ultraviolet rays	(iv)	Absorbed by the ozone layer of the atmosphere

	1	2	3	4
(a)	(iv)	(iii)	(ii)	(i)
(b)	(i)	(ii)	(iv)	(iii)
(c)	(iii)	(ii)	(i)	(iv)
(d)	(i)	(ii)	(iii)	(iv)

19. If microwaves, X rays, infrared, gamma rays, ultra-violet, radio waves and visible parts of the electromagnetic spectrum are denoted by M, X, I, G, U, R and V then which of the following is the arrangement in ascending order of wavelength ? **[Online April 19, 2014]**
(a) R, M, I, V, U, X and G
(b) M, R, V, X, U, G and I
(c) G, X, U, V, I, M and R
(d) I, M, R, U, V, X and G

20. Match the List-I (Phenomenon associated with electromagnetic radiation) with List-II (Part of electromagnetic spectrum) and select the correct code from the choices given below this lists: **[Online April 11, 2014]**

	List I		List II
I	Doublet of sodium	(A)	Visible radiation
II	Wavelength corresponding to temperature associated with the isotropic radiation filling all space	(B)	Microwave
III	Wavelength emitted by atomic hydrogen in interstellar space	(C)	Short radio wave
IV	Wavelength of radiation arising from two close energy levels in hydrogen	(D)	X-rays

(a) (I)-(A), (II)-(B), (III)-(B), (IV)-(C)
(b) (I)-(A), (II)-(B), (III)-(C), (IV)-(C)
(c) (I)-(D), (II)-(C), (III)-(A), (IV)-(B)
(d) (I)-(B), (II)-(A), (III)-(D), (IV)-(A)

21. Match List I (Wavelength range of electromagnetic spectrum) with List II (Method of production of these waves) and select the correct option from the options given below the lists. **[Online April 9, 2014]**

	List I		List II
(1)	700 nm to 1 mm	(i)	Vibration of atoms and molecules.
(2)	1 nm to 400 nm	(ii)	Inner shell electrons in atoms moving from one energy level to a lower level.
(3)	$< 10^{-3}$ nm	(iii)	Radioactive decay of the nucleus.
(4)	1 mm to 0.1 m	(iv)	Magnetron valve.

(a) (1)-(iv), (2)-(iii), (3)-(ii), (4)-(i)
(b) (1)-(iii), (2)-(iv), (3)-(i), (4)-(ii)
(c) (1)-(ii), (2)-(iii), (3)-(iv), (4)-(i)
(d) (1)-(i), (2)-(ii), (3)-(iii), (4)-(iv)

22. Photons of an electromagnetic radiation has an energy 11 keV each. To which region of electromagnetic spectrum does it belong ? **[Online April 9, 2013]**

(a) X-ray region
(b) Ultra violet region
(c) Infrared region
(d) Visible region

23. The frequency of *X*-rays; γ-rays and ultraviolet rays are respectively *a*, *b* and *c* then **[Online May 26, 2012]**

(a) $a < b; b > c$
(b) $a > b; b > c$
(c) $a < b < c$
(d) $a = b = c$

Hints & Solutions

TOPIC-1 : Electromagnetic Waves, Conduction and Displacement Current

1. (c) Given, Electric field component of monochromatic radiation, $(\vec{E}) = 2E_0\hat{i}\cos kz \cos\omega t$

We know that, $\frac{dE}{dz} = -\frac{dB}{dt}$

$\frac{dE}{dz} = -2E_0 k \sin kz \cos\omega t = -\frac{dB}{dt}$

$dB = +2E_0 k \sin kz \cos\omega t\, dt$ ..... (i)

Integrating eq^n (i), we have

$B = +2E_0 k \sin kz \int \cos\omega t\, dt$

Magnetic field is given by,

$= +2E_0 \frac{k}{\omega} \sin kz \sin\omega t$

We also know that,

$\frac{E_0}{B_0} = \frac{\omega}{k} = c$

Magnetic field vector,

$\vec{B} = \frac{2E_0}{c}\hat{j} \sin kz \sin\omega t$

2. (a) Speed of EM wave in force space (c) $= \frac{E_0}{B_0}$

or $\vec{E} = cB_0 \sin(kx + \omega t)\hat{k}$

3. (d) Wave in X-direction means E and B should be function of x and t.

$\hat{y} - \hat{z} \perp \hat{y} + \hat{z}$

4. (b) As we know, $\vec{E}.\vec{B} = 0 \quad \because [\vec{E} \perp \vec{B}]$

and $\vec{E} \times \vec{B}$ should be along Z direction

As $(-2\hat{i} - 3\hat{j}) \times (3\hat{i} - 2\hat{j}) = 5\hat{k}$

Hence option (b) is the correct answer.

5. (d) As we know,

$B_0 = \frac{E_0}{C} = \frac{27}{3\times10^8} = 9\times10^{-8}$ tesla

Oscillation of B can be only along $\hat{j}$ or $\hat{k}$ direction.

$\omega = 2\pi f = 2\pi \times 2 \times 10^{14}$ Hz

$\therefore \vec{B}(x,t) = (9\times10^{-8}T)\hat{k}\sin[2\pi(1.5\times10^{-6}\, x - 2\times10^{4}t)]$

6. (c) $E_0 = CB_0$ and $C = \frac{1}{\sqrt{\mu_0 \varepsilon_0}}$

Electric energy density $= \frac{1}{2}\varepsilon_0 E_0^2 = \mu_E$

Magnetic energy density $= \frac{1}{2}\frac{Bo^2}{\mu_0} = \mu_B$

Thus, $\mu_E = \mu_B$

Energy is equally divided between electric and magnetic field

7. (b) Wavelength of monochromatic green light $= 5.5 \times 10^{-5}$ cm

Intensity $I = \frac{\text{Power}}{\text{Area}}$

$= \frac{100\times(3/100)}{4\pi(5)^2} = \frac{3}{100\pi}\text{Wm}^{-2}$

Now, half of this intensity (I) belongs to electric field and half of that to magnetic field, therefore,

$\frac{I}{2} = \frac{1}{4}\varepsilon_0 E_0^2 C$

or $E_0 = \sqrt{\frac{2I}{\varepsilon_0 C}}$

$= \sqrt{\frac{2\times\left(\frac{3}{100}\pi\right)}{\left(\frac{1}{4\pi\times9\times10^9}\right)\times(3\times10^8)}}$

$= \sqrt{\frac{6}{25}\times30} = \sqrt{7.2}$

$\therefore \quad E_0 = 2.68$ V/m

8. (c) **Given:** Amplitude of electric field,

$E_0 = 4$ v/m

Absolute permitivity,

$\varepsilon_0 = 8.8 \times 10^{-12}$ c^2/N-m^2

Average energy density u_E = ?

Applying formula,

Average energy density $u_E = \frac{1}{4}\varepsilon_0 E^2$

$\Rightarrow \quad u_E = \frac{1}{4}\times 8.8\times10^{-12}\times(4)^2$

$= 35.2 \times 10^{-12}$ J/m^3

9. (b) From question,

$B_0 = 20$ nT $= 20 \times 10^{-9}$T

($\because$ velocity of light in vacuum $C = 3 \times 10^8$ ms^{-1})

$\vec{E}_0 = \vec{B}_0 \times \vec{C}$

$|\vec{E}_0| = |\vec{B}|.|\vec{C}| = 20\times10^{-9}\times3\times10^8$

$= 6$ V/m.

10. (b)

11. (d) Electromagnetic waves do not required any medium to propagate. They can travel in vacuum. They are transverse in nature like light. They carry both energy and momentum.
A changing electric field produces a changing magnetic field and vice-versa. Which gives rise to a transverse wave known as electromagnetic wave.

12. (b) ∵ The E.M. wave are transverse in nature i.e.,

$$= \frac{\vec{k}\times\vec{E}}{\mu\omega} = \vec{H} \qquad \ldots(i)$$

where $\vec{H} = \frac{\vec{B}}{\mu}$

and $\frac{\vec{k}\times\vec{H}}{\omega\varepsilon} = -\vec{E} \qquad \ldots(ii)$

$\vec{k}$ is $\perp$ $\vec{H}$ and $\vec{k}$ is also $\perp$ to $\vec{E}$

or In other words $\vec{X} \parallel \vec{E}$ and $\vec{k} \parallel \vec{E}\times\vec{B}$

13. (c) In an electromagnetic wave electric field and magnetic field are perpendicular to the direction of propagation of wave. The vector equation for the electric field is

$$\vec{E} = E_0 \cos\left(\omega t - \frac{2\pi}{\lambda} y\right)\hat{z}$$

14. (a) Frequency remains constant during refraction

$$v_{med} = \frac{1}{\sqrt{\mu_0 \in_0 \times 4}} = \frac{c}{2}$$

$$\frac{\lambda_{med}}{\lambda_{air}} = \frac{v_{med}}{v_{air}} = \frac{c/2}{c} = \frac{1}{2}$$

∴ wavelength is halved and frequency remains unchanged

15. (a) The phenomenon of polarisation is shown only by transverse waves.

TOPIC-2 : Electromagnetic Spectrum

16. (c)

E, Decreases →

γ-rays X-rays uv-rays Visible rays VIBGYOR IR rays Microwaves Radio waves

Radio wave < yellow light < blue light < X-rays
(Increasing order of energy)

17. (c) Microwave oven acts on the principle of giving vibrational energy to water molecules.

18. (d)
(1) Infrared rays are used to treat muscular strain because these are heat rays.
(2) Radio waves are used for broadcasting because these waves have very long wavelength ranging from few centimeters to few hundred kilometers
(3) X-rays are used to detect fracture of bones because they have high penetrating power but they can't penetrate through denser medium like dones.
(4) Ultraviolet rays are absorbed by ozone of the atmosphere.

19. (c) Gamma rays < X-rays < Ultra violet < Visible rays < Infrared rays < Microwaves < Radio waves.

20. (d) Wavelength emitted by atomic hydrogen in interstellar space - Part of short radio wave of electromagnetic spectrum.
Doublet of sodium - visible radiation.

21. (d) Vibration of atoms and molecules 700 nm to 1 mm
Radioactive decay of the nucleus < 10^{-3} nm
Magnetron valve 1 mm to 0.1 m

22. (a) $E = \frac{hc}{\lambda} \Rightarrow \lambda = \frac{hc}{E}$

$$\Rightarrow \lambda = \frac{6.6\times10^{-34}\times3\times10^{8}}{11\times1000\times1.6\times10^{-19}}$$

$= 12.4$ Å

Increasing order of frequency →

x-rays u-v rays visible Infrared

wavelength range of visible region is 4000Å to 7800Å.

23. (a) Frequency range of γ-ray,
$b = 10^{18} - 10^{23}$ Hz
Frequency range of X-ray,
$a = 10^{16} - 10^{20}$ Hz
Frequency range of ultraviolet ray,
$c = 10^{15} - 10^{17}$ Hz
$\therefore a < b;\ b > c$

Chapter 23

Ray Optics and Optical Instruments

TOPIC - 1: Plane Mirror, Spherical Mirror and Reflection of Light

1. You are asked to design a shaving mirror assuming that a person keeps it 10 cm from his face and views the magnified image of the face at the closest comfortable distance of 25 cm. The radius of curvature of the mirror would then be : **[Online April 10, 2015]**

(a) 60 cm (b) –24 cm
(c) – 60 cm (d) 24 cm

2. A car is fitted with a convex side-view mirror of focal length 20 cm. A second car 2.8 m behind the first car is overtaking the first car at a relative speed of 15 m/s. The speed of the image of the second car as seen in the mirror of the first one is : **[2011]**

(a) $\frac{1}{15}$ m/s (b) 10 m/s (c) 15 m/s (d) $\frac{1}{10}$ m/s

3. To get three images of a single object, one should have two plane mirrors at an angle of **[2003]**

(a) 60° (b) 90° (c) 120° (d) 30°

4. If two plane mirrors are kept at 60° to each other, then the number of images formed by them is **[2002]**

(a) 5 (b) 6 (c) 7 (d) 8

TOPIC - 2: Refraction of Light at Plane Surface and Total Internal Reflection

5. Let the refractive index of a denser medium with respect to a rarer medium be n_{12} and its critical angle be θ_C. At an angle of incidence A when light is travelling from denser medium to rarer medium, a part of the light is reflected and the rest is refracted and the angle between reflected and refracted rays is 90°. Angle A is given by : **[Online April 8, 2017]**

(a) $\frac{1}{\cos^{-1}(\sin\theta_C)}$ (b) $\frac{1}{\tan^{-1}(\sin\theta_C)}$
(c) $\cos^{-1}(\sin\theta_C)$ (d) $\tan^{-1}(\sin\theta_C)$

6. A diver looking up through the water sees the outside world contained in a circular horizon. The refractive index of water is $\frac{4}{3}$, and the diver's eyes are 15 cm below the surface of water. Then the radius of the circle is: **[Online April 9, 2014]**

(a) $15\times3\times\sqrt{5}$ cm (b) $15\times3\sqrt{7}$ cm
(c) $\frac{15\times\sqrt{7}}{3}$ cm (d) $\frac{15\times3}{\sqrt{7}}$ cm

7. A printed page is pressed by a glass of water. The refractive index of the glass and water is 1.5 and 1.33, respectively. If the thickness of the bottom of glass is 1 cm and depth of water is 5 cm, how much the page will appear to be shifted if viewed from the top ? **[Online April 25, 2013]**

(a) 1.033 cm (b) 3.581 cm
(c) 1.3533 cm (d) 1.90 cm

8. A light ray falls on a square glass slab as shown in the diagram. The index of refraction of the glass, if total internal reflection is to occur at the vertical face, is equal to : **[Online April 23, 2013]**

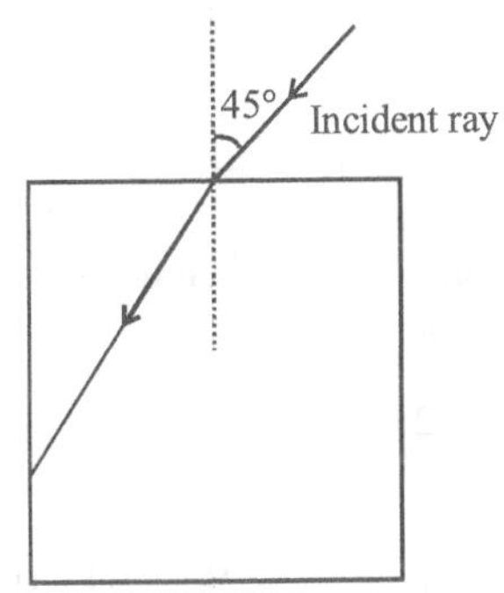

(a) $\frac{(\sqrt{2}+1)}{2}$ (b) $\sqrt{\frac{5}{2}}$
(c) $\frac{3}{2}$ (d) $\sqrt{\frac{3}{2}}$

9. Light is incident from a medium into air at two possible angles of incidence (A) 20° and (B) 40°. In the medium light travels 3.0 cm in 0.2 ns. The ray will : **[Online April 9, 2013]**

(a) suffer total internal reflection in both cases (A) and (B)
(b) suffer total internal reflection in case (B) only
(c) have partial reflection and partial transmission in case (B)
(d) have 100% transmission in case (A)

10. Let the *x-z* plane be the boundary between two transparent media. Medium 1 in $z \geq 0$ has a refractive index of $\sqrt{2}$ and medium 2 with $z < 0$ has a refractive index of $\sqrt{3}$. A ray of light in medium 1 given by the vector $\vec{A} = 6\sqrt{3}\hat{i} + 8\sqrt{3}\hat{j} - 10\hat{k}$ is incident on the plane of separation. The angle of refraction in medium 2 is: **[2011]**

(a) 45° (b) 60° (c) 75° (d) 30°

11. A beaker contains water up to a height h_1 and kerosene of height h_2 above water so that the total height of (water + kerosene) is $(h_1 + h_2)$. Refractive index of water is μ_1 and that of kerosene is μ_2. The apparent shift in the position of the bottom of the beaker when viewed from above is **[2011 RS]**

(a) $\left(1+\frac{1}{\mu_1}\right)h_1 - \left(1+\frac{1}{\mu_2}\right)h_2$

(b) $\left(1-\frac{1}{\mu_1}\right)h_1 + \left(1-\frac{1}{\mu_2}\right)h_2$

(c) $\left(1+\frac{1}{\mu_1}\right)h_2 - \left(1+\frac{1}{\mu_2}\right)h_1$

(d) $\left(1-\frac{1}{\mu_1}\right)h_2 + \left(1-\frac{1}{\mu_2}\right)h_1$

12. A transparent solid cylindrical rod has a refractive index of $\frac{2}{\sqrt{3}}$. It is surrounded by air. A light ray is incident at the mid-point of one end of the rod as shown in the figure.

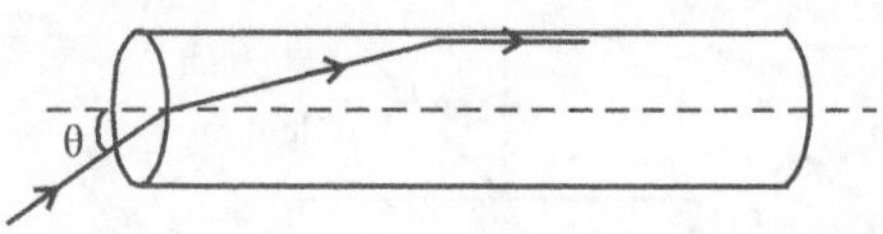

The incident angle θ for which the light ray grazes along the wall of the rod is : **[2009]**

(a) $\sin^{-1}(\sqrt{3}/2)$ (b) $\sin^{-1}\left(\frac{2}{\sqrt{3}}\right)$

(c) $\sin^{-1}\left(\frac{1}{\sqrt{3}}\right)$ (d) $\sin^{-1}(1/2)$

13. A fish looking up through the water sees the outside world contained in a circular horizon. If the refractive index of water is $\frac{4}{3}$ and the fish is 12 cm below the surface, the radius of this circle in cm is **[2005]**

(a) $\frac{36}{\sqrt{7}}$ (b) $36\sqrt{7}$ (c) $4\sqrt{5}$ (d) $36\sqrt{5}$

14. Consider telecommunication through optical fibres. Which of the following statements is **not** true? **[2003]**
(a) Optical fibres can be of graded refractive index
(b) Optical fibres are subject to electromagnetic interference from outside
(c) Optical fibres have extremely low transmission loss
(d) Optical fibres may have homogeneous core with a suitable cladding.

15. Which of the following is used in optical fibres? **[2002]**
(a) total internal reflection
(b) scattering
(c) diffraction
(d) refraction.

TOPIC - 3: Refraction at Curved Surface Lenses and Power of Lens

16. In an experiment a convex lens of focal length 15 cm is placed coaxially on an optical bench in front of a convex mirror at a distance of 5 cm from it. It is found that an object and its image coincide, if the object is placed at a distance of 20 cm from the lens. The focal length of the convex mirror is : **[Online April 9, 2017]**
(a) 27.5 cm (b) 20.0 cm (c) 25.0 cm (d) 30.5 cm

17. A hemispherical glass body of radius 10 cm and refractive index 1.5 is silvered on its curved surface. A small air bubble is 6 cm below the flat surface inside it along the axis. The position of the iamge of the air bubble made by the mirror is seen : **[Online April 10, 2016]**

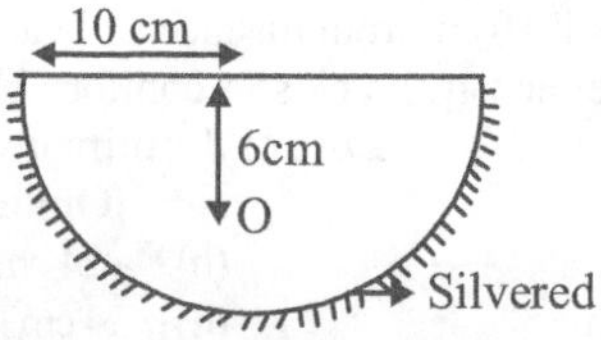

(a) 14 cm below flat surface
(b) 20 cm below flat surface
(c) 16 cm below flat surface
(d) 30 cm below flat surface

18. A convex lens, of focal length 30 cm, a concave lens of focal length 120 cm, and a plane mirror are arranged as shown. For an object kept at a distance of 60 cm from the convex lens, the final image, formed by the combination, is a real image, at a distance of: **[Online April 9, 2016]**

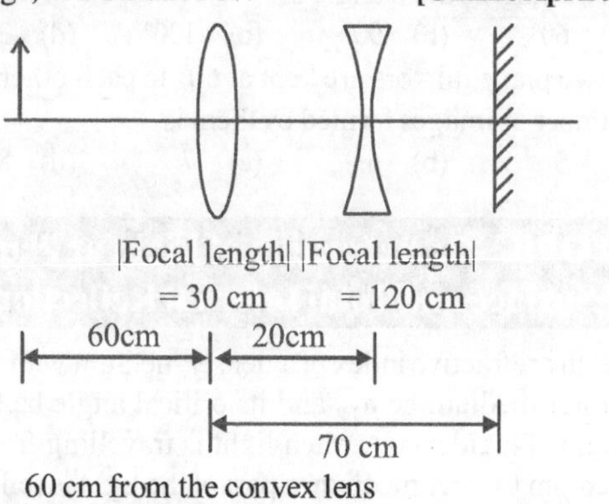

(a) 60 cm from the convex lens
(b) 60 cm from the concave lens
(c) 70 cm from the convex lens
(d) 70 cm from the concave lens

19. To find the focal length of a convex mirror, a student records the following data : **[Online April 9, 2016]**

Object Pin	Convex Lens	Convex Mirror	Image Pin
22.2cm	32.2cm	45.8cm	71.2cm

The focal length of the convex lens is f_1 and that of mirror is f_2. Then taking index correction to be negligibly small, f_1 and f_2 are close to :
(a) $f_1 = 7.8$ cm $f_2 = 12.7$ cm
(b) $f_1 = 12.7$ cm $f_2 = 7.8$ cm
(c) $f_1 = 15.6$ cm $f_2 = 25.4$ cm
(d) $f_1 = 7.8$ cm $f_2 = 25.4$ cm

20. A thin convex lens of focal length 'f' is put on a plane mirror as shown in the figure. When an object is kept at a distance 'a' from the lens - mirror combination, its image is formed at a distance $\frac{a}{3}$ in front of the combination. The value of 'a' is : **[Online April 11, 2015]**

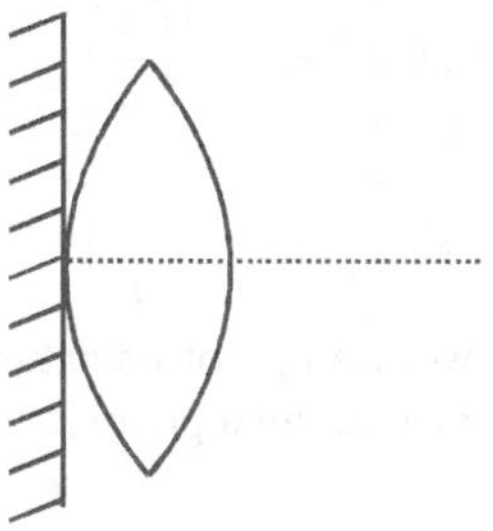

(a) 3f (b) $\frac{3}{2}$f
(c) f (d) 2f

21. A thin convex lens made from crown glass $\left(\mu = \frac{3}{2}\right)$ has focal length f. When it is measured in two different liquids having refractive indices $\frac{4}{3}$ and $\frac{5}{3}$, it has the focal lengths f_1 and f_2 respectively. The correct relation between the focal lengths is: **[2014]**
(a) $f_1 = f_2 < f$
(b) $f_1 > f$ and f_2 becomes negative
(c) $f_2 > f$ and f_1 becomes negative
(d) f_1 and f_2 both become negative

22. The refractive index of the material of a concave lens is μ. It is immersed in a medium of refractive index μ_1. A parallel beam of light is incident on the lens. The path of the emergent rays when $\mu_1 > \mu$ is: **[Online April 12, 2014]**

(a)
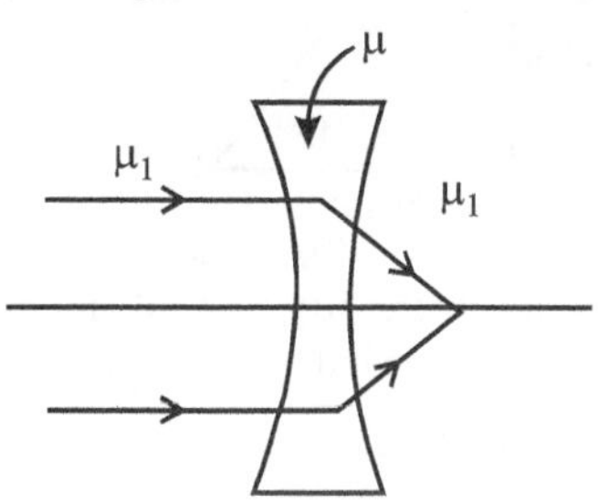

(b)
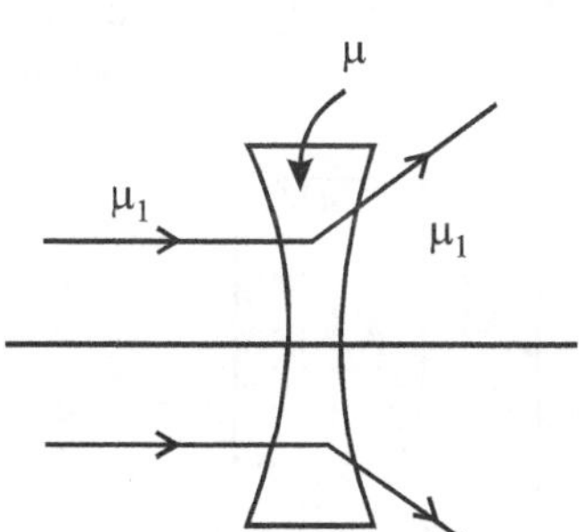

(c)
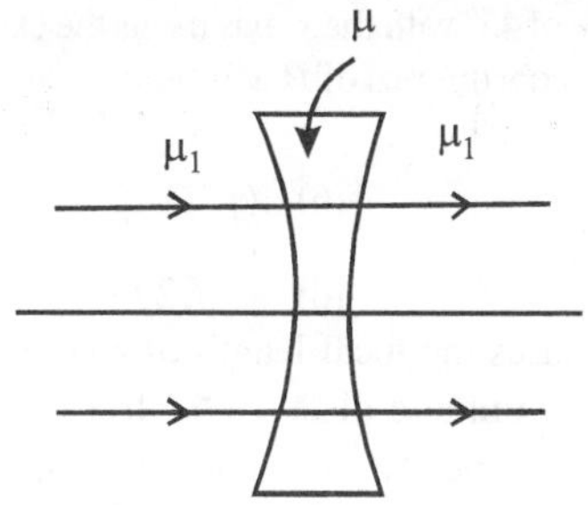

(d)
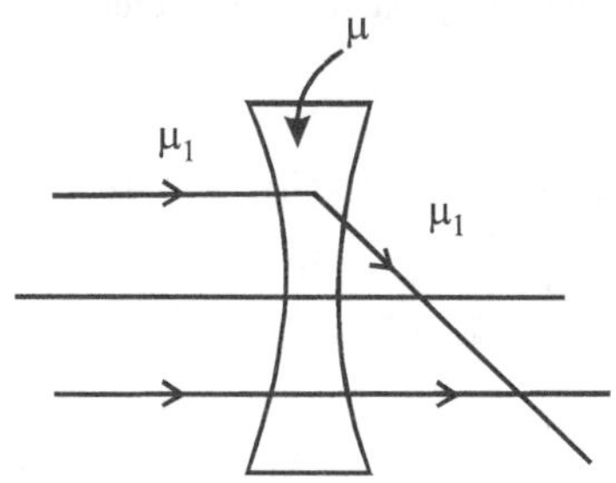

23. An object is located in a fixed position in front of a screen. Sharp image is obtained on the screen for two positions of a thin lens separated by 10 cm. The size of the images in two situations are in the ratio 3 : 3. What is the distance between the screen and the object? **[Online April 11, 2014]**
(a) 124.5 cm (b) 144.5 cm
(c) 65.0 cm (d) 99.0 cm

24. Diameter of a plano-convex lens is 6 cm and thickness at the centre is 3 mm. If speed of light in material of lens is 2×10^8 m/s, the focal length of the lens is **[2013]**
(a) 15 cm (b) 20 cm (c) 30 cm (d) 10 cm

25. The image of an illuminated square is obtained on a screen with the help of a converging lens. The distance of the square from the lens is 40 cm. The area of the image is 9 times that of the square. The focal length of the lens is : **[Online April 22, 2013]**
(a) 36 cm (b) 27 cm (c) 60 cm (d) 30 cm

26. An object at 2.4 m in front of a lens forms a sharp image on a film 12 cm behind the lens. A glass plate 1 cm thick, of refractive index 1.50 is interposed between lens and film with its plane faces parallel to film. At what distance (from lens) should object shifted to be in sharp focus of film? **[2012]**
(a) 7.2 m (b) 2.4 m (c) 3.2 m (d) 5.6 m

27. When monochromatic red light is used instead of blue light in a convex lens, its focal length will **[2011 RS]**
(a) increase
(b) decrease
(c) remain same
(d) does not depend on colour of light

28. In an optics experiment, with the position of the object fixed, a student varies the position of a convex lens and for each position, the screen is adjusted to get a clear image of the object. A graph between the object distance *u* and the image distance *v*, from the lens, is plotted using the same scale for the two axes. A straight line passing through the origin and making an angle of 45° with the x-axis meets the experimental curve at P. The coordinates of P will be **[2009]**

(a) $\left(\frac{f}{2},\frac{f}{2}\right)$ (b) (f, f)

(c) $(4f, 4f)$ (d) $(2f, 2f)$

29. A student measures the focal length of a convex lens by putting an object pin at a distance 'u' from the lens and measuring the distance 'v' of the image pin. The graph between 'u' and 'v' plotted by the student should look like **[2008]**

(a) 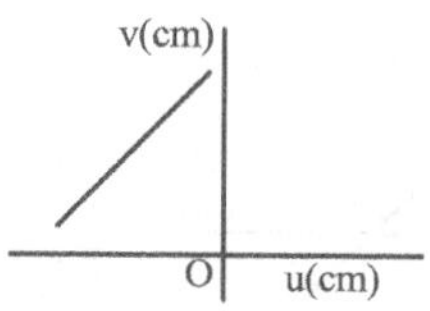

(b) 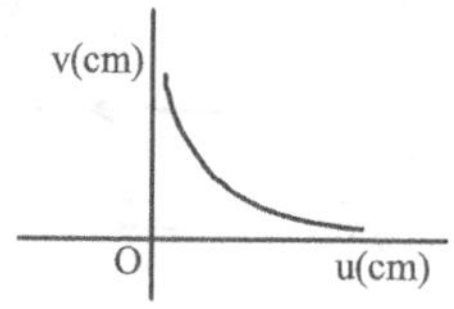

(c) 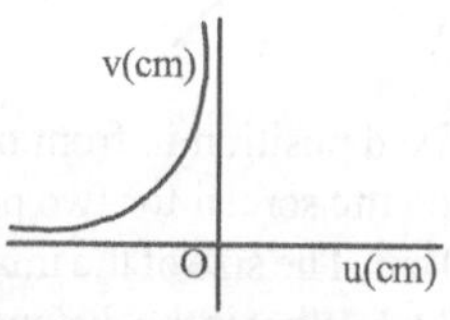

(d) 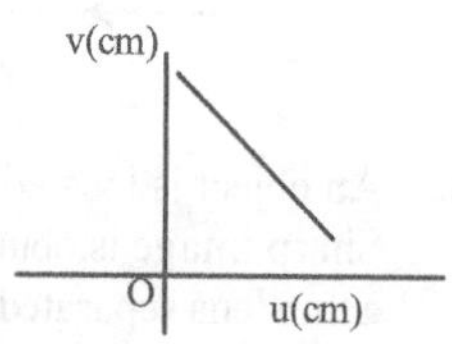

30. Two lenses of power $-15\,D$ and $+5\,D$ are in contact with each other. The focal length of the combination is **[2007]**

(a) $+10$ cm (b) -20 cm

(c) -10 cm (d) $+20$ cm

31. A thin glass (refractive index 1.5) lens has optical power of $-5\,D$ in air. Its optical power in a liquid medium with refractive index 1.6 will be **[2005]**

(a) $-1D$ (b) $1D$ (c) $-25D$ (d) $25D$

32. A plano convex lens of refractive index 1.5 and radius of curvature 30 cm. Is silvered at the curved surface. Now this lens has been used to form the image of an object. At what distance from this lens an object be placed in order to have a real image of size of the object **[2004]**

(a) 60 cm (b) 30 cm (c) 20 cm (d) 80 cm

TOPIC - 4: Prism and Dispersion of Light

33. In an experiment for determination of refractive index of glass of a prism by $i-\delta$, plot it was found thata ray incident at angle 35°, suffers a deviation of 40° and that it emerges at angle 79°. In that case which of the following is closest to the maximum possible value of the refractive index? **[2016]**

(a) 1.7 (b) 1.8 (c) 1.5 (d) 1.6

34. Monochromatic light is incident on a glass prism of angle A. If the refractive index of the material of the prism is μ, a ray, incident at an angle θ, on the face AB would get transmitted through the face AC of the prism provided : **[2015]**

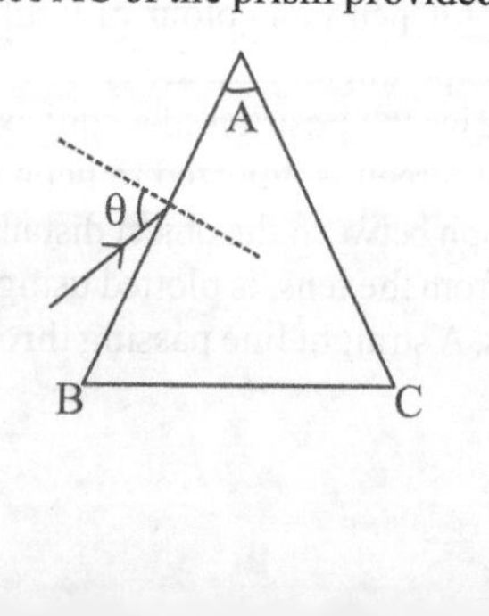

(a) $\theta > \cos^{-1}\left[\mu\sin\left(A+\sin^{-1}\left(\frac{1}{\mu}\right)\right)\right]$

(b) $\theta < \cos^{-1}\left[\mu\sin\left(A+\sin^{-1}\left(\frac{1}{\mu}\right)\right)\right]$

(c) $\theta > \sin^{-1}\left[\mu\sin\left(A-\sin^{-1}\left(\frac{1}{\mu}\right)\right)\right]$

(d) $\theta < \sin^{-1}\left[\mu\sin\left(A-\sin^{-1}\left(\frac{1}{\mu}\right)\right)\right]$

35. The graph between angle of deviation (δ) and angle of incidence (i) for a triangular prism is represented by **[2013]**

(a) 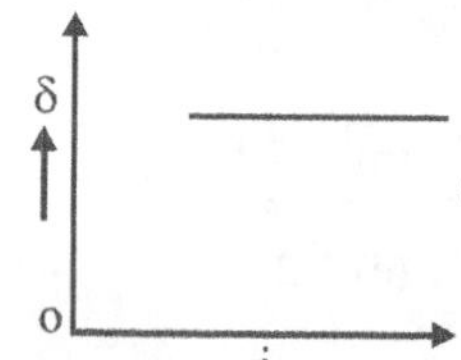

(b) 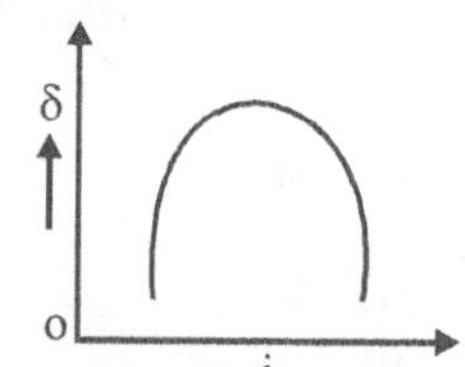

(c) 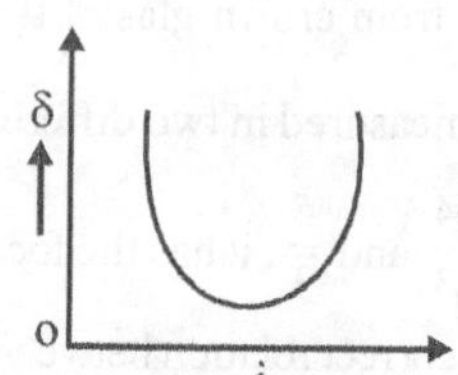

(d) 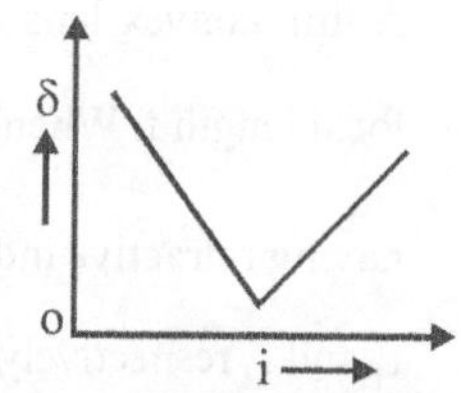

36. A beam of light consisting of red, green and blue colours is incident on a right-angled prism on face AB. The refractive indices of the material for the above red, green and blue colours are 1.39, 1.44 and 1.47 respectively. A person looking on surface AC of the prism will see **[Online May 26, 2012]**

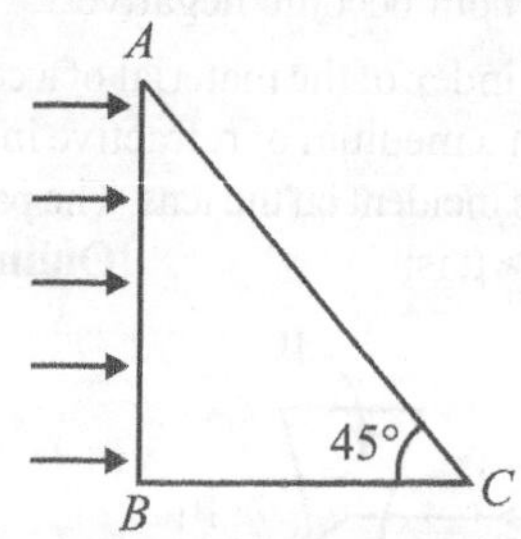

(a) no light (b) green and blue colours

(c) red and green colours (d) red colour only

37. A glass prism of refractive index 1.5 is immersed in water (refractive index $\frac{4}{3}$) as shown in figure. A light beam incident normally on the face AB is totally reflected to reach the face BC, if **[Online May 19, 2012]**

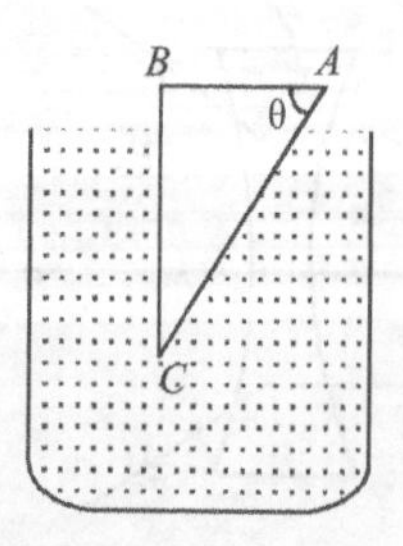

(a) $\sin\theta > \frac{5}{9}$ (b) $\sin\theta > \frac{2}{3}$

(c) $\sin\theta > \frac{8}{9}$ (d) $\sin\theta > \frac{1}{3}$

38. Which of the following processes play a part in the formation of a rainbow? **[Online May 7, 2012]**
(i) Refraction (ii) Total internal reflection
(iii) Dispersion (iv) Interference
(a) (i), (ii) and (iii) (b) (i) and (ii)
(c) (i), (ii) and (iv) (d) (iii) and (iv)

39. The refractive index of a glass is 1.520 for red light and 1.525 for blue light. Let D_1 and D_2 be angles of minimum deviation for red and blue light respectively in a prism of this glass. Then, **[2006]**
(a) $D_1 < D_2$ (b) $D_1 = D_2$
(c) D_1 can be less than or greater than D_2 depending upon the angle of prism
(d) $D_1 > D_2$

40. A light ray is incident perpendicularly to one face of a 90° prism and is totally internally reflected at the glass-air interface. If the angle of reflection is 45°, we conclude that the refractive index n **[2004]**

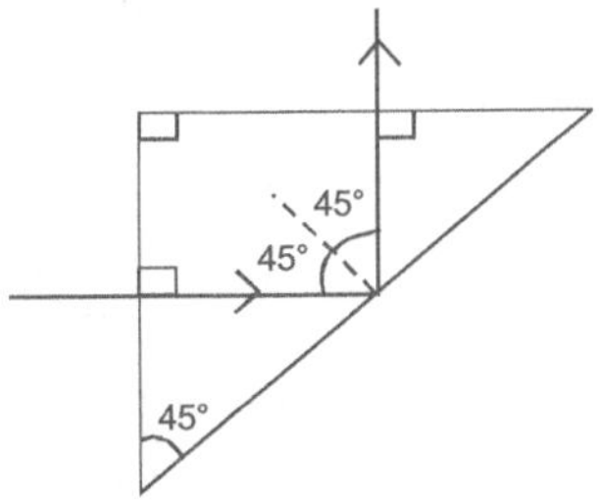

(a) $n > \frac{1}{\sqrt{2}}$ (b) $n > \sqrt{2}$

(c) $n < \frac{1}{\sqrt{2}}$ (d) $n < \sqrt{2}$

TOPIC - 5: Optical Instruments

41. An observer looks at a distant tree of height 10 m with a telescope of magnifying power of 20. To the observer the tree appears : **[2016]**
(a) 20 times taller (b) 20 times nearer
(c) 10 times taller (d) 10 times nearer

42. To determine refractive index of glass slab using a travelling microscope, minimum number of readings required are : **[Online April 10, 2016]**
(a) Two (b) Four (c) Three (d) Five

43. A telescope has an objective lens of focal length 150 cm and an eyepiece of focal length 5 cm. If a 50 m tall tower at a distance of 1 km is observed through this telescope in normal setting, the angle formed by the image of the tower is θ, then θ is close to : **[Online April 10, 2015]**
(a) 30° (b) 15° (c) 60° (d) 1°

44. In a compound microscope, the focal length of objective lens is 1.2 cm and focal length of eye piece is 3.0 cm. When object is kept at 1.25 cm in front of objective, final image is formed at infinity. Magnifying power of the compound microscope should be: **[Online April 11, 2014]**
(a) 200 (b) 100 (c) 400 (d) 150

45. The focal lengths of objective lens and eye lens of a Galilean telescope are respectively 30 cm and 3.0 cm. telescope produces virtual, erect image of an object situated far away from it at least distance of distinct vision from the eye lens. In this condition, the magnifying power of the Galilean telescope should be: **[Online April 9, 2014]**
(a) +11.2 (b) −11.2 (c) −8.8 (d) +8.8

46. This question has Statement-1 and Statement-2. Of the four choices given after the Statements, choose the one that best describes the two Statements.
Statement 1: Very large size telescopes are reflecting telescopes instead of refracting telescopes.
Statement 2: It is easier to provide mechanical support to large size mirrors than large size lenses. **[Online April 23, 2013]**
(a) Statement-1 is true and Statement-2 is false.
(b) Statement-1 is false and Statement-2 is true.
(c) Statement-1 and statement-2 are true and Statement-2 is correct explanation for statement-1.
(d) Statements-1 and statement-2 are true and Statement-2 is not the correct explanation for statement-1.

47. The focal length of the objective and the eyepiece of a telescope are 50 cm and 5 cm respectively. If the telescope is focussed for distinct vision on a scale distant 2 m from its objective, then its magnifying power will be : **[Online April 22, 2013]**
(a) −4 (b) −8 (c) +8 (d) −2

48. A telescope of aperture 3×10^{-2} m diameter is focused on a window at 80 m distance fitted with a wire mesh of spacing 2×10^{-3} m. Given: $\lambda = 5.5 \times 10^{-7}$ m, which of the following is true for observing the mesh through the telescope? **[Online May 26, 2012]**
(a) Yes, it is possible with the same aperture size.
(b) Possible also with an aperture half the present diameter.
(c) No, it is not possible.
(d) Given data is not sufficient.

49. We wish to make a microscope with the help of two positive lenses both with a focal length of 20 mm each and the object is positioned 25 mm from the objective lens. How far apart the lenses should be so that the final image is formed at infinity? **[Online May 12, 2012]**
(a) 20mm (b) 100mm
(c) 120mm (d) 80mm

50. An experment is performed to find the refractive index of glass using a travelling microscope. In this experiment distances are measured by **[2008]**
(a) a vernier scale provided on the microscope
(b) a standard laboratory scale
(c) a meter scale provided on the microscope
(d) a screw gauge provided on the microscope

51. The image formed by an objective of a compound microscope is **[2003]**
(a) virtual and diminished (b) real and diminished
(c) real and enlarged (d) virtual and enlarged

52. An astronomical telescope has a large aperture to **[2002]**
(a) reduce spherical aberration
(b) have high resolution
(c) increase span of observation
(d) have low dispersion

Hints & Solutions

TOPIC - 1: Plane Mirror, Spherical Mirror and Reflection of Light

1. (c) Convex morror is used as a shaving mirror.

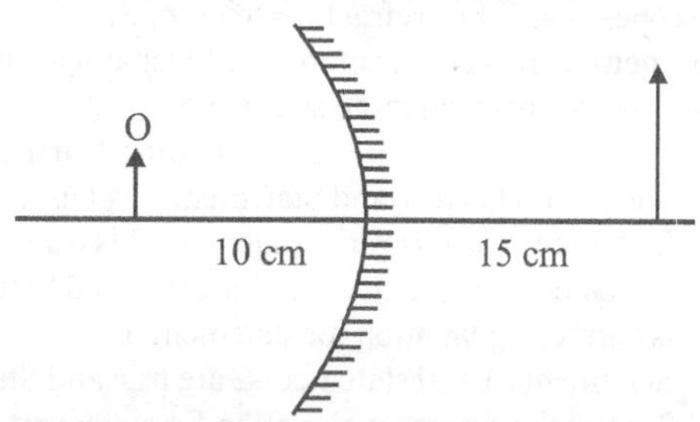

From question : $v = 15$ cm, $u = -10$ cm

Radius of curvature, $R = 2f = ?$

Using mirror formula, $\frac{1}{v}+\frac{1}{u}=\frac{1}{f}$

$$\frac{1}{15}+\frac{1}{(-10)}=\frac{1}{f} \Rightarrow f = -30 \text{ cm}$$

Therefore radius of curvature,
$R = 2f = -60$ cm

2. (a) From mirror formula

$\frac{1}{v}+\frac{1}{u}=\frac{1}{f}$ so, $\frac{dv}{dt}=-\frac{v^2}{u^2}\left(\frac{du}{dt}\right)$

$$\Rightarrow \frac{dv}{dt}=-\left(\frac{f}{u-f}\right)^2\frac{du}{dt}$$

$$\Rightarrow \frac{dv}{dt}=\frac{1}{15} \text{ m/s}$$

3. (b) When $\theta = 90°$ then $\frac{360}{\theta}=\frac{360}{90}=4$ is an even number. The number of images formed is given by

$$n=\frac{360}{\theta}-1=\frac{360}{90}-1=4-1=3$$

4. (a) When two plane mirrors are inclined at each other at an angle θ then the number of the images of a point object placed between the plane mirrors is $\frac{360°}{\theta}-1$, if $\frac{360°}{\theta}$ is even

$\therefore$ Number of images formed $=\frac{360°}{60°}-1=5$

TOPIC - 2: Refraction of Light at Plane Surface and Total Internal Reflection

5. (d)

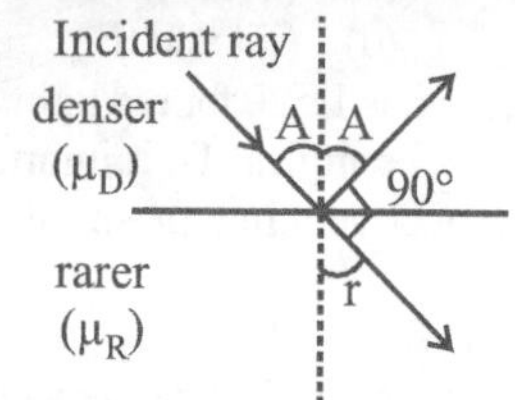

From Snell's law, $\frac{\mu_R}{\mu_D}=\frac{\sin i}{\sin r}$ ..... (i)

$\because \angle i = A$ and $\angle r = (90° - A)$

We also know that, $\sin\theta_C=\frac{\mu_R}{\mu_D}$

From eq^n (i), $\sin\theta_C=\frac{\sin A}{\sin(90°-A)}$

$$\sin\theta_C=\frac{\sin A}{\cos A}$$

$$\sin\theta_C=\tan A$$

or $A=\tan^{-1}(\sin\theta_c)$

6. (d) Given, $\mu=\frac{4}{3}$

h = 15 cm

R = ?

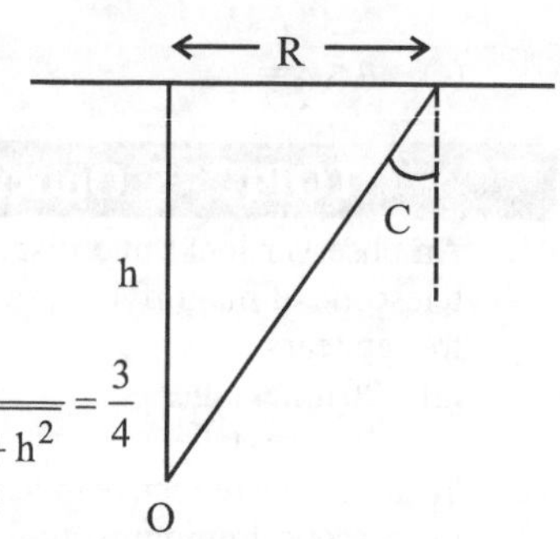

$$\frac{\sin 90°}{\sin C}=\mu$$

$$\Rightarrow \sin C=\frac{1}{\mu}=\frac{R}{\sqrt{R^2+h^2}}=\frac{3}{4}$$

$\Rightarrow$ $16R^2=9R^2+9h^2$

or, $7R^2=9h^2$

or, $R=\frac{3}{\sqrt{7}}h=\frac{3}{\sqrt{7}}\times 15\text{cm}$

7. (c) Real depth = 5 cm + 1cm = 6 cm

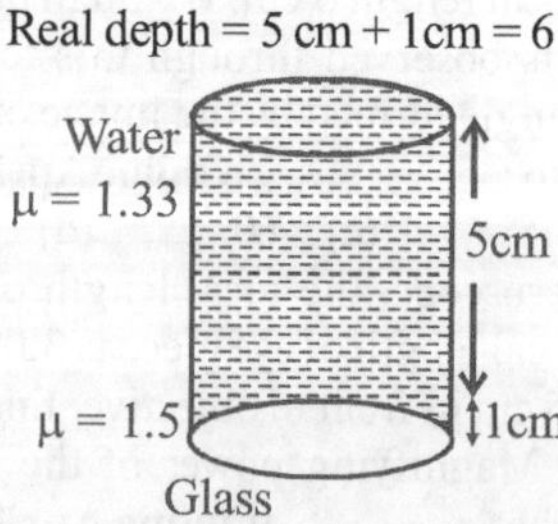

Apparent depth $= \frac{d_1}{\mu_1} + \frac{d_2}{\mu_2} + ...$

$= \frac{5}{1.33} + \frac{1}{1.5}$

$\simeq 3.8 + 0.7 \simeq 4.5$ cm

$\therefore$ Shift $= 6$ cm $- 4.5$ cm $\cong 1.5$ cm

8. **(d)** At point A by Snell's law

$$\mu = \frac{\sin 45°}{\sin r} \Rightarrow \sin r = \frac{1}{\mu\sqrt{2}} \quad ...(i)$$

At point B, for total internal reflection,

$$\sin i_1 = \frac{1}{\mu}$$

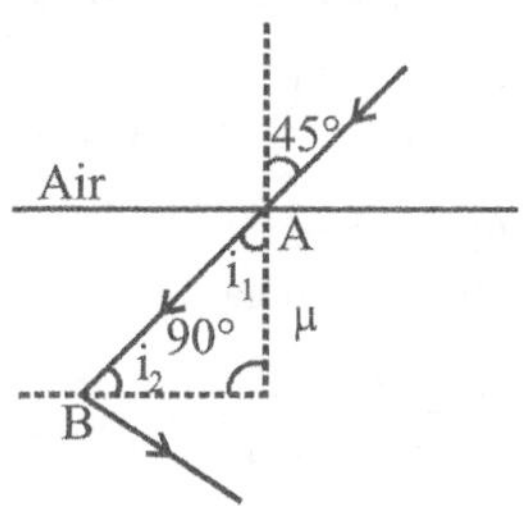

From figure, $i_1 = 90° - r$

$$\therefore (\sin 90° - r) = \frac{1}{\mu}$$

$$\Rightarrow \cos r = \frac{1}{\mu} \quad ...(ii)$$

Now $\cos r = \sqrt{1 - \sin^2 r} = \sqrt{1 - \frac{1}{2\mu^2}}$

$$= \sqrt{\frac{2\mu^2 - 1}{2\mu^2}} \quad ...(iii)$$

From eqs (ii) and (iii)

$$\frac{1}{\mu} = \sqrt{\frac{2\mu^2 - 1}{2\mu^2}}$$

Squaring both sides and then solving, we get

$$\mu = \sqrt{\frac{3}{2}}$$

9. **(b)** Velocity of light in medium

$$V_{med} = \frac{3\text{ cm}}{0.2\text{ns}} = \frac{3 \times 10^{-2}\text{ m}}{0.2 \times 10^{-9}\text{ s}} = 1.5 \text{ m/s}$$

Refractive index of the medium

$$\mu = \frac{V_{air}}{V_{med}} = \frac{3 \times 10^8}{1.5} = 2 \text{ m/s}$$

As $\mu = \frac{1}{\sin C}$

$$\therefore \sin C = \frac{1}{\mu} = \frac{1}{2} = 30°$$

Condition of TIR is angle of incidence i must be greater than critical angle. Hence ray will suffer TIR in case of (B) $(i = 40° > 30°)$ only.

10. **(a)** Angle of incidence is given by

$$\cos(\pi - i) = \frac{(6\sqrt{3}\hat{i} + 8\sqrt{3}\hat{j} - 10\hat{k}).\hat{k}}{20}$$

$$-\cos i = -\frac{1}{2}$$

$\angle i = 60°$

From Snell's law,

$\sqrt{2} \sin i = \sqrt{3} \sin r$

$\angle r = 45°$

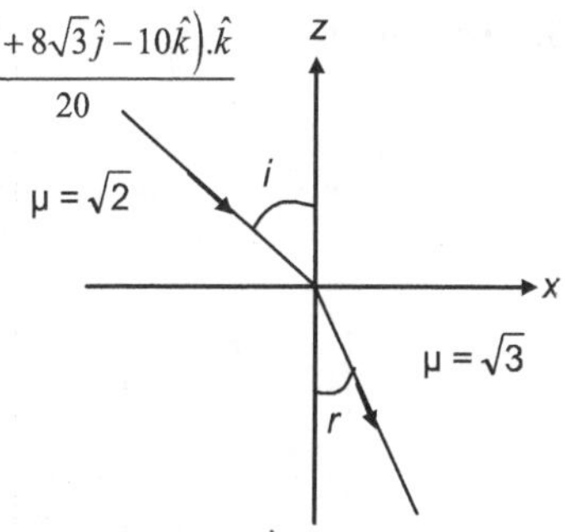

11. **(b)**

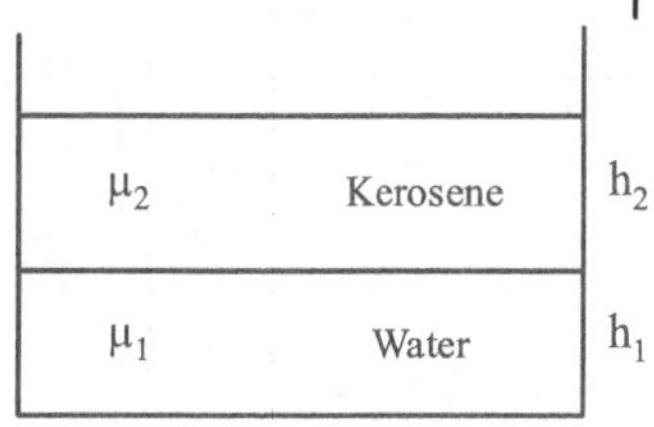

Apparent shift due to water $= h_1\left[1 - \frac{1}{\mu_1}\right]$

Apparent shift due to kerosene

$= h_2\left[1 - \frac{1}{\mu_2}\right]$

Thus, total apparent shift :

$= h_1\left(1 - \frac{1}{\mu_1}\right) + h_2\left(1 - \frac{1}{\mu_2}\right)$

12. **(c)**

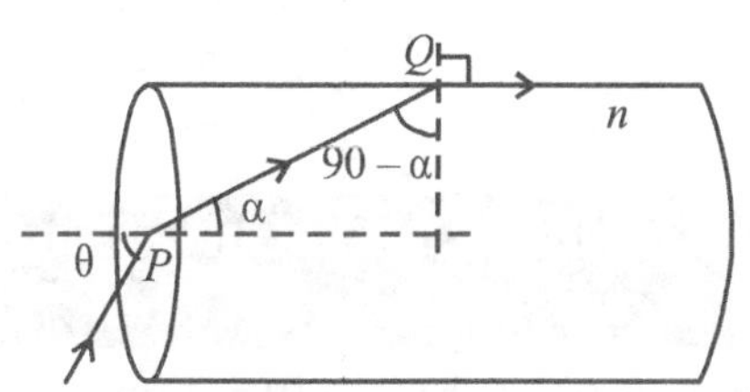

Applying Snell's law at Q

$$n = \frac{\sin 90°}{\sin(90° - \alpha)} = \frac{1}{\cos\alpha}$$

$$\therefore \cos\alpha = \frac{1}{n}$$

$\therefore \sin\alpha = \sqrt{1-\cos^2\alpha} = \sqrt{1-\frac{1}{n^2}} = \frac{\sqrt{n^2-1}}{n}$ ...(1)

Applying Snell's Law at *P*

$n = \frac{\sin\theta}{\sin\alpha} \Rightarrow \sin\theta = n\times\sin\alpha = \sqrt{n^2-1}$; from (1)

$\therefore \sin\theta = \sqrt{\left(\frac{2}{\sqrt{3}}\right)^2 - 1} = \sqrt{\frac{4}{3}-1} = \frac{1}{\sqrt{3}}$

or $\theta = \sin^{-1}\left(\frac{1}{\sqrt{3}}\right)$

13. (a) $\sin\theta_c = \frac{1}{\mu} = \frac{3}{4}$

or $\tan\theta_c = \frac{3}{\sqrt{16-9}} = \frac{3}{\sqrt{7}} = \frac{R}{12}$

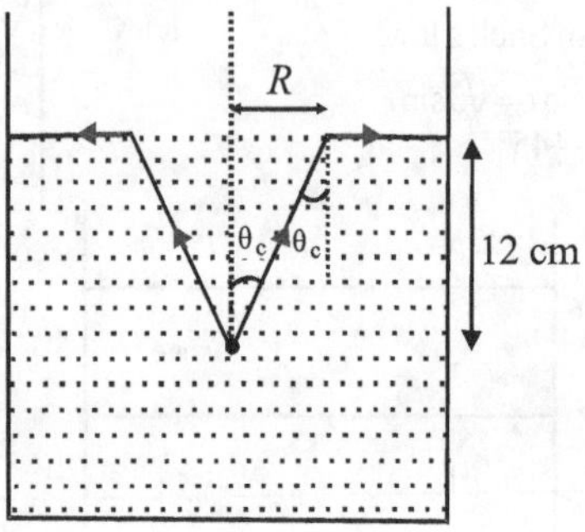

$\Rightarrow R = \frac{36}{\sqrt{7}}$ cm

14. (b) Optical fibres form a dielectric wave guide and are free from electromagnetic interference or radio frequency interference.

15. (a) In an optical fibre, light is sent through the fibre without any loss by the phenomenon of total internal reflection as shown in the figure.

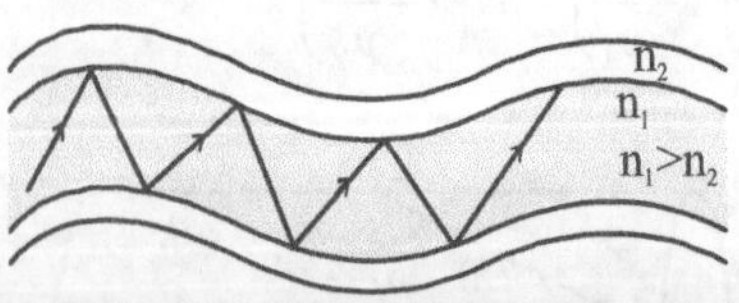

TOPIC - 3: Refraction at Curved Surface Lenses and Power of Lens

16. (a) Given, focal length of lens (f) = 15 cm
object is placed at a distance (u) = – 20 cm
By lens formula,

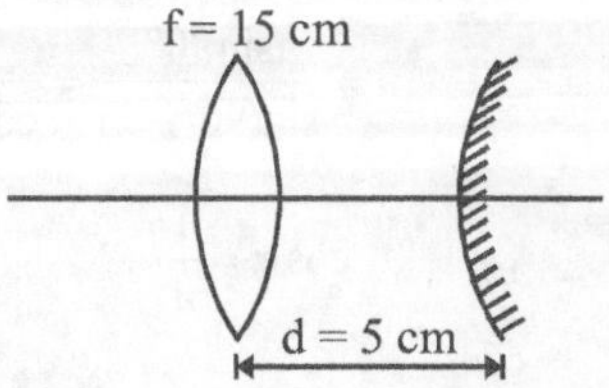

$\frac{1}{f} = \frac{1}{v} - \frac{1}{u}$

$\frac{1}{v} = \frac{1}{f} + \frac{1}{u} = \frac{1}{15} - \frac{1}{20}$

$\frac{1}{v} = \frac{4-3}{60}$

v = 60 cm

The image I gets formed at 60 cm to the right of the lens and it will be inverted.

The rays from the image (I) formed further falls on the convex mirror forms another image. This image should formed in such a way that it coincide with object at the same point due to reflection takes place by convex mirror.

Distance between lens and mirror will be

d = image distance (v) – radius of curvature of convex mirror.

5 = 60 – 2f

2f = 60 – 5

$f = \frac{55}{2} = 27.5$ cm (convex mirror)

17. (b) Given, radius of hemispherical glass R = 10 cm

$\therefore$ Focal length $f = \frac{10}{2} = -5$ cm

u = (10 – 6) = –4 cm.

By using mirror formula,

$\frac{1}{v} + \frac{1}{u} = \frac{1}{f} \Rightarrow \frac{1}{v} + \frac{1}{-4} = \frac{1}{-5} \Rightarrow v = 20$ cm.

Apparent height, $h_a = h_r \frac{\mu_1}{\mu_2} = 30 \times \frac{1}{1.5} = 20$ cm below flat surface.

18. (a) Len's formula is given by

$\frac{1}{f} = \frac{1}{v} - \frac{1}{u}$

For convex lens,

$\frac{1}{30} = \frac{1}{v} + \frac{1}{60} \Rightarrow \frac{1}{60} = \frac{1}{v}$

Similarly for concave lens

$\frac{1}{-120} = \frac{1}{v} - \frac{1}{40} \Rightarrow \frac{1}{v} = \frac{1}{60}$

Virtual object 10 cm behind plane mirror.

Hence real image 10 cm infront of mirror or, 60 cm from convex lens.

19. (a) Taking $f_2 = 12.07$

Using Mirror's formula

$\frac{1}{f} = \frac{1}{v} + \frac{1}{u}$

$\Rightarrow \frac{1}{12.7} = \frac{1}{25.4} + \frac{1}{u} \Rightarrow \frac{1}{12.7} - \frac{1}{25.4} = \frac{1}{u}$

u = 25.4 = v'

Now using Len's formula

$\frac{1}{f} = \frac{1}{v} - \frac{1}{u} \Rightarrow \frac{1}{f_1} = \frac{1}{25.4+13.6} + \frac{1}{10}$

$$\Rightarrow \frac{1}{f_1} = \frac{1}{39} + \frac{1}{10} \Rightarrow f_1 = \frac{390}{49} = 7.96$$

The closest answers is (a) as option (c) and (d) are not possible.

20. (d) When object is kept at a distance 'a' from thin covex lens

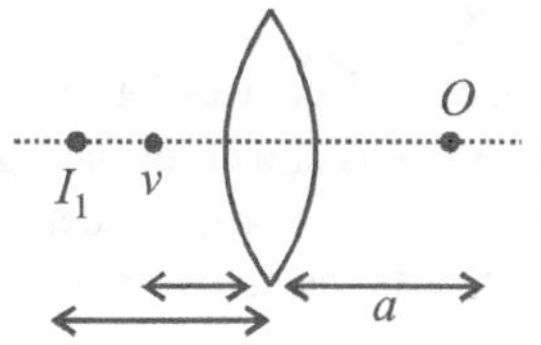

By lens formula : $\frac{1}{v} - \frac{1}{u} = \frac{1}{f}$

$$\frac{1}{V} - \frac{1}{(-a)} = \frac{1}{f}$$

or, $\frac{1}{v} = \frac{1}{f} - \frac{1}{a}$ ...(i)

Mirror forms image at equal distance from mirror

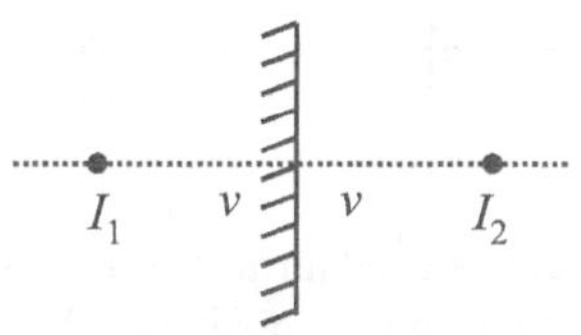

Now, again from lens formula

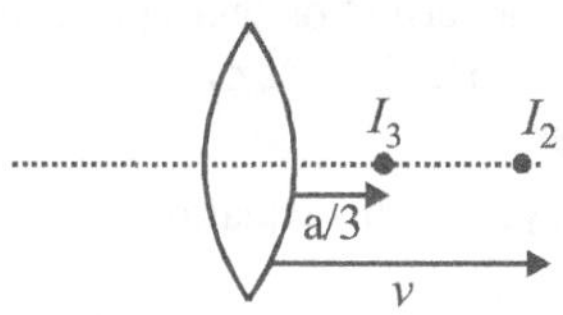

$$\frac{3}{a} - \frac{1}{V} = \frac{1}{f}$$

$$\frac{3}{a} - \frac{1}{f} + \frac{1}{a} = \frac{1}{f} \quad \text{[From eqn. (i)]}$$

Hence, $a = 2f$

21. (b) By Lens maker's formula for convex lens

$$\frac{1}{f} = \left(\frac{\mu}{\mu_L} - 1\right)\left(\frac{2}{R}\right)$$

for, $\mu_{L_1} = \frac{4}{3}, f_1 = 4R$

for $\mu_{L_2} = \frac{5}{3}, f_2 = -5R$

$\Rightarrow f_2 = (-)$ ve

22. (a) If a lens of refractive index μ is immersed in a medium of refractive index μ_1, then its focal length in medium is given by

$$\frac{1}{f_m} = ({}_m\mu_l - 1)\left(\frac{1}{R_1} - \frac{1}{R_2}\right)$$

If f_a is the focal length of lens in air, then

$$\frac{1}{f_a} = ({}_a\mu_l - 1)\left(\frac{1}{R_1} - \frac{1}{R_2}\right)$$

$$\Rightarrow \frac{f_m}{f_a} = \frac{({}_a\mu_l - 1)}{({}_m\mu_l - 1)}$$

If $\mu_1 > \mu$, then f_m and f_a have opposite signs and the nature of lens changes i.e. a convex lens diverges the light rays and concave lens converges the light rays. Thus given option (a) is correct.

23. (d) **Given:** Separation of lens for two of its position, $d = 10$ cm

Ratio of size of the images in two positions

$$\frac{I_1}{I_2} = \frac{3}{2}$$

Distance of object from the screen, $D = ?$

Applying formula,

$$\frac{I_1}{I_2} = \frac{(D+d)^2}{(D-d)^2}$$

$$\Rightarrow \frac{3}{2} = \frac{(D+10)^2}{(D-10)^2}$$

$$\Rightarrow \frac{3}{2} = \frac{D^2+100+20D}{D^2+100-20D}$$

$\Rightarrow 3D^2 + 300 - 60D = 2D^2 + 200 + 40D$

$\Rightarrow D^2 - 100D + 100 = 0$

On solving, we get $D = 99$ cm

Hence the distance between the screen and the object is 99 cm.

24. (c) $\therefore n = \frac{\text{Velocity of light in vacuum}}{\text{Velocity of light in medium}}$

$\therefore n = \frac{3}{2}$

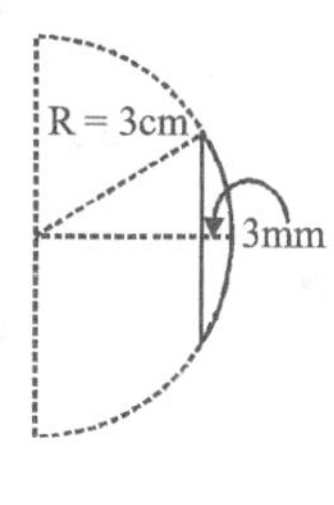

$3^2 + (R - 3mm)^2 = R^2$

$\Rightarrow 3^2 + R^2 - 2R(3mm) + (3mm)^2 = R^2$

$\Rightarrow R \approx 15$ cm

$$\frac{1}{f} = \left(\frac{3}{2} - 1\right)\left(\frac{1}{15}\right) \Rightarrow f = 30 \text{ cm}$$

25. (d) If side of object square $= \ell$

and side of image square $= \ell'$

From question, $\frac{\ell'^2}{\ell} = 9$

or $\frac{\ell'}{\ell} = 3$

i.e., magnification m = 3

u = – 40 cm

v = 3 × 40 = 120 cm

f = ?

From formula, $\frac{1}{v} - \frac{1}{u} = \frac{1}{f}$

$$\frac{1}{120} - \frac{1}{-40} = \frac{1}{f}$$

or, $\frac{1}{f} = \frac{1}{120} + \frac{1}{40} = \frac{1+3}{120}$ $\therefore$ f = 30 cm

26. (d) The focal length of the lens

$$\frac{1}{f} = \frac{1}{v} - \frac{1}{u} = \frac{1}{12} + \frac{1}{240} = \frac{20+1}{240} = \frac{21}{240}$$

$$f = \frac{240}{21}\text{cm}$$

$$\text{Shift} = t\left(1 - \frac{1}{\mu}\right)$$

$$1\left(1 - \frac{1}{3/2}\right) = 1 \times \frac{1}{3}$$

$$\text{Now } v' = 12 - \frac{1}{3} = \frac{35}{3}\text{ cm}$$

Now the object distance u.

$$\frac{1}{u} = \frac{3}{35} - \frac{21}{240} = \frac{1}{5}\left[\frac{3}{7} - \frac{21}{48}\right]$$

$$\frac{1}{u} = \frac{1}{5}\left[\frac{48-49}{7 \times 16}\right]$$

$$u = -7 \times 16 \times 5 = -560 \text{ cm} = -5.6 \text{ m}$$

27. (a) We know that $\mu_R < \mu_B$

and $\frac{1}{f} = (\mu - 1)\left(\frac{1}{R_1} - \frac{1}{R_2}\right)$

$$\Rightarrow \frac{1}{f_B} > \frac{1}{f_R} \Rightarrow f_R > f_B.$$

28. (d)

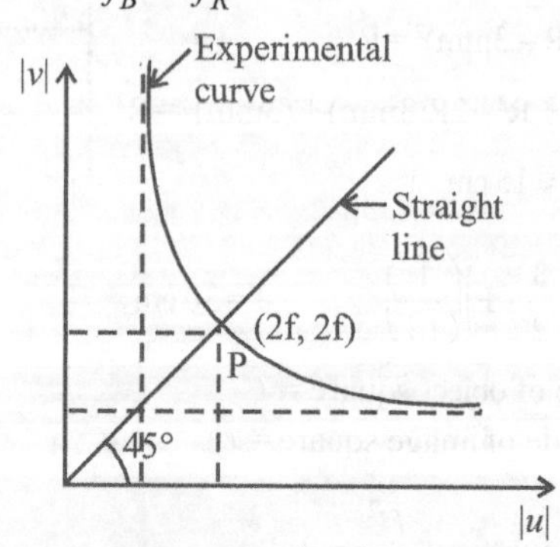

For a convex lens $\frac{1}{v} - \frac{1}{u} = \frac{1}{f}$

when $u = -\alpha$, $v = +f$

when $u = -f$, $v = +\alpha$

Then $u = -2f, v = 2f$

Also $v = \frac{f}{1 + \frac{f}{u}}$

As $|u|$ increases, v decreases for $|u| > f$. The graph between $|v|$ and $|u|$ is shown in the figure. A straight line passing through the origin and making an angle of 45°with the x-axis meets the experimental curve at $P(2f, 2f)$.

29. (c) This graph suggest that when $u = -f, v = + \propto$

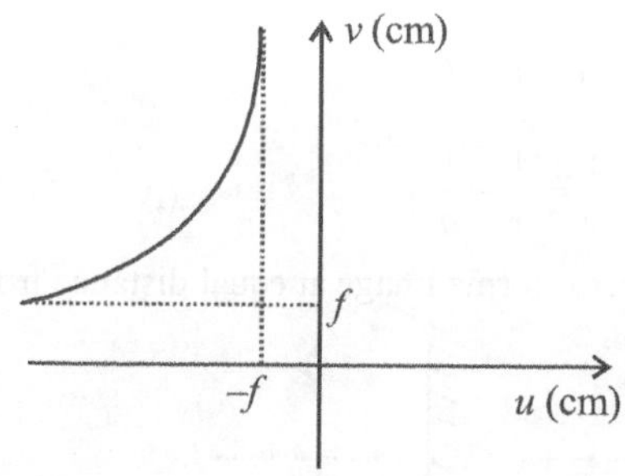

When the object is moved further away from the lens, v decreases but remains positive. When u is at $-\propto$, $v = f$.

This is how image formation takes place for different positions of the object in case of a convex lens.

ALTERNATE SOLUTION

This graph obeys the lens equation

$$\frac{1}{v} - \frac{1}{u} = \frac{1}{f}$$

where f is a positive constant for a given convex lens.

30. (c) Power of combination is given by

$P = P_1 + P_2 = (-15+5)D = -10D.$

Now, $P = \frac{1}{f} \Rightarrow f = \frac{1}{P} = \frac{1}{-10}$ metre

$$\therefore f = -\left(\frac{1}{10} \times 100\right) \text{cm} = -10 \text{ cm}.$$

31. (b) $\frac{1}{f_a} = \left(\frac{1.5}{1} - 1\right)\left(\frac{1}{R_1} - \frac{1}{R_2}\right)$ .... (i)

$$\frac{1}{f_m} = \left(\frac{\mu_g}{\mu_m} - 1\right)\left(\frac{1}{R_1} - \frac{1}{R_2}\right)$$

$\frac{1}{f_m} = \left(\frac{1.5}{1.6} - 1\right)\left(\frac{1}{R_1} - \frac{1}{R_2}\right)$ .... (ii)

Dividing (i) by (ii), $\frac{f_m}{f_a} = \left(\frac{1.5-1}{\frac{1.5}{1.6}-1}\right) = -8$

$$P_a = -5 = \frac{1}{f_a} \Rightarrow f_a = -\frac{1}{5}$$

$$\Rightarrow f_m = -8 \times f_a = -8 \times -\frac{1}{5} = \frac{8}{5}$$

$$P_m = \frac{\mu}{f_m} = \frac{1.6}{8} \times 5 = 1\text{D}$$

32. **(c)** The focal length(F) of the final mirror is

$$\frac{1}{F} = \frac{2}{f_\ell} + \frac{1}{f_m}$$

Here $\frac{1}{f_\ell} = (\mu-1)\left(\frac{1}{R_1} - \frac{1}{R_2}\right)$

$$= (1.5-1)\left[\frac{1}{\alpha} - \frac{1}{-30}\right] = \frac{1}{60}$$

$$\therefore \frac{1}{F} = 2 \times \frac{1}{60} + \frac{1}{30/2} = \frac{1}{10}$$

$\therefore F = 10$ cm

The combination acts as a converging mirror. For the object to be of the same size of mirror,

$u = 2F = 20$ cm

TOPIC - 4: Prism and Dispersion of Light

33. **(c)** We know that $i + e - A = \delta$

$35° + 79° - A = 40° \quad \therefore \quad A = 74°$

But $\mu = \frac{\sin\left(\frac{A+\delta_m}{2}\right)}{\sin A/2} = \frac{\sin\left(\frac{74+\delta_m}{2}\right)}{\sin\frac{74}{2}}$

$$= \frac{5}{3}\sin\left(37° + \frac{\delta_m}{2}\right)$$

μ_{max} can be $\frac{5}{3}$. That is μ_{max} is less than $\frac{5}{3} = 1.67$

But δ_m will be less than 40° so

$$\mu < \frac{5}{3}\sin 57° < \frac{5}{3}\sin 60° \Rightarrow \mu = 1.45$$

34. **(c)** When $r_2 = C, \angle N_2Rc = 90°$

Where C = critical angle

As $\sin C = \frac{1}{v} = \sin r_2$

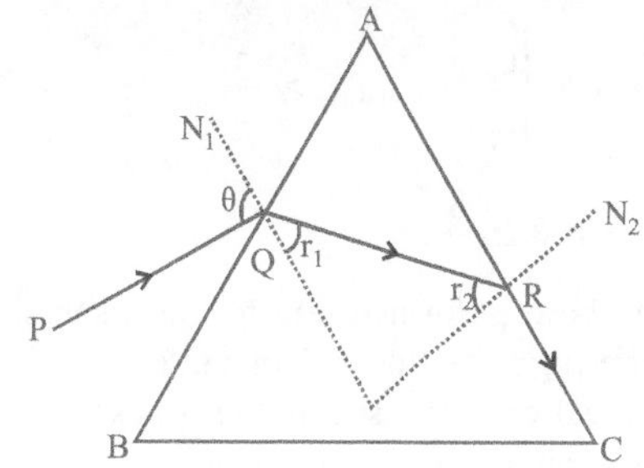

Applying snell's law at 'R'

$\mu \sin r_2 = 1 \sin 90°$ ...(i)

Applying snell's law at 'Q'

$1 \times \sin\theta = \mu \sin r_1$ ...(ii)

But $r_1 = A - r_2$

So, $\sin\theta = \mu \sin(A - r_2)$

$\sin\theta = \mu \sin A \cos r_2 - \cos A$ ...(iii) [using (i)]

From (1)

$\cos r_2 = \sqrt{1-\sin^2 r_2} = \sqrt{1-\frac{1}{\mu^2}}$ ...(iv)

By eq. (iii) and (iv)

$$\sin\theta = \mu \sin A\sqrt{1-\frac{1}{\mu^2}} - \cos A$$

on further solving we can show for ray not to transmitted through face AC

$$\theta = \sin^{-1}\left[u \sin(A - \sin^{-1}\left(\frac{1}{\mu}\right)\right]$$

So, for transmission through face AC

$$\theta > \sin^{-1}\left[u \sin(A - \sin^{-1}\left(\frac{1}{\mu}\right)\right]$$

35. **(c)** For the prism as the angle of incidence (i) increases, the angle of deviation (δ) first decreases goes to minimum value and then increases.

36. **(d)** For light to come out through face 'AC', total internal reflection must not take place.

i.e., $\theta < c \Rightarrow \sin\theta < \sin c$

$$\Rightarrow \sin\theta < \frac{1}{\mu}$$

or $\mu < \frac{1}{\sin\theta} \Rightarrow \mu < \frac{1}{\sin 45°}$

$$\Rightarrow \mu < \sqrt{2} \Rightarrow \mu < 1.414$$

37. **(c)** For total internal reflection on face AC

$\theta >$ critical angle (C)

and $\sin\theta \geq \sin C$

$$\sin\theta \geq \frac{1}{{}^w\mu_g}$$

$\sin\theta \ge \frac{\mu_w}{\mu_g} \Rightarrow \sin\theta \ge \frac{\frac{4}{3}}{\frac{3}{2}}$

$\therefore \sin\theta \ge \frac{8}{9}$.

38. (a) Rainbow is formed due to the dispersion of light suffering refraction and total internal reflection (TIR) in the droplets present in the atmosphere.

39. (a) For a thin prism, $D = (\mu - 1)A$
Since $\lambda_b < \lambda_r \Rightarrow \mu_r < \mu_b \Rightarrow D_1 < D_2$

40. (b) The incident angle is 45°.
Incident angle > critical angle, $i > i_c$

$\therefore \sin i > \sin i_c$ or $\sin 45 > \sin i_c$

$\sin i_c = \frac{1}{n}$

$\therefore \sin 45° > \frac{1}{n}$ or $\frac{1}{\sqrt{2}} > \frac{1}{n} \Rightarrow n > \sqrt{2}$

TOPIC - 5: Optical Instruments

41. (b) A telescope magnifies by making the object appearing closer.

42. (c) Reading one ⇒ without slab
Reading two ⇒ with slab
Reading three ⇒ with saw dust
Minimum three readings are required to determine refractive index of glass slab using a travelling microscope.

43. (c) Magnifying power of telescope,

$$MP = \frac{\beta \text{ (angle subtended by image at eye piece)}}{\alpha \text{ (angle subtended by object on objective)}}$$

Also, $MP = \frac{f_o}{f_e} = \frac{150}{5} = 30$

$\alpha = \frac{50}{1000} = \frac{1}{20}$ rad

$\therefore \quad \beta = \theta = MP \times \alpha = 30 \times \frac{1}{20} = \frac{3}{2} = 1.5$ rad

or, $\beta = 1.5 \times \frac{180°}{\pi} \simeq 84°$

44. (a) **Given:** $f_0 = 1.2$ cm; $f_e = 3.0$ cm
$u_0 = 1.25$ cm; $M_\infty = ?$

From $\frac{1}{f_0} = \frac{1}{v_0} - \frac{1}{u_0}$

$\Rightarrow \frac{1}{1.2} = \frac{1}{v_0} - \frac{1}{(-1.25)}$

$\Rightarrow \frac{1}{v_0} = \frac{1}{1.2} - \frac{1}{1.25}$

$\Rightarrow v_0 = 30$ cm

Magnification at infinity,

$M_\infty = -\frac{v_0}{u_0} \times \frac{D}{f_e}$

$= \frac{30}{1.25} \times \frac{25}{3}$

($\because D = 25$ cm least distance of distinct vision) = 200
Hence the magnifying power of the compound microscope is 200

45. (d) Given, Focal length of objective, $f_0 = 30$ cm
focal length of eye lens, $f_e = 3.0$ cm
Magnifying power, M = ?
Magnifying power of the Galilean telescope,

$M_D = \frac{f_0}{f_e}\left(1 - \frac{f_e}{D}\right)$

$= \frac{30}{3}\left(1 - \frac{3}{25}\right)$ [$\because$ D = 25 cm]

$= 10 \times \frac{22}{25} = 8.8$ cm

46. (c) One side of mirror is opaque and another side is reflecting this is not in case of lens hence, it is easier to provide mechanical support to large size mirrors than large size lenses. Reflecting telescopes are based on the same principle except that the formation of images takes place by reflection instead of refraction.

47. (d) Given: $f_0 = 50$ cm, $f_e = 5$ cm
d = 25 cm, $u_0 = -200$ cm
Magnification M = ?

As $\frac{1}{v_0} - \frac{1}{u_0} = \frac{1}{f_0}$

$\Rightarrow \frac{1}{v_0} = \frac{1}{f_0} + \frac{1}{u_0} = \frac{1}{50} - \frac{1}{200} = \frac{4-1}{200} = \frac{3}{200}$

or $v_0 = \frac{200}{3}$ cm

Now $v_e = d = -25$ cm

From, $\frac{1}{v_e} - \frac{1}{u_e} = \frac{1}{f_e}$

$-\frac{1}{u_e} = \frac{1}{f_e} - \frac{1}{v_e}$

$= \frac{1}{5} + \frac{1}{25} = \frac{6}{25}$

or, $v_e = \frac{-25}{6}$ cm

Magnification $M = M_0 \times M_e$

$$= \frac{v_0}{u_0} \times \frac{v_e}{u_e} = \frac{-200/3}{200} \times \frac{-25}{-25/6}$$

$$= -\frac{1}{3} \times 6 = -2$$

48. **(a)** Given : $d = 3 \times 10^{-2}$ m
$\lambda = 5.5 \times 10^{-7}$ m

Limit of resolution, $\Delta\theta = \frac{1.22\lambda}{d}$

$$= \frac{1.22 \times 5.5 \times 10^{-7}}{3 \times 10^{-2}} = 2.23 \times 10^{-5} \text{ rad.}$$

At a distance of 80 m , the telescope is able to resolve between two points which are separated by $2.23 \times 10^{-5} \times 80$ m
$= 1.78 \times 10^{-3}$ m

49. **(c)**

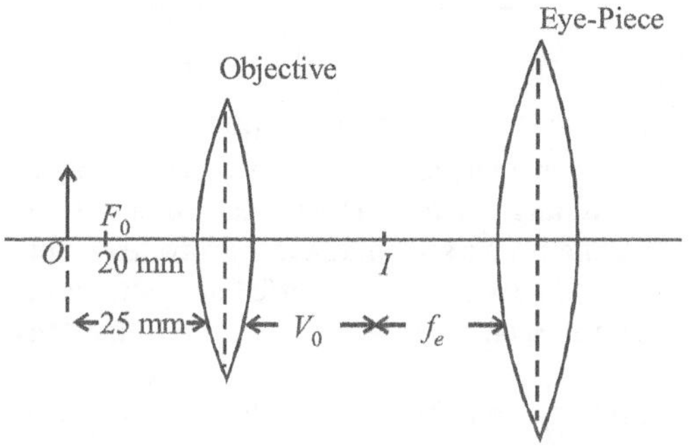

To obtain final image at infinity, object which is the image formed by objective should be at focal distance of eye-piece.
By lens formula (for objective)

$$\frac{1}{v_0} - \frac{1}{u_0} = \frac{1}{f_0}$$

or, $\frac{1}{v_0} - \frac{1}{-25} = \frac{1}{20}$

$$\Rightarrow \frac{1}{v_0} = \frac{1}{20} - \frac{1}{25} = \frac{5-4}{100} = \frac{1}{100} \text{mm}$$

$\therefore$ $v_0 = 100$ mm
Therefore the distance between the lenses
$= v_0 + f_e = 100 \text{ mm} + 20 \text{ mm} = 120 \text{ mm}$

50. **(a)** To find the refractive index of glass using a travelling microscope, a vernier scale is provided on the microscope

51. **(c)** A real, inverted and enlarged image of the object is formed by the objective lens of a compound microscope.

52. **(b)** The resolving power of a telescope

$$R.P = \frac{D}{1.22\lambda}$$

where D = diameter of the objective lens
λ = wavelength of light.
Clearly, larger the aperture, larger is the value of D, more is the resolving power or resolution.

Chapter 24

Wave Optics

TOPIC - 1: Wavefront, Interference of Light, Coherent and Incoherent Sources

1. On a hot summer night, the refractive index of air is smallest near the ground and increases with height from the ground. When a light beam is directed horizontally, the Huygens' principle leads us to conclude that as it travels, the light beam : **[2015]**
   (a) bends downwards
   (b) bends upwards
   (c) becomes narrower
   (d) goes horizontally without any deflection
2. Interference pattern is observed at 'P' due to superimposition of two rays coming out from a source 'S' as shown in the figure. The value of 'l' for which maxima is obtained at 'P' is:
   (R is perfect reflecting surface) **[Online April 12, 2014]**

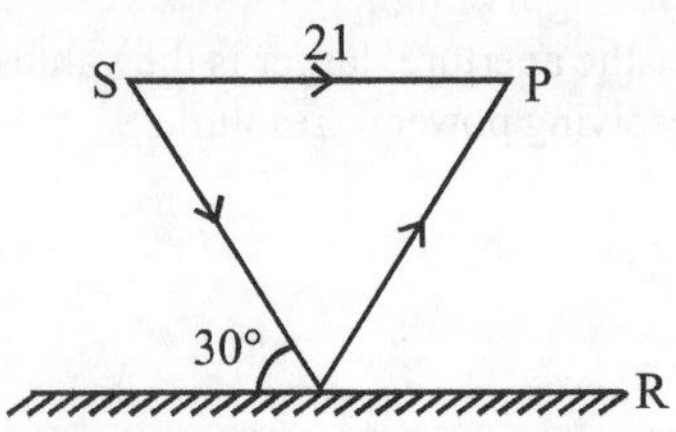

   (a) $l=\frac{2n\lambda}{\sqrt{3}-1}$ (b) $l=\frac{(2n-1)\lambda}{2(\sqrt{3}-1)}$
   (c) $l=\frac{(2n-1)\lambda\sqrt{3}}{4(2-\sqrt{3})}$ (d) $l=\frac{(2n-1)\lambda}{\sqrt{3}-1}$
3. Two monochromatic light beams of intensity 16 and 9 units are interfering. The ratio of intensities of bright and dark parts of the resultant pattern is: **[Online April 11, 2014]**
   (a) $\frac{16}{9}$ (b) $\frac{4}{3}$ (c) $\frac{7}{1}$ (d) $\frac{49}{1}$
4. n identical waves each of intensity I_0 interfere with each other. The ratio of maximum intensities if the interference is (i) coherent and (ii) incoherent is : **[Online April 23, 2013]**
   (a) n^2 (b) $\frac{1}{n}$ (c) $\frac{1}{n^2}$ (d) n
5. A ray of light of intensity I is incident on a parallel glass slab at point A as shown in diagram. It undergoes partial reflection and refraction. At each reflection, 25% of incident energy is reflected. The rays AB and A'B' undergo interference. The ratio of I_{max} and I_{min} is : **[Online April 9, 2013]**

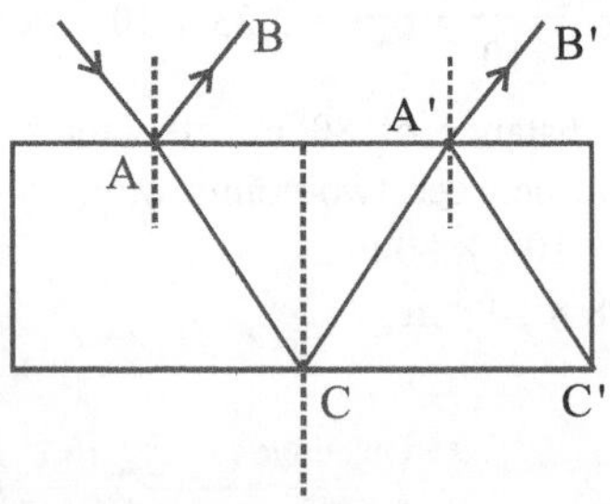

   (a) 49 : 1 (b) 7 : 1 (c) 4 : 1 (d) 8 : 1
6. Two coherent plane light waves of equal amplitude makes a small angle α ($<<1$) with each other. They fall almost normally on a screen. If λ is the wavelength of light waves, the fringe width Δx of interference patterns of the two sets of waves on the screen is **[Online May 19, 2012]**
   (a) $\frac{2\lambda}{\alpha}$ (b) $\frac{\lambda}{\alpha}$ (c) $\frac{\lambda}{(2\alpha)}$ (d) $\frac{\lambda}{\sqrt{\alpha}}$
7. This question has a paragraph followed by two statements, Statement – 1 and Statement – 2. Of the given four alternatives after the statements, choose the one that describes the statements.
   A thin air film is formed by putting the convex surface of a plane-convex lens over a plane glass plate. With monochromatic light, this film gives an interference pattern due to light reflected from the top (convex) surface and the bottom (glass plate) surface of the film.
   Statement – 1 : When light reflects from the air-glass plate interface, the reflected wave suffers a phase change of π.
   Statement – 2 : The centre of the interference pattern is dark. **[2011]**
   (a) Statement – 1 is true, Statement – 2 is true, Statement – 2 is the correct explanation of Statement – 1.
   (b) Statement – 1 is true, Statement – 2 is true, Statement – 2 is not the correct explanation of Statement – 1.
   (c) Statement – 1 is false, Statement – 2 is true.
   (d) Statement – 1 is true, Statement – 2 is false.

Directions : Questions number 10-12 are based on the following paragraph.

An initially parallel cylindrical beam travels in a medium of refractive index $\mu(I)=\mu_0+\mu_2 I$, where μ_0 and μ_2 are positive constants and I is the intensity of the light beam. The intensity of the beam is decreasing with increasing radius

8. As the beam enters the medium , it will **[2010]**
   (a) diverge

(b) converge
(c) diverge near the axis and converge near the periphery
(d) travel as a cylindrical beam

9. The initial shape of the wavefront of the beam is **[2010]**
(a) convex
(b) concave
(c) convex near the axis and concave near the periphery
(d) planar

10. The speed of light in the medium is **[2010]**
(a) minimum on the axis of the beam
(b) the same everywhere in the beam
(c) directly proportional to the intensity I
(d) maximum on the axis of the beam

11. To demonstrate the phenomenon of interference, we require two sources which emit radiation **[2003]**
(a) of nearly the same frequency
(b) of the same frequency
(c) of different wavelengths
(d) of the same frequency and having a definite phase relationship

TOPIC - 2: Young's Double Slit Experiment

12. In a Young's double slit experiment, slits are separated by 0.5 mm, and the screen is placed 150 cm away. A beam of light consisting of two wavelengths, 650 nm and 520 nm, is used to obtain interference fringes on the screen. The least distance from the common central maximum to the point where the bright fringes due to both the wavelengths coincide is : **[2017]**
(a) 9.75 mm (b) 15.6 mm
(c) 1.56 mm (d) 7.8 mm

13. A single slit of width b is illuminated by a coherent monochromatic light of wavelength λ. If the second and fourth minima in the diffraction pattern at a distance 1 m from the slit are at 3 cm and 6 cm respectively from the central maximum, what is the width of the central maximum? (i.e. distance between first minimum on either side of the central maximum) **[Online April 8, 2017]**
(a) 1.5 cm (b) 3.0 cm (c) 4.5 cm (d) 6.0 cm

14. In a Young's double slit experiment with light of wavelength λ the separation of slits is d and distance of screen is D such that $D >> d >> \lambda$. If the fringe width is β, the distance from point of maximum intensity to the point where intensity falls to half of maximum intensity on either side is: **[Online April 11, 2015]**
(a) $\frac{\beta}{6}$ (b) $\frac{\beta}{3}$ (c) $\frac{\beta}{4}$ (d) $\frac{\beta}{2}$

15. In a Young's double slit experiment, the distance between the two identical slits is 6.1 times larger than the slit width. Then the number of intensity maxima observed within the central maximum of the single slit diffraction pattern is: **[Online April 19, 2014]**
(a) 3 (b) 6 (c) 12 (d) 24

16. Using monochromatic light of wavelength λ, an experimentalist sets up the Young's double slit experiment in three ways as shown.
If she observes that $y = \beta'$, the wavelength of light used is: **[Online April 9, 2014]**

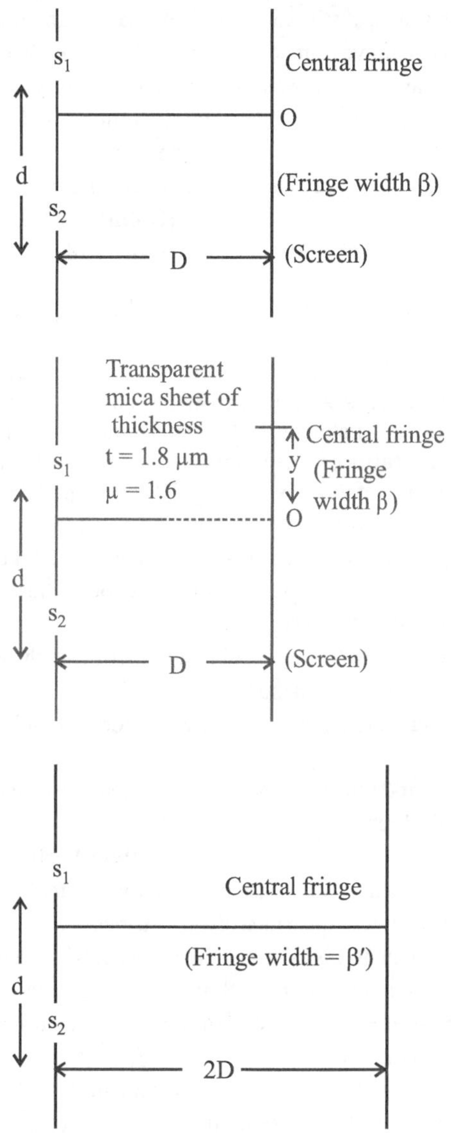

(a) 520 nm (b) 540 nm (c) 560 nm (d) 580 nm

17. Two coherent point sources S_1 and S_2 are separated by a small distance 'd' as shown. The fringes obtained on the screen will be **[2013]**

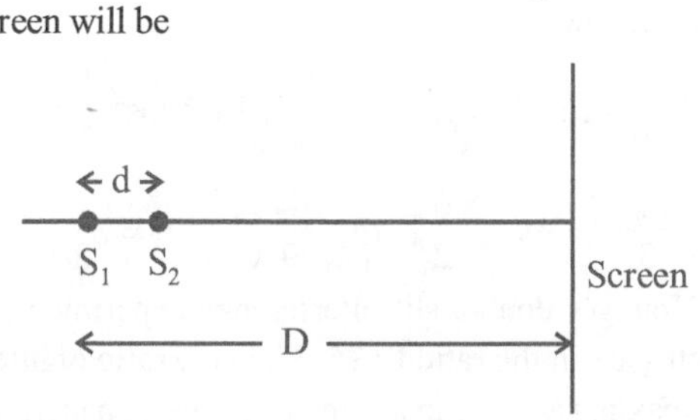

(a) points (b) straight lines
(c) semi-circles (d) concentric circles

18. The source that illuminates the double - slit in 'double - slit interference experiment' emits two distinct monochromatic waves of wavelength 500 nm and 600 nm, each of them producing its own pattern on the screen. At the central point of the pattern when path difference is zero, maxima of both the patterns coincide and the resulting interference pattern is most distinct at the region of zero path difference. But as one moves out of this central region, the two fringe systems are gradually out of step such that maximum due to on wavelength coincides with the minimum due to the other and the combined fringe system becomes completely indistinct. This may happen when path difference in nm is: **[Online April 25, 2013]**

(a) 2000 (b) 3000 (c) 1000 (d) 1500

19. A thin glass plate of thickness is $\frac{2500}{3}\lambda$ (λ is wavelength of light used) and refractive index $\mu = 1.5$ is inserted between one of the slits and the screen in Young's double slit experiment. At a point on the screen equidistant from the slits, the ratio of the intensities before and after the introduction of the glass plate is : **[Online April 25, 2013]**

(a) 2 : 1 (b) 1 : 4 (c) 4 : 1 (d) 4 : 3

20. This question has Statement-1 and Statement-2. Of the four choices given after the Statements, choose the one that best describes the two Statements.

Statement-1: In Young's double slit experiment, the number of fringes observed in the field of view is small with longer wavelength of light and is large with shorter wavelength of light.

Statement-2: In the double slit experiment the fringe width depends directly on the wavelength of light.

[Online April 22, 2013]

(a) Statement-1 is true, Statement-2 is true and the Statement-2 is correct explanation of the Statement-1.
(b) Statement-1 is false and the Statement-2 is true.
(c) Statement-1 is true Statement-2 is true and the Statement-2 is not correct explanation of the Statement-1.
(d) Statement-1 is true and the Statement-2 is false.

21. In Young's double slit experiment, one of the slit is wider than other, so that amplitude of the light from one slit is double of that other slit. If I_m be the maximum intensity, the resultant intensity I when they interfere at phase difference ϕ is given by : **[2012]**

(a) $\frac{I_m}{9}(4+5\cos\phi)$ (b) $\frac{I_m}{3}\left(1+2\cos^2\frac{\phi}{2}\right)$

(c) $\frac{I_m}{5}\left(1+4\cos^2\frac{\phi}{2}\right)$ (d) $\frac{I_m}{9}\left(1+8\cos^2\frac{\phi}{2}\right)$

22. In Young's double slit interference experiment, the slit widths are in the ratio 1 : 25. Then the ratio of intensity at the maxima and minima in the interference pattern is **[Online May 26, 2012]**

(a) 3 : 2 (b) 1 : 25 (c) 9 : 4 (d) 1 : 5

23. The maximum number of possible interference maxima for slit separation equal to 1.8λ, where λ is the wavelength of light used, in a Young's double slit experiment is **[Online May 12, 2012]**

(a) zero (b) 3 (c) infinite (d) 5

24. In a Young's double slit experiment with light of wavelength λ, fringe pattern on the screen has fringe width β. When two thin transparent glass (refractive index μ) plates of thickness t_1 and t_2 ($t_1 > t_2$) are placed in the path of the two beams respectively, the fringe pattern will shift by a distance **[Online May 7, 2012]**

(a) $\frac{\beta(\mu-1)}{\lambda}\left(\frac{t_1}{t_2}\right)$ (b) $\frac{\mu\beta}{\lambda}\frac{t_1}{t_2}$

(c) $\frac{\beta(\mu-1)}{\lambda}(t_1-t_2)$ (d) $(\mu-1)\frac{\lambda}{\beta}(t_1+t_2)$

25. At two points P and Q on screen in Young's double slit experiment, waves from slits S_1 and S_2 have a path difference of 0 and $\frac{\lambda}{4}$, respectively. The ratio of intensities at P and Q will be : **[2011 RS]**

(a) 2 : 1 (b) $\sqrt{2}$: 1 (c) 4 : 1 (d) 3 : 2

26. In a Young's double slit experiment, the two slits act as coherent sources of wave of equal amplitude A and wavelength λ. In another experiment with the same arrangement the two slits are made to act as incoherent sources of waves of same amplitude and wavelength. If the intensity at the middle point of the screen in the first case is I_1 and in the second case is I_2, then the ratio $\frac{I_1}{I_2}$ is **[2011 RS]**

(a) 2 (b) 1 (c) 0.5 (d) 4

27. A mixture of light, consisting of wavelength 590 nm and an unknown wavelength, illuminates Young's double slit and gives rise to two overlapping interference patterns on the screen. The central maximum of both lights coincide. Further, it is observed that the third bright fringe of known light coincides with the 4th bright fringe of the unknown light. From this data, the wavelength of the unknown light is: **[2009]**

(a) 885.0 nm (b) 442.5 nm (c) 776.8 nm (d) 393.4 nm

28. In a Young's double slit experiment the intensity at a point where the path difference is $\frac{\lambda}{6}$ (λ being the wavelength of light used) is I. If I_0 denotes the maximum intensity, $\frac{I}{I_0}$ is equal to **[2007]**

(a) $\frac{3}{4}$ (b) $\frac{1}{\sqrt{2}}$ (c) $\frac{\sqrt{3}}{2}$ (d) $\frac{1}{2}$

29. A Young's double slit experiment uses a monochromatic source. The shape of the interference fringes formed on a screen is **[2005]**

(a) circle (b) hyperbola
(c) parabola (d) straight line

30. The maximum number of possible interference maxima for slit-separation equal to twice the wavelength in Young's double-slit experiment is **[2004]**

(a) three (b) five (c) infinite (d) zero

TOPIC - 3: Diffraction, Polarisation of Light and Resolving Power

31. An observer is moving with half the speed of light towards a stationary microwave source emitting waves at frequency 10 GHz. What is the frequency of the microwave measured by the observer? (speed of light = $3 \times 10^8 ms^{-1}$) **[2017]**

(a) 17.3 GHz (b) 15.3 GHz
(c) 10.1 GHz (d) 12.1 GHz

32. A single slit of width 0.1 mm is illuminated by a parallel beam of light of wavelength 6000 Å and diffraction bands are observed on a screen 0.5 m from the slit. The distance of the third dark band from the central bright band is : **[Online April 9, 2017]**

(a) 3mm (b) 9mm (c) 4.5mm (d) 1.5mm

33. The box of a pin hole camera, of length L, has a hole of radius a. It is assumed that when the hole is illuminated by a parallel beam of light of wavelength λ the spread of the spot (obtained on the opposite wall of the camera) is the sum of its geometrical spread and the spread due to diffraction. The spot would then have its minimum size (say b_{min}) when : **[2016]**

(a) $a = \sqrt{\lambda L}$ and $b_{min} = \sqrt{4\lambda L}$

(b) $a = \frac{\lambda^2}{L}$ and $b_{min} = \sqrt{4\lambda L}$

(c) $a = \frac{\lambda^2}{L}$ and $b_{min} = \left(\frac{2\lambda^2}{L}\right)$

(d) $a = \sqrt{\lambda l}$ and $b_{min} = \left(\frac{2\lambda^2}{L}\right)$

34. Two stars are 10 light years away from the earth. They are seen through a telescope of objective diameter 30 cm. The wavelength of light is 600 nm. To see the stars just resolved by the telescope, the minimum distance between them should be (1 light year = 9.46×10^{15} m) of the order of: **[Online April 10, 2016]**

(a) 10^8 km (b) 10^{10} km (c) 10^{11} km (d) 10^6 km

35. In Young's double slit experiment, the distance between slits and the screen is 1.0 m and monochromatic light of 600 nm is being used. A person standing near the slits is looking at the fringe pattern. When the separation between the slits is varied, the interference pattern disappears for a particular distance d_0 between the slits. If the angular resolution of the eye is $\frac{1°}{60}$, the value of d_0 is close to : **[Online April 9, 2016]**

(a) 1mm (b) 3mm (c) 2mm (d) 4mm

36. Assuming human pupil to have a radius of 0.25 cm and a comfortable viewing distance of 25 cm, the minimum separation between two objects that human eye can resolve at 500 nm wavelength is : **[2015]**

(a) 100 μm (b) 300 μm (c) 1 μm (d) 30 μm

37. Unpolarized light of intensity I_0 is incident on surface of a block of glass at Brewster's angle. In that case, which one of the following statements is true ? **[Online April 11, 2015]**

(a) reflected light is completely polarized with intensity less than $\frac{I_0}{2}$

(b) transmitted light is completely polarized with intensity less than $\frac{I_0}{2}$

(c) transmitted light is partially polarized with intensity $\frac{I_0}{2}$

(d) reflected light is partially polarized with intensity $\frac{I_0}{2}$

38. Two beams, A and B, of plane polarized light with mutually perpendicular planes of polarization are seen through a polaroid. From the position when the beam A has maximum intensity (and beam B has zero intensity), a rotation of polaroid through 30° makes the two beams appear equally bright. If the initial intensities of the two beams are I_A and I_B respectively, then $\frac{I_A}{I_B}$ equals: **[2014]**

(a) 3 (b) $\frac{3}{2}$ (c) 1 (d) $\frac{1}{3}$

39. The diameter of the objective lens of microscope makes an angle β at the focus of the microscope. Further, the medium between the object and the lens is an oil of refractive index n. Then the resolving power of the microscope **[Online April 19, 2014]**

(a) increases with decreasing value of n
(b) increases with decreasing value of β
(c) increases with increasing value of n sin 2β
(d) increases with increasing value of $\frac{1}{n \sin 2\beta}$

40. A ray of light is incident from a denser to a rarer medium. The critical angle for total internal reflection is θ_{iC} and Brewster's angle of incidence is θ_{iB}, such that $\sin\theta_{iC}/\sin\theta_{iB} = \eta = 1.28$. The relative refractive index of the two media is: **[Online April 19, 2014]**

(a) 0.2 (b) 0.4 (c) 0.8 (d) 0.9

41. In an experiment of single slit diffraction pattern, first minimum for red light coincides with first maximum of some other wavelength. If wavelength of red light is 6600 Å, then wavelength of first maximum will be: **[Online April 12, 2014]**

(a) 3300Å (b) 4400Å (c) 5500Å (d) 6600Å

42. A beam of unpolarised light of intensity I_0 is passed through a polaroid A and then through another polaroid B which is oriented so that its principal plane makes an angle of 45° relative to that of A. The intensity of the emergent light is **[2013]**

(a) I_0 (b) $I_0/2$ (c) $I_0/4$ (d) $I_0/8$

43. This question has Statement-1 and Statements-2. Of the four choices given after the Statements, choose the one that best describes the two Statements.

Statement-1 : Out of radio waves and microwaves, the radio waves undergo more diffraction.

Statement-2 : Radio waves have greater frequency compared to microwaves. **[Online April 25, 2013]**

(a) Statement-l is true, Statement-2 is true and Statement-2 is the correct explanation of Statement-1
(b) Statement-1 is false , Statement-2 is true.
(c) Statement-1 is true, Statement-2 is false.
(d) Statement-1 is true, Statement-2 is true but Statement-2 is not the correct explanation of Statement-1

44. A person lives in a high-rise building on the bank of a river 50 m wide. Across the river is a well lit tower of height 40 m. When the person, who is at a height of 10 m, looks through a polarizer at an appropriate angle at light of the tower reflecting from the river surface, he notes that intensity of light coming from distance X from his building is the least and this corresponds to the light coming from light bulbs at height 'Y' on the tower. The values of X and Y are respectively close to (refractive index of water $\approx \frac{4}{3}$) **[Online April 9, 2013]**

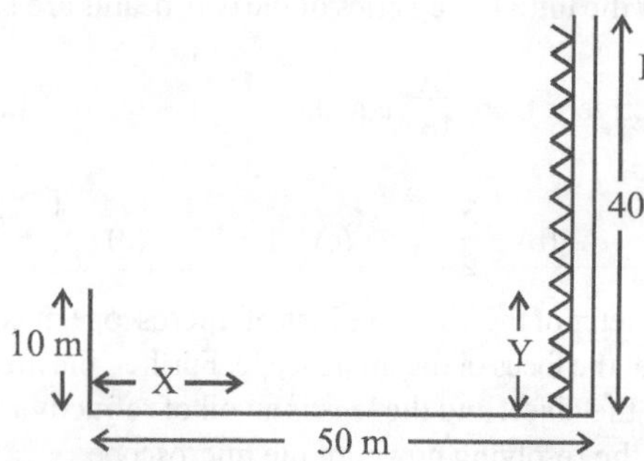

(a) 25 m, 10 m (b) 13 m, 27 m
(c) 22 m, 13 m (d) 17 m, 20 m

45. The first diffraction minimum due to the single slit diffraction is seen at θ = 30° for a light of wavelength 5000 Å falling perpendicularly on the slit. The width of the slit is **[Online May 12, 2012]**

(a) 2.5×10^{-5} cm (b) 1.25×10^{-5} cm
(c) 10×10^{-5} cm (d) 5×10^{-5} cm

46. Two polaroids have their polarizing directions parallel so that the intensity of a transmitted light is maximum. The angle through which either polaroid must be turned if the intensity is to drop by one-half is **[Online May 7, 2012]**

(a) 135° (b) 90° (c) 120° (d) 180°

47. Statement - 1: On viewing the clear blue portion of the sky through a Calcite Crystal, the intensity of transmitted light varies as the crystal is rotated.

Statement - 2: The light coming from the sky is polarized due to scattering of sun light by particles in the atmosphere. The scattering is largest for blue light. **[2011 RS]**

(a) Statement -1 is true, statement-2 is false.
(b) Statement-1 is true, statement-2 is true, statement-2 is the correct explanation of statement-1
(c) Statement-1 is true, statement-2 is true, statement-2 is not the correct explanation of statement-1
(d) Statement-1 is false, statement-2 is true.

48. In an experiment, electrons are made to pass through a narrow slit of width '*d*' comparable to their de Broglie wavelength. They are detected on a screen at a distance '*D*' from the slit (see figure).

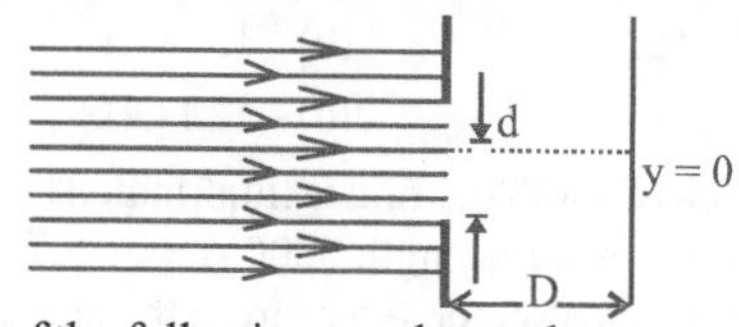

Which of the following graphs can be expected to represent the number of electrons '*N*' detected as a function of the detector position '*y*'(*y* = 0 corresponds to the middle of the slit) **[2008]**

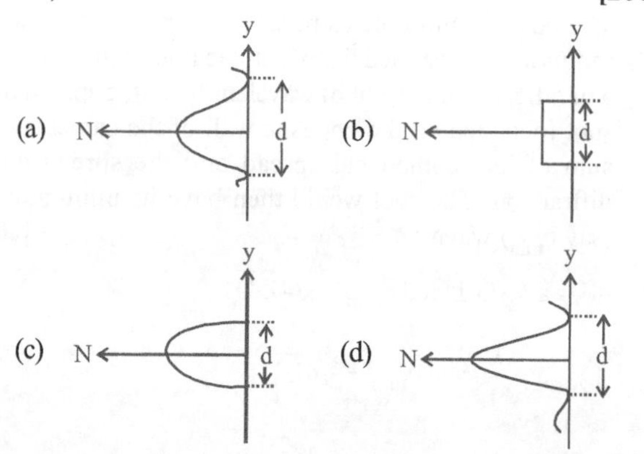

49. If I_0 is the intensity of the principal maximum in the single slit diffraction pattern, then what will be its intensity when the slit width is doubled? **[2005]**

(a) $4I_0$ (b) $2I_0$ (c) $\frac{I_0}{2}$ (d) I_0

50. When an unpolarized light of intensity I_0 is incident on a polarizing sheet, the intensity of the light which does not get transmitted is **[2005]**

(a) $\frac{1}{4}I_0$ (b) $\frac{1}{2}I_0$ (c) I_0 (d) zero

51. Two point white dots are 1 mm apart on a black paper. They are viewed by eye of pupil diameter 3 mm. Approximately, what is the maximum distance at which these dots can be resolved by the eye?
[Take wavelength of light = 500 nm] **[2005]**

(a) 1 m (b) 5 m (c) 3 m (d) 6 m

52. The angle of incidence at which reflected light is totally polarized for reflection from air to glass (refractive index *n*), is **[2004]**

(a) $\tan^{-1}(1/n)$ (b) $\sin^{-1}(1/n)$
(c) $\sin^{-1}(n)$ (d) $\tan^{-1}(n)$

53. Wavelength of light used in an optical instrument are $\lambda_1 = 4000$ Å and $\lambda_2 = 5000$ Å, then ratio of their respective resolving powers (corresponding to λ_1 and λ_2) is **[2002]**

(a) 16 : 25 (b) 9 : 1 (c) 4 : 5 (d) 5 : 4

Hints & Solutions

TOPIC - 1: Wavefront, Interference of Light, Coherent and Incoherent Sources

1. (b)

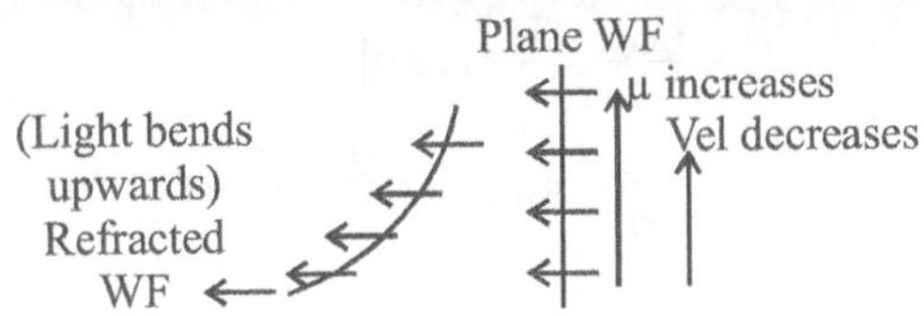

2. (c)

3. (d) Intensity ∝ (amplitude)^2

$$\frac{I_1}{I_2}=\frac{16}{9}=\frac{a_1^2}{a_2^2}$$

$\Rightarrow$ $a_1=4;\ a_2=3$

Therefore the ratio of intensities of bright and dark parts

$$\frac{I_{Bright}}{I_{Dark}}=\frac{(a_1+a_2)^2}{(a_1-a_2)^2}=\frac{(4+3)^2}{(4-3)^2}=\frac{49}{1}$$

4. (d) $\frac{\text{(Maximum intensity) coherent interference}}{\text{(Maximum intensity) in coherent interference}}$

$$=\frac{n^2 I_0}{nI_0}=n$$

5. (a)

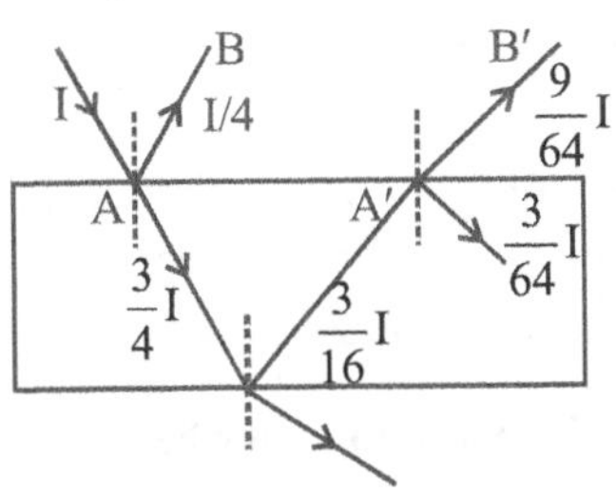

From figure $I_1=\frac{I}{4}$ and $I_2=\frac{9I}{64}$

$$\Rightarrow \frac{I_2}{I_1}=\frac{9}{16}$$

By using $\frac{I_{max}}{I_{min}}=\left(\frac{\sqrt{\frac{I_2}{I_1}}+1}{\sqrt{\frac{I_2}{I_1}}-1}\right)^2$

$$=\left(\frac{\sqrt{\frac{9}{16}}+1}{\sqrt{\frac{9}{16}}-1}\right)^2=\frac{49}{1}$$

6. (c) $\Delta x=\frac{\lambda}{(2\alpha)}$

7. (b) A phase change of π rad appears when the ray reflects at the glass-air interface. Also, the centre of the interference pattern is dark.

8. (b) In the medium, the refractive index will decrease from the axis towards the periphery of the beam. Therefore, the beam will move as one move from the axis to the periphery and hence the beam will converge.

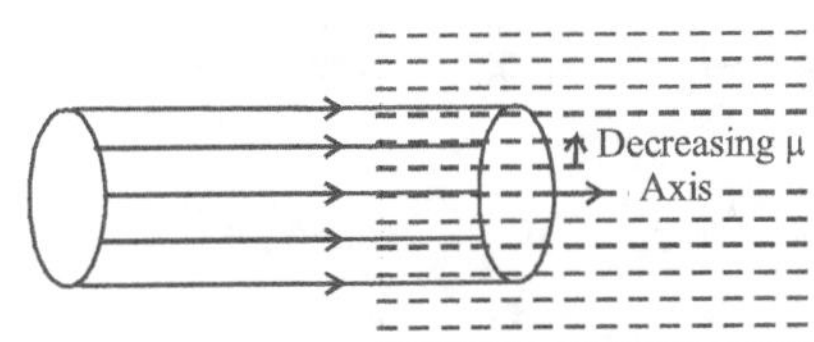

9. (d) Initially the parallel beam is cylindrical . Therefore, the wavefront will be planar.

10. (a) The speed of light (c) in a medium of refractive index (μ) is given by

$\mu=\frac{c_0}{c}$, where c_0 is the speed of light in vacuum

$$\therefore c=\frac{c_0}{\mu}$$

$$=\frac{c_0}{\mu_0+\mu_2(I)}$$

As I is decreasing with increasing radius, it is maximum on the axis of the beam. Therefore, c is minimum on the axis of the beam.

11. (d) For the phenomenon of interference we require two sources of light of same frequency and having a definite phase relationship (a phase relationship that does not change with time)

TOPIC - 2: Young's Double Slit Experiment

12. (d) For common maxima, $n_1\lambda_1=n_2\lambda_2$

$$\Rightarrow \frac{n_1}{n_2}=\frac{\lambda_2}{\lambda_1}=\frac{520\times10^{-9}}{650\times10^{-9}}=\frac{4}{5}$$

For λ_1

$$y=\frac{n_1\lambda_1 D}{d},\lambda_1=650\,\text{nm}$$

$$y=\frac{4\times650\times10^{-9}\times1.5}{0.5\times10^{-3}}\quad \text{or,}\quad y=7.8\,\text{mn}$$

13. (b) For secondary minima,

$$b\sin\theta=n\lambda\Rightarrow\sin\theta=\frac{n\lambda}{b}$$

Distance of nth secondary minima $x=D\sin\theta$

or $\sin\theta_1=\frac{x_1}{D}$

$\sin\theta_1 = \frac{2\lambda}{b}$

n = 4

$\sin\theta_2 = \frac{4\lambda}{b} = \frac{x_2}{D}$

$x_2 - x_1 = \frac{4\lambda}{b} - \frac{2\lambda}{b} = \frac{2\lambda}{b}$

$3 = \frac{2\lambda}{b} \Rightarrow b = \frac{2\lambda}{3}$ ..... (i)

Width of central maxima $= \frac{2\lambda}{b}$

$= \frac{2\lambda}{\frac{2\lambda}{3}} = 3$ cm. .. from eq. (i)

14. (c) $2I_0 = 4I_0\cos^2\left(\frac{\Delta\phi}{2}\right)$ here, $\Delta\phi = \frac{\pi}{2}$

But, $\Delta\phi = \frac{2\pi}{\lambda}\Delta x$ so, $\Delta x = \frac{\lambda}{4}$

$\frac{dy}{D} = \frac{\lambda}{4}$ ....(i)

$\frac{\lambda D}{d} = \beta$ ....(ii)

Multiplying equation (i) and (ii) we get,

$y = \frac{\beta}{4}$

15. (c)

16. (b) Given $t = 1.8 \times 10^{-6}$m

$\mu = 1.6$

n = 2 (from figure)

Applying formula $(\mu - 1)t = n\lambda$

$(1.6 - 1) \times 1.8 \times 10^{-6} = 2\lambda$

or, $\lambda = \frac{1.8\times10^{-6}\times0.6}{2}$

= 540 nm

17. (d) It will be concentric circles.

18. (d)

19. (c)

20. (c) Fringe width $B = \frac{D}{d}\lambda$

And number of fringes observed in the field of view is obtained by $\frac{d}{\lambda}$

21. (d) Let $a_1 = a, I_1 = a_1^2 = a^2$

$a_2 = 2a, I_2 = a_2^2 = 4a^2$

$I_2 = 4I_1$

$I_r = a_1^2 + a_2^2 + 2a_1a_2\cos\phi$

$= I_1 + I_2 + 2\sqrt{I_1I_2}\cos\phi$

$I_r = I_1 + 4I_1 + 2\sqrt{4I_1^2}\cos\phi$

$\Rightarrow I_r = 5I_1 + 4I_1\cos\phi$ ...(1)

Now, $I_{max} = (a_1 + a_2)^2 = (a + 2a)^2 = 9a^2$

$I_{max} = 9I_1 \Rightarrow I_1 = \frac{I_{max}}{9}$

Substituting in equation (1)

$I_r = \frac{5I_{max}}{9} + \frac{4I_{max}}{9}\cos\phi$

$I_r = \frac{I_{max}}{9}[5 + 4\cos\phi]$

$I_r = \frac{I_{max}}{9}\left[5 + 8\cos^2\frac{\phi}{2} - 4\right]$

$I_r = \frac{I_{max}}{9}\left[1 + 8\cos^2\frac{\phi}{2}\right]$

22. (c) We know that,

$$\frac{I_{max}}{I_{min}} = \frac{\left(\sqrt{\frac{\omega_1}{\omega_2}} + 1\right)^2}{\left(\sqrt{\frac{\omega_1}{\omega_2}} - 1\right)^2}$$

I_{max} and I_{min} are maximum and minium intensity ω_1 and ω_2 are widths of two slits

$$\therefore \frac{I_{max}}{I_{min}} = \frac{\left(\sqrt{\frac{1}{25}} + 1\right)^2}{\left(\sqrt{\frac{1}{25}} - 1\right)^2} \quad \left(\frac{\omega_1}{\omega_2} = \frac{1}{25}\text{given}\right)$$

On solving we get,

$$\frac{I_{max}}{I_{min}} = \frac{\frac{36}{25}}{\frac{16}{25}} = \frac{9}{4} = 9:4$$

23. (b) As $\sin\theta = \frac{n\lambda}{d}$ and sinθ cannot be $\not>1$

$\therefore 1 = \frac{n\lambda}{1.8\lambda}$

or $n = 1.8$

Hence maximum number of possible interference maximas, 0, ±1 i.e. 3

24. (c) Shift $= \frac{\beta(\mu-1)}{\lambda}t_1 - \frac{\beta(\mu-1)}{\lambda}t_2$

$= \frac{\beta(\mu-1)}{\lambda}(t_1 - t_2)$

25. (a) Path difference at p

$\Delta x_1 = 0$

$\therefore$ Phase difference at P

$\Delta\phi_1 = 0°$

Intensity at p

$I_1 = I_0 + I_0 + 2I_0 \cos 0° = 4I_0$

Path difference at Q

$\Delta x_2 = \frac{\lambda}{4}$

$\therefore$ Phase difference at Q

$\Delta\phi_2 = \frac{2\pi}{\lambda} \cdot \frac{\lambda}{4} = \left(\frac{\pi}{2}\right)$

Intensity at Q.

$I_2 = I_0 + I_0 + 2I_0 \cos\frac{\pi}{2} = 2I_0$

Thus, $\frac{I_1}{I_2} = \frac{4I_0}{2I_0} = \frac{2}{1}$

26. (a) For coherent sources :

$I_1 = 4I_0$

For incoherent sources

$I_2 = 2I_0 \quad \therefore \frac{I_1}{I_2} = \frac{2}{1}$

27. (b) Third bright fringe of known light coincides with the 4th bright fringe of the unknown light.

$\therefore \frac{3(590)D}{d} = \frac{4\lambda D}{d}$

$\Rightarrow \lambda = \frac{3}{4} \times 590 = 442.5 \text{ nm}$

28. (a) For path difference of λ, the phase difference is 2π

For path difference of $\frac{\lambda}{6}$, the phase difference is

$\frac{2\pi \times \lambda/6}{\lambda} = \frac{\pi}{3}$

$\therefore$ Intensity $I = I_1 + I_2 + 2\sqrt{I_1}\sqrt{I_2}\cos\frac{\pi}{3}$

$\therefore I = I_1 + I_2 + \sqrt{I_1}\sqrt{I_2}$

when $I_1 = I_2 = I'$ (say) then $I = 3I'$

$I_{max} = \left(\sqrt{I_1} + \sqrt{I_2}\right)^2$

$= \left(\sqrt{I'} + \sqrt{I'}\right)^2 = \left(2\sqrt{I'}\right)^2 = 4I'$

$\therefore \frac{I}{I_{max}} = \frac{3}{4}$

ALTERNATE SOLUTION

The intensity of light at any point of the screen where the phase difference due to light coming from the two slits is ϕ is given by

$I = I_0 \cos^2\left(\frac{\phi}{2}\right)$ where I_0 is the maximum intensity.

NOTE This formula is applicable when $I_1 = I_2$. Here $\phi = \pi/3$

$\therefore \frac{I}{I_0} = \cos^2\frac{\pi}{6} = \left(\frac{\sqrt{3}}{2}\right)^2 = \frac{3}{4}$

29. (d) The shape of interference fringes formed on a screen in case of a monochromatic source is a straight line. Remember for double hole experiment a hyperbola is generated.

30. (b) For constructive interference $d\sin\theta = n\lambda$

given $d = 2\lambda \Rightarrow \sin\theta = \frac{n}{2}$

$n = 0, 1, -1, 2, -2$ hence five maxima are possible

TOPIC - 3: Diffraction, Polarisation of Light and Resolving Power

31. (a) Use relativistic doppler's effect as velocity of observer is not small as compared to light

$f = f_0\sqrt{\frac{c+v}{c+v}}$; V = relative speed of approach

$f_0 = 10$ GHz

$\therefore f = 10\sqrt{\frac{c+\frac{c}{2}}{c-\frac{c}{2}}} = 10\sqrt{3} = 17.3 \text{ GHz}$

32. (b) a = 0.1 mm = 10^{-4} cm,

$\lambda = 6000 \times 10^{-10}$ cm $= 6 \times 10^{-7}$ cm, D = 0.5 m

for 3rd dark band, a sin $\theta = 3\lambda$

or $\sin\theta = \frac{3\lambda}{a} = \frac{x}{D}$

The distance of the third dark band from the central bright band

$x = \frac{3\lambda D}{a} = \frac{3 \times 6 \times 10^{-7} \times 0.5}{10^{-4}} = 9 \text{ mm}$

33. (a) Given geometrical spread = a

Diffraction spread $= \frac{\lambda}{a} \times L = \frac{\lambda L}{a}$

The sum $b = a + \frac{\lambda L}{a}$

For b to be minimum $\frac{db}{da} = 0 \quad \frac{d}{da}\left(a + \frac{\lambda L}{a}\right) = 0$

$a = \sqrt{\lambda L}$

$b\min = \sqrt{\lambda L} + \sqrt{\lambda L} = 2\sqrt{\lambda L} = \sqrt{4\lambda L}$

34. (a) We know that $\Delta\theta = \frac{0.61\lambda}{4} = \frac{l}{R}$

The minimum distance between them

$$l = \frac{R}{9} 0.61 \times \lambda = \frac{9.46 \times 10^{15} \times 10 \times 0.61 \times 600 \times 10^{-9}}{0.3}$$

$= 1.15 \times 10^{11}$ m

$\Rightarrow 1.115 \times 10^{8}$ km.

35. (c) Given D = 1.0m, wavelength of monochromatic light λ = 600 nm.

$$d : D\theta = 1 \times \frac{\pi}{180} \times \frac{1}{60}$$

$$d_0 = 2 \times 10^{-3} = 2\,\text{mm}$$

36. (d) $\sin\theta = \frac{0.25}{25} = \frac{1}{100}$

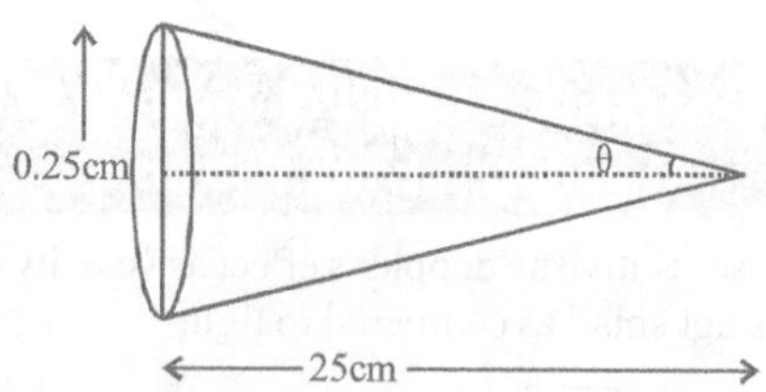

Resolving power $= \frac{1.22\lambda}{2\mu \sin\theta} = 30\ \mu\text{m}$.

37. (a) When unpolarised light is incident at Brewster's angle then reflected light is completely polarized and the intensity of the reflected light is less than half of the incident light.

38. (d) According to malus law, intensity of emerging beam is given by,

$I = I_0 \cos^2\theta$

Now, $I_{A'} = I_A \cos^2 30°$

$I_{B'} = I_B \cos^2 60°$

As $I_{A'} = I_{B'}$

$$\Rightarrow \quad I_A \times \frac{3}{4} = I_B \times \frac{1}{4}$$

$$\frac{I_A}{I_B} = \frac{1}{3}$$

39. (c) Resolving power of microscope,

$$\text{R.P.} = \frac{2n\sin\theta}{\lambda}$$

λ = Wavelength of light used to illuminate the object

n = Refractive index of the medium between object and objective

θ = Angle

40. (c) Here, $\sin\theta_{ic} / \sin\theta_{iB} = 1.28$

As we know,

$$\mu = \frac{\sin\theta_{iB}}{\sin\left(\frac{\pi}{2} - \theta_{iB}\right)}$$

where, θ_{iB} is Brewster's angle of incidence,

And, $\mu = \frac{1}{\sin\theta_{ic}}$

On solving we get, relative refractive index of the two media.

41. (b) In a single slit experiment,

For diffraction maxima,

$$a\sin\theta = (2n+1)\frac{\lambda}{2}$$

and for diffraction minima,

$a\sin\theta = n\lambda$

According to question,

$$(2 \times 1 + 1)\frac{\lambda}{2} = 1 \times 6600$$

$$(\because \lambda_R = 6600\text{Å})$$

$$\lambda = \frac{6600 \times 2}{3}$$

$$\lambda = 4400\text{Å}$$

42. (c) Relation between intensities

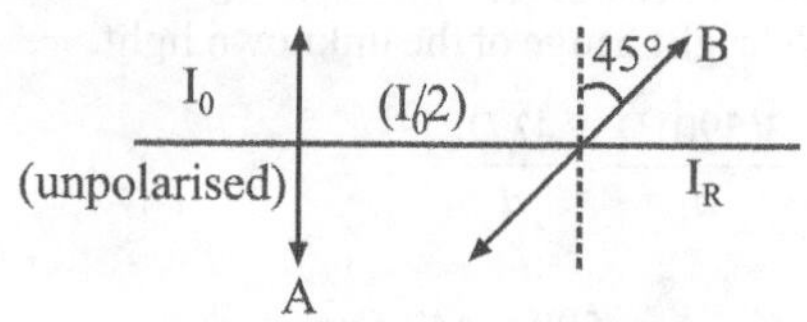

$$I_r = \left(\frac{I_0}{2}\right)\cos^2(45°) = \frac{I_0}{2} \times \frac{1}{2} = \frac{I_0}{4}$$

43. (c) Wavelength of radio waves is greater than microwaves hence frequency of radio waves is less than microwaves.

The degree of diffraction is greater whose wavelength is greater.

44. (b)

45. (c) For first minimum,

$d\sin\theta = \lambda$

$$\Rightarrow \quad d = \frac{\lambda}{\sin\theta} = \frac{5000 \times 10^{-8}\ \text{cm}}{\sin 30°}$$

$$= \frac{5000 \times 10^{-8}\ \text{cm}}{1/2} = 10 \times 10^{-5}\ \text{cm}$$

46. (a) For $I = \frac{I_0}{2}$ and $I = I_0\cos^2\theta = \frac{I_0}{2}$

$\therefore \theta = 45°$

Therefore the angle through which either polaroids turned is 135° (= 180° − 45°)

47. (b) When viewed through a polaroid which is rotated then the light from a clear blue portion of the sky shows a rise and fall of intensity.

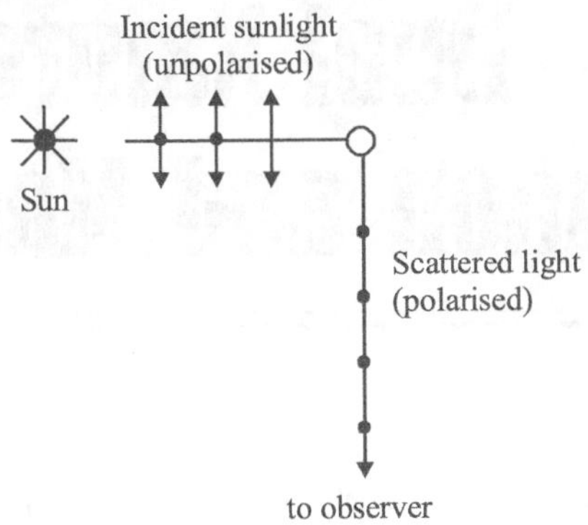

48. **(d)** The electron beam will be diffracted and the maxima is obtained at $y = 0$. Also the distance between the first minima on both side will be greater than d.

49. **(a)** $I = I_0\left(\frac{\sin\phi}{\phi}\right)^2$ and $\phi = \frac{\pi}{\lambda}(b\sin\theta)$

When the slit width is doubled, the amplitude of the wave at the centre of the screen is doubled, so the intensity at the centre is increased by a factor 4.

50. **(b)** $I = I_0\cos^2\theta$

Intensity of polarized light $= \frac{I_0}{2}$

$\Rightarrow$ Intensity of untransmitted light

$$= I_0 - \frac{I_0}{2} = \frac{I_0}{2}$$

51. **(b)** $\frac{y}{D} \geq 1.22\frac{\lambda}{d}$

$$\Rightarrow D \leq \frac{yd}{(1.22)\lambda} = \frac{10^{-3}\times 3\times 10^{-3}}{(1.22)\times 5\times 10^{-7}}$$

$$= \frac{30}{6.1} \approx 5\text{m}$$

$\therefore D_{max} = 5\text{m}$

52. **(d)** The angle of incidence for total polarization is given by $\tan\theta = n \Rightarrow \theta = \tan^{-1} n$

Where n is the refractive index of the glass

53. **(d)** The resolving power of an optical instrument is inversely proportional to the wavelength of light used.

$$\frac{(R.P)_1}{(R.P)_2} = \frac{\lambda_2}{\lambda_1} = \frac{5}{4}$$

Chapter 25

Dual Nature of Radiation and Matter

TOPIC - 1: Matter Waves, Cathode and Positive Rays

1. A particle A of mass m and initial velocity v collides with a particle B of mass $\frac{m}{2}$ which is at rest. The collision is head on, and elastic. The ratio of the de-Broglie wavelengths λ_A to λ_B after the collision is **[2017]**

(a) $\frac{\lambda_A}{\lambda_B}=\frac{2}{3}$ (b) $\frac{\lambda_A}{\lambda_B}=\frac{1}{2}$

(c) $\frac{\lambda_A}{\lambda_B}=\frac{1}{3}$ (d) $\frac{\lambda_A}{\lambda_B}=2$

2. A parallel beam of electrons travelling in x-direction falls on a slit of width d (see figure). If after passing the slit, an electron acquires momentum p_y in the y-direction then for a majority of electrons passing through the slit (h is Planck's constant) : **[Online April 10, 2015]**

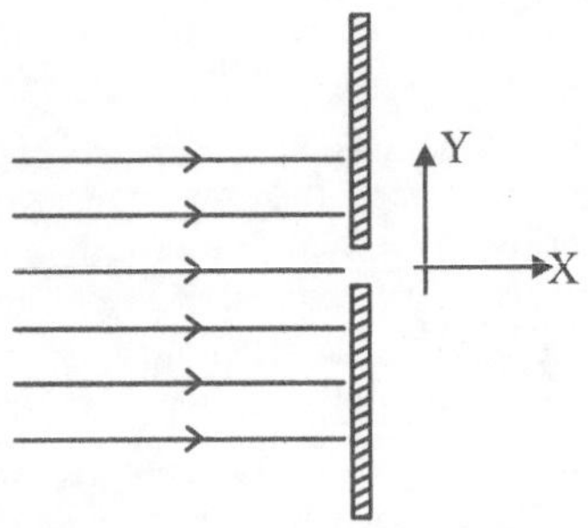

(a) $|P_y| d > h$ (b) $|P_y| d < h$

(c) $|P_y| d \simeq h$ (d) $|P_y| d >> h$

3. de-Broglie wavelength of an electron accelerated by a voltage of 50 V is close to ($|e| = 1.6 \times 10^{-19}$ C, $m_e = 9.1 \times 10^{-31}$ kg, $h = 6.6 \times 10^{-34}$ Js) : **[Online April 10, 2015]**

(a) 2.4 Å (b) 0.5 Å

(c) 1.7 Å (d) 1.2 Å

4. For which of the following particles will it be most difficult to experimentally verify the de-Broglie relationship? **[Online April 9, 2014]**

(a) an electron (b) a proton

(c) an α-particle (d) a dust particle

5. Electrons are accelerated through a potential difference V and protons are accelerated through a potential difference 4 V. The de-Broglie wavelengths are λ_e and λ_p for electrons and protons respectively. The ratio of $\frac{\lambda_e}{\lambda_p}$ is given by : (given m_e is mass of electron and m_p is mass of proton). **[Online April 23, 2013]**

(a) $\frac{\lambda_e}{\lambda_p}=\sqrt{\frac{m_p}{m_e}}$ (b) $\frac{\lambda_e}{\lambda_p}=\sqrt{\frac{m_e}{m_p}}$

(c) $\frac{\lambda_e}{\lambda_p}=\frac{1}{2}\sqrt{\frac{m_e}{m_p}}$ (d) $\frac{\lambda_e}{\lambda_p}=2\sqrt{\frac{m_p}{m_e}}$

6. If the kinetic energy of a free electron doubles, it's de-Broglie wavelength changes by the factor **[2005]**

(a) 2 (b) $\frac{1}{2}$ (c) $\sqrt{2}$ (d) $\frac{1}{\sqrt{2}}$

7. Formation of covalent bonds in compounds exhibits **[2002]**

(a) wave nature of electron

(b) particle nature of electron

(c) both wave and particle nature of electron

(d) none of these

TOPIC - 2: Photon, Photoelectric Effect X-rays and Davisson-Germer Experiment

8. An electron beam is accelerated by a potential difference V to hit a metallic target to produce X-rays. It produces continuous as well as characteristic X-rays. If λ_{min} is the smallest possible wavelength of X-ray in the spectrum, the variation of log λ_{min} with log V is correctly represented in : **[2017]**

(a) 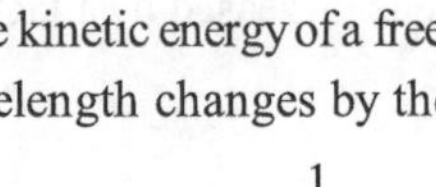

(b) 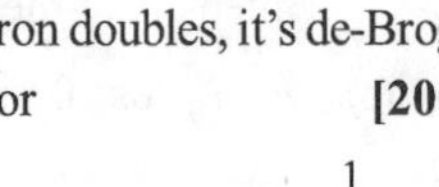

(c) 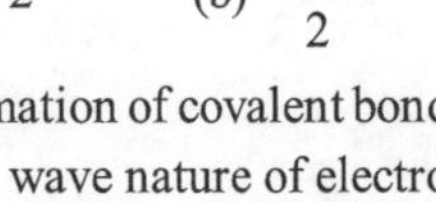

(d) 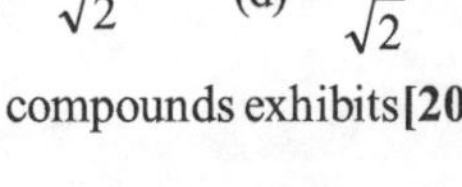

9. A Laser light of wavelength 660 nm is used to weld Retina detachment. If a Laser pulse of width 60 ms and power 0.5 kW is used the approximate number of photons in the pulse are : [Take Planck's constant $h = 6.62 \times 10^{-34}$ Js] **[Online April 9, 2017]**

(a) 10^{20} (b) 10^{18} (c) 10^{22} (d) 10^{19}

10. The maximum velocity of the photoelectrons emitted from the surface is v when light of frequency n falls on a metal surface. If the incident frequency is increased to 3n, the maximum velocity of the ejected photoelectrons will be : **[Online April 8, 2017]**

(a) less than $\sqrt{3}v$ (b) v

(c) more than $\sqrt{3}v$ (d) equal to $\sqrt{3}v$

11. Radiation of wavelength λ, is incident on a photocell. The fastest emitted electron has speed v. If the wavelength is changed to $\frac{3\lambda}{4}$, the speed of the fastest emitted electron will be: **[2016]**

(a) $= v\left(\frac{4}{3}\right)^{\frac{1}{2}}$ (b) $= v\left(\frac{3}{4}\right)^{\frac{1}{2}}$

(c) $> v\left(\frac{4}{3}\right)^{\frac{1}{2}}$ (d) $< v\left(\frac{4}{3}\right)^{\frac{1}{2}}$

12. A photoelectric surface is illuminated successively by monochromatic light of wavelengths λ and $\frac{\lambda}{2}$. If the maximum kinetic energy of the emitted photoelectrons in the second case is 3 times that in the first case, the work function of the surface is : **[Online April 10, 2016]**

(a) $\frac{hc}{2\lambda}$ (b) $\frac{hc}{\lambda}$

(c) $\frac{hc}{3\lambda}$ (d) $\frac{3hc}{\lambda}$

13. When photons of wavelength λ_1 are incident on an isolated sphere, the corresponding stopping potential is found to be V. When photons of wavelength λ_2 are used, the corresponding stopping potential was thrice that of the above value. If light of wavelength λ_3 is used then find the stopping potential for this case : **[Online April 9, 2016]**

(a) $\frac{hc}{e}\left[\frac{1}{\lambda_3}+\frac{1}{\lambda_2}-\frac{1}{\lambda_1}\right]$ (b) $\frac{hc}{e}\left[\frac{1}{\lambda_3}+\frac{1}{2\lambda_2}-\frac{1}{\lambda_1}\right]$

(c) $\frac{hc}{e}\left[\frac{1}{\lambda_3}-\frac{1}{\lambda_2}-\frac{1}{\lambda_1}\right]$ (d) $\frac{hc}{e}\left[\frac{1}{\lambda_3}+\frac{1}{2\lambda_2}-\frac{3}{2\lambda_1}\right]$

14. Match **List - I** (Fundamental Experiment) with **List - II** (its conclusion) and select the correct option from the choices given below the list: **[2015]**

List-I	List-II
A. Franck-Hertz Experiment	(i) Particle nature of light
B. Photo-electric experiment	(ii) Discrete energy levels of atom
C. Davison-Germer experiment	(iii) Wave nature of electron
	(iv) Structure of atom

(a) (A)-(ii); (B)-(i); (C)-(iii)

(b) (A)-(iv); (B)-(iii); (C)-(ii)

(c) (A)-(i); (B)-(iv); (C)-(iii)

(d) (A)-(ii); (B)-(iv); (C)-(iii)

15. A beam of light has two wavelengths of 4972Å and 6216Å with a total intensity of 3.6×10^{-3} Wm^{-2} equally distributed among the two wavelengths. The beam falls normally on an area of 1 cm^2 of a clean metallic surface of work function 2.3 eV. Assume that there is no loss of light by reflection and that each capable photon ejects one electron. The number of photoelectrons liberated in 2s is approximately: **[Online April 12, 2014]**

(a) 6×10^{11} (b) 9×10^{11}

(c) 11×10^{11} (d) 15×10^{11}

16. A photon of wavelength λ is scattered from an electron, which was at rest. The wavelength shift $\Delta\lambda$ is three times of λ and the angle of scattering θ is 60°. The angle at which the electron recoiled is ϕ. The value of tan ϕ is : (electron speed is much smaller than the speed of light) **[Online April 11, 2014]**

(a) 0.16 (b) 0.22 (c) 0.25 (d) 0.28

17. The anode voltage of a photocell is kept fixed. The wavelength λ of the light falling on the cathode is gradually changed. The plate current I of the photocell varies as follows : **[2013]**

(a) 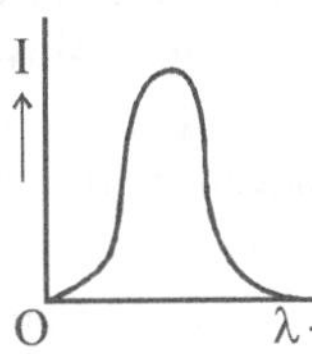

(b) 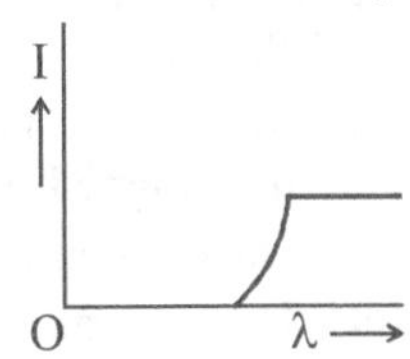

(c) 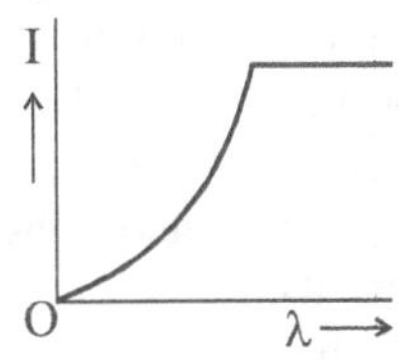

(d) 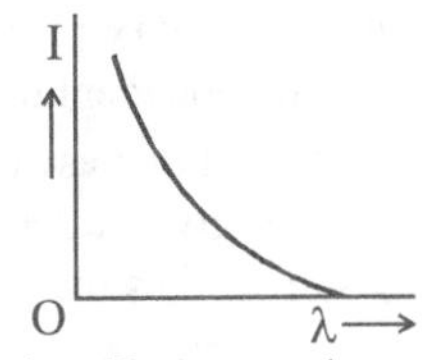

18. In an experiment on photoelectric effect, a student plots stopping potential V_0 against reciprocal of the wavelength λ of the incident light for two different metals A and B. These are shown in the figure. **[Online April 25, 2013]**

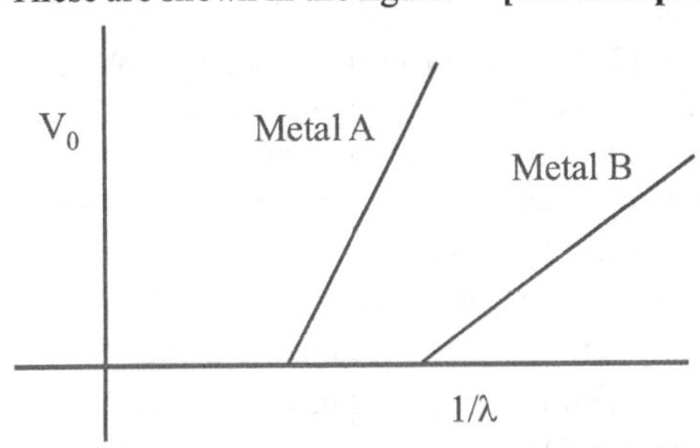

Looking at the graphs, you can most appropriately say that:

(a) Work function of metal B is greater than that of metal A

(b) For light of certain wavelength falling on both metal, maximum kinetic energy of electrons emitted from A will be greater than those emitted from B.

(c) Work function of metal A is greater than that of metal B

(d) Students data is not correct

19. A copper ball of radius 1 cm and work function 4.47eV is irradiated with ultraviolet radiation of wavelength 2500 Å. The effect of irradiation results in the emission of electrons from the ball. Further the ball will acquire charge and due to this there will be a finite value of the potential on the ball. The charge acquired by the ball is : **[Online April 25, 2013]**

(a) 5.5×10^{-13}C (b) 7.5×10^{-13}C

(c) 4.5×10^{-12}C (d) 2.5×10^{-11}C

20. This equation has statement 1 and statement 2. Of the four choices given after the statements, choose the one that describes the two statements.

Statement 1: Davisson-Germer experiment established the wave nature of electrons.

Statement 2 : If electrons have wave nature, they can interfere and show diffraction. **[2012]**

(a) Statement 1 is false, Statement 2 is true.

(b) Statement 1 is true, Statement 2 is false

(c) Statement 1 is true, Statement 2 is true, Statement 2 is the correct explanation of statement 1

(d) Statement 1 is true, Statement 2 is true, Statement 2 is not the correct explanation of Statement 1

21. Photoelectrons are ejected from a metal when light of frequency υ falls on it. Pick out the wrong statement from the following. **[Online May 26, 2012]**

(a) No electrons are emitted if υ is less than W/h, where W is the work function of the metal

(b) The ejection of the photoelectrons is instantaneous.

(c) The maximum energy of the photoelectrons is $h\upsilon$.

(d) The maximum energy of the photoelectrons is independent of the intensity of the light.

22. This question has Statement 1 and Statement 2. Of the four choices given after the Statements, choose the one that best describes the two Statements.

Statement 1: A metallic surface is irradiated by a monochromatic light of frequency $\upsilon > \upsilon_0$ (the threshold frequency). If the incident frequency is now doubled, the photocurrent and the maximum kinetic energy are also doubled.

Statement 2: The maximum kinetic energy of photoelectrons emitted from a surface is linearly dependent on the frequency of the incident light. The photocurrent depends only on the intensity of the incident light. **[Online May 19, 2012]**

(a) Statement 1 is true, Statement 2 is true, Statement 2 is the correct explanation of Statement 1.

(b) Statement 1 is false, Statement 2 is true.

(c) Statement 1 is true, Statement 2 is false.

(d) Statement 1 is true, Statement 2 is true, Statement 2 is not the correct explanation of Statement 1.

23. This question has Statement – 1 and Statement – 2. Of the four choices given after the statements, choose the one that best describes the two statements. **[2011]**

Statement – 1: A metallic surface is irradiated by a monochromatic light of frequency $v > v_0$ (the threshold frequency). The maximum kinetic energy and the stopping potential are K_{max} and V_0 respectively. If the frequency incident on the surface is doubled, both the K_{max} and V_0 are also doubled.

Statement – 2 : The maximum kinetic energy and the stopping potential of photoelectrons emitted from a surface are linearly dependent on the frequency of incident light.

(a) Statement–1 is true, Statement–2 is true, Statement – 2 is the correct explanation of Statement – 1.

(b) Statement–1 is true, Statement–2 is true, Statement – 2 is not the correct explanation of Statement – 1.

(c) Statement – 1 is false, Statement – 2 is true.

(d) Statement – 1 is true, Statement – 2 is false.

24. **Statement -1 :** When ultraviolet light is incident on a photocell, its stopping potential is V_0 and the maximum kinetic energy of the photoelectrons is K_{max}. When the ultraviolet light is replaced by X-rays, both V_0 and K_{max} increase.

Statement -2 : Photoelectrons are emitted with speeds ranging from zero to a maximum value because of the range of frequencies present in the incident light. **[2010]**

(a) Statement -1 is true, Statement -2 is true ; Statement -2 is the correct explanation of Statement -1.

(b) Statement -1 is true, Statement -2 is true; Statement -2 is **not** the correct explanation of Statement -1

(c) Statement -1 is false, Statement -2 is true.

(d) Statement -1 is true, Statement -2 is false.

25. The surface of a metal is illuminted with the light of 400 nm. The kinetic energy of the ejected photoelectrons was found to be 1.68 eV. The work function of the metal is : **[2009]**

(hc = 1240 eV.nm)

(a) 1.41 eV (b) 1.51 eV

(c) 1.68 eV (d) 3.09 eV

Directions: Question No. 13 and 14 are based on the following paragraph.

Wave property of electrons implies that they will show diffraction effects. Davisson and Germer demonstrated this by diffracting electrons from crystals. The law governing the diffraction from a crystal is obtained by requiring that electron waves reflected from the planes of atoms in a crystal interfere constructively (see figure).

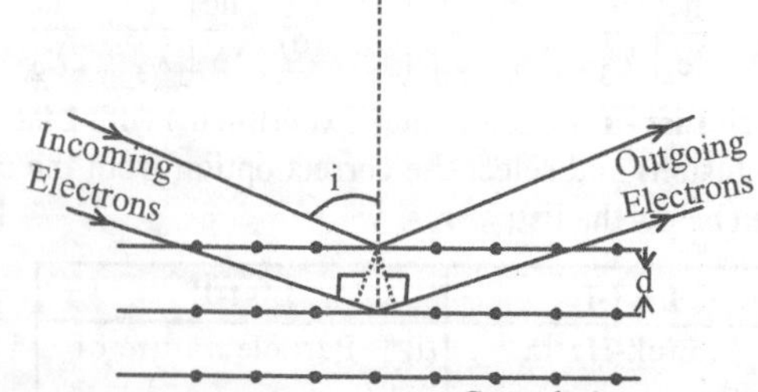

26. Electrons accelerated by potential V are diffracted from a crystal. If d = 1Å and i = 30°, V should be about **[2008]**

($h = 6.6 \times 10^{-34}$ Js, $m_e = 9.1 \times 10^{-31}$ kg, $e = 1.6 \times 10^{-19}$ C)

(a) 2000 V (b) 50 V (c) 500 V (d) 1000 V

27. If a strong diffraction peak is observed when electrons are incident at an angle 'i' from the normal to the crystal planes with distance 'd' between them (see figure), de Broglie wavelength λ_{dB} of electrons can be calculated by the relationship (n is an integer) [2008]

(a) $d \sin i = n\lambda_{dB}$ (b) $2d \cos i = n\lambda_{dB}$

(c) $2d \sin i = n\lambda_{dB}$ (d) $d \cos i = n\lambda_{dB}$

28. Photon of frequency ν has a momentum associated with it. If c is the velocity of light, the momentum is [2007]

(a) $h\nu / c$ (b) ν / c (c) $h \nu c$ (d) $h\nu / c^2$

29. The threshold frequency for a metallic surface corresponds to an energy of 6.2 eV and the stopping potential for a radiation incident on this surface is 5 V. The incident radiation lies in [2006]

(a) ultra-violet region (b) infra-red region
(c) visible region (d) *X*-ray region

30. The time taken by a photoelectron to come out after the photon strikes is approximately [2006]

(a) 10^{-4} s (b) 10^{-10} s (c) 10^{-16} s (d) 10^{-1} s

31. The anode voltage of a photocell is kept fixed. The wavelength λ of the light falling on the cathode is gradually changed. The plate current I of the photocell varies as follows [2006]

(a) 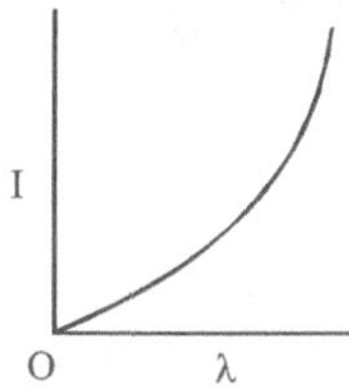

(b) 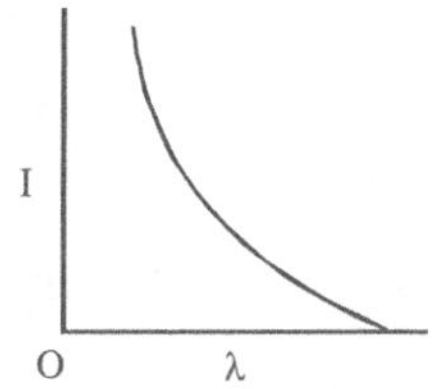

(c) 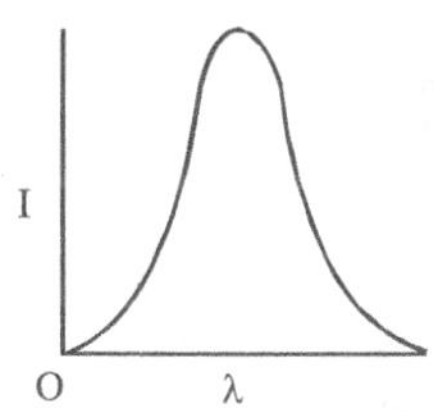

(d) 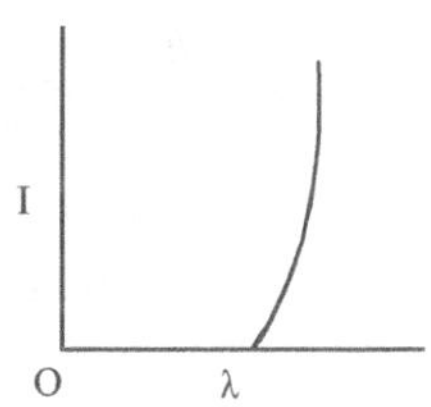

32. A photocell is illuminated by a small bright source placed 1 m away. When the same source of light is placed $\frac{1}{2}$ m away, the number of electrons emitted by photocathode would

(a) increase by a factor of 4 [2005]
(b) decrease by a factor of 4
(c) increase by a factor of 2
(d) decrease by a factor of 2

33. A radiation of energy E falls normally on a perfectly reflecting surface. The momentum transferred to the surface is [2004]

(a) Ec (b) $2E/c$ (c) E/c (d) E/c^2

34. According to Einstein's photoelectric equation, the plot of the kinetic energy of the emitted photo electrons from a metal Versus the frequency, of the incident radiation gives a straight line whose slope [2004]

(a) depends both on the intensity of the radiation and the metal used
(b) depends on the intensity of the radiation
(c) depends on the nature of the metal used
(d) is the same for the all metals and independent of the intensity of the radiation

35. The work function of a substance is 4.0 eV. The longest wavelength of light that can cause photoelectron emission from this substance is approximately [2004]

(a) 310 nm (b) 400 nm (c) 540 nm (d) 220 nm

36. Two identical photocathodes receive light of frequencies f_1 and f_2. If the velocites of the photo electrons (of mass m) coming out are respectively v_1 and v_2, then [2003]

(a) $v_1^2 - v_2^2 = \frac{2h}{m}(f_1 - f_2)$

(b) $v_1 + v_2 = \left[\frac{2h}{m}(f_1 + f_2)\right]^{1/2}$

(c) $v_1^2 + v_2^2 = \frac{2h}{m}(f_1 + f_2)$

(d) $v_1 - v_2 = \left[\frac{2h}{m}(f_1 - f_2)\right]^{1/2}$

37. Sodium and copper have work functions 2.3 eV and 4.5 eV respectively. Then the ratio of the wavelengths is nearest to [2002]

(a) 1 : 2 (b) 4 : 1 (c) 2 : 1 (d) 1 : 4

Hints & Solutions

TOPIC - 1: Matter Waves, Cathode and Positive Rays

1. **(d)** From question, $m_A = M; m_B = \frac{m}{2}$

$u_A = V \quad u_B = 0$

Let after collision velocity of $A = V_1$ and velocity of $B = V_2$

Applying law of conservation of momentum,

$$mu = mv_1 + \left(\frac{m}{2}\right)v_2$$

$$\text{or, } 24 = 2v_1 + v_2 \quad ....(i)$$

By law of collision

$$e = \frac{v_2 - v_1}{u - 0}$$

$$\text{or, } u = v_2 - v_1 \quad ....(ii)$$

$[\because$ collision is elastic, $e = 1]$

using eqns (i) and (ii)

$$v_1 = \frac{4}{3} \text{ and } v_2 = \frac{4}{3}u$$

de-Broglie wavelength $\lambda = \frac{h}{p}$

$$\therefore \frac{\lambda_A}{\lambda_B} = \frac{P_B}{P_A} = \frac{\frac{m}{2} \times \frac{4}{3}u}{m \times \frac{4}{3}} = 2$$

2. **(a)** From Bragg's equation

$d \sin\theta = \lambda$

$$\sin\theta = \frac{\lambda}{d} < 1$$

$$\therefore \lambda < d$$

$$\frac{h}{|p_y|} < d \qquad \left[\because \lambda = \frac{h}{|p_y|}\right]$$

$$\therefore h < |p_y| d$$

3. **(c)** de-Broglie wavelength,

$$\lambda = \frac{h}{P} = \frac{h}{mv} = \frac{h}{\sqrt{2mqV}}$$

$$\text{or, } \lambda = \frac{6.6 \times 10^{-34}}{\sqrt{2 \times 9.1 \times 10^{-31} \times 1.6 \times 10^{-19} \times 50}}$$

$$= 1.7 \text{ Å}$$

4. **(d)** Among the given particles most difficult to experimentally verify the de-broglie relationship is for a dust particle.

5. **(d)** Energy in joule (E)

= charge × potential diff. in volt

$E_{electron} = q_e V$ and $E_{proton} = q_p 4V$

de-Broglie wavelength $\lambda = \frac{h}{P} = \frac{h}{\sqrt{2mE}}$

$$\lambda_e = \frac{h}{\sqrt{2m_e eV}} \text{ and } \lambda_P = \frac{h}{\sqrt{2m_P e4V}} \quad (\because q_e = q_P)$$

$$\therefore \frac{\lambda_e}{\lambda_P} = \frac{\frac{h}{\sqrt{2m_e eV}}}{\frac{h}{\sqrt{2m_P e4V}}} = \sqrt{\frac{2m_P e4V}{2m_e eV}}$$

$$= 2\sqrt{\frac{m_P}{m_e}}$$

6. **(d)** de-Broglie wavelength,

$$\lambda = \frac{h}{p} = \frac{h}{\sqrt{2.m.(K.E)}}$$

$$\therefore \lambda \propto \frac{1}{\sqrt{K.E}}$$

If K.E is doubled, wavelength becomes $\frac{\lambda}{\sqrt{2}}$

7. **(a)** Formation of covalent bond is best explained by molecular orbital theory.

TOPIC - 2: Photon, Photoelectric Effect X-rays and Davisson-Germer Experiment

8. **(c)** In X-ray tube, $\lambda_{min} = \frac{hc}{eV}$

$$\ln \lambda_{min} = \ln\left(\frac{hc}{e}\right) - \ln V$$

Clearly, log λ_{min} versus log V graph slope is negative hence option (3) correctly depicts.

9. **(a)** Given, $\lambda = 660$ nm, Power = 0.5 kW, t = 60 ms

$$\text{Power } P = \frac{nhc}{\lambda t} \Rightarrow n = \frac{p\lambda t}{hc}$$

$$= 0.5 \times 10^3 \times \frac{660 \times 10^{-9} \times 60 \times 10^{-3}}{6.6 \times 10^{-34} \times 3 \times 10^8}$$

$$= 100 \times 10^{18} = 10^{20}$$

10. **(c)** As the metal surface is same, work function (ϕ) is same for both the case.

Initially $KE_{max} = nh - \phi$ .....(i)

After increase

$KE'_{max} = 3\,nh - \phi$ ....(ii)

For work function ϕ – not to be –ve or zero, $v' > \sqrt{3}v$

11. **(c)** $h\nu_0{}^2 - h\nu_0 = \frac{1}{2}mv^2$

$\therefore \frac{4}{3}h\nu_0 - h\nu_0 = \frac{1}{2}mv'^2$

$\therefore \frac{v'^2}{v^2} = \frac{\frac{4}{3}\nu - \nu_0}{\nu - \nu_0}$ $\therefore v' = v\sqrt{\frac{\frac{4}{3}\nu - \nu_0}{\nu - \nu_0}}$

$\therefore v' > v\sqrt{\frac{4}{3}}$

12. **(a)** From Einstein's photoelectric equation

$K.E._\lambda = \frac{hc}{\lambda} - \phi$ ...(i)

(for monochromatic light of wavelength λ)

where ϕ is work function

$K.E._{\lambda/2} = \frac{hc}{\lambda/2} - \phi$ ...(ii)

(for monochromatic light of wavelength $\lambda/2$)

From question,

$K.E._{\lambda/2} = 3(K.E._\lambda) \Rightarrow \frac{hc}{\lambda/2} - \phi = 3\left(\frac{hc}{\lambda} - \phi\right)$

$\frac{2hc}{\lambda} - \phi = 3\frac{hc}{\lambda} - 3\phi$

$\Rightarrow 2\phi = \frac{hc}{\lambda} \therefore \phi = \frac{hc}{2\lambda}$

13. **(None)**

From Einstein's photoelectric equation, we have

$\frac{hc}{\lambda_1} = \frac{hc}{\lambda_0} + eV$ ...(1)

$\frac{hc}{\lambda_2} = \frac{hc}{\lambda_0} + eV$ ...(2)

$\frac{hc}{\lambda_3} = \frac{hc}{\lambda_0} + 3eV'$ ...(3)

From equation (1) & (2)

$\frac{3}{2\lambda_1} - \frac{2}{2\lambda_2} = \frac{1}{\lambda_0}$

$\frac{hc}{\lambda_1} - hc\left[\frac{3}{2\lambda_1} - \frac{1}{2\lambda_2}\right] = eV'$

$\frac{hc}{e}\left[\frac{1}{\lambda_3} - \frac{3}{2\lambda_1} + \frac{1}{2\lambda_2}\right] = V'$

14. **(a)** Frank-Hertz experiment - Discrete energy levels of atom

Photoelectric effect - Particle nature of light

Davison - Germer experiment - wave nature of electron.

15. **(b)** Given, $\lambda_1 = 4972Å$

and $\lambda_2 = 6216Å$

and $I = 3.6 \times 10^{-3}\,Wm^{-2}$

Intensity associated with each wavelength

$= \frac{3.6\times10^{-3}}{2}$

$= 1.8 \times 10^{-3}\,Wm^{-2}$

work function $\phi = h\nu$

$= \frac{hc}{\lambda}$

$= \frac{(6.62\times10^{-34})(3\times10^8)}{\lambda}$

$= \frac{12.4\times10^3}{\lambda}\,ev$

for different wavelengths

$\phi_1 = \frac{12.4\times10^3}{\lambda_1} = \frac{12.4\times10^3}{4972} = 2.493\,eV$

$= 3.984 \times 10^{-19}\,J$

$\phi_2 = \frac{12.4\times10^3}{\lambda_2} = \frac{12.4\times10^3}{6216} = 1.994\,eV$

$= 3.184 \times 10^{-19}\,J$

Work function for metallic surface $\phi = 2.3$ eV (given)

$\phi_2 < \phi$

Therefore, ϕ_2 will not contribute in this process.

Now, no. of electrons per m^2-s = no. of photons per m^2-s

no. of electrons per m^2-s $= \frac{1.8\times10^{-3}}{3.984\times10^{-19}} \times 10^{-4}$

$(\because 1\,cm^2 = 10^{-4}\,m^2)$

$= 0.45 \times 10^{12}$

So, the number of photo electrons liberated in 2 sec.

$= 0.45 \times 10^{12} \times 2$

$= 9 \times 10^{11}$

16. **(b)**

17. **(d)** As λ is increased, there will be a value of λ above which photoelectrons will be cease to come out so photocurrent will become zero. Hence (d) is correct answer.

18. (d) $\frac{hc}{\lambda} - \phi = eV_0$

$V_0 = \frac{hc}{e\lambda} - \frac{\phi}{e}$

For metal A $\frac{\phi A}{hc} = \frac{1}{\lambda}$ For metal B $\frac{\phi B}{hc} = \frac{1}{\lambda}$

As the value of $\frac{1}{\lambda}$ (increasing and decreasing) is not specified hence we cannot say that which metal has comparatively greater or lesser work function (ϕ).

19. (a)

20. (c)

21. (c) According to photo-electric equation :
$K.E_{max} = h\nu - h\nu_0$ (Work function)
Some sort of energy is used in ejecting the photoelectrons.

22. (b) The maximum kinetic energy of photoelectrons depends upon frequency on incident light and photo current depends upon intensity of incident light.

23. (c) By Einstein photoelectric equation,
$K_{max} = eV_0 = h\nu - h\nu_0$
When ν is doubled, K_{max} and V_0 become more than double.

24. (d) We know that

$eV_0 = K_{max} = h\nu - \phi$

where, ϕ is the work function.

Hence, as ν increases (note that frequency of X-rays is greater than that of U.V. rays), both V_0 and K_{max} increase. So statement - 1 is correct

25. (a) $\lambda = 400$ nm, $hc = 1240$ eV.nm, K.E. $= 1.68$ eV

We know that,

$\frac{hc}{\lambda} - W = K.E \Rightarrow W = \frac{hc}{\lambda} - K.E$

$\Rightarrow W = \frac{1240}{400} - 1.68 = 3.1 - 1.68 = 1.42$ eV

26. (b) The path difference between the rays APB and CQD is
$\Delta x = MQ + QN = d\cos i + d\cos i$
$\Delta x = 2d\cos i$

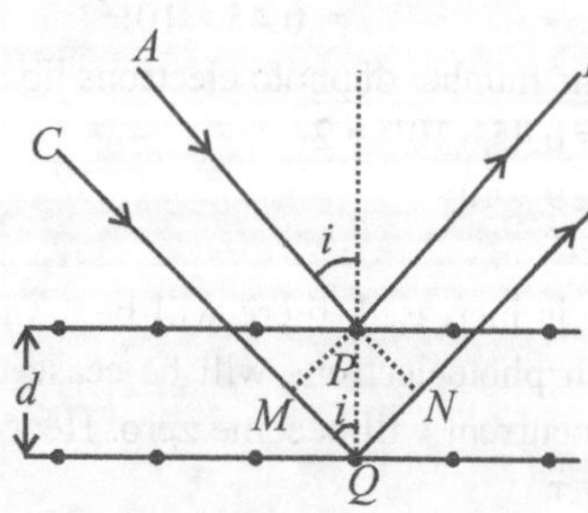

We know that for constructive interference the path difference is $n\lambda$

$\therefore \quad n\lambda = 2d\cos i$

Also by de-broglie concept

$\lambda = \frac{h}{p} = \frac{h}{\sqrt{2mK.E}} = \frac{h}{\sqrt{2meV}}$

$\therefore \quad \frac{nh}{\sqrt{2meV}} = 2d\cos i$

Here $n = 1$: $V = \frac{h^2}{8med^2\cos^2 i}$

$= \frac{(6.6\times10^{-34})^2}{8\times9.1\times10^{-31}\times1.6\times10^{-19}\times(10^{-10})^2\times\cos^2 30}$

$= 50$ V

27. (b) $2d\cos i = n\lambda_{dB}$

28. (a) Energy of a photon of frequency ν is given by $E = h\nu$.
Also, $E = mc^2$, $mc^2 = h\nu$

$\Rightarrow mc = \frac{h\nu}{c} \quad \Rightarrow p = \frac{h\nu}{c}$

29. (a) $\phi = 6.2$ eV $= 6.2\times1.6\times10^{-19}$ J

$V = 5$ volt

$\frac{hc}{\lambda} - \phi = eV_0$

$\Rightarrow \lambda = \frac{hc}{\phi + eV_0}$

$= \frac{6.6\times10^{-34}\times3\times10^8}{1.6\times10^{-19}(6.2+5)} \approx 10^{-7}$ m

This range lies in ultra violet range.

30. (b) The order of time is nano second.

31. (b) As λ decreases, ν increases and hence the speed of photoelectron increases. The chances of photo electron to meet the anode increases and hence photo electric current increases.

32. (a) $I \propto \frac{I}{r^2}$; $\frac{I_1}{I_2} = \left(\frac{r_2}{r_1}\right)^2 = \frac{1}{4}$

$I_2 \rightarrow 4$ times I_1

When intensity becomes 4 times, no. of photoelectrons emitted would increase by 4 times, since number of electrons emitted per second is directly proportional to intensity.

33. (b) Momentum of photon $= \frac{E}{c}$

Change in momentum $= \frac{2E}{c}$

= momentum transferred to the surface
(the photon will reflect with same magnitude of momentum in opposite direction)

34. **(d)** From Equation $K.E = h\nu - \phi$
slope of graph of K.E & ν is h (Plank's constant) which is same for all metals

35. **(a)** For the longest wavelength to emit photo electron

$$\frac{hc}{\lambda} = \phi \Rightarrow \lambda = \frac{hc}{\phi}$$

$$\Rightarrow \lambda = \frac{6.63\times10^{-34}\times3\times10^{8}}{40\times1.6\times10^{-16}} = 310\,\text{nm}$$

36. **(a)** For one photocathode

$$hf_1 - W = \frac{1}{2}mv_1^2 \qquad \text{....(i)}$$

For another photo cathode

$$hf_2 - W = \frac{1}{2}mv_2^2 \qquad \text{....(ii)}$$

Subtracting (ii) from (i) we get

$$(hf_1 - W) - (hf_2 - W) = \frac{1}{2}mv_1^2 - \frac{1}{2}mv_2^2$$

$$\therefore\ h(f_1 - f_2) = \frac{m}{2}(v_1^2 - v_2^2)$$

$$\therefore\ v_1^2 - v_2^2 = \frac{2h}{m}(f_1 - f_2)$$

37. **(c)** We know that work function is the energy required and energy $E = h\upsilon$

$$\therefore\ \frac{E_{Na}}{E_{Cu}} = \frac{h\upsilon_{Na}}{h\upsilon_{Cu}} = \frac{\lambda_{Cu}}{\lambda_{Na}}$$

$$\left[\because\ \upsilon \propto \frac{1}{\lambda}\ \text{for light}\right]$$

$$\therefore\ \frac{\lambda_{Na}}{\lambda_{Cu}} = \frac{E_{Cu}}{E_{Na}} = \frac{4.5}{2.3} \approx \frac{2}{1}$$

Chapter 26

Atoms

TOPIC - 1: Atomic Structure and Rutherford's Nuclear Model

1. In the Rutherford experiment, α-particles are scattered from a nucleus as shown. Out of the four paths, which path is not possible? **[Online May 7, 2012]**

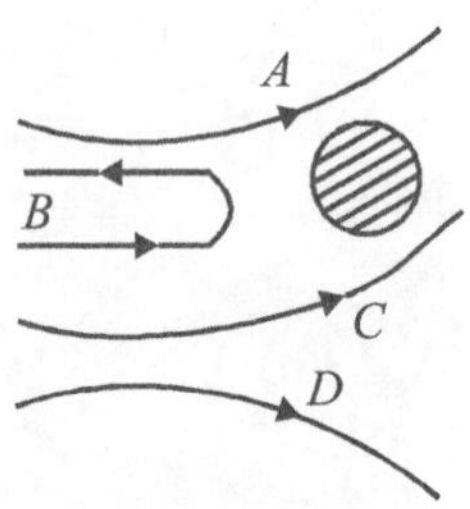

(a) D (b) B (c) C (d) A

2. An alpha nucleus of energy $\frac{1}{2}mv^2$ bombards a heavy nuclear target of charge Ze. Then the distance of closest approach for the alpha nucleus will be proportional to **[2006]**

(a) v^2 (b) $\frac{1}{m}$ (c) $\frac{1}{v^2}$ (d) $\frac{1}{Ze}$

3. An α-particle of energy 5 MeV is scattered through 180° by a fixed uranium nucleus. The distance of closest approach is of the order of **[2004]**

(a) 10^{-12} cm (b) 10^{-10} cm
(c) 10^{-14} cm (d) 10^{-15} cm

TOPIC - 2 : Bohr's Model and the Spectra of the Hydrogen Atom

4. Some energy levels of a molecule are shown in the figure. The ratio of the wavelengths $r = \lambda_1 / \lambda_2$, is given by

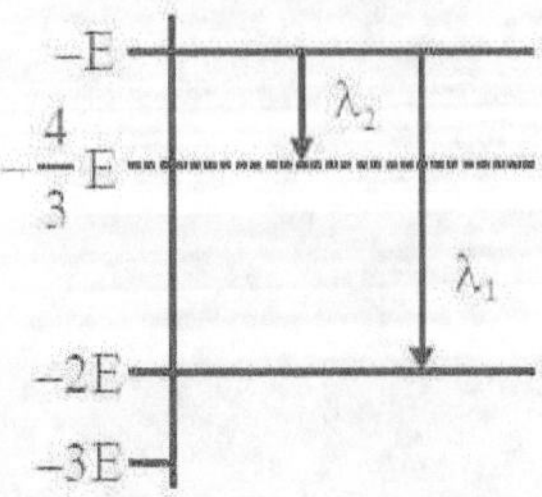

(a) $r = \frac{3}{4}$ (b) $r = \frac{1}{3}$

(c) $r = \frac{4}{3}$ (d) $r = \frac{2}{3}$

5. The acceleration of an electron in the first orbit of the hydrogen atom (z = 1) is : **[Online April 9, 2017]**

(a) $\frac{h^2}{\pi^2 m^2 r^3}$ (b) $\frac{h^2}{8\pi^2 m^2 r^3}$

(c) $\frac{h^2}{4\pi^2 m^2 r^3}$ (d) $\frac{h^2}{4\pi m^2 r^3}$

6. According to Bohr's theory, the time averaged magnetic field at the centre (i.e. nucleus) of a hydrogen atom due to the motion of electrons in the nth orbit is proportional to : (n = principal quantum number) **[Online April 8, 2017]**

(a) n^{-4} (b) n^{-5} (c) n^{-3} (d) n^{-2}

7. A hydrogen atom makes a transition from n = 2 to n = 1 and emits a photon. This photon strikes a doubly ionized lithium atom (z = 3) in excited state and completely removes the orbiting electron. The least quantum number for the excited state of the ion for the process is : **[Online April 9, 2016]**

(a) 2 (b) 4
(c) 5 (d) 3

8. As an electron makes a transition from an excited state to the ground state of a hydrogen - like atom/ion : **[2015]**

(a) kinetic energy decreases, potential energy increases but total energy remains same
(b) kinetic energy and total energy decrease but potential energy increases
(c) its kinetic energy increases but potential energy and total energy decrease
(d) kinetic energy, potential energy and total energy decrease

9. The de–Broglie wavelength associated with the electron in the n = 4 level is : **[Online April 11, 2015]**

(a) $\frac{1}{4}$ th of the de–Broglie wavelength of the electron in the ground state.
(b) four times the de–Broglie wavelength of the electron in the ground state

(c) two times the de–Broglie wavelength of the electron in the ground state

(d) half of the de–Broglie wavelength of the electron in the ground state

10. If one were to apply Bohr model to a particle of mass 'm' and charge 'q' moving in a plane under the influence of a magnetic field 'B', the energy of the charged particle in the nth level will be : **[Online April 10, 2015]**

(a) $n\left(\frac{hqB}{2\pi m}\right)$ (b) $n\left(\frac{hqB}{8\pi m}\right)$

(c) $n\left(\frac{hqB}{4\pi m}\right)$ (d) $n\left(\frac{hqB}{\pi m}\right)$

11. The radiation corresponding to $3 \to 2$ transition of hydrogen atom falls on a metal surface to produce photoelectrons. These electrons are made to enter a magnetic field of 3×10^{-4} T. If the radius of the largest circular path followed by these electrons is 10.0 mm, the work function of the metal is close to: **[2014]**

(a) 1.8 eV (b) 1.1 eV (c) 0.8 eV (d) 1.6 eV

12. Hydrogen $\left({}_1H^1\right)$, Deuterium $\left({}_1H^2\right)$, singly ionised Helium $\left({}_2He^4\right)^+$ and doubly ionised lithium $\left({}_3Li^6\right)^{++}$ all have one electron around the nucleus. Consider an electron transition from n = 2 to n = 1. If the wavelengths of emitted radiation are $\lambda_1, \lambda_2, \lambda_3$ and λ_4 respectively then approximately which one of the following is correct? **[2014]**

(a) $4\lambda_1 = 2\lambda_2 = 2\lambda_3 = \lambda_4$

(b) $\lambda_1 = 2\lambda_2 = 2\lambda_3 = \lambda_4$

(c) $\lambda_1 = \lambda_2 = 4\lambda_3 = 9\lambda_4$

(d) $\lambda_1 = 2\lambda_2 = 3\lambda_3 = 4\lambda_4$

13. Match List - I (Experiment performed) with List-II (Phenomena discovered/associated) and select the correct option from the options given below the lists: **[Online April 19, 2014]**

List - I		List - II	
(1)	Davisson and Germer experiment	(i)	Wave nature of electrons
(2)	Millikan's oil drop experiment	(ii)	Charge of an electron
(3)	Rutherford experiment	(iii)	Quantisation of energy levels
(4)	Franck-Hertz experiment	(iv)	Existence of nucleus

(a) (1)-(i), (2)-(ii), (3)-(iii), (4)-(iv)

(b) (1)-(i), (2)-(ii), (3)-(iv), (4)-(iii)

(c) (1)-(iii), (2)-(iv), (3)-(i), (4)-(ii)

(d) (1)-(iv), (2)-(iii), (3)-(ii), (4)-(i)

14. The binding energy of the electron in a hydrogen atom is 13.6 eV, the energy required to remove the electron from the first excited state of Li^{++} is: **[Online April 9, 2014]**

(a) 122.4 eV (b) 30.6 eV

(c) 13.6 eV (d) 3.4 eV

15. Ina hydrogen like atom electron make transition from an energy level with quantum number n to another with quantum number (n – 1). If n>>1, the frequency of radiation emitted is proportional to : **[2013]**

(a) $\frac{1}{n}$ (b) $\frac{1}{n^2}$ (c) $\frac{1}{n^{3/2}}$ (d) $\frac{1}{n^3}$

16. A 12.5 eV electron beam is used to bombard gaseous hydrogen at room temperature. It will emit : **[Online April 25, 2013]**

(a) 2 lines in the Lyman series and 1 line in the Balmar series

(b) 3 lines in the Lyman series

(c) 1 line in the Lyman series and 2 lines in the Balmar series

(d) 3 lines in the Balmer series

17. In the Bohr's model of hydrogen-like atom the force between the nucleus and the electron is modified as $F = \frac{e^2}{4\pi\varepsilon_0}\left(\frac{1}{r^2}+\frac{\beta}{r^3}\right)$, where β is a constant. For this atom, the radius of the nth orbit in terms of the Bohr radius $\left(a_0 = \frac{\varepsilon_0 h^2}{m\pi e^2}\right)$ is : **[Online April 23, 2013]**

(a) $r_n = a_0 n - \beta$ (b) $r_n = a_0 n^2 + \beta$

(c) $r_n = a_0 n^2 - \beta$ (d) $r_n = a_0 n + \beta$

18. Orbits of a particle moving in a circle are such that the perimeter of the orbit equals an integer number of de-Broglie wavelengths of the particle. For a charged particle moving in a plane perpendicular to a magnetic field, the radius of the nth orbital will therefore be proportional to : **[Online April 22, 2013]**

(a) n^2 (b) n (c) $n^{1/2}$ (d) $n^{1/4}$

19. In the Bohr model an electron moves in a circular orbit around the proton. Considering the orbiting electron to be a circular current loop, the magnetic moment of the hydrogen atom, when the electron is in n^{th} excited state, is : **[Online April 9, 2013]**

(a) $\left(\frac{e}{2m}\frac{n^2h}{2\pi}\right)$ (b) $\left(\frac{e}{m}\right)\frac{nh}{2\pi}$

(c) $\left(\frac{e}{2m}\right)\frac{nh}{2\pi}$ (d) $\left(\frac{e}{m}\right)\frac{n^2h}{2\pi}$

20. Hydrogen atom is excited from ground state to another state with principal quantum number equal to 4. Then the number of spectral lines in the emission spectra will be : **[2012]**
(a) 2 (b) 3 (c) 5 (d) 6

21. A diatomic molecule is made of two masses m_1 and m_2 which are separated by a distance r. If we calculate its rotational energy by applying Bohr's rule of angular momentum quantization, its energy will be given by: (n is an integer) **[2012]**

(a) $\frac{(m_1+m_2)^2n^2h^2}{2m_1^2m_2^2r^2}$ (b) $\frac{n^2h^2}{2(m_1+m_2)r^2}$

(c) $\frac{2n^2h^2}{(m_1+m_2)r^2}$ (d) $\frac{(m_1+m_2)n^2\hbar^2}{2m_1m_2r^2}$

22. Which of the plots shown in the figure represents speed (v_n) of the electron in a hydrogen atom as a function of the principal quantum number (n)? **[Online May 26, 2012]**

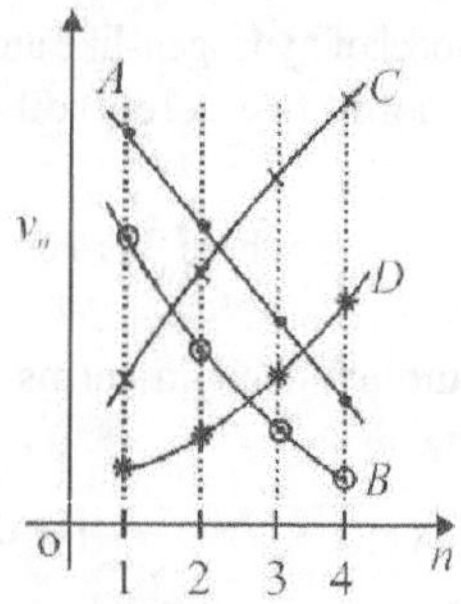

(a) B (b) D (c) C (d) A

23. A doubly ionised Li atom is excited from its ground state(n = 1) to n = 3 state. The wavelengths of the spectral lines are given by λ_{32}, λ_{31} and λ_{21}. The ratio $\lambda_{32}/\lambda_{31}$ and $\lambda_{21}/\lambda_{31}$ are, respectively **[Online May 12, 2012]**
(a) 8.1, 0.67 (b) 8.1, 1.2
(c) 6.4, 1.2 (d) 6.4, 0.67

24. A hypothetical atom has only three energy levels. The ground level has energy, E_1 = – 8 eV. The two excited states have energies, E_2 = – 6 eV and E_3 = – 2 eV. Then which of the following wavelengths will not be present in the emission spectrum of this atom? **[Online May 12, 2012]**
(a) 207 nm (b) 465 nm (c) 310 nm (d) 620 nm

25. The electron of a hydrogen atom makes a transition from the $(n + 1)^{th}$ orbit to the nth orbit. For large n the wavelength of the emitted radiation is proportional to **[Online May 7, 2012]**
(a) n (b) n^3 (c) n^4 (d) n^2

26. Energy required for the electron excitation in Li^{++} from the first to the third Bohr orbit is : **[2011]**
(a) 36.3 eV (b) 108.8 eV (c) 122.4 eV (d) 12.1 eV

27. The transition from the state n = 4 to n = 3 in a hydrogen like atom results in ultraviolet radiation. Infrared radiation will be obtained in the transition from : **[2009]**
(a) $3\rightarrow2$ (b) $4\rightarrow2$ (c) $5\rightarrow4$ (d) $2\rightarrow1$

28. Suppose an electron is attracted towards the origin by a force $\frac{k}{r}$ where 'k' is a constant and 'r' is the distance of the electron from the origin. By applying Bohr model to this system, the radius of the nth orbital of the electron is found to be 'r_n' and the kinetic energy of the electron to be 'T_n'. Then which of the following is true? **[2008]**

(a) $T_n \propto \frac{1}{n^2}, r_n \propto n^2$

(b) T_n independent of n, $r_n \propto n$

(c) $T_n \propto \frac{1}{n}, r_n \propto n$

(d) $T_n \propto \frac{1}{n^3}, r_n \propto n^2$

29. Which of the following transitions in hydrogen atoms emit photons of highest frequency? **[2007]**
(a) n = 1 to n = 2 (b) n = 2 to n = 6
(c) n = 6 to n = 2 (d) n = 2 to n = 1

30. The diagram shows the energy levels for an electron in a certain atom. Which transition shown represents the emission of a photon with the most energy? **[2005]**

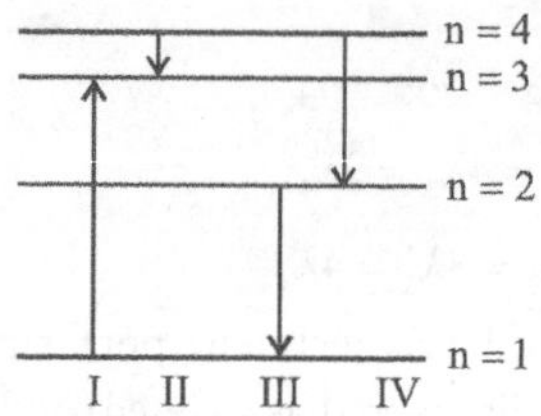

(a) IV (b) III (c) II (d) I

31. The wavelengths involved in the spectrum of deuterium $\left({}_1^2D\right)$ are slightly different from that of hydrogen spectrum, because **[2003]**
(a) the size of the two nuclei are different
(b) the nuclear forces are different in the two cases
(c) the masses of the two nuclei are different
(d) the attraction between the electron and the nucleus is differernt in the two cases

32. If 13.6 eV energy is required to ionize the hydrogen atom, then the energy required to remove an electron from n = 2 is **[2002]**
(a) 10.2 eV (b) 0 eV (c) 3.4 eV (d) 6.8 eV

Hints & Solutions

TOPIC - 1: Atomic Structure, Rutherford's Nuclear Model of Atom

1. **(c)** As α-particles are doubly ionised helium He^{++} i.e. Positively charged and nucleus is also positively charged and we know that like charges repel each other.

2. **(b)** Work done to stop the α particle is equal to K.E.

$$\therefore qV = \frac{1}{2}mv^2 \Rightarrow q \times \frac{K(Ze)}{r} = \frac{1}{2}mv^2$$

$$\Rightarrow r = \frac{2(2e)K(Ze)}{mv^2} = \frac{4KZe^2}{mv^2}$$

$$\Rightarrow r \propto \frac{1}{v^2} \text{ and } r \propto \frac{1}{m}.$$

3. **(a)** Distance of closest approach

$$r_0 = \frac{Ze(2e)}{4\pi\varepsilon_0\left(\frac{1}{2}mv^2\right)}$$

Energy, $E = 5\times10^6 \times 1.6\times10^{-19}$ J

$$\therefore r_0 = \frac{9\times10^9 \times (92\times1.6\times10^{-19})(2\times1.6\times10^{-19})}{5\times10^6\times1.6\times10^{-19}}$$

$$\Rightarrow r_h = 5.2\times10^{-14}\, m = 5.3\times10^{-12} \text{ cm}$$

TOPIC - 2 : Bohr's Model and the Spectra of the Hydrogen Atom

4. **(b)** From energy level diagram, using $\Delta E = \frac{hc}{\lambda}$

For wavelength λ_1 $\Delta E = -E-(-2E) = \frac{hc}{\lambda_1}$

$$\therefore \quad \lambda_1 = \frac{hc}{E}$$

For wavelength λ_2 $\Delta E = -E - \left(-\frac{4E}{3}\right) = \frac{hc}{\lambda_2}$

$$\therefore \quad \lambda_2 = \frac{hc}{\left(\frac{E}{3}\right)} \qquad \therefore \quad r = \frac{\lambda_1}{\lambda_2} = \frac{1}{3}$$

5. **(c)** Speed of electron in first orbit (n = 1) of hydrogen atom (z = 1),

$$v = \frac{e^2}{2\varepsilon_0 h}$$

radius of Bohr's first orbit,

$$r = \frac{h^2\varepsilon_0}{\pi me^2} \Rightarrow \varepsilon_0 = \frac{r\pi me^2}{h^2} \quad \text{....... (i)}$$

Acceleration of electron,

$$\frac{v^2}{r} = \frac{e^4}{4\varepsilon_0^2h^2} \times \frac{\pi me^2}{h^2\varepsilon_0}$$

$$= \frac{e^4 \times \pi me^2}{4h^4\varepsilon_0^3} \quad \text{....... (ii)}$$

eliminating ε_0 from eq (ii),

$$= \frac{e^4\, \pi me^2h^6}{4h^4r^3\pi^3m^3e^6} \quad \text{from eq}^n\text{ (i)}$$

$$= \frac{h^2}{4\pi^2m^2r^3}$$

6. **(d)** Magnetic field at the centre of nucleus of H-atom,

$$B = \frac{\mu_0 I}{2r} \quad \text{..... (i)}$$

According to Bohr's model, radius of orbit $r \propto n^2$ from eq. (i) we can also write as $B \propto n^{-2}$

7. **(b)** A hydrogen atom makes a transition from n = 2 to n = 1

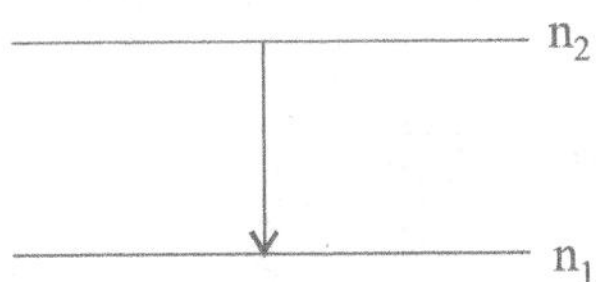

$$\text{Then wavelength} = Rcz^2\left[\frac{1}{n_1^2} - \frac{1}{n_2^2}\right] = Rc(1)^2\left[1 - \frac{1}{4}\right]$$

$$\lambda = Rc\left[\frac{3}{4}\right] \quad \text{...(1)}$$

For ionized lithium

$$\lambda = Rc(3)^2\left[\frac{1}{n^2}\right] = Rc9\left[\frac{1}{n^2}\right] \quad \text{...(2)}$$

$$Rc\left[\frac{3}{4}\right] = Rc9\left[\frac{1}{n^2}\right]$$

$$\Rightarrow \frac{3}{4} = \frac{9}{n^2} \Rightarrow n = \sqrt{12} = 2\sqrt{3}$$

$\therefore$ The least quantum number must be 4.

8. (c) $U = -K\frac{ze^2}{r}$; $T.E = -\frac{k\ ze^2}{2\ r}$

$K.E = \frac{k\ ze^2}{2\ r}$. Here r decreases

9. (b) De-Broglie wavelength of electron $\lambda = \frac{h}{mV}$

As we know, $V \propto \frac{1}{n}$

So, $\lambda \propto n$

$\lambda_4 = 4\lambda_1$

λ_1 is the de-Broglie wavelength of the electron in the ground state.

10. (c) $qVB = \frac{mv^2}{r}$ ....(i)

$\frac{nh}{2\pi} = mvr$ ....(ii)

Multiplying equation (i) and (ii),

$$\frac{qBnh}{2\pi} = m^2v^2$$

Now multiplying both sides by $\frac{1}{2m}$,

$$n\frac{qBh}{4\pi m} = \frac{1}{2}mv^2$$

i.e. $KE = n\left[\frac{qBh}{4\pi m}\right]$

11. (b) Radius of circular path followed by electron is given by,

$$r = \frac{m\upsilon}{qB} = \frac{\sqrt{2meV}}{eB} = \frac{1}{B}\sqrt{\frac{2m}{e}V}$$

$$\Rightarrow V = \frac{B^2r^2e}{2m} = 0.8V$$

For transition between 3 to 2.

$$E = 13.6\left(\frac{1}{4} - \frac{1}{9}\right) = \frac{13.6 \times 5}{36} = 1.88eV$$

Work function = 1.88 eV – 0.8 eV = 1.08 eV ≈ 1.1eV

12. (c) Wave number $\frac{1}{\lambda} = RZ^2\left[\frac{1}{n_1^2} - \frac{1}{n^2}\right]$

$$\Rightarrow \lambda \propto \frac{1}{Z^2}$$

By question n = 1 and $n_1 = 2$

Then, $\lambda_1 = \lambda_2 = 4\lambda_3 = 9\lambda_4$

13. (b) (1) Davisson and Gemner experiment-wave nature of electrons.

(2) Millikan's oil drop experiment - charge of an electron.

(3) Rutherford experiment - Existance of nucleus.

(4) Frank-Hertz experiment - Quantisation of energy levels.

14. (b) For first excited state, n = 2 and for Li^{++} Z = 3

$$E_n = \frac{13.6}{n^2} \times Z^2 = \frac{13.6}{4} \times 9 = 30.6\ eV$$

15. (d) $\Delta E = hv$

$$v = \frac{\Delta E}{h} = k\left[\frac{1}{(n-1)^2} - \frac{1}{n^2}\right] = \frac{k(2n-1)}{n^2(n-1)^2}$$

$$\approx \frac{2k}{n^3} \quad \text{or} \quad v \propto \frac{1}{n^3}$$

16. (a) $E = \frac{hc}{\lambda} \Rightarrow \lambda = \frac{hc}{E} = \frac{6.62 \times 10^{-34} \times 3 \times 10^8}{12.5 \times 1.6 \times 10^{-19}}$

$$= 993\ A^\circ$$

$$\frac{1}{\lambda} = R\left(\frac{1}{n_1^2} - \frac{1}{n_2^2}\right)$$

(where Rydberg constant, $R = 1.097 \times 10^7$)

or, $\frac{1}{993 \times 10^{-10}} = 1.097 \times 10^7\left(\frac{1}{1^2} - \frac{1}{n_2^2}\right)$

Solving we get $n_2 = 3$

Spectral lines

Total number of spectral lines = 3

Two lines in Lyman series for $n_1 = 1, n_2 = 2$ and $n_1 = 1, n_2 = 3$ and one in Balmer series for $n_1 = 2, n_2 = 3$

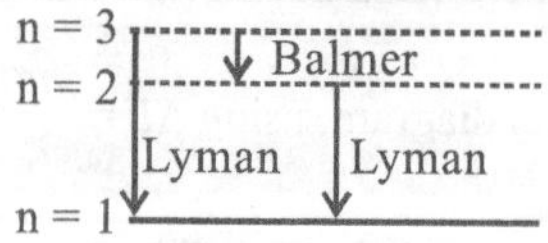

17. (c) As $F = \frac{mv^2}{r} = \frac{e^2}{4\pi \epsilon_0}\left(\frac{1}{r^2} + \frac{\beta}{r^3}\right)$

and $mvr = \frac{nh}{2\pi} \Rightarrow v = \frac{nh}{2\pi mr}$

$$\therefore m\left(\frac{nh}{2\pi mr}\right)^2 \times \frac{1}{r} = \frac{e^2}{4\pi \epsilon_0}\left(\frac{1}{r^2} + \frac{\beta}{r^3}\right)$$

or, $\frac{1}{r^2} + \frac{\beta}{r^3} = \frac{mn^2h^2 4\pi \epsilon_0}{4\pi^2m^2e^2r^3}$

or, $\frac{a_0 n^2}{r^3} = \frac{1}{r^2} + \frac{\beta}{r^3}$ $\left(\because a_0 = \frac{\epsilon_0 h^2}{m\pi e^2} \text{ Given}\right)$

For n^{th} atom

$\therefore r_n = a_0 n^2 - \beta$

18. (c) According to the question,

$$2\pi r = n\lambda = \frac{nh}{p} = \frac{nh}{mv}$$

or $mvr = \frac{nh}{2\pi}$ or $mv = \frac{nh}{2\pi r}$

$$F = qv_B = \frac{mv^2}{r}$$

or, $q_B = \frac{mv}{r} = \frac{nh}{2\pi r.r}$

or, $r^2 = \frac{nh}{2\pi qB}$

or, $r = \sqrt{\frac{nh}{2\pi qB}}$

i.e., $r \propto n^{1/2}$

19. (c) Magnetic moment of the hydrogen atom, when the electron is in n^{th} excited state, i.e., $n' = (n+1)$

As magnetic moment $M_n = I_n A = i_n(\pi r_n^2)$

$$i_n = eV_n = \frac{mz^2e^5}{4\varepsilon_0^2 n^3 h^3}$$

$$r_n = \frac{n^2h^2}{4\pi^2 kzme^2}\left(k = \frac{1}{4\pi\epsilon_0}\right)$$

Solving we get magnetic moment of the hydrogen atom for n^{th} excited state

$$M_{n'} = \left(\frac{e}{2m}\right)\frac{nh}{2\pi}$$

20. (d) For ground state, the principal quantum no. $(n) = 1$. There is a 3rd excited state for principal quantum number.

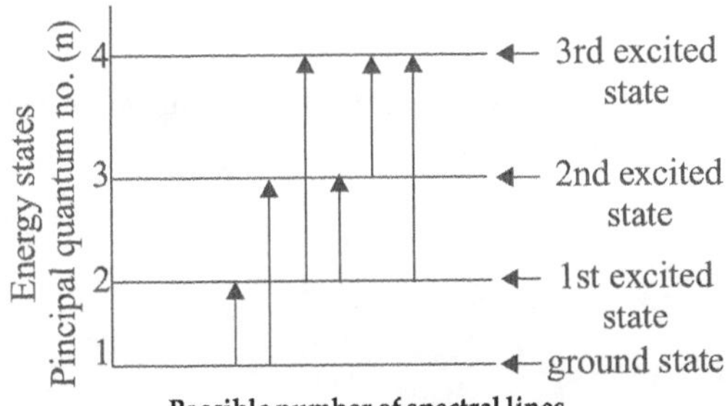

Possible number of spectral lines

The possible number of the spectral lines is given

$$= \frac{n(n-1)}{2} = \frac{4(4-1)}{2} = 6$$

21. (d) The energy of the system of two atoms of diatomic molecule $E = \frac{1}{2}I\omega^2$

where I = moment of inertia

ω = Angular velocity = $\frac{L}{I}$,

L = Angular momentum

$$I = \frac{1}{2}(m_1 r_1^2 + m^2 r_2^2)$$

Thus, $E = \frac{1}{2}(m_1 r_1^2 + m_2 r_2^2)\omega^2$ ... (i)

$$E = \frac{1}{2}(m_1 r_1^2 + m_2 r_2^2)\frac{L^2}{I^2}$$

$L = n\hbar$

(According to Bohr's Hypothesis)

$$E = \frac{1}{2}(m_1 r_1^2 + m_2 r_2^2)\frac{L^2}{(m_1 r_1^2 + m_2 r_2^2)^2}$$

$$E = \frac{1}{2}\frac{L^2}{(m_1 r_1^2 + m_2 r_2^2)}$$

$$= \frac{n^2 h^2}{8\pi^2(m_1 r_1^2 + m_2 r_2^2)}$$

$$E = \frac{(m_1 + m_2)n^2 h^2}{8\pi^2 r^2 m_1 m_2}$$

22. (a) Velocity of electron in n^{th} orbit of hydrogen atom is given by :

$$V_n = \frac{2\pi KZe^2}{nh}$$

Substituting the values we get,

$V_n = \frac{2.2 \times 10^6}{n}$ m/s or $V_n \propto \frac{1}{n}$

As principal quantum number increases, velocity decreases.

23. (c) $\frac{1}{\lambda} = R\left(\frac{1}{n_1^2} - \frac{1}{n_2^2}\right)$ where R = Rydberg constant

$$\frac{1}{\lambda_{32}} = \left(\frac{1}{4} - \frac{1}{9}\right) = \frac{5}{36}$$

$$\Rightarrow \lambda_{32} = \frac{36}{5}$$

Similarly solving for λ_{31} and λ_{21}

$$\lambda_{31} = \frac{9}{8} \text{ and } \lambda_{21} = \frac{4}{3}$$

$$\therefore \quad \frac{\lambda_{32}}{\lambda_{31}} = 6.4 \text{ and } \frac{\lambda_{21}}{\lambda_{31}} = 1.2$$

24. **(b)** $E = \frac{hc}{\lambda}$

25. **(b)** If $n_1 = n$ and $n_2 = n + 1$

Maximum wavelength $\lambda_{max} = \frac{n^2(n+1)^2}{(2n+1)R}$

Therefore, for large n, $\lambda_{max} \propto n^3$

26. **(b)** Energy of excitation,

$$\Delta E = 13.6\, \pi^2 \left(\frac{1}{\eta_1} - \frac{1}{\eta_2}\right) eV$$

$$\Rightarrow \Delta E = 13.6\,(3)^2 \left(\frac{1}{1^2} - \frac{1}{3^2}\right) = 108.8\, eV$$

27. **(c)** It is given that transition from the state $n = 4$ to $n = 3$ in a hydrogen like atom result in ultraviolet radiation. For infrared radiation the energy gap should be less. The only option is $5 \rightarrow 4$.

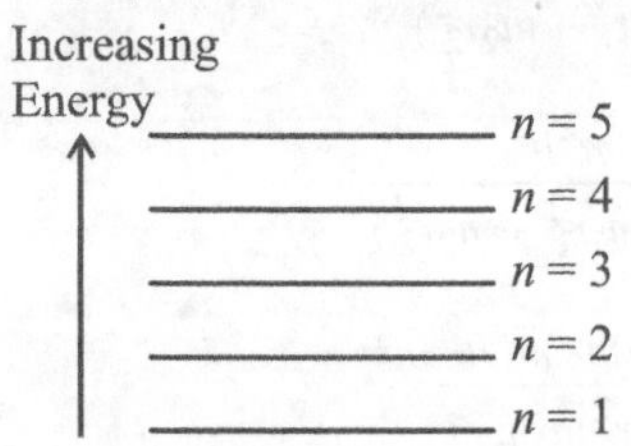

28. **(b)** When $F = \frac{k}{r}$ = centripetal force, then $\frac{k}{r} = \frac{mv^2}{r}$

$\Rightarrow mv^2$ = constat $\Rightarrow$ kinetic energy is constant $\Rightarrow T$ is independent of n.

29. **(d)** We have to find the frequency of emitted photons. For emission of photons the transition must take place from a higher energy level to a lower energy level which are given only in options (c) and (d).

Frequency is given by

$$h\nu = -13.6\left(\frac{1}{n_2^2} - \frac{1}{n_1^2}\right)$$

For transition from $n = 6$ to $n = 2$,

$$\nu_1 = \frac{-13.6}{h}\left(\frac{1}{6^2} - \frac{1}{2^2}\right) = \frac{2}{9} \times \left(\frac{13.6}{h}\right)$$

For transition from n = 2 to n = 1,

$$\nu_2 = \frac{-13.6}{h}\left(\frac{1}{2^2} - \frac{1}{1^2}\right) = \frac{3}{4} \times \left(\frac{13.6}{h}\right).$$

$$\therefore \nu_1 > \nu_2$$

30. **(b)** $E = Rhc\left[\frac{1}{n_1^2} - \frac{1}{n_2^2}\right]$

E will be maximum for the transition for which $\left[\frac{1}{n_1^2} - \frac{1}{n_2^2}\right]$ is maximum. Here n_2 is the higher energy level.

Clearly, $\left[\frac{1}{n_1^2} - \frac{1}{n_2^2}\right]$ is maximum for the third transition, i.e. $2 \rightarrow 1$. I transition represents the absorption of energy.

31. **(c)** The wavelength of spectrum is given by

$$\frac{1}{\lambda} = Rz^2\left(\frac{1}{n_1^2} - \frac{1}{n_2^2}\right) \quad \text{where } R = \frac{1.097 \times 10^7}{1 + \frac{m}{M}}$$

where m = mass of electron

M = mass of nucleus.

For different M, R is different and therefore λ is different

32. **(c)** The energy of nth orbit of hydrogen is given by

$$E_n = -\frac{13.6}{n^2} \text{ eV/atom}$$

For $n = 2$, $E_n = \frac{-13.6}{4} = -3.4\, eV$

Therefore the energy required to remove electron from $n = 2$ is $+3.4$ eV.

Chapter 27

Nuclei

TOPIC - 1: Composition and Size of the Nuclei

1. Which of the following are the constituents of the nucleus? **[2007]**
   (a) Electrons and protons
   (b) Neutrons and protons
   (c) Electrons and neutrons
   (d) Neutrons and positrons

2. If radius of the $^{27}_{13}Al$ nucleus is estimated to be 3.6 fermi then the radius of $^{125}_{52}Te$ nucleus be nearly **[2005]**
   (a) 8 fermi (b) 6 fermi
   (c) 5 fermi (d) 4 fermi

TOPIC - 2: Mass-Energy Equivalence and Nuclear Reactions

3. Imagine that a reactor converts all given mass into energy and that it operates at a power level of 10^9 watt. The mass of the fuel consumed per hour in the reactor will be : (velocity of light, c is 3×10^8 m/s) **[Online April 9, 2017]**
   (a) 0.96 gm (b) 0.8 gm
   (c) 4×10^{-2} gm (d) 6.6×10^{-5} gm

4. Two deuterons undergo nuclear fusion to form a Helium nucleus. Energy released in this process is : (given binding energy per nucleon for deuteron=1.1 MeV and for helium=7.0 MeV) **[Online April 8, 2017]**
   (a) 30.2 MeV (b) 32.4 MeV
   (c) 23.6 MeV (d) 25.8 MeV

5. When Uranium is bombarded with neutrons, it undergoes fission. The fission reaction can be written as :

   $${}_{92}U^{235} + {}_{0}n^{1} \rightarrow {}_{56}Ba^{141} + {}_{36}Kr^{92} + 3x + Q(\text{energy})$$

   where three particles named x are produced and energy Q is released. What is the name of the particle x ? **[Online April 9, 2013]**
   (a) electron (b) α-particle
   (c) neutron (d) neutrino

6. Assume that a neutron breaks into a proton and an electron. The energy released during this process is : (mass of neutron = 1.6725×10^{-27} kg, mass of proton = 1.6725×10^{-27} kg, mass of electron = 9×10^{-31} kg). **[2012]**
   (a) 0.51 MeV (b) 7.10 MeV
   (c) 6.30 MeV (d) 5.4 MeV

7. Ionisation energy of Li (Lithium) atom in ground state is 5.4 eV. Binding energy of an electron in Li^+ ion in ground state is 75.6 eV. Energy required to remove all three electrons of Lithium (Li) atom is **[Online May 19, 2012]**
   (a) 81.0 eV (b) 135.4 eV
   (c) 203.4 eV (d) 156.6 eV

8. After absorbing a slowly moving neutron of mass m_N (momentum ≈ 0) a nucleus of mass M breaks into two nuclei of masses m_1 and $5m_1$ $(6m_1 = M + m_N)$ respectively. If the de Broglie wavelength of the nucleus with mass m_1 is λ, the de Broglie wavelength of the nucleus will be **[2011]**
   (a) 5λ (b) $\lambda/5$ (c) λ (d) 25λ

DIRECTIONS: Questions number 9-10 are based on the following paragraph.

A nucleus of mass $M + \Delta m$ is at rest and decays into two daughter nuclei of equal mass $\frac{M}{2}$ each. Speed of light is c. **[2010]**

9. The binding energy per nucleon for the parent nucleus is E_1 and that for the daughter nuclei is E_2. Then
   (a) $E_2 = 2E_1$ (b) $E_1 > E_2$
   (c) $E_2 > E_1$ (d) $E_1 = 2E_2$

10. The speed of daughter nuclei is
    (a) $c\frac{\Delta m}{M + \Delta m}$ (b) $c\sqrt{\frac{2\Delta m}{M}}$
    (c) $c\sqrt{\frac{\Delta m}{M}}$ (d) $c\sqrt{\frac{\Delta m}{M + \Delta m}}$

11. This question contains Statement-1 and statement-2. Of the four choices given after the statements, choose the one that best describes the two statements. **[2008]**
    Statement-1:
    Energy is released when heavy nuclei undergo fission or light nuclei undergo fusion and
    Statement-2 :
    For heavy nuclei, binding energy per nucleon increases with increasing Z while for light nuclei it decreases with increasing Z.
    (a) Statement-1 is false, Statement-2 is true
    (b) Statement-1 is true, Statement-2 is true; Statement-2 is a correct explanation for Statement-1
    (c) Statement-1 is true, Statement-2 is true; Statement-2 is not a correct explanation for Statement-1
    (d) Statement-1 is true, Statement-2 is false

12. If M_O is the mass of an oxygen isotope ${}_8O^{17}$, M_P and M_N are the masses of a proton and a neutron respectively, the nuclear binding energy of the isotope is **[2007]**
(a) $(M_O-17M_N)c^2$ (b) $(M_O-8M_P)c^2$
(c) $(M_O-8M_P-9M_N)c^2$ (d) M_Oc^2

13. When ${}_3Li^7$ nuclei are bombarded by protons, and the resultant nuclei are ${}_4Be^8$, the emitted particles will be **[2006]**
(a) alpha particles (b) beta particles
(c) gamma photons (d) neutrons

14. If the binding energy per nucleon in ${}_3^7Li$ and ${}_2^4He$ nuclei are 5.60 MeV and 7.06 MeV respectively, then in the reaction

$$p + {}_3^7Li \longrightarrow 2\,{}_2^4He$$

energy of proton must be **[2006]**
(a) 28.24 MeV (b) 17.28 MeV
(c) 1.46 MeV (d) 39.2 MeV

15. A nuclear transformation is denoted by $X(n, \alpha)\,{}_3^7Li$. Which of the following is the nucleus of element X? **[2005]**
(a) ${}_5^{10}B$ (b) ${}^{12}C_6$ (c) ${}_4^{11}Be$ (d) ${}_5^9B$

16. A nucleus disintegrated into two nuclear parts which have their velocities in the ratio of 2 : 1. The ratio of their nuclear sizes will be **[2004]**
(a) $3^{1/2}:1$ (b) $1:2^{1/3}$ (c) $2^{1/3}:1$ (d) $1:3^{1/2}$

17. The binding energy per nucleon of deuteron $\left({}_1^2H\right)$ and helium nucleus $\left({}_2^4He\right)$ is 1.1 MeV and 7 MeV respectively. If two deuteron nuclei react to form a single helium nucleus, then the energy released is **[2004]**
(a) 23.6 MeV (b) 26.9 MeV
(c) 13.9 MeV (d) 19.2 MeV

18. When a U^{238} nucleus originally at rest, decays by emitting an alpha particle having a speed 'u', the recoil speed of the residual nucleus is **[2003]**
(a) $\frac{4u}{238}$ (b) $-\frac{4u}{234}$ (c) $\frac{4u}{234}$ (d) $-\frac{4u}{238}$

19. In the nuclear fusion reaction

$${}_1^2H + {}_1^3H \rightarrow {}_2^4He + n$$

given that the repulsive potential energy between the two nuclei is $\sim 7.7\times10^{-14}$ J, the temperature at which the gases must be heated to initiate the reaction is nearly [Boltzmann's Constant $k = 1.38\times10^{-23}$ J/K] **[2003]**
(a) 10^7 K (b) 10^5 K (c) 10^3 K (d) 10^9 K

TOPIC - 3: Radioactivity

20. A radioactive nucleus A with a half life T, decays into a nucleus B. At t = 0, there is no nucleus B. At sometime t, the ratio of the number of B to that of A is 0.3. Then, t is given by **[2017]**
(a) $t = T\log(1.3)$ (b) $t = \frac{T}{\log(1.3)}$
(c) $t = T\frac{\log 2}{\log 1.3}$ (d) $t = \frac{\log 1.3}{\log 2}$

21. Half-lives of two radioactive elements A and B are 20 minutes and 40 minutes, respectively. Initially, the samples have equal number of nuclei. After 80 minutes, the ratio of decayed number of A and B nuclei will be : **[2016]**
(a) 1 : 4 (b) 5 : 4
(c) 1 : 16 (d) 4 : 1

22. Let N_β be the number of β particles emitted by 1 gram of Na^{24} radioactive nuclei (half life = 15 hrs) in 7.5 hours, N_β is close to (Avogadro number = 6.023×10^{23}/g. mole): **[Online April 11, 2015]**
(a) 6.2×10^{21} (b) 7.5×10^{21}
(c) 1.25×10^{22} (d) 1.75×10^{22}

23. A piece of wood from a recently cut tree shows 20 decays per minute. A wooden piece of same size placed in a museum (obtained from a tree cut many years back) shows 2 decays per minute. If half life of C^{14} is 5730 years, then age of the wooden piece placed in the museum is approximately: **[Online April 19, 2014]**
(a) 10439 years (b) 13094 years
(c) 19039 years (d) 39049 years

24. A piece of bone of an animal from a ruin is found to have ^{14}C activity of 12 disintegrations per minute per gm of its carbon content. The ^{14}C activity of a living animal is 16 disintegrations per minute per gm. How long ago nearly did the animal die? (Given half life of ^{14}C is $t_{1/2}$ = 5760 years) **[Online April 12, 2014]**
(a) 1672 years (b) 2391 years
(c) 3291 years (d) 4453 years

25. A radioactive nuclei with decay constant 0.5/s is being produced at a constant rate of 100 nuclei/s. If at t = 0 there were no nuclei, the time when there are 50 nuclei is: **[Online April 11, 2014]**
(a) 1s (b) $2\ln\left(\frac{4}{3}\right)$ s
(c) $\ln 2$ s (d) $\ln\left(\frac{4}{3}\right)$ s

26. The half-life of a radioactive element A is the same as the mean-life of another radioactive element B. Initially both substances have the same number of atoms, then : **[Online April 22, 2013]**
(a) A and B decay at the same rate always.
(b) A and B decay at the same rate initially.
(c) A will decay at a faster rate than B.
(d) B will decay at a faster rate than A.

27. The counting rate observed from a radioactive source at $t = 0$ was 1600 counts s^{-1}, and $t = 8$ s, it was 100 counts s^{-1}. The counting rate observed as counts s^{-1} at $t = 6$ s will be **[Online May 26, 2012]**
(a) 250 (b) 400 (c) 300 (d) 200

28. The decay constants of a radioactive substance for α and β emission are λ_α and λ_β respectively. If the substance emits α and β simultaneously, then the average half life of the material will be **[Online May 19, 2012]**

(a) $\frac{2T_\alpha T_\beta}{T_\alpha + T_\beta}$ (b) $T_\alpha + T_\beta$

(c) $\frac{T_\alpha T_\beta}{T_\alpha + T_\beta}$ (d) $\frac{1}{2}(T_\alpha + T_\beta)$

29. Which of the following Statements is correct? **[Online May 12, 2012]**

(a) The rate of radioactive decay cannot be controlled but that of nuclear fission can be controlled.
(b) Nuclear forces are short range, attractive and charge dependent.
(c) Nuclei of atoms having same number of neutrons are known as isobars.
(d) Wavelength of matter waves is given by de Broglie formula but that of photons is not given by the same formula

30. A sample originally contained 10^{20} radioactive atoms, which emit α-particles. The ratio of α-particles emitted in the third year to that emitted during the second year is 0.3. How many α-particles were emitted in the first year? **[Online May 7, 2012]**

(a) 3×10^{18} (b) 3×10^{19}
(c) 5×10^{18} (d) 7×10^{19}

31. The half life of a radioactive substance is 20 minutes. The approximate time interval $(t_2 - t_1)$ between the time t_2 when $\frac{2}{3}$ of it had decayed and time t_1 when $\frac{1}{3}$ of it had decayed is: **[2011]**

(a) 14min (b) 20min (c) 28min (d) 7min

32. **Statement - 1 :** A nucleus having energy E_1 decays by β^- emission to daughter nucleus having energy E_2, but the β^- rays are emitted with a continuous energy spectrum having end point energy $E_1 - E_2$.
Statement - 2 : To conserve energy and momentum in β^- decay at least three particles must take part in the transformation. **[2011 RS]**

(a) Statement-1 is correct but statement-2 is not correct.
(b) Statement-1 and statement-2 both are correct and statement-2 is the correct explanation of statement-1.
(c) Statement-1 is correct, statement-2 is correct and statement-2 is not the correct explanation of Statement-1
(d) Statement-1 is incorrect, statement-2 is correct.

33. A radioactive nucleus (initial mass number A and atomic number Z emits 3 α - particles and 2 positrons. The ratio of number of neutrons to that of protons in the final nucleus will be **[2010]**

(a) $\frac{A-Z-8}{Z-4}$ (b) $\frac{A-Z-4}{Z-8}$

(c) $\frac{A-Z-12}{Z-4}$ (d) $\frac{A-Z-4}{Z-2}$

34. The half-life period of a radio-active element X is same as the mean life time of another radio-active element Y. Initially they have the same number of atoms. Then **[2007]**

(a) X and Y decay at same rate always
(b) X will decay faster than Y
(c) Y will decay faster than X
(d) X and Y have same decay rate initially

35. The energy spectrum of β-particles [number N(E) as a function of β-energy E] emitted from a radioactive source is **[2006]**

(a) 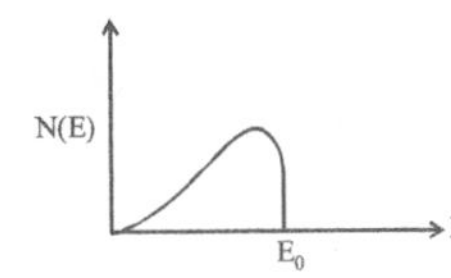

(b) 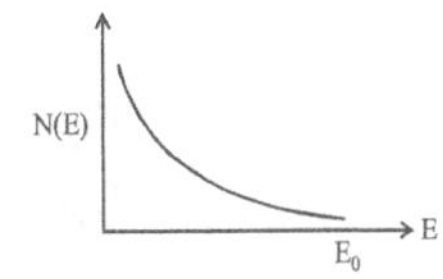

(c) 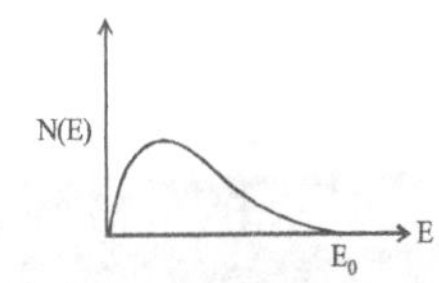

(d) 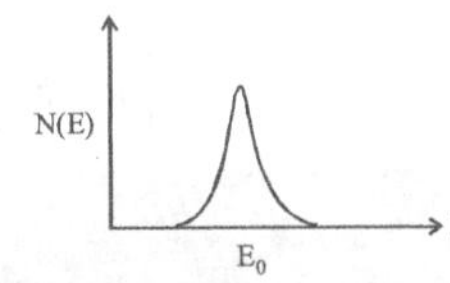

36. Starting with a sample of pure ^{66}Cu, $\frac{7}{8}$ of it decays into Zn in 15 minutes. The corresponding half life is **[2005]**

(a) 15 minutes (b) 10 minutes
(c) $7\frac{1}{2}$ minutes (d) 5 minutes

37. The intensity of gamma radiation from a given source is I. On passing through 36 mm of lead, it is reduced to $\frac{I}{8}$. The thickness of lead which will reduce the intensity to $\frac{I}{2}$ will be **[2005]**

(a) 9mm (b) 6mm
(c) 12mm (d) 18mm

38. Which of the following **cannot** be emitted by radioactive substances during their decay? **[2003]**

(a) Protons (b) Neutrinoes
(c) Helium nuclei (d) Electrons

39. A nucleus with $Z = 92$ emits the following in a sequence:
$\alpha, \beta^-, \beta^- \alpha, \alpha, \alpha, \alpha, \alpha, \beta^-, \beta^-, \alpha, \beta^+, \beta^+, \alpha$
Then Z of the resulting nucleus is **[2003]**

(a) 76 (b) 78 (c) 82 (d) 74

40. A radioactive sample at any instant has its disintegration rate 5000 disintegrations per minute. After 5 minutes, the rate is 1250 disintegrations per minute. Then, the decay constant (per minute) is **[2003]**

(a) 0.4 ln 2 (b) 0.2 ln 2
(c) 0.1 ln 2 (d) 0.8 ln 2

41. At a specific instant emission of radioactive compound is deflected in a magnetic field. The compound can emit

(i) electrons (ii) protons
(iii) He^{2+} (iv) neutrons

The emission at instant can be **[2002]**

(a) i, ii, iii (b) i, ii, iii, iv
(c) iv (d) ii, iii

42. If N_0 is the original mass of the substance of half-life period $t_{1/2} = 5$ years, then the amount of substance left after 15 years is **[2002]**

(a) $N_0/8$ (b) $N_0/16$ (c) $N_0/2$ (d) $N_0/4$

Hints & Solutions

TOPIC - 1: Composition and Size of the Nuclei

1. (b)

2. (b) $R = R_0(A)^{1/3}$

$$\therefore \frac{R_1}{R_2} = \left(\frac{A_1}{A_2}\right)^{1/3} = \left(\frac{27}{125}\right)^{1/3} = \frac{3}{5}$$

$$R_2 = \frac{5}{3} \times 3.6 = 6 \text{ fermi}$$

TOPIC - 2: Mass-Energy Equivalence and Nuclear Reactions

3. (c) Power level of reactor, $P = \frac{E}{\Delta t} = \frac{\Delta mc^2}{\Delta t}$

mass of the fuel consumed per hour in the reactor,

$$\frac{\Delta m}{\Delta t} = \frac{P}{c^2} = \frac{10^9}{(3 \times 10^8)^2} = 4 \times 10^{-2} \text{ gm}$$

4. (c) ${}_1H^2 + {}_1H^2 \to {}_2He^4$

Total binding energy of two deuterium nuclei $= 1.1 \times 4 = 4.4$ MeV

Binding energy of a (${}_2He^4$) nuclei $= 4 \times 7 = 28$ MeV

Energy released in this process $= 28 - 4.4 = 23.6$ MeV

5. (c) Nuclear fission equation

$$_{92}U^{135} + {}_0n^1 \longrightarrow {}_{56}Ba^{141} + {}_{36}Kr^{92} + 3\,{}_0n^1 + Q(\text{energy})$$

Hence particle x is neutron.

6. (a) ${}_0^1n \longrightarrow {}_1^1H + {}_{-1}e^0 + \bar{v} + Q$

The mass defect during the process

$$\Delta m = m_n - m_H - m_e = 1.6725 \times 10^{-27} - (1.6725 \times 10^{-27} + 9 \times 10^{-31} \text{kg})$$

$$= -9 \times 10^{-31} \text{ kg}$$

The energy released during the process

$E = \Delta mc^2$

$E = 9 \times 10^{-31} \times 9 \times 10^{16} = 81 \times 10^{-15}$ Joules

$$E = \frac{81 \times 10^{-15}}{1.6 \times 10^{-19}} = 0.511 \text{MeV}$$

7. (d)

8. (c) $p_i = 0$

$$p_f = p_1 + p_2$$

$$p_i = p_f$$

$$0 = p_1 + p_2$$

$$p_1 = -p_2$$

$$\lambda_1 = \frac{h}{p_1}$$

$$\lambda_2 = \frac{h}{p_2}$$

$$|\lambda_1| = |\lambda_2|$$

$$\lambda_1 = \lambda_2 = \lambda.$$

9. (c) In nuclear fission, the binding energy per nucleon of daughter nuclei is always greater than the parent nucleus.

10. (b) By conservation of energy,

$$(M + \Delta m)c^2 = \frac{2.M}{2}c^2 + \frac{1}{2}.\frac{2M}{2}v^2,$$

where v is the speed of the daughter nuclei

$$\Rightarrow \Delta mc^2 = \frac{M}{2}v^2 \qquad \therefore v = c\sqrt{\frac{2\Delta m}{M}}$$

11. (d) We know that energy is released when heavy nuclei undergo fission or light nuclei undergo fusion. Therefore statement (1) is correct.

The second statement is false because for heavy nuclei the binding energy per nucleon decreases with increasing Z and for light nuclei, B.E/nucleon increases with increasing Z.

12. (c) Binding energy

$= [ZM_P + (A - Z)M_N - M]c^2$

$= [8M_P + (17 - 8)M_N - M]c^2$

$= [8M_P + 9M_N - M]c^2$

$= [8M_P + 9M_N - M_o]c^2$

13. (c) ${}_3^7Li + {}_1^1p \longrightarrow {}_4^8Be + {}_0^0\gamma$

14. (b) Let E be the energy of proton, then

$E+7\times 5.6=2\times[4\times 7.06]$

$\Rightarrow E=56.48-39.2=17.28\text{MeV}$

15. (a) ${}_{Z}X^{A}+{}_{0}n^{1}\longrightarrow {}_{3}Li^{7}+{}_{2}He^{4}$

On comparison,

$A=7+4-1=10, z=3+2-0=5$

It is boron ${}_{5}B^{10}$

16. (b) From conservation of momentum $m_1v_1=m_2v_2$

$\Rightarrow \left(\frac{m_1}{m_2}\right)=\left(\frac{v_2}{v_1}\right)$ given $\frac{v_1}{v_2}=2$

$\Rightarrow \frac{m_1}{m_2}=\frac{1}{2}\Rightarrow \frac{r_1^3}{r_2^3}=\frac{1}{2}\Rightarrow\left(\frac{r_1}{r_2}\right)=\left(\frac{1}{2}\right)^{1/3}$

17. (a) The chemical reaction of process is $2{}_1^2H\rightarrow{}_2^4He$

Energy released $=4\times(7)-4(1.1)=23.6\text{ MeV}$

18. (c) Here, conservation of linear momentum can be applied

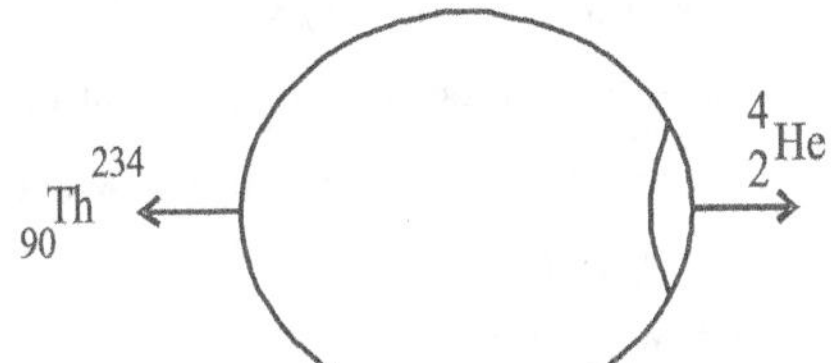

$238\times 0=4u+234v$

$\therefore\ v=-\frac{4}{234}u$

$\therefore$ speed $=|\vec{v}|=\frac{4}{234}u$

19. (d) The average kinetic energy per molecule $=\frac{3}{2}kT$

This kinetic energy should be able to provide the repulsive potential energy

$\therefore\ \frac{3}{2}kT=7.7\times 10^{-14}$

$\Rightarrow T=\frac{2\times 7.7\times 10^{-14}}{3\times 1.38\times 10^{-23}}=3.7\times 10^{9}$

TOPIC - 3: Radioactivity

20. (d) Let initially there are total N_0 number of nuclei

At time t $\frac{N_B}{N_A}=0.3$(given)

$\Rightarrow\ N_B=0.3N_A$

$N_0=N_A+N_B=N_A+0.3N_A$

$\therefore\ N_A=\frac{N_0}{1.3}$

As we know $N_t=N_0e^{-\lambda t}$

or, $\frac{N_0}{1.3}=N_0e^{-\lambda t}$

$\frac{1}{1.3}=e^{-\lambda t}\Rightarrow ln(1.3)=\lambda t$

or, $t=\frac{ln(1.3)}{\lambda}\ \Rightarrow\ t=\frac{ln(1.3)}{\frac{ln(2)}{T}}=\frac{ln(1.3)}{ln(2)}T$

21. (b) For $A_{t_{1/2}}=20$ min, t = 80 min, number of half lifes n = 4

$\therefore$ Nuclei remaining $=\frac{N_0}{2^4}$. Therefore nuclei decayed

$=N_0-\frac{N_0}{2^4}$

For $B_{t_{1/2}}=40$ min., t = 80 min, number of half lifes n = 2

$\therefore$ Nuclei remaining $=\frac{N_0}{2^2}$. Therefore nuclei decayed

$=N_0-\frac{N_0}{2^2}$

$\therefore$Required ratio $=\frac{No-\frac{No}{2^4}}{No-\frac{No}{2^2}}=\frac{1-\frac{1}{16}}{1-\frac{1}{4}}=\frac{15}{16}\times\frac{4}{3}=\frac{5}{4}$

22. (b) We know that $N_\beta=N_0(1-e^{-\lambda t})$

$N_\beta=\frac{6.023\times 10^{23}}{24}\left[1-e^{\frac{\ell n2}{15}\times 7.5}\right]$

on solving we get,

$N_\beta=7.4\times 10^{21}$

23. (c) **Given:** $\frac{dN_0}{dt}=20$ decays/min

$\frac{dN}{dt}=2$ decays/min

$T_{1/2}=5730$ years

As we know,

$N=N_0e^{-\lambda t}$

$\text{Log}\frac{N_0}{N}=\lambda t$

$\therefore\ t=\frac{1}{\lambda}\text{Log}\frac{N_0}{N}$

$$= \frac{2.303 \times T_{1/2}}{0.693} \times \text{Log}_{10} \frac{N_0}{N}$$

$$\text{But } \frac{\frac{dN_0}{dt}}{\frac{dN}{dt}} = \frac{N_0}{N} = \frac{20}{2} = 10$$

$$\therefore\ t = \frac{2.303 \times 5730}{0.693} \times 1$$

$$= 19039 \text{ years}$$

24. (b) Given, for ^{14}C

$A_0 = 16$ dis min^{-1} g^{-1}

$A = 12$ dis min^{-1} g^{-1}

$t_{1/2} = 5760$ years

$$\text{Now, } \lambda = \frac{0.693}{t_{1/2}}$$

$$\lambda = \frac{0.693}{5760} \text{ per year}$$

$$\text{Then, from, } t = \frac{2.303}{\lambda} \log_{10} \frac{A_0}{A}$$

$$= \frac{2.303 \times 5760}{0.693} \log_{10} \frac{16}{12}$$

$$= \frac{2.303 \times 5760}{0.693} \log_{10} 1.333$$

$$= \frac{2.303 \times 5760 \times 0.1249}{0.693} = 2390.81 \approx 2391 \text{ years.}$$

25. (b) Let N be the number of nuclei at any time t then,

$$\frac{dN}{dt} = 100 - \lambda N$$

$$\text{or } \int_0^N \frac{dN}{(100 - \lambda N)} = \int_0^t dt$$

$$-\frac{1}{\lambda}[\log(100 - \lambda N)]_0^N = t$$

$$\log(100 - \lambda N) - \log 100 = -\lambda t$$

$$\log \frac{100 - \lambda N}{100} = -\lambda t$$

$$\frac{100 - \lambda N}{100} = e^{-\lambda t}$$

$$1 - \frac{\lambda N}{100} = e^{-\lambda t}$$

$$N = \frac{100}{\lambda}(1 - e^{-\lambda t})$$

As, $N = 50$ and $\lambda = 0.5$/sec

$$\therefore\ 50 = \frac{100}{0.5}(1 - e^{-0.5t})$$

Solving we get,

$$t = 2\ln\left(\frac{4}{3}\right) \text{ sec}$$

26. (d) $(T_{1/2})_A = (t_{mean})_B$

$$\Rightarrow \frac{0.693}{\lambda_A} = \frac{1}{\lambda_B} \Rightarrow \lambda_A = 0.693\lambda_B$$

or $\lambda_A < \lambda_B$

Also rate of decay $= \lambda N$

Initially number of atoms (N) of both are equal but since $\lambda_B > \lambda_A$, therefore B will decay at a faster rate than A

27. (d) As we know,

$$\left[\frac{N}{N_0}\right] = \left[\frac{1}{2}\right]^n \quad \text{...(i)}$$

n = no. of half life

N - no. of atoms left

N_0 - initial no. of atoms

By radioactive decay law,

$$\frac{dN}{dt} = kN$$

k - disintegration constant

$$\therefore \frac{\frac{dN}{dt}}{\frac{dN_0}{dt}} = \frac{N}{N_0} \quad \text{...(ii)}$$

From (i) and (ii) we get

$$\frac{\frac{dN}{dt}}{\frac{dN_0}{dt}} = \left[\frac{1}{2}\right]^n$$

$$\text{or, } \left[\frac{100}{1600}\right] = \left[\frac{1}{2}\right]^n \Rightarrow \left[\frac{1}{2}\right]^4 = \left[\frac{1}{2}\right]^n$$

$\therefore n = 4$, Therefore, in 8 seconds 4 half life had occurred in which counting rate reduces to 100 counts s^{-1}.

$\therefore$ Half life, $T_{\frac{1}{2}} = 2$ sec

In 6 sec, 3 half life will occur

$$\therefore \left[\frac{\frac{dN}{dt}}{1600}\right] = \left[\frac{1}{2}\right]^3$$

$$\Rightarrow \frac{dN}{dt} = 200 \text{ counts s}^{-1}$$

28. (c) $T_{av} = \dfrac{T_\alpha T_\beta}{T_\alpha + T_\beta}$

If α and B are emitted simultaneously.

29. (a) Radioactive decay is a continuous process. Rate of radioactive decay cannot be controlled. Nuclear fission can be controlled but not of nuclear fusion.

30. (b)

31. (b) Number of undecayed atom after time t_2;

$$\frac{N_0}{3} = N_0 e^{-\lambda t_2} \quad ...(i)$$

Number of undecayed atom after time t_1;

$$\frac{2N_0}{3} = N_0 e^{-\lambda t_1} \quad ...(ii)$$

From (i), $e^{-\lambda t_2} = \dfrac{1}{3}$

$$\Rightarrow -\lambda t_2 = \log_e\left(\frac{1}{3}\right) \quad ...(iii)$$

From (ii) $- e^{-\lambda t_2} = \dfrac{2}{3}$

$$\Rightarrow -\lambda t_1 = \log_e\left(\frac{2}{3}\right) \quad ...(iv)$$

Solving (iii) and (iv), we get

$t_2 - t_1 = 20$ min

32. (b) **Statement-1:** Energy of β-particle from 0 to maximum so $E_1 - E_2$ is the continuous energy spectrum.

Statement-2: For energy conservation and momentum conservation at least three particles, daughter nucleus, β^{-1} and anti-neutron are required.

33. (b) As a result of emission of 1 α-particle, the mass number decreases by 4 units and atomic number decreases by 2 units. And by the emission of 1 positron the atomic number decreases by 1 unit but mass number remains constant.

$\therefore$ Mass number of final nucleus $= A - 12$

Atomic number of final nucleus $= Z - 8$

$\therefore$ Number of neutrons $= (A - 12) - (Z - 8)$
$= A - Z - 4$

Number of protons $= Z - 8$

$\therefore$ Required ratio $= \dfrac{A - Z - 4}{Z - 8}$

34. (c) According to question,

Half life of X, $T_{1/2} = \tau_{av}$, average life of Y

$$\Rightarrow \frac{0.693}{\lambda_X} = \frac{1}{\lambda_Y}$$

$$\Rightarrow \lambda_X = (0.693).\lambda_Y$$

$$\therefore \lambda_X < \lambda_Y.$$

Now, the rate of decay is given by

$$-\left(\frac{dN}{dt}\right)_x = \lambda_X N_0$$

$$-\left(\frac{dN}{dt}\right)_y = \lambda_y N_0$$

Y will decay faster than X.

35. (c) The range of energy of β-particles is from zero to some maximum value.

36. (d) $\dfrac{7}{8}$ of Cu decays in 15 minutes.

$$\therefore \text{Cu undecayed} = N = 1 - \frac{7}{8} = \frac{1}{8} = \left(\frac{1}{2}\right)^3$$

$\therefore$ No. of half lifes = 3

$$n = \frac{t}{T} \text{ or } 3 = \frac{15}{T}$$

$$\Rightarrow T = \text{half life period} = \frac{15}{3} = 5 \text{ minutes}$$

ALTERNATE SOLUTION

$N = N_0 (1 - e^{-\lambda t})$

$$\Rightarrow \frac{N_0 - N}{N_0} = e^{-\lambda t} \qquad \therefore \frac{1}{8} = e^{-\lambda t}$$

$$3\, \ell n\, 2 = \lambda t \text{ or } \lambda = \frac{3 \times 0.693}{15} = 0.1386$$

Half-lifeperiod,

$$t_{½} = \frac{0.693}{\lambda} = \frac{0.693}{0.1386} = 5 \text{ minutes}$$

37. (c) Intensity $I = I_0.e^{-\mu d}$,

Applying logarithm on both sides,

$$-\mu d = \log\left(\frac{I}{I_0}\right)$$

$$-\mu \times 36 = \log\left(\frac{I/8}{I}\right) \text{ ....(i)}$$

$$-\mu \times d = \log\left(\frac{I/2}{I}\right) \text{ ....}(ii)$$

Dividing (i) by (ii),

$$\frac{36}{d} = \frac{\log\left(\frac{1}{8}\right)}{\log\left(\frac{1}{2}\right)} = \frac{3\log\left(\frac{1}{2}\right)}{\log\left(\frac{1}{2}\right)} = 3 \text{ or } d = \frac{36}{3} = 12 \text{ mm}$$

38. (a) The radioactive substances emit α -particles (Helium nucleus), β –particles (electrons) and neutrinoes.

39. (b) The number of α - particles released =8

Therefore the atomic number should decrease by 16

The number of β^- -particles released = 4

Therefore the atomic number should increase by 4.

Also the number of β^+ particles released is 2, which should decrease the atomic number by 2.

Therefore the final atomic number

$= Z–16+4–2 = Z–14$

$= 92 – 14 = 78$

40. (a) $\lambda = \frac{1}{t}\log_e\frac{A_o}{A} = \frac{1}{5}\log_e\frac{5000}{1250}$

$$= \frac{2}{5}\log_e 2 = 0.4\log_e 2$$

41. (a) Charged particles are deflected in magnetic field.

42. (a) After every half-life, the mass of the substance reduces to half its initial value.

$$N_0 \xrightarrow{5\text{ years}} \frac{N_0}{2} \xrightarrow{5\text{ years}} \frac{N_0/2}{2}$$

$$= \frac{N_0}{4} \xrightarrow{5\text{years}} \frac{N_0/4}{2} = \frac{N_0}{8}$$

Chapter 28 Semiconductor Electronics : Materials, Devices and Simple Circuits

TOPIC - 1: Solids, Semiconductors and P-N Junction Diode

1. What is the conductivity of a semiconductor sample having electron concentration of 5×10^{18} m^{-3}, hole concentration of 5×10^{19} m^{-3}, electron mobility of 2.0 m^{2} V^{-1} s^{-1} and hole mobility of 0.01 m^{2} V^{-1} s^{-1}? **[Online April 8, 2017]**

   (Take charge of electron as 1.6×10^{-19} C)

   (a) $1.68\,(\Omega-\text{m})^{-1}$ (b) $1.83\,(\Omega-\text{m})^{-1}$
   (c) $0.59\,(\Omega-\text{m})^{-1}$ (d) $1.20\,(\Omega-\text{m})^{-1}$

2. The V–I characteristic of a diode is shown in the figure. The ratio of forward to reverse bias resistance is : **[Online April 8, 2017]**

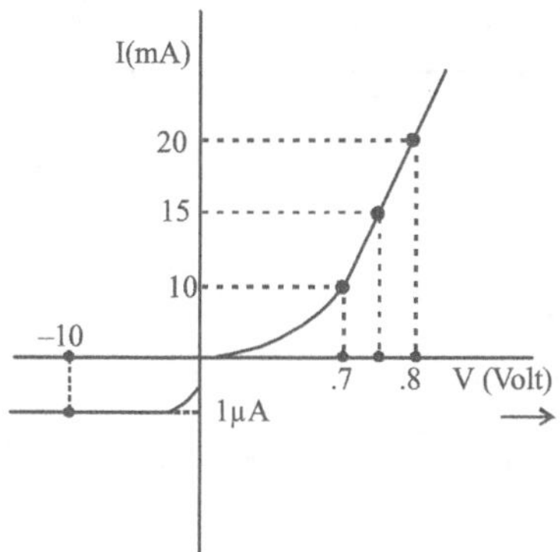

   (a) 10 (b) 10^{-6} (c) 10^{6} (d) 100

3. Identify the semiconductor devices whose characteristics are given below, in the order (i), (ii), (iii), (iv) : **[2016]**

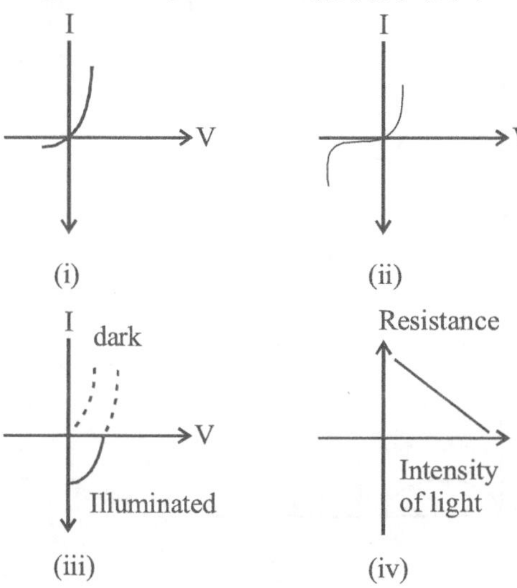

   (a) Solar cell, Light dependent resistance, Zener diode, simple diode
   (b) Zener diode, Solar cell, simple diode, Light dependent resistance
   (c) Simple diode, Zener diode, Solar cell, Light dependent resistance
   (d) Zener diode, Simple diode, Light dependent resistance, Solar cell

4. The temperature dependence of resistances of Cu and undoped Si in the temperature range 300-400 K, is best described by : **[2016]**

   (a) Linear increase for Cu, exponential decrease of Si.
   (b) Linear decrease for Cu, linear decrease for Si.
   (c) Linear increase for Cu, linear increase for Si.
   (d) Linear increase for Cu, exponential increase for Si.

5. An experiment is performed to determine the 1–V characteristics of a Zener diode, which has a protective resistance of R = 100 Ω, and a maximum power of dissipation rating of 1 W. The minimum voltage range of the DC source in the circuit is : **[Online April 9, 2016]**

   (a) 0 – 5V (b) 0 – 24 V
   (c) 0 – 12 V (d) 0 – 8V

6. A red LED emits light at 0.1 watt uniformly around it. The amplitude of the electric field of the light at a distance of 1 m from the diode is : **[2015]**

   (a) 5.48 V/m (b) 7.75 V/m
   (c) 1.73 V/m (d) 2.45 V/m

7. A 2V battery is connected across AB as shown in the figure. The value of the current supplied by the battery when in one case battery's positive terminal is connected to A and in other case when positive terminal of battery is connected to B will respectively be: **[Online April 11, 2015]**

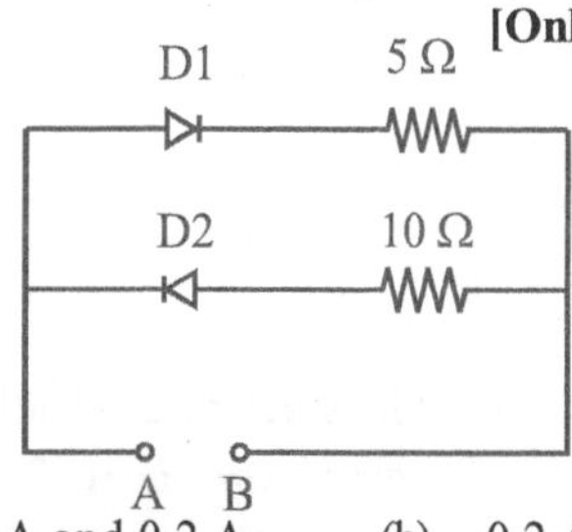

   (a) 0.4 A and 0.2 A (b) 0.2 A and 0.4 A
   (c) 0.1 A and 0.2 A (d) 0.2 A and 0.1 A

8. In an unbiased n-p junction electrons diffuse from n-region to p-region because : **[Online April 10, 2015]**

   (a) holes in p-region attract them

(b) electrons travel across the junction due to potential difference
(c) only electrons move from n to p region and not the vice-versa
(d) electron concentration in n-region is more compared to that in p-region

9. The forward biased diode connection is: **[2014]**

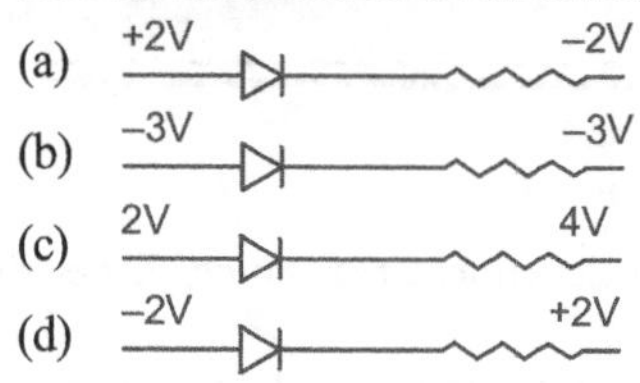

10. For LED's to emit light in visible region of electromagnetic light, it should have energy band gap in the range of: **[Online April 12, 2014]**

(a) 0.1 eV to 0.4 eV (b) 0.5 eV to 0.8 eV
(c) 0.9 eV to 1.6 eV (d) 1.7 eV to 3.0 eV

11. A Zener diode is connected to a battery and a load as show below: **[Online April 11, 2014]**

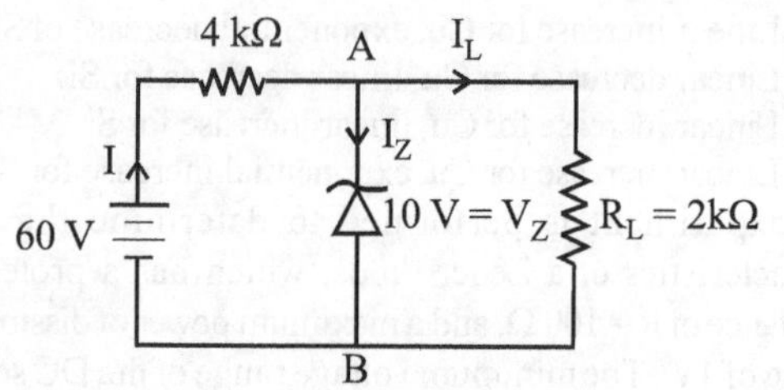

The currents, I, I_Z and I_L are respectively.

(a) 15 mA, 5 mA, 10 mA
(b) 15 mA, 7.5 mA, 7.5 mA
(c) 12.5 mA, 5 mA, 7.5 mA
(d) 12.5 mA, 7.5 mA, 5 mA

12. The I-V characteristic of an LED is **[2013]**

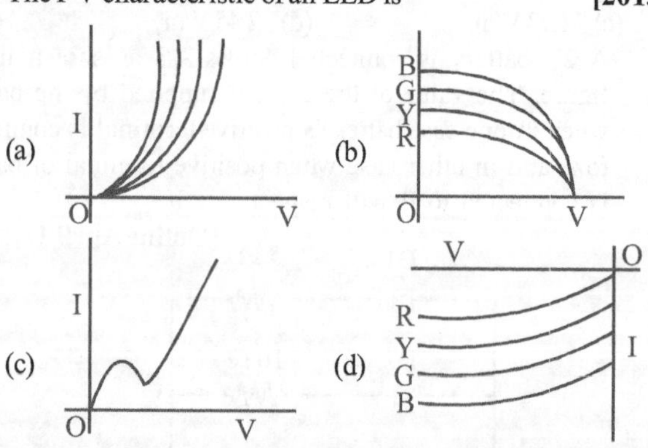

13. Figure shows a circuit in which three identical diodes are used. Each diode has forward resistance of 20 Ω and infinite backward resistance. Resistors $R_1 = R_2 = R_3 = 50\ \Omega$. Battery voltage is 6 V. The current through R_3 is : **[Online April 22, 2013]**

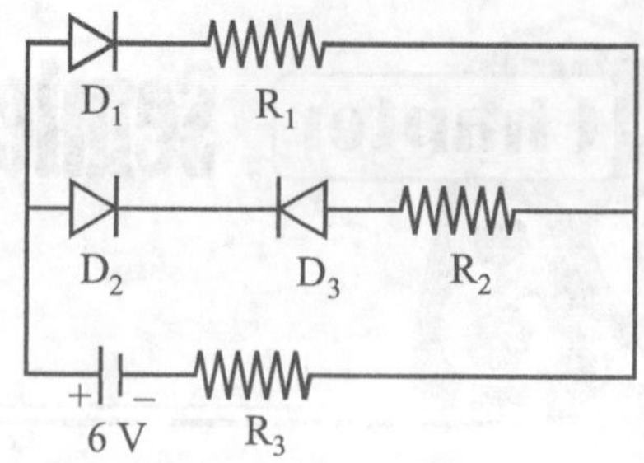

(a) 50 mA (b) 100 mA (c) 60 mA (d) 25 mA

14. This question has Statement 1 and Statement 2. Of the four choices given after the Statements, choose the one that best describes the two Statements.

Statement 1: A pure semiconductor has negative temperature coefficient of resistance.

Statement 2: On raising the temperature, more charge carriers are released into the conduction band. **[Online May 12, 2012]**

(a) Statement 1 is false, Statement 2 is true.
(b) Statement 1 is true, Statement 2 is false.
(c) Statement 1 is true, Statement 2 is true, Statement 2 is not a correct explanation of Statement 1.
(d) Statement 1 is true, Statement 2 is true, Statement 2 is the correct explanation of Statement 1.

15. A *p-n* junction (*D*) shown in the figure can act as a rectifier. An alternating current source (*V*) is connected in the circuit.

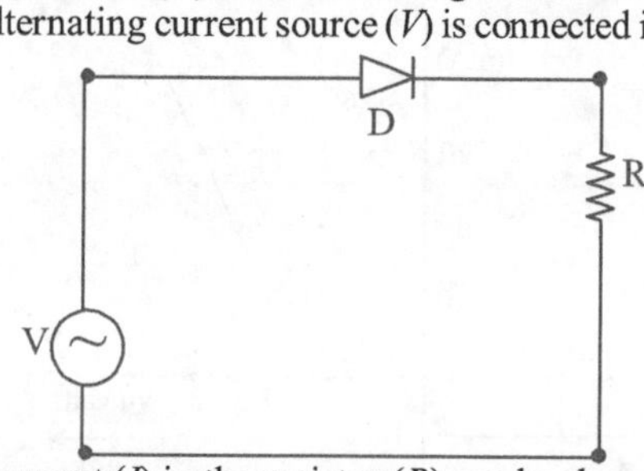

The current (*I*) in the resistor (*R*) can be shown by : **[2009]**

(a)
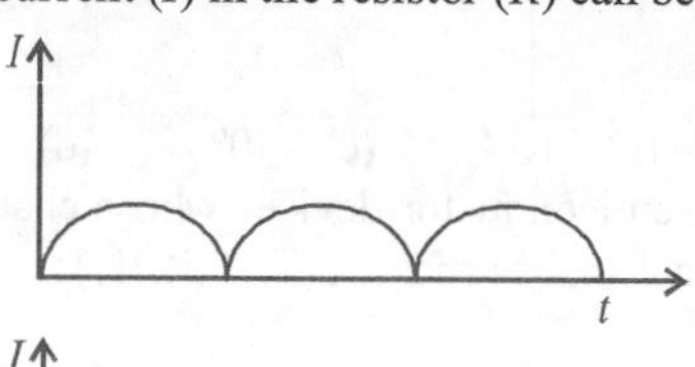

(b)
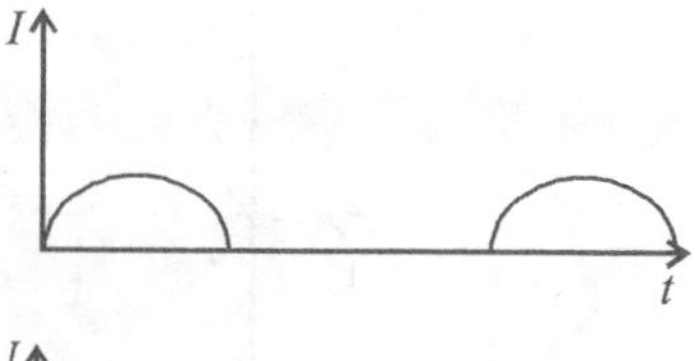

(c)
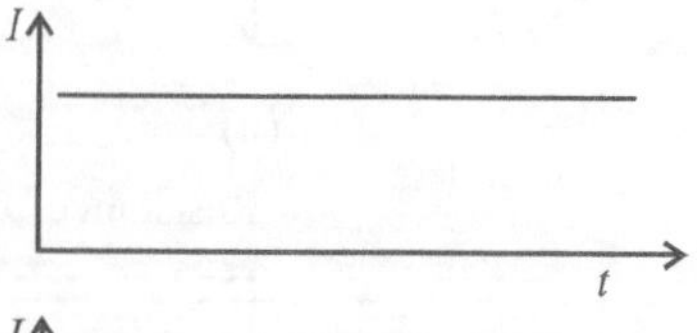

(d)
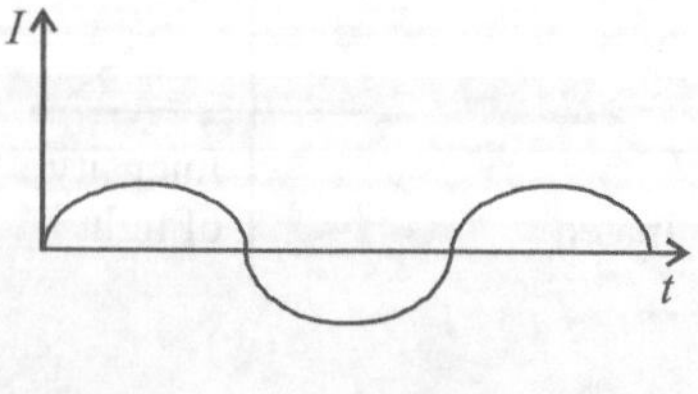

16. If in a p-n junction diode, a square input signal of 10 V is applied as shown **[2007]**

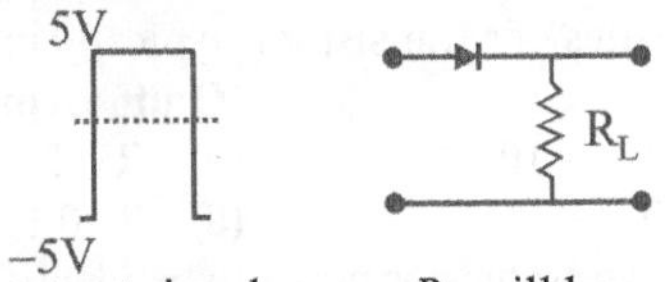

Then the output signal across R_L will be

(a) 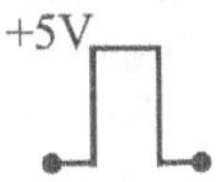

(b) 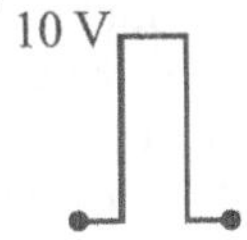

(c) 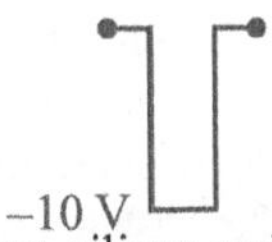

(d) 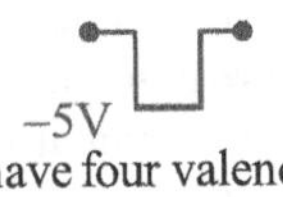

17. Carbon, silicon and germanium have four valence electrons each. At room temperature which one of the following statements is most appropriate ? **[2007]**
(a) The number of free electrons for conduction is significant only in Si and Ge but small in C.
(b) The number of free conduction electrons is significant in C but small in Si and Ge.
(c) The number of free conduction electrons is negligibly small in all the three.
(d) The number of free electrons for conduction is significant in all the three.

18. If the lattice constant of this semiconductor is decreased, then which of the following is correct? **[2006]**

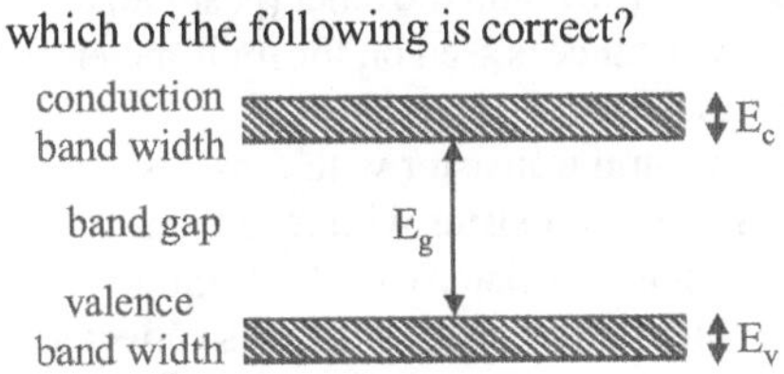

(a) All E_c, E_g, E_v increase
(b) E_c and E_v increase, but E_g decreases
(c) E_c and E_v decrease, but E_g increases
(d) All E_c, E_g, E_v decrease

19. A solid which is not transparent to visible light and whose conductivity increases with temperature is formed by **[2006]**
(a) Ionic bonding
(b) Covalent bonding
(c) Vander Waals bonding
(d) Metallic bonding

20. If the ratio of the concentration of electrons to that of holes in a semiconductor is $\frac{7}{5}$ and the ratio of currents is $\frac{7}{4}$, then what is the ratio of their drift velocities? **[2006]**

(a) $\frac{5}{8}$ (b) $\frac{4}{5}$ (c) $\frac{5}{4}$ (d) $\frac{4}{7}$

21. The circuit has two oppositively connected ideal diodes in parallel. What is the current flowing in the circuit? **[2006]**

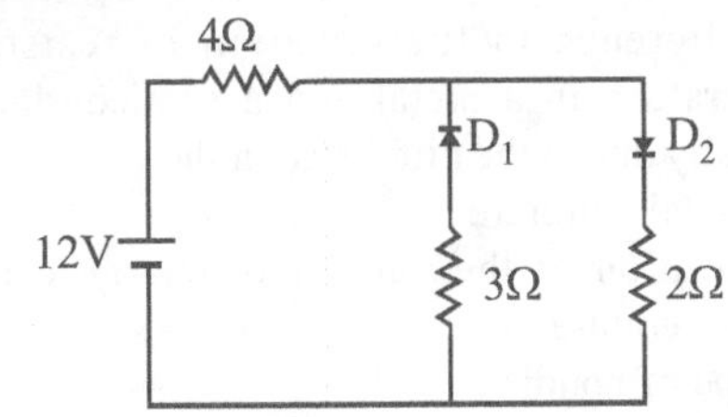

(a) 1.71A (b) 2.00A (c) 2.31A (d) 1.33A

22. In the following, which one of the diodes reverse biased? **[2006]**

(a) 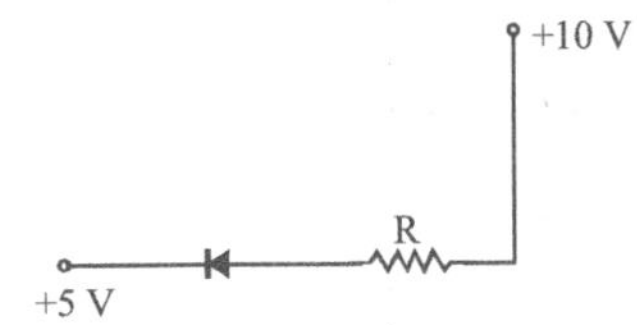

(b) 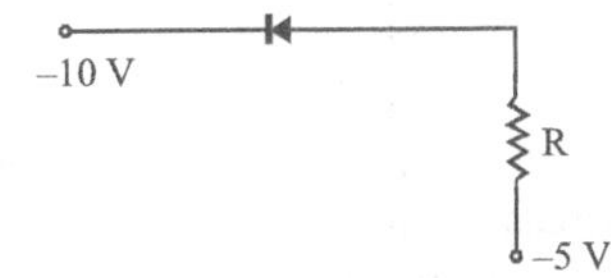

(c) 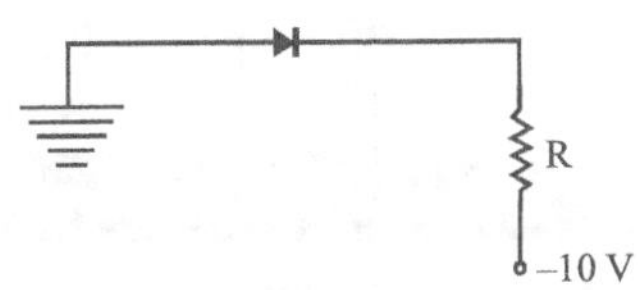

(d) 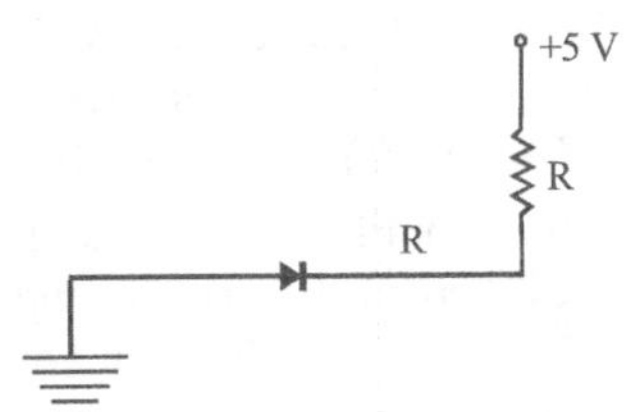

23. The electrical conductivity of a semiconductor increases when electromagnetic radiation of wavelength shorter than 2480 nm is incident on it. The band gap in (eV) for the semiconductor is **[2005]**
(a) 2.5 eV (b) 1.1 eV (c) 0.7 eV (d) 0.5 eV

24. When p-n junction diode is forward biased then **[2004]**
(a) both the depletion region and barrier height are reduced
(b) the depletion region is widened and barrier height is reduced
(c) the depletion region is reduced and barrier height is increased
(d) Both the depletion region and barrier height are increased

25. A strip of copper and another of germanium are cooled from room temperature to 80K. The resistance of **[2003]**
(a) each of these decreases
(b) copper strip increases and that of germanium decreases
(c) copper strip decreases and that of germanium increases
(d) each of these increases

26. The difference in the variation of resistance with temeperature in a metal and a semiconductor arises essentially due to the difference in the **[2003]**
(a) crystal sturcture
(b) variation of the number of charge carriers with temperature
(c) type of bonding
(d) variation of scattering mechanism with temperature

27. In the middle of the depletion layer of a reverse- biased *p-n* junction, the **[2003]**
(a) electric field is zero
(b) potential is maximum
(c) electric field is maximum
(d) potential is zero

28. At absolute zero, Si acts as **[2002]**
(a) non-metal (b) metal
(c) insulator (d) none of these

29. By increasing the temperature, the specific resistance of a conductor and a semiconductor **[2002]**
(a) increases for both (b) decreases for both
(c) increases, decreases (d) decreases, increases

30. The energy band gap is maximum in **[2002]**
(a) metals (b) superconductors
(c) insulators (d) semiconductors.

TOPIC - 2: Junction Transistor

31. The current gain of a common emitter amplifier is 69. If the emitter current is 7.0 mA, collector current is : **[Online April 9, 2017]**
(a) 9.6 mA (b) 6.9 mA (c) 0.69 mA (d) 69 mA

32. In a common emitter amplifier circuit using an n-p-n transistor, the phase difference between the input and the output voltages will be : **[Online April 2, 2017]**
(a) 135° (b) 180° (c) 45° (d) 90°

33. For a common emitter configuration, if α and β have their usual meanings, the incorrect relationship between α and β is : **[2016]**
(a) $\alpha = \dfrac{\beta}{1+\beta}$ (b) $\alpha = \dfrac{\beta^2}{1+\beta^2}$
(c) $\dfrac{1}{\alpha} = \dfrac{1}{\beta} + 1$ (d) None of these

34. A realistic graph depicting the variation of the reciprocal of input resistance in an input characteristics measurement in a common emitter transistor configuration is : **[Online April 10, 2016]**

(a)
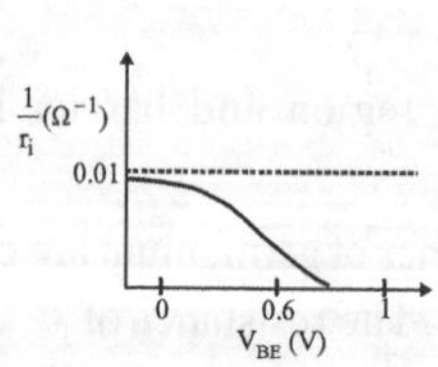

(b)
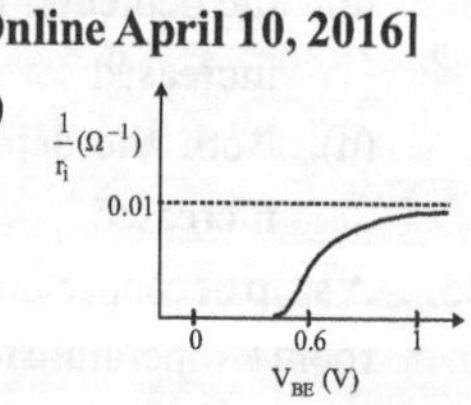

(c)
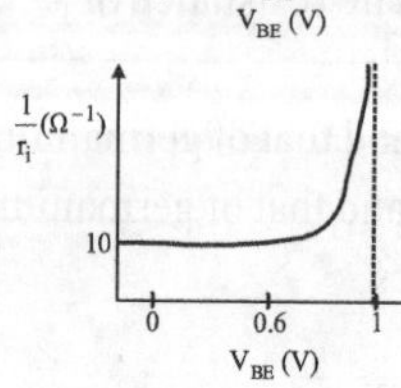

(d)
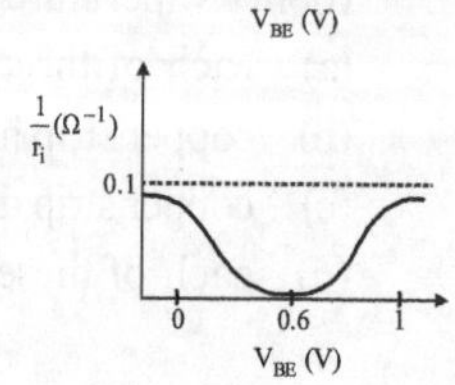

35. The ratio (R) of output resistance r_0, and the input resistance r_i in measurements of input and output characteristics of a transistor is typically in the range : **[Online April 10, 2016]**
(a) $R \sim 10^2 - 10^3$ (b) $R \sim 1 - 10$
(c) $R \sim 0.1 - 1.0$ (d) $R \sim 0.1 - 0.01$

36. An unknown transistor needs to be identified as a npn or pnp type. A multimeter, with +ve and –ve terminals, is used to measure resistance between different terminals of transistor. If terminal 2 is the base of the transistor then which of the following is correct for a pnp transistor? **[Online April 9, 2016]**
(a) +ve terminal 2, –ve terminal 3, resistance low
(b) +ve terminal 2, –ve terminal 1, resistane high
(c) +ve terminal 1, –ve terminal 2, resistance high
(d) +ve terminal 3, –ve terminal 2, resistance high

37. An n-p-n transistor has three leads A, B and C. Connecting B and C by moist fingers, A to the positive lead of an ammeter, and C to the negative lead of the ammeter, one finds large deflection. Then, A, B and C refer respectively to: **[Online April 9, 2014]**
(a) Emitter, base and collector
(b) Base, emitter and collector
(c) Base, collector and emitter
(d) Collector, emitter and base.

38. A working transistor with its three legs marked *P*, *Q* and *R* is tested using a multimeter. No conduction is found between *P* and *Q*. By connecting the common (negative) terminal of the multimeter to *R* and the other (positive) terminal to *P* or *Q*, some resistance is seen on the multimeter. Which of the following is true for the transistor? **[2008]**
(a) It is an npn transistor with *R* as base
(b) It is a pnp transistor with *R* as base
(c) It is a pnp transistor with *R* as emitter
(d) It is an npn transistor with *R* as collector

39. In a common base mode of a transistor, the collector current is 5.488 mA for an emitter current of 5.60 mA. The value of the base current amplification factor (β) will be **[2006]**
(a) 49 (b) 50 (c) 51 (d) 48

40. In a common base amplifier, the phase difference between the input signal voltage and output voltage is **[2005]**
(a) π (b) $\dfrac{\pi}{4}$ (c) $\dfrac{\pi}{2}$ (d) 0

41. When npn transistor is used as an amplifier **[2004]**
(a) electrons move from collector to base
(b) holes move from emitter to base
(c) electrons move from base to collector
(d) holes move from base to emitter

42. For a transistor amplifier in common emitter configuration for load impedance of 1kΩ ($h_{fe} = 50$ and $h_{oe} = 25$) the current gain is **[2004]**
(a) –24.8 (b) – 15.7 (c) –5.2 (d) –48.78

43. The part of a transistor which is most heavily doped to produce large number of majority carriers is **[2002]**
(a) emmiter
(b) base
(c) collector
(d) can be any of the above three.

TOPIC - 3: Digital Electronics and Logic Gates

44. If a, b, c, d are inputs to a gate and x is its output, then, as per the following time graph, the gate is : **[2016]**

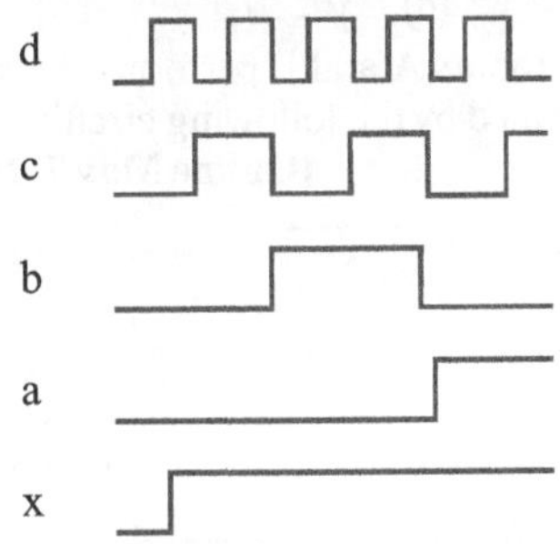

(a) OR (b) NAND
(c) NOT (d) AND

45. To get an output of 1 from the circuit shown in figure the input must be : **[Online April 10, 2016]**

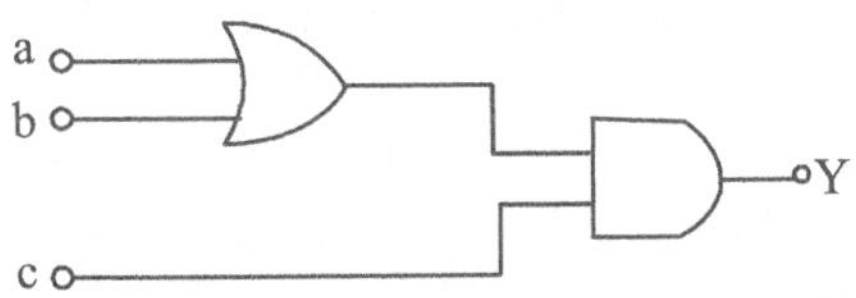

(a) $a = 0, b = 0, c = 1$ (b) $a = 1, b = 0, c = 0$
(c) $a = 1, b = 0, c = 1$ (d) $a = 0, b = 1, c = 0$

46. The truth table given in fig. represents : **[Online April 9, 2016]**

A	B	Y
0	0	0
0	1	1
1	0	1
1	1	1

(a) OR – Gate (b) NAND– Gate
(c) AND– Gate (d) NOR– Gate

47.

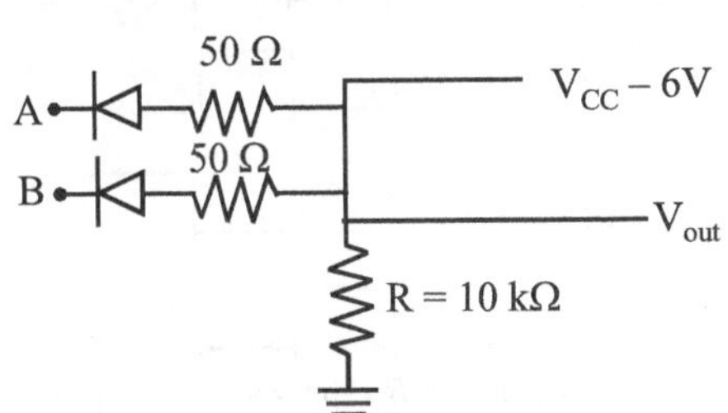

Given: A and B are input terminals.
Logic 1 = > 5 V
Logic 0 = < 1 V
Which logic gate operation, the above circuit does? **[Online April 19, 2014]**

(a) AND Gate (b) OR Gate
(c) XOR Gate (d) NOR Gate

48. Identify the gate and match A, B, Y in bracket to check. **[Online April 9, 2014]**

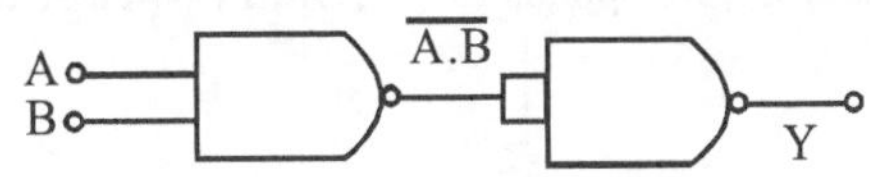

(a) AND $(A = 1, B = 1, Y = 1)$
(b) OR $(A = 1, B = 1, Y = 0)$
(c) NOT $(A = 1, B = 1, Y = 1)$
(d) XOR $(A = 0, B = 0, Y = 0)$

49. Which of the following circuits correctly represents the following truth table ? **[Online April 25, 2013]**

A	*B*	*C*
0	0	0
0	1	0
1	0	1
1	1	0

(a) 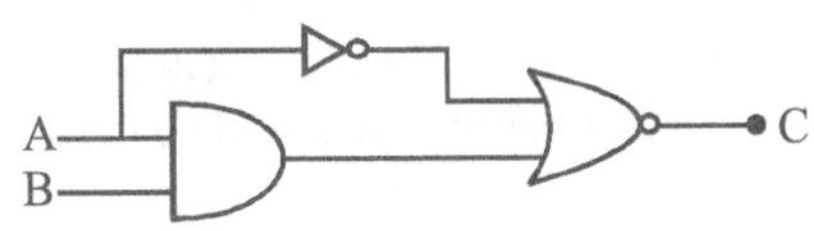

(b) 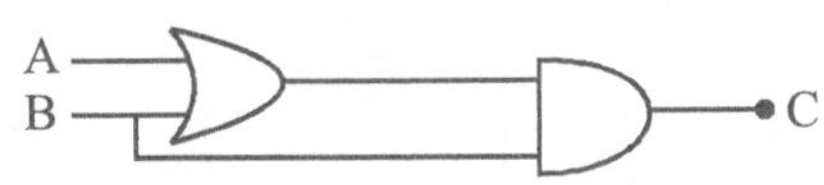

(c) 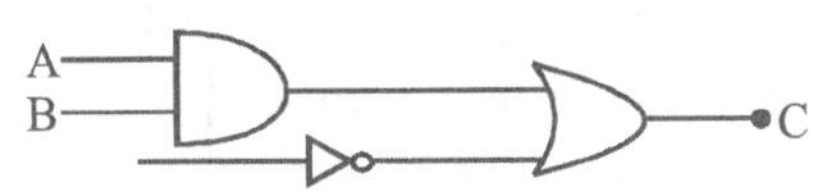

(d) 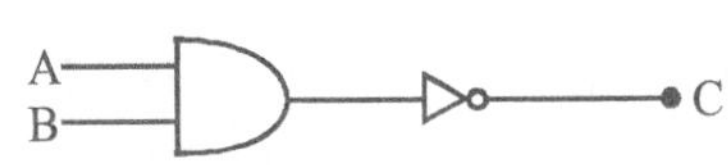

50. A system of four gates is set up as shown. The 'truth table' corresponding to this system is : **[Online April 23, 2013]**

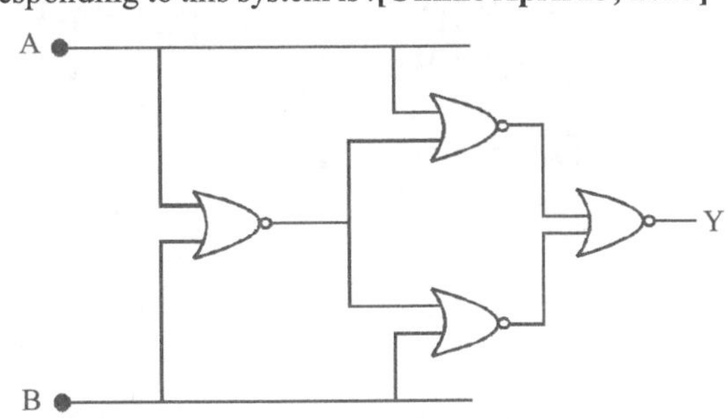

(a)

A	B	Y
0	0	1
0	1	0
1	0	0
1	1	1

(b)

A	B	Y
0	0	0
0	1	0
1	0	1
1	1	0

(c)

A	B	Y
0	0	1
0	1	0
1	0	1
1	1	0

(d)

A	B	Y
0	0	1
0	1	1
1	0	0
1	1	0

51. Consider two *npn* transistors as shown in figure. If 0 Volts corresponds to false and 5 Volts correspond to true then the output at C corresponds to : **[Online April 9, 2013]**

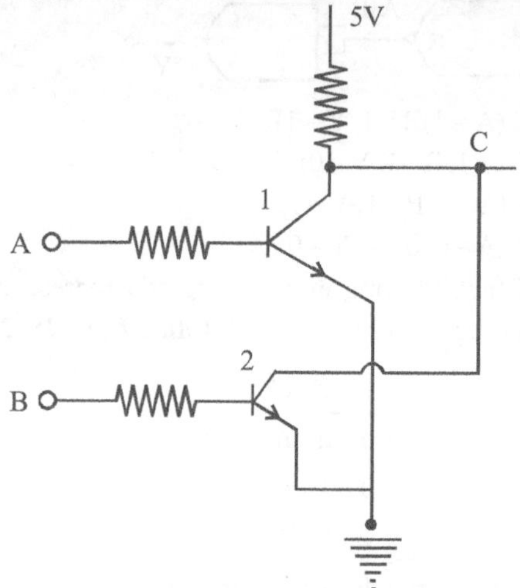

(a) A NAND B (b) A OR B
(c) A AND B (d) A NOR B

52. Truth table for system of four NAND gates as shown in figure is : **[2012]**

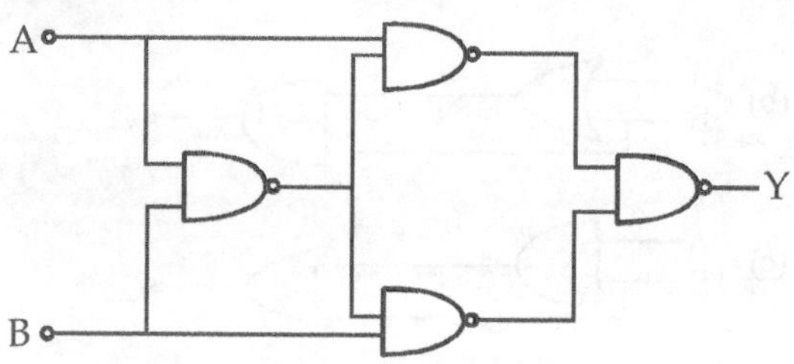

(a)

A	B	Y
0	0	0
0	1	1
1	0	1
1	1	0

(b)

A	B	Y
0	0	0
0	1	0
1	0	1
1	1	1

(c)

A	B	Y
0	0	1
0	1	1
1	0	0
1	1	0

(d)

A	B	Y
0	0	1
0	1	0
1	0	1
1	1	1

53. The figure shows a combination of two NOT gates and a NOR gate. **[Online May 26, 2012]**

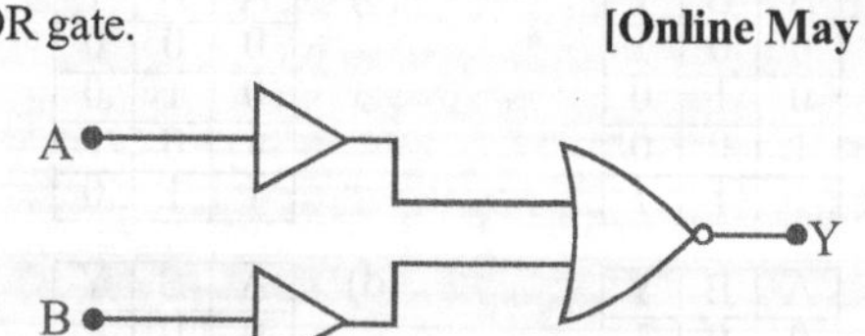

The combination is equivalent to a
(a) NAND gate (b) NOR gate
(c) AND gate (d) OR gate

54. Which one of the following is the Boolean expression for NOR gate? **[Online May 19, 2012]**
(a) $Y = \overline{A+B}$ (b) $Y = \overline{A.B}$
(c) $Y = A.B$ (d) $Y = \overline{A}$

55. Which logic gate with inputs A and B performs the same operation as that performed by the following circuit? **[Online May 7, 2012]**

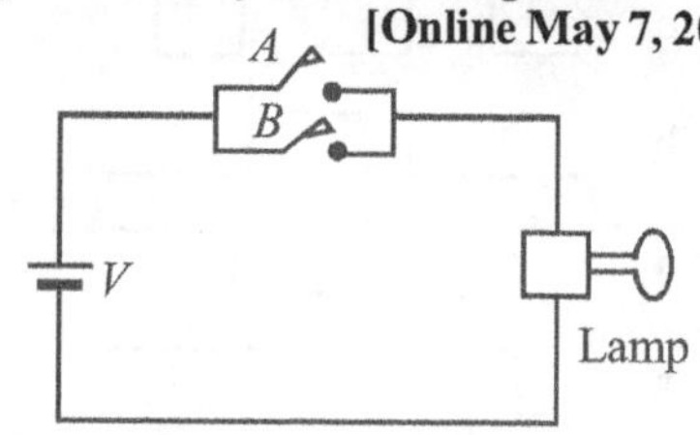

(a) NAND gate
(b) OR gate
(c) NOR gate
(d) AND gate

56. The output of an OR gate is connected to both the inputs of a NAND gate. The combination will serve as a: **[2011 RS]**
(a) NOT gate (b) NOR gate
(c) AND gate (d) OR gate

57. The combination of gates shown below yields **[2010]**

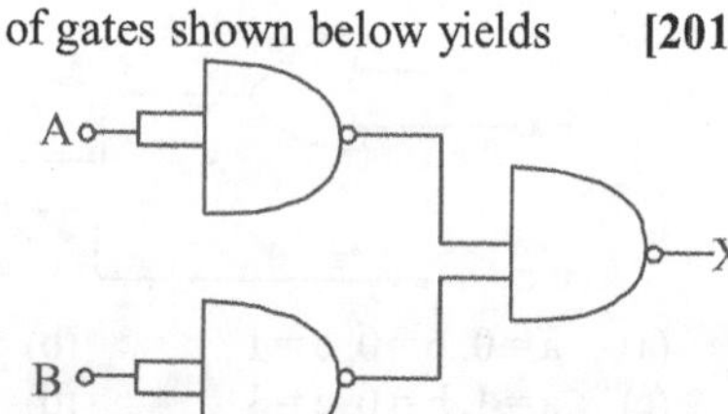

(a) OR gate
(b) NOT gate
(c) XOR gate
(d) NAND gate

58. The logic circuit shown below has the input waveforms '*A*' and '*B*' as shown. Pick out the correct output waveform. **[2009]**

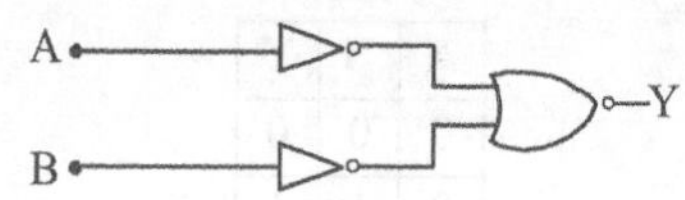

Input A
Input B

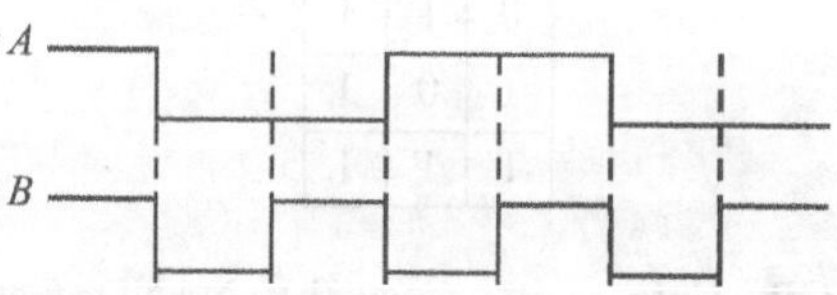

Output is

(a)

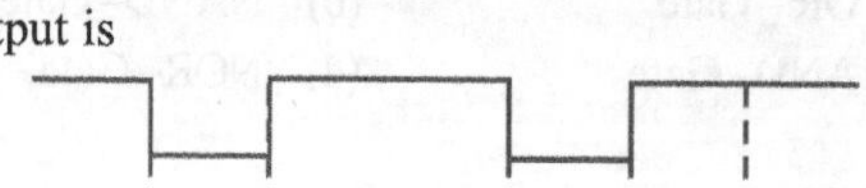

(b)

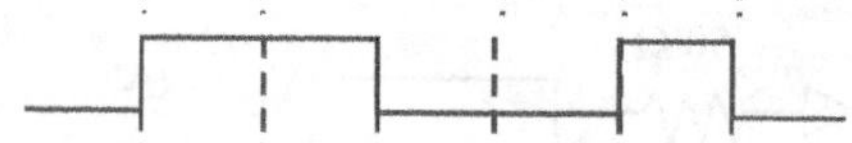

(c)

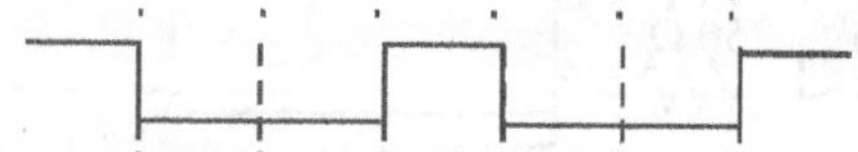

(d)

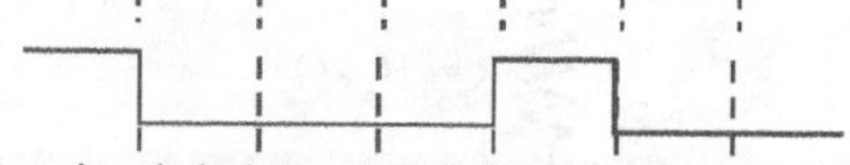

59. In the circuit below, *A* and *B* represent two inputs and *C* represents the output. **[2008]**

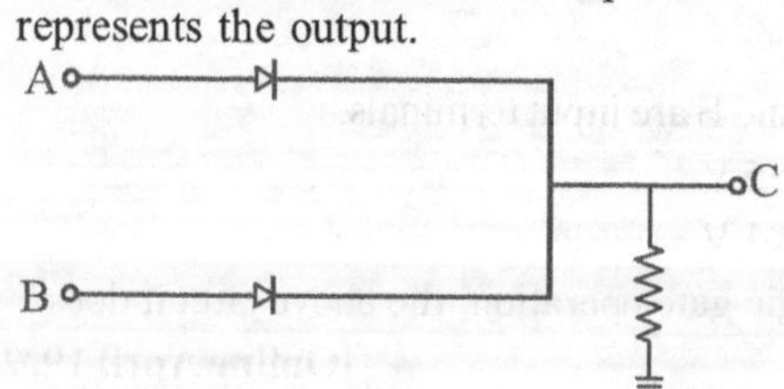

The circuit represents
(a) NOR gate (b) AND gate
(c) NAND gate (d) OR gate

Hints & Solutions

TOPIC - 1: Solids, Semiconductors and P-N Junction Diode

1. (a) The conductivity of semiconductor

$\sigma = e(\eta_e\mu_e + \eta_h\mu_h)$

$= 1.6 \times 10^{-19}(5 \times 10^{18} \times 2 + 5 \times 10^{19} \times 0.01)$

$= 1.6 \times 1.05 = 1.68$

2. (b) Forward bias resistance $= \dfrac{\Delta V}{\Delta I} = \dfrac{0.1}{10 \times 10^{-3}} = 10\,\Omega$

Reverse bias resistance $= \dfrac{10}{10^{-6}} = 10^7\,\Omega$

Ratio of resistances $= \dfrac{\text{Forward bias resistance}}{\text{Reverse bias resistance}} = 10^{-6}$

3. (c) Graph (a) is for a simple diode.
Graph (b) is showing the V Break down used for zener diode.
Graph (c) is for solar cell which shows cut-off voltage and open circuit current.
Graph (d) shows the variation of resistance h and hence current with intensity of light.

4. (a)

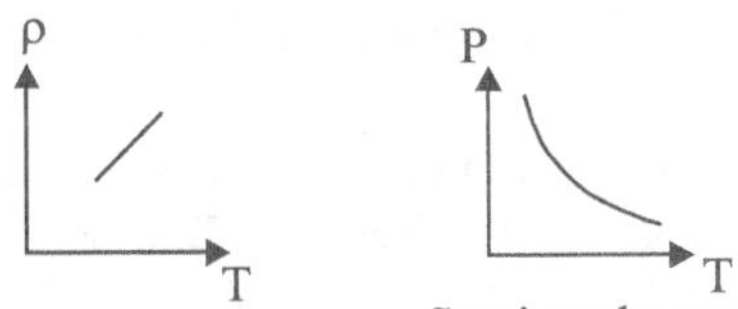

Metal (for limited range of temperature) Semiconductor $\rho = \rho_o e^{\frac{-E_g}{K_BT}}$

5. (c) The minimum voltage range of DC source is given by

$V^2 = PR$ $\quad\because P = 1$ watt, $R = 100\Omega$

$= 1 \times 100$

$\therefore V = 10$ volt.

6. (d) Using $U_{av} = \dfrac{1}{2}\varepsilon_0 E^2$

But $U_{av} = \dfrac{P}{4\pi r^2 \times c}$

$\therefore \dfrac{P}{4\pi r^2} = \dfrac{1}{2}\varepsilon_0 E^2 \times c$

$$E_0^2 = \frac{2P}{4\pi r^2 \varepsilon_0 c} = \frac{2 \times 0.1 \times 9 \times 10^9}{1 \times 3 \times 10^8}$$

$\therefore E_0 = \sqrt{6} = 2.45$ V/m

7. (a) When positive terminal connected to A then diode D_1 is forward biased, current, $I = \dfrac{2}{5} = 0.4A$

When positive terminal connected to B then diode D_2 is forward biased, current, $I = \dfrac{2}{10} = 0.2A$

8. (d) Electrons in an unbiased *p-n* junction, diffuse from *n* -region i.e. higher electron concentration to *p*-region i.e. low electron concentration region.

9. (a) P —▷|— n

For forward bias, p-side must be at higher potential than *n*-side. $\Delta V = (+)Ve$

10. (d) Energy band gap range is given by,

$$E_g = \frac{hc}{\lambda}$$

For visible region $\lambda = \left(4 \times 10^{-7} \sim 7 \times 10^{-7}\right)$m

$$E_g = \frac{6.6 \times 10^{-34} \times 3 \times 10^8}{7 \times 10^{-7}}$$

$$= \frac{19.8 \times 10^{-26}}{7 \times 10^{-7}}$$

$$= \frac{2.8 \times 10^{-19}}{1.6 \times 10^{-19}}$$

$E_g = 1.75$ eV

11. (d) Here, $R = 4\,k\Omega = 4 \times 10^3\,\Omega$

$V_i = 60$ V

Zener voltage $V_z = 10$ V

$R_L = 2\,k\Omega = 2 \times 10^3\,\Omega$

Load current, $I_L = \dfrac{V_Z}{R_L} = \dfrac{10}{2 \times 10^3} = 5$ mA

Current through R, $I = \dfrac{V_i - V_Z}{R}$

$= \dfrac{60 - 10}{4 \times 10^3} = \dfrac{50}{4 \times 10^3} = 12.5$ mA

Fom circuit diagram,

$I = I_Z + I_L$

$\Rightarrow 12.5 = I_Z + 5$

$\Rightarrow I_Z = 12.5 - 5 = 7.5$ mA

12. (a) For same value of current higher value of voltage is required for higher frequency hence (a) is correct answer.

13. (a) Here, diodes D_1 and D_2 are forward biased and D_3 is reverse biased.
Therefore current through R_3

$$i = \frac{V}{R'} = \frac{6}{120} = \frac{1}{20} A = 50 mA$$

14. (d) Temperature coefficient of resistance is negative for pure semiconductor. And no. of charge carriers in conduction band increases with increase in temperature.

15. (b) We know that a single *p-n* junction diode connected to an *a-c* source acts as a half wave rectifier [Forward biased in one half cycle and reverse biased in the other half cycle].

16. (a) The current will flow through R_L when the diode is forward biased.

17. (a) Si and Ge are semiconductors but C is an insulator. Also, the conductivity of Si and Ge is more than C because the valence electrons of Si, Ge and C lie in third, fourth and second orbit respectively.

18. (c) A crystal structure is composed of a unit cell, a set of atoms arranged in a particular way; which is periodically repeated in three dimensions on a lattice. The spacing between unit cells in various directions is called its lattice parameters or constants. Increasing these lattice constants will increase or widen the band-gap (E_g), which means more energy would be required by electrons to reach the conduction band from the valence band. Automatically E_c and E_v decreases.

19. (b) Van der Waal's bonding is attributed to the attractive forces between molecules of a liquid. The conductivity of semiconductors (covalent bonding) and insulators (ionic bonding) increases with increase in temperature while that of metals (metallic bonding) decreases.

20. (c) $$\frac{I_e}{I_h} = \frac{n_e A v_e}{n_h e A v_h} \Rightarrow \frac{7}{4} = \frac{7}{5} \times \frac{v_e}{v_h} \Rightarrow \frac{v_e}{v_h} = \frac{5}{4}$$

21. (b) D_2 is forward biased whereas D_1 is reversed biased.
So effective resistance of the circuit
$R = 4 + 2 = 6\Omega$

$$\therefore i = \frac{12}{6} = 2 \text{ A}$$

22. (d) *p*-side connected to low potential and *n*-side is connected to high potential.

23. (d) Band gap = energy of photon of wavelength 2480 nm.
So,

$$\Delta E = \frac{hc}{\lambda} = \left(\frac{6.63 \times 10^{-34} \times 3 \times 10^8}{2480 \times 10^{-9}}\right) \times \frac{1}{1.6 \times 10^{-19}} eV$$

$= 0.5$ eV

24. (a) Both the depletion region and barrier height is reduced.

25. (c) The resistance of metal (like Cu) decreases with decrease in temperature whereas the resistance of a semi-conductor (like Ge) increases with decrease in temperature.

26. (b) When the temperature increases, certain bounded electrons become free which tend to promote conductivity. Simultaneously number of collisions between electrons and positive kernels increases

27. (c) It can be seen from the following graph -

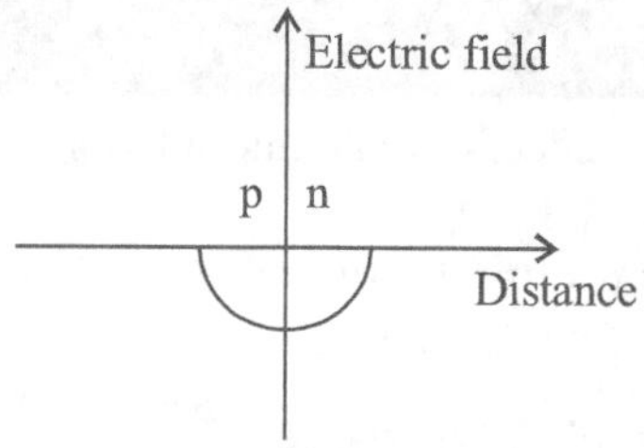

28. (c) Pure silicon, at absolute zero, will contain all the electrons in bounded state. The conduction band will be empty. So there will be no free electrons (in conduction band) and holes (in valence band) due to thermal agitation. Pure silicon will act as insulator.

29. (c) Specific resistance is resistivity which is given by

$$\rho = \frac{m}{ne^2 \tau}$$

where n = no. of free electrons per unit volume
and τ = average relaxation time

For a conductor with rise in temperature n increases and τ decreases. But the decrease in τ is more dominant than increase in n resulting an increase in the value of ρ.

For a semiconductor with rise in temperature, n increases and τ decreases. But the increase in n is more dominant than decrease in τ resulting in a decrease in the value of ρ.

30. (c) The energy band gap is maximum in insulators. Because of this the conduction band of insulators is empty.

TOPIC - 2: Junction Transistor

31. (b) Given, current gain of CE amplifier $\beta = 69$, $I_E = 7$ mA

or $\frac{I_C}{I_B} = 69$

We know that, $\alpha = \frac{\beta}{1+\beta} = \frac{69}{70} = \frac{I_C}{I_E}$

$$I_C = I_E \times \frac{69}{70} = \frac{69}{70} \times 7$$

Collector current, $I_C = 6.9$ mA

32. (b) In common emitter configuration for *n-p-n* transistor input and output signals are 180° out of phase *i.e.*, phase difference between output and input voltage is 180°.

33. (b) We know that $\alpha = \frac{I_c}{I_e}$ and $\beta = \frac{I_c}{I_b}$

Also $I_e = I_b + I_c$

$$\therefore\ \alpha = \frac{I_c}{I_b + I_c} = \frac{\frac{I_c}{I_b}}{1+\frac{I_c}{I_b}} = \frac{\beta}{1+\beta}$$

Option (2) and (4) are therefore correct.

34. (c)

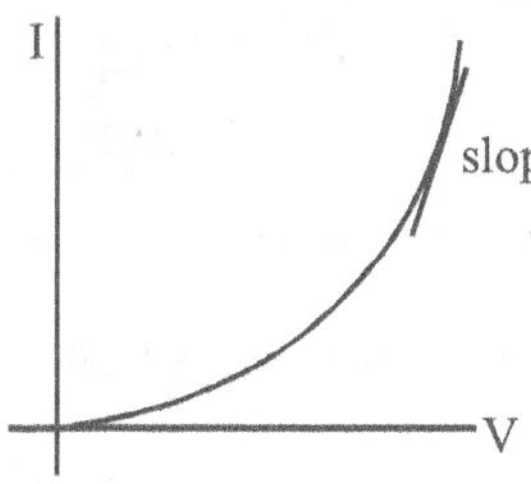

$\Rightarrow$

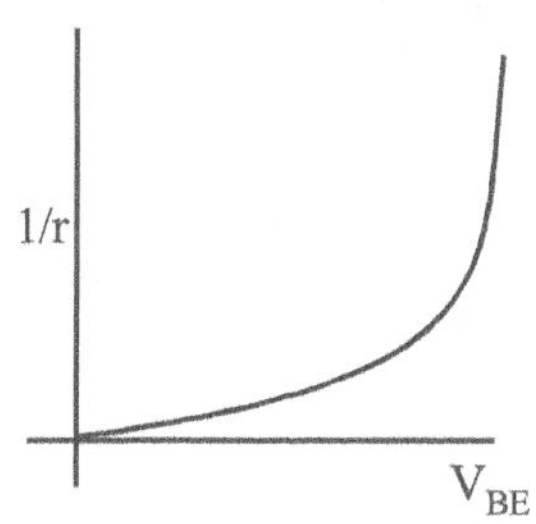

35. (c) For C.B. configuration $\frac{r_i}{r_o} \simeq 0.1\Omega$

For CE and CC-configuration

$\frac{r_i}{r_0} \approx 1\Omega$.

36. (c) Connecting circuit according to question, it is clear

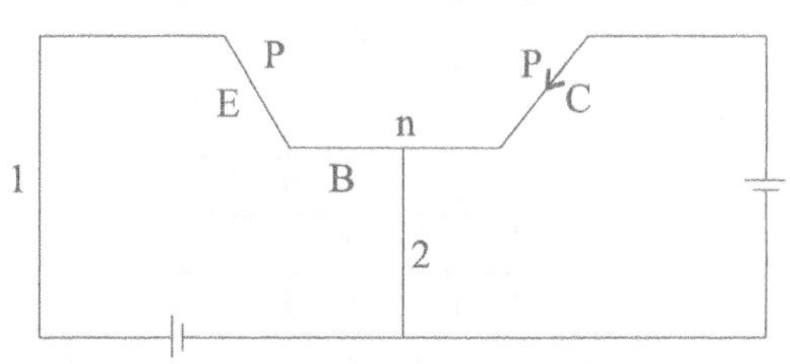

+ve terminal 1, –ve terminal 2, resistance high.

37. (c) In the given question, A, B and C refer base, collector and emitter respectively.

38. (b) It is a *p-n-p* transistor with *R* as base. None of the option is correct.

39. (a) $I_C = 5.488$ mA, $I_e = 5.6$ mA

$$\alpha = \frac{5.488}{5.6},\ \beta = \frac{\alpha}{1-\alpha} = 49$$

40. (d) Zero; In common base amplifier circuit, input and output voltage are in the same phase.

41. (d) Holes move from base to emmitter.

42. (d) In common emitter configuration current gain

$$A_i = \frac{-hf_e}{1+b_{oe}R_L}$$

$$= \frac{-50}{1+25\times10^{-6}\times1\times10^3}$$

$$= -48.78$$

43. (a) Emitter sends the majority charge carrriers towards the collector. Therefore emitter is most heavily doped.

TOPIC - 3: Digital Electronics and Logic Gates

44. (a) In case of an 'OR' gate the input is zero when all inputs are zero. If any one input is ' 1', then the output is '1'.

45. (c) Truth table for given logical circuit

a	b	(a + b)	c	Y = (a + b) .c
0	0	0	0	0
0	1	1	1	1
1	0	1	1	1
1	1	1	0	0

Output of OR gate must be 1 and c = 1

So, a = 1, b = 0 or a = 0, b = 1.

46. (a) It represents OR-Gate.

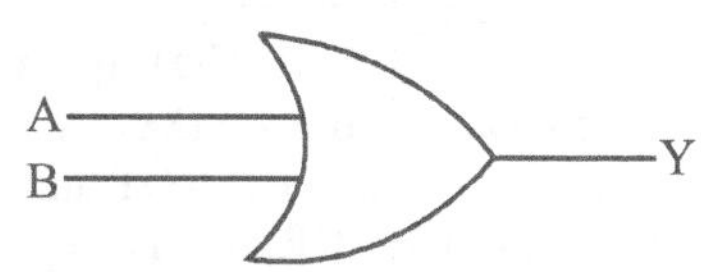

A	B	A+B=Y
0	0	0
0	1	1
1	0	1
1	1	1

47. (a) AND Gate

48. (a)

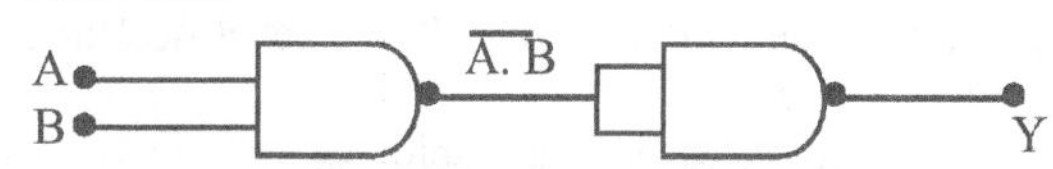

$$Y = \overline{\overline{AB}.\overline{AB}} = \overline{\overline{AB}} + \overline{\overline{AB}} = AB + AB = AB$$

In this case output Y is equivalent to AND gate.

49. (a) For circuit 1

$A.B = \overline{Y+\bar{A}} = C$

A	B	$\overline{Y+\bar{A}}$		= C
0	0	0	1	0
0	1	0	1	0
1	0	0	0	1
1	1	1	0	0

50. (a) In the given system all four gate is NOR gate

Truth Table

A	B	$(y' = \overline{A+B})$	$y'' = \overline{(A+y')}$	$y''' = \overline{(A+y'')}$	$y = \overline{y''+y'''}$
0	0	1	0	0	1
0	1	0	1	0	0
1	0	0	0	1	0
1	1	0	0	0	1

i.e.,

A	B	y
0	0	1
0	1	0
1	0	0
1	1	1

51. **(a)** The output at C corresponds to A NAND B or $\overline{A \cdot B} = C$

52. **(a)**

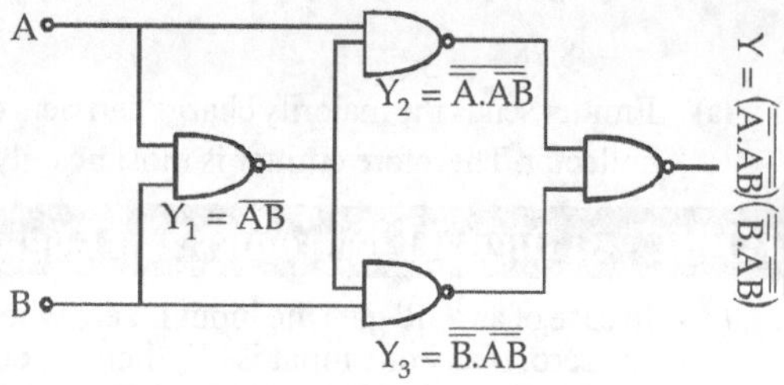

By expanding this Boolen expression

$$Y = A\overline{B} + B.\overline{A}$$

Thus the truth table for this expression should be (a).

53. **(c)** Truth table is as shown :

A	B	$\overline{A}$	$\overline{B}$	$\overline{A}+\overline{B}$	$\overline{\overline{A}+\overline{B}}$
0	0	1	1	1	0
0	1	1	0	1	0
1	0	0	1	1	0
1	1	0	0	0	1

Thus the combination of two NOT gates and one NOR gate is equivalent to a AND gate.

54. **(a)** NOR gate is the combination of NOT and OR gate. Boolean expression for NOR gate is

$Y = \overline{A+B}$

55. **(b)** When either of A or B is 1 i.e. closed then lamp will glow.
In this case, Truth table

Inputs		Output
A	B	Y
0	0	0
0	1	1
1	0	1
1	1	1

This represents OR gate.

56. **(b)** $\overline{(A+B)}$ = NOR gate

When both inputs of NAND gate are connected, it behaves as NOT gate

OR + NOT = NOR.

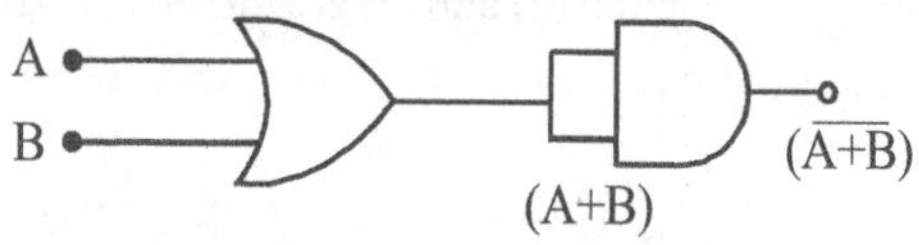

57. **(a)** The final boolean expression is,

$$X = \overline{(\overline{A}.\overline{B})} = \overline{\overline{A}} + \overline{\overline{B}} = A + B \Rightarrow \text{OR gate}$$

58. **(d)** Here $Y = \overline{(\overline{A}+\overline{B})} = \overline{\overline{A}}.\overline{\overline{B}} = A \cdot B$. Thus, it is an AND gate for which truth table is

A	B	Y
0	0	0
0	1	0
1	0	0
1	1	1

59. **(d)**

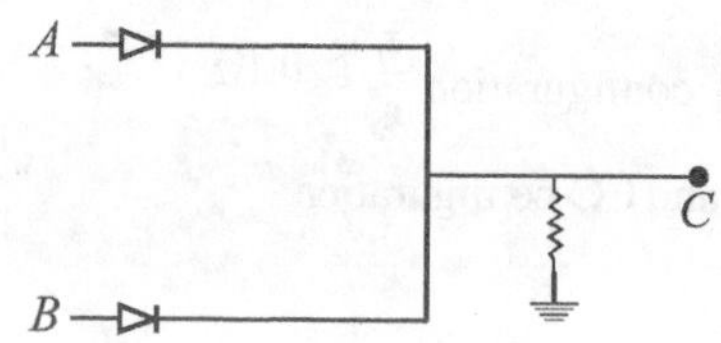

The truth table for the above logic gate is :

A	B	C
1	1	1
1	0	1
0	1	1
0	0	0

This truth table follows the boolean algebra $C = A + B$ which is for OR gate.

Chapter 29

Communication Systems

TOPIC-1 : Communication Systems

1. In amplitude modulation, sinusoidal carrier frequency used is denoted by ω_c and the signal frequency is denoted by ω_m. The bandwidth ($\Delta\omega_m$) of the signal is such that $\Delta\omega_m < \omega_c$. Which of the following frequencies is not contained in the modulated wave ? **[2017]**
   (a) $\omega_m + \omega_c$ (b) $\omega_c - \omega_m$
   (c) ω_m (d) ω_c

2. A signal is to be transmitted through a wave of wavelength λ, using a linear antenna. The length 1 of the antenna and effective power radiated P_{eff} will be given respectively as : (K is a constant of proportionality) **[Online April 9, 2017]**
   (a) $\lambda, P_{eff} = K\left(\frac{1}{\lambda}\right)^2$ (b) $\frac{\lambda}{8}, P_{eff} = K\left(\frac{1}{\lambda}\right)$
   (c) $\frac{\lambda}{16}, P_{eff} = K\left(\frac{1}{\lambda}\right)^3$ (d) $\frac{\lambda}{5}, P_{eff} = K\left(\frac{1}{\lambda}\right)^{\frac{1}{2}}$

3. A signal of frequency 20 kHz and peak voltage of 5 Volt is used to modulate a carrier wave of frequency 1.2 MHz and peak voltage 25 Volts. Choose the correct statement. **[Online April 8, 2017]**
   (a) Modulation index = 5, side frequency bands are at 1400 kHz and 1000 kHz
   (b) Modulation index = 5, side frequency bands are at 21.2 kHz and 18.8 kHz
   (c) Modulation index=0.8, side frequency bands are at 1180 kHz and 1220 kHz
   (d) Modulation index=0.2, side frequency bands are at 1220 kHz and 1180 kHz

4. Choose the correct statement : **[2016]**
   (a) In frequency modulation the amplitude of the high frequency carrier wave is made to vary in proportion to the amplitude of the audio signal.
   (b) In frequency modulation the amplitude of the high frequency carrier wave is made to vary in proportion to the frequency of the audio signal.
   (c) In amplitude modulation the amplitude of the high frequency carrier wave is made to vary in proportion to the amplitude of the audio signal.
   (d) In amplitude modulation the frequency of the high frequency carrier wave is made to vary in proportion to the amplitude of the audio signal.

5. A modulated signal $C_m(t)$ has the form $C_m(t) = 30 \sin 300\pi t + 10 (\cos 200\pi t - \cos 400\pi t)$. The carrier frequency f_c, the modulating frequency (message frequency) f_ω and the modulation indix μ are respectively given by : **[Online April 10, 2016]**
   (a) $f_c = 200$ Hz; $f_w = 50$ Hz; $\mu = \frac{1}{2}$
   (b) $f_c = 150$ Hz; $f_w = 50$ Hz; $\mu = \frac{2}{3}$
   (c) $f_c = 150$ Hz; $f_w = 30$ Hz; $\mu = \frac{1}{3}$
   (d) $f_c = 200$ Hz; $f_w = 30$ Hz; $\mu = \frac{1}{2}$

6. An audio signal consists of two distinct sounds: one a human speech signal in the frequency band of 200 Hz to 2700 Hz, while the other is a high frequency music signal in the frequency band of 10200 Hz to 15200 Hz. The ratio of the AM signal bandwidth required to send both the signals together to the AM signal bandwidth requried to send just the human speech is : **[Online April 9, 2016]**
   (a) 2 (b) 5 (c) 6 (d) 3

7. A signal of 5 kHz frequency is amplitude modulated on a carrier wave of frequency 2 MHz. The frequencies of the resultant signal is/are : **[2015]**
   (a) 2005 kHz, 2000 kHz and 1995 kHz
   (b) 2000 kHz and 1995 kHz
   (c) 2 MHz only
   (d) 2005 kHz and 1995 kHz

8. Long range radio transmission is possible when the radio waves are reflected from the ionosphere. For this to happen the frequency of the radio waves must be in the range: **[Online April 19, 2014]**
   (a) 80 - 150 MHz (b) 8 - 25 MHz
   (c) 1 - 3 MHz (d) 150 - 1500 kHz

9. For sky wave propagation, the radio waves must have a frequency range in between: **[Online April 12, 2014]**
   (a) 1 MHz to 2 MHz (b) 5 MHz to 25 MHz
   (c) 35 MHz to 40 MHz (d) 45 MHz to 50 MHz

10. A transmitting antenna at the top of a tower has height 32 m and height of the receiving antenna is 50 m. What is the maximum distance between them for satisfactory communication in line of sight (LOS) mode? **[Online April 9, 2014]**
   (a) 55.4 km (b) 45.5 km (c) 54.5 km (d) 455 km

11. A diode detector is used to detect an amplitudemodulated wave of 60% modulation by using a condenser of capacity 250 picofarad in parallel with a load resistance 100 kilo ohm. Find the maximum modulated frequency which could be detected by it. **[2013]**

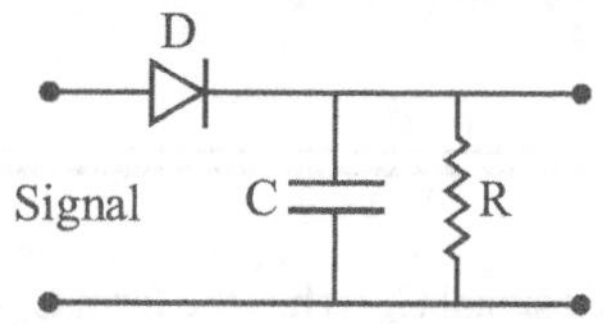

(a) 10.62 MHz (b) 10.62 kHz
(c) 5.31 MHz (d) 5.31 kHz

12. Which of the following modulated signal has the best noise-tolerance ? **[Online April 25, 2013]**
(a) Long-wave (b) Short-wave
(c) Medium-wave (d) Amplitude-modulated

13. Which of the following statement is NOT correct? **[Online April 23, 2013]**
(a) Ground wave signals are more stable than the sky wave signals.
(b) The critical frequency of an ionospheric layer is the highest frequency that will be reflected back by the layer when it is vertically incident.
(c) Electromagnetic waves of frequencies higher than about 30 MHz cannot penetrate the ionosphere.
(d) Sky wave signals in the broadcast frequency range are stronger at night than in the day time.

14. This question has Statement-1 and Statement-2. Of the four choices given after the Statements, choose the one that best describes the two Statements.
Statement-1: Short wave transmission is achieved due to the total internal reflection of the e-m wave from an appropriate height in the ionosphere.
Statement-2: Refractive index of a plasma is independent of the frequency of e-m waves. **[Online April 22, 2013]**
(a) Statement-1 is true, Statement-2 is false.
(b) Statement-1 is false, Statement-2 is true.
(c) Statement-1 is true, Statement-2 is true but Statement -2 is **not** the correct explanation of statement-1.
(d) Statement-1 is true, Statement-2 is true and Statement -2 is the correct explanation of Statement-1.

15. If a carrier wave c(t) = A sin ω_ct is amplitude modulated by a modulator signal m(t) = A sin ω_mt then the equation of modulated signal [C_m(t)] and its modulation index are respectively **[Online April 9, 2013]**
(a) $C_m(t) = A(1 + \sin\omega_m t)\sin\omega_c t$ and 2
(b) $C_m(t) = A(1 + \sin\omega_m t)\sin\omega_m t$ and 1
(c) $C_m(t) = A(1 + \sin\omega_m t)\sin\omega_c t$ and 1
(d) $C_m(t) = A(1 + \sin\omega_c t)\sin\omega_m t$ and 2

16. A radar has a power of 1kW and is operating at a frequency of 10 GHz. It is located on a mountain top of height 500 m. The maximum distance upto which it can detect object located on the surface of the earth
(Radius of earth = 6.4×10^6m) is : **[2012]**
(a) 80 km (b) 16 km (c) 40 km (d) 64 km

17. A radio transmitter transmits at 830 kHz. At a certain distance from the transmitter magnetic field has amplitude 4.82×10^{-11}T. The electric field and the wavelength are respectively **[Online May 26, 2012]**
(a) 0.014 N/C, 36 m (b) 0.14 N/C, 36 m
(c) 0.14 N/C, 360 m (d) 0.014 N/C, 360 m

18. Given the electric field of a complete amplitude modulated wave as

$$\vec{E} = \hat{i}E_c\left(1 + \frac{E_m}{E_c}\cos\omega_m t\right)\cos\omega_c t.$$

Where the subscript c stands for the carrier wave and m for the modulating signal. The frequencies present in the modulated wave are **[Online May 19, 2012]**
(a) ω_c and $\sqrt{\omega_c^2 + \omega_m^2}$
(b) $\omega_c, \omega_c + \omega_m$ and $\omega_c - \omega_m$
(c) ω_c and ω_m
(d) ω_c and $\sqrt{\omega_c \omega_m}$

19. A 10 kW transmitter emits radio waves of wavelength 500 m. The number of photons emitted per second by the transmitter is of the order of **[Online May 12, 2012]**
(a) 10^{37} (b) 10^{31} (c) 10^{25} (d) 10^{43}

20. This question has Statement – 1 and Statement – 2. Of the four choices given after the statements, choose the one that best describes the two statements. **[2011]**
Statement – 1 : Sky wave signals are used for long distance radio communication. These signals are in general, less stable than ground wave signals.
Statement – 2 : The state of ionosphere varies from hour to hour, day to day and season to season.
(a) Statement–1 is true, Statement–2 is true, Statement–2 is the correct explanation of Statement–1.
(b) Statement–1 is true, Statement–2 is true, Statement–2 is not the correct explanation of Statement – 1.
(c) Statement – 1 is false, Statement – 2 is true.
(d) Statement – 1 is true, Statement – 2 is false.

21. Which of the following four alternatives is not correct ? We need modulation : **[2011 RS]**
(a) to reduce the time lag between transmission and reception of the information signal
(b) to reduce the size of antenna
(c) to reduce the fractional band width, that is the ratio of the signal band width to the centre frequency
(d) to increase the selectivity

Hints & Solutions

TOPIC-1 : Communication Systems

1. (c) Modulated carrier wave contains frequency w_c and $w_c \pm w_m$

2. (a) Length of antenna = comparable to λ
Power radiated by linear antenna inversely depends on the square of wavelength and directly on the length of the antenna. Hence,

$$\text{Power } P = \mu\left(\frac{1}{\lambda}\right)^2$$

here $\mu = K$

3. (d) Modulation index (m) $= \frac{V_m}{V_0} = \frac{5}{25} = 0.2$
Given, frequency of carrier wave $(f_c) = 1.2 \times 10^6$ Hz
$= 1200$ kHz.
Frequency of signal $(f_0) = 20$ kHz.
Side frequency bands $= f_c \pm f_0$
$f_1 = 1200 - 20 = 1180$ kHz
$f_2 = 1200 + 20 = 1220$ kHz

4. (c) In amplitude modulation, the amplitude of the high frequency carrier wave made to vary in proportional to the amplitude of audio signal.

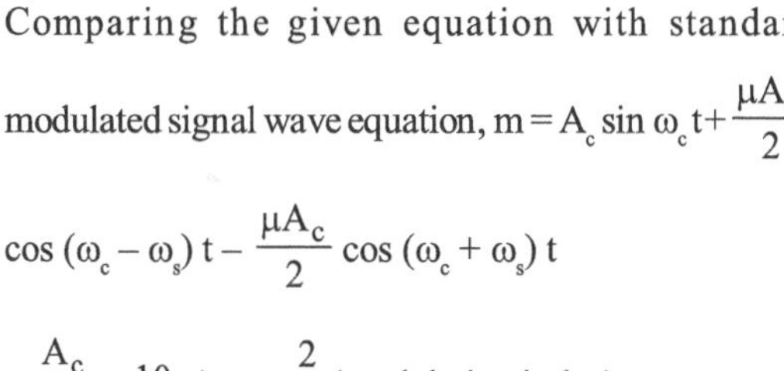

5. (b) Comparing the given equation with standard modulated signal wave equation, $m = A_c \sin \omega_c t + \frac{\mu A_c}{2}$

$\cos(\omega_c - \omega_s)t - \frac{\mu A_c}{2}\cos(\omega_c + \omega_s)t$

$$\mu\frac{A_c}{2} = 10 \Rightarrow \mu = \frac{2}{3} \text{ (modulation index)}$$

$A_c = 30$
$\omega_c - \omega_s = 200\pi$
$\omega_c + \omega_s = 400\pi$
$\Rightarrow f_c = 150,\ f_s = 50$ Hz.

6. (c) Ratio of AM signal Bandwidths

$$= \frac{15200 - 200}{2700 - 200} = \frac{15000}{2500} = 6.$$

7. (a) Amplitude modulated wave consists of three frequencies are $\omega_c + \omega_m, \omega, \omega_c - \omega_m$
i.e. 2005 KHz, 2000KHz, 1995 KHz

8. (b) Frequency of radio waves for sky wave propagation is 2 MHZ to 30 MHZ.

9. (b) Sky wave propagation is suitable for frequency range 5 MHz to 25 MHz.

10. (b) Given : $h_R = 32$ m
$h_T = 50$ m
Maximum distance, $d_M = ?$
Applying, $d_M = \sqrt{2Rh_T} + \sqrt{2Rh_R}$

$$= \sqrt{2\times 6.4\times 10^6 \times 50} + \sqrt{2\times 6.4\times 10^6\times 32} = 45.5 \text{ km}$$

11. (b) **Given :** Resistance R = 100 kilo ohm
$= 100 \times 10^3\ \Omega$
Capacitance C = 250 picofarad
$= 250 \times 10^{-12}$F
$\tau = RC = 100 \times 10^3 \times 250 \times 10^{-12}$ sec
$= 2.5 \times 10^7 \times 10^{-12}$ sec
$= 2.5 \times 10^{-5}$ sec
The higher frequency whcih can be detected with tolerable distortion is

$$f = \frac{1}{2\pi m_a RC} = \frac{1}{2\pi\times 0.6\times 2.5\times 10^{-5}} Hz$$

$$= \frac{100\times 10^4}{25\times 1.2\pi} Hz = \frac{4}{1.2\pi}\times 10^4 Hz$$

$= 10.61$ KHz
This condition is obtained by applying the condition that rate of decay of capacitor voltage must be equal or less than the rate of decay modulated singnal voltage for proper detection of mdoulated signal.

12. (b) Short-wave has the best noise tolerance.

13. (c) Above critical frequency (f_c), an electromagnetic wave penetrates the ionosphere and is not reflected by it.

14. (a) Effective refractive index of the ionosphere

$$n_{eff} = n_0\left[1 - \frac{80.5N}{f^2}\right]^{1/2}$$

where f is the frequency of em waves

15. (c) Modulation index

$$m_a = \frac{E_m}{E_c} = \frac{A}{A} = 1$$

Equation of modulated signal $[C_m(t)]$

$= E_{(C)} + m_a E_{(C)} \sin \omega_m t$

$= A(1 + \sin w_c t) \sin \omega_m t$

(As $E_{(C)} = A \sin\omega_c t$)

16. (a) Let *d* is the maximum distance, upto which it can detect the objects

From ΔAOC

$$OC^2 = AC^2 + AO^2$$

$$(h+R)^2 = d^2 + R^2$$

$$\Rightarrow d^2 = (h+R)^2 - R^2$$

$$d = \sqrt{(h+R)^2 - R^2}$$

$$d = \sqrt{h^2 + 2hR}$$

$$d = \sqrt{500^2 + 2 \times 6.4 \times 10^6} = 80\,\text{km}$$

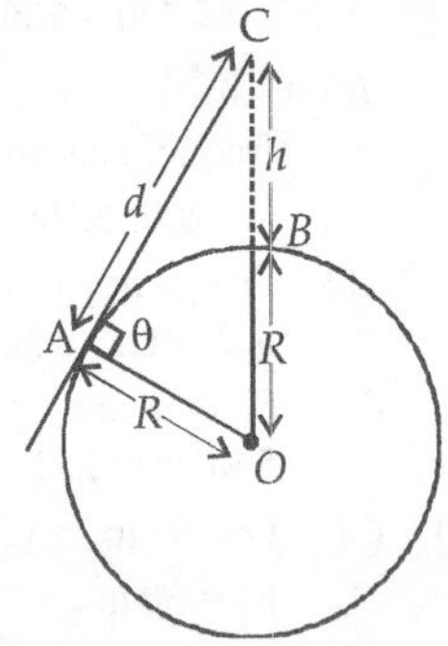

17. (d) Frequency of EM wave υ = 830 KHz

= 830×10^3 Hz.

Magnetic field, $B = 4.82 \times 10^{-11}$ T

As we know, frequency, $\upsilon = \frac{c}{\lambda}$

or $\lambda = \frac{c}{\nu} = \frac{3 \times 10^8}{830 \times 10^3}$

$\lambda \simeq 360$ m

And, $E = BC = 4.82 \times 10^{-11} \times 3 \times 10^8$

= 0.014 N/C

18. (b) The frequencies present in amplitude modulated wave are :

Carrier frequency = ω_c

Upper side band frequency = $\omega_c + \omega_m$

Lower side band frequency = $\omega_c - \omega_m$.

19. (b) Power $= \frac{nhc}{\lambda}$

(where, n = no. of photons per second)

$$\Rightarrow n = \frac{10 \times 10^3 \times 500}{6.6 \times 10^{-34} \times 3 \times 10^8} \simeq 10^{31}$$

20. (b) For long distance communication, sky wave signals are used.

Also, the state of ionosphere varies every time.

So, both statements are correct.

21. (a) Low frequencies cannot be transmitted to long distances. Therefore, they are super imposed on a high frequency carrier signal by a process known as modulation.

Speed of electro-magnetic waves will not change due to modulation. So there will be time lag between transmission and reception of the information signal.